NEUROLOGY OF HEREDITARY METABOLIC DISEASES OF CHILDREN

Notice

Medicine is an ever-changing science. As new research and clinical experience broaden our knowledge, changes in treatment and drug therapy are required. The authors and the publisher of this work have checked with sources believed to be reliable in their efforts to provide information that is complete and generally in accord with the standards accepted at the time of publication. However, in view of the possibility of human error or changes in medical sciences, neither the authors nor the publisher nor any other party who has been involved in the preparation or publication of this work warrants that the information contained herein is in every respect accurate or complete, and they are not responsible for any errors or omissions or for the results obtained from use of such information. Readers are encouraged to confirm the information contained herein with other sources. For example and in particular, readers are advised to check the product information sheet included in the package of each drug they plan to administer to be certain that the information contained in this book is accurate and that changes have not been made in the recommended dose or in the contraindications for administration. This recommendation is of particular importance in connection with new or infrequently used drugs.

NEUROLOGY OF HEREDITARY METABOLIC DISEASES OF CHILDREN

Second Edition

Gilles Lyon, M.D.

Professor of Child Neurology and Chief of Child Neurology Service (Emeritus), University of Louvain School of Medicine, Brussels, Belgium
Formerly Associate Professor of Child Neurology, René Descartes University School of Medicine, Paris, France
Adjunct Professor of Neurology, New York University School of Medicine
New York, New York

Raymond D. Adams, M.A., M.D.
M.A. (Hon.), D.Sc. (Hon.), M.D. (Hon.), F.R.C.P. (Hon.)

Bullard Professor Emeritus, Neuropathology, Harvard Medical School
Senior Neurologist and Formerly Chief of Neurology Service
Massachusetts General Hospital
Founder and Director Emeritus, Eunice K. Shriver Center
Boston, Massachusetts
Adjunct Professor, Karolinska University, Stockholm, Sweden
Adjunct Physician, Université de Lausanne, Switzerland

Edwin H. Kolodny, M.D.

Bernard A. and Charlotte Marden Professor and Chairman
Department of Neurology
New York University School of Medicine
New York, New York

McGraw-Hill
Health Professions Division

New York   St. Louis   San Francisco   Auckland   Bogotá   Caracas   Lisbon
London   Madrid   Mexico City   Milan   Montreal   New Delhi   San Juan
Singapore   Sydney   Tokyo   Toronto

McGraw-Hill

A Division of The McGraw·Hill Companies

NEUROLOGY OF HEREDITARY METABOLIC DISEASES OF CHILDREN

Copyright © 1996 by The **McGraw-Hill** Companies, Inc. Copyright © 1982 by Hemisphere Publishing Corporation. All rights reserved. Printed in the United States of America. Except as permitted under the United States Copyright Act of 1976, no part of this publication may be reproduced or distributed in any form or by any means, or stored in a data base or retrieval system, without the prior written permission of the publisher.

234567890 DOCDOC 9876

ISBN 0-07-000389-0

This book was set in Times Roman by Keyword Publishing Services Ltd; the editors were Joseph Hefta and Muza Navrozov; the production supervisor was Richard Ruzycka. The cover was designed by Robert Freese. The index was prepared by Information Index. R. R. Donnelley & Sons Company was printer and binder.

This book was printed on acid-free paper.

Library of Congress Cataloging-in-Publication Data

Lyon, Gilles.
  Neurology of hereditary metabolic diseases of children / Gilles Lyon, Raymond D. Adams, Edwin H. Kolodny—2nd ed.
    p. cm.
  Adams' name appears first on the earlier edition.
  Includes bibliographical references and index.
  ISBN 0-07-000389-0 (alk. paper)
  1. Pediatric neurology. 2. Metabolism, Inborn errors of. 3. Metabolic disorders in children. I. Adams. Raymond D. (Raymond Delacy), date. II. Kolodny, Edwin H. III. Title.
  [DNLM: 1. Nervous System Diseases—in infancy & childhood.
2. Metabolism, Inborn Errors. WS 340 L9915n 1996]
RJ486.A3 1996
618.92$'$0042—dc20
DNLM/DLC
for Library of Congress

CONTENTS

Preface   xi

**1 General Aspects of Hereditary Metabolic Diseases
    of the Nervous System**   1

MATTERS PERTAINING TO ETIOLOGIES   2

MATTERS PERTAINING TO CLASSIFICATION   3

CLINICAL CRITERIA OF AN HMD. QUESTIONS OF DEVELOPMENTAL
ARREST AND REGRESSION   3

PLAN OF THIS BOOK   5

2 The Neurology of Neonatal Hereditary Metabolic Diseases   6

GENERAL SYMPTOMATOLOGY, CHARACTERISTIC FEATURES OF
NEONATAL HMDs, AND DIAGNOSTIC TESTS   6
General Symptomatology of Neonatal Neurologic Disorders   7
Clinical and Radiological Characteristics of HMDs   9
Diagnostic Laboratory Tests   9

CLASSIFICATION OF HMDs IN THE NEONATAL PERIOD   12
Inherited Disorders of Amino Acid and Organic Acid Metabolism   12
Neonatal Mitochondrial Encephalopathies   22
Disorders of Biotin Metabolism   30
Neonatal Peroxisomal Disorders   30
Disorders of Carbohydrate Metabolism   39
Pyridoxine (Vitamin B$_6$) Dependency   40
Other Metabolic Disorders with a Possible Neonatal Onset   41

CONCLUSIONS   41

**3 Early Infantile Progressive Metabolic Encephalopathies:
    Clinical Problems and Diagnostic Considerations**   45

MAIN FEATURES AND DIAGNOSTIC GUIDELINES   45
Evidence of Neurological Regression   46
Delay in Motor Development   46
Neurologic Signs   46
Nonneurologic Abnormalities   47
Neurologic Disorders in the Family   47

The Confirmatory Standard Laboratory Tests   47
Neuroradiologic Imaging   48

EARLY INFANTILE NEUROMETABOLIC DISORDERS
WITH A RELENTLESSLY PROGRESSIVE COURSE   48
The Sphingolipidoses   48
Sialidoses and Sialic Acid Storage Disorders   61
Glycogenesis Type II   64
The Genetic Early Infantile Leukodystrophies   66
Hereditary Metabolic Disorders with Cutaneous Signs
    and Frequent Seizures   76
Syndromes with Severe Seizures as a Constant Sign   81
An Oculocerebrorenal Syndrome: Lowe Syndrome   84
Organoacidopathies with Dystonia or Choreoathetosis   85
Disorders of Amino Acids or Organic Acids with Ataxia   86
Inborn Errors of Amino Acids, Organic Acids, and Carbohydrate
    Metabolism with Isolated Cognitive and Behavioral Abnormalities   86
Disorders of Valine Catabolism with Prenatal Developmental Defects
    of the Brain   91

HMDs WITH ACUTE AND REMITTING NEUROLOGIC DISORDERS   92
Disorders with Lactic Acidosis as a Major Metabolic Sign   92
Disorders with Episodic Nonketotic Hypoglycemia   100
Disorders with Intermittent Episodes of Ketoacidosis   104
Disorders with Hyperammonemia and Respiratory Alkalosis   107
Reye-like Syndromes   108

OTHER DISORDERS WITH CLINICAL EXPRESSION IN THE EARLY
INFANTILE PERIOD   109

CONCLUSIONS   109

4   Late Infantile Progressive Genetic Encephalopathies (Metabolic
    Encephalopathies of the Second Year of Life)   124

    GENERAL CONSIDERATIONS   124

    PROGRESSIVE WALKING DIFFICULTIES RELATED TO LESIONS OF
    THE CENTRAL AND/OR PERIPHERAL MOTOR NEURONS (SPASTIC
    PARAPLEGIA AND/OR PERIPHERAL NEUROPATHY)   125
    HMDs Which Cause Spastic Paraplegia and/or Peripheral Neuropathy   128
    Spastic Paraplegia, Mental Deterioration, and Seizures   140

    UNSTEADY GAIT AND INCOORDINATE MOVEMENTS RESULTING
    FROM CEREBELLAR ATAXIA, DYSTONIA, CHOREOATHETOSIS,
    OR SOME COMBINATION THEREOF   142

    INTENTION MYOCLONUS (POLYMYOCLONUS) VARIABLY
    ASSOCIATED WITH EPILEPSY AND CEREBELLAR ATAXIA   145

INTERMITTENT EPISODES OF ACUTE NEUROLOGICAL
DYSFUNCTION AND COMA   150

MENTAL RETARDATION AND REGRESSION WITH PARALLEL
DEVELOPMENT OF SKELETAL AND OTHER SOMATIC
ABNORMALITIES   150
The Mucopolysaccharidoses   151
Disorders with the Hurler Phenotype and no Mucopolysacchariduria:
  Mucolipidoses, Disorders of Glycoprotein Degradation   161
Concluding Remarks   171

PSYCHOMOTOR RETARDATION AND ARREST OF PSYCHIC
FUNCTION   172

5   Childhood and Adolescent Hereditary Metabolic Disorders   177

GENERAL FEATURES   177

COMMON CLINICAL SYNDROMES   178

PROGRESSIVE SPASTIC PARAPLEGIAS   179

PREDOMINANTLY PROGRESSIVE CEREBELLAR ATAXIAS   186

HMDs PRESENTING WITH ACTION MYOCLONUS, SEIZURES,
AND ATAXIA   192

HEREDITARY, PREDOMINANTLY EXTRAPYRAMIDAL DISORDERS
OF LATE CHILDHOOD AND ADOLESCENCE   199

FAMILIAL POLYNEUROPATHIES IN JUVENILE METABOLIC
DISEASE   219

PROGRESSIVE VISUAL LOSS AS AN INITIAL MANIFESTATION IN
JUVENILE HEREDITARY METABOLIC DISORDERS   234

FAMILIAL METABOLIC ENCEPHALOPATHIES WITH CLINICAL
EVIDENCE OF DIFFUSE CNS DISORDER   235
Disorders with a Mendelian Mode of Inheritance   235
Diseases with a Maternal Mode of Inheritance: Defects in Mitochondrial DNA   254

PROGRESSIVE METABOLIC AND DEGENERATIVE DISEASES
WITH SPECIAL NEUROLOGIC AND SOMATIC (ESSENTIALLY
CUTANEOUS) FEATURES   258

PROGRESSIVE GENETIC ENCEPHALOPATHIES
LEADING TO STROKE   264

METABOLIC DISORDERS WITH INTERMITTENT
NEUROLOGIC SIGNS   268

FAMILIAL ENCEPHALOPATHIES IN WHICH PERSONALITY
CHANGES, BEHAVIORAL DISTURBANCES, AND DEMENTIA
MAY BE A PRESENTING SIGN   270

ISOLATED DELAY IN MENTAL AND MOTOR DEVELOPMENT   272

6   **Distinction between Hereditary Metabolic Diseases
    and Other Diseases of the Child's Nervous System**   **282**

DIFFERENTIAL DIAGNOSIS OF GENETIC NEUROMETABOLIC
DISEASES IN THE NEONATAL PERIOD   283
Perinatal Hypoxia and Circulatory Insufficiency: Hypoxic-Ischemic
  Encephalopathy of the Newborn   283
Intracranial Hemorrhage   283
Kernicterus   284
Prenatal Encephalitis; Neonatal Bacterial Meningitis   284
Prenatal Developmental Abnormalities of the Brain   284
Other Neonatal Conditions   285

DIFFERENTIATION OF HEREDITARY METABOLIC DISEASES
FROM STATIC ENCEPHALOPATHIES AND DEVELOPMENTAL
ABNORMALITIES IN INFANCY AND EARLY CHILDHOOD   286
Cerebral Palsies and Their Differentiation from HMDs   286
Prenatal Developmental Brain Defects   288
Psychomotor Retardation, Developmental Delay, Mental Retardation 291
Behavioral Syndromes: Autism and Rett Syndrome   292

DIFFERENTIAL DIAGNOSIS OF NEUROLOGIC SYNDROMES
ENCOUNTERED IN THE HEREDITARY METABOLIC AND
DEGENERATIVE ENCEPHALOPATHIES OF CHILDHOOD
AND ADOLESCENCE   293
Ataxias   293
Basal Ganglia Disorders   297
Spastic Paraplegia   300
Hemiplegias   302
Epilepsy   303
Differential Diagnostic of Action Myoclonus (Polymyoclonus)   309

PRINCIPAL FEATURES AND DIFFERENTIAL DIAGNOSIS OF
HEREDITARY METABOLIC AND DEGENERATIVE
NEUROPATHIES   310
Sensorimotor Neuropathies   311
Lower Motor Neuronopathies in HMDs   315
Involvement of Cranial Nerves in HMDs   315

OCULAR ABNORMALITIES   321
Visual Failure   321
Derangement of Ocular Movements   323
Characteristic Morphological Changes of the Eyes   324

DEAFNESS   324

**7   Visceral and Other Tissue Abnormalities That Are Associated
     with the Hereditary Metabolic Encephalopathies   327**

LIVER AND SPLEEN   328

CARDIOVASCULAR SYSTEM   328

KIDNEYS   329

ADRENAL INSUFFICIENCY   332

DIABETES MELLITUS   332

SKELETAL SYSTEM   332

ALTERATIONS OF SKIN AND HAIR   332

HEMATOLOGIC CHANGES   332

FACIAL DYSMORPHIAS. SOMATIC MALFORMATIONS   332

RESPIRATORY TRACT   336

GASTROINTESTINAL SIGNS, MALNUTRITION, AND GROWTH
FAILURE   336

**8   Laboratory Tests for the Diagnosis of Hereditary
     Metabolic Encephalopathies   340**

BIOCHEMISTRY AND MOLECULAR BIOLOGY   340
Common Clinical Tests in Urine, Blood, and CSF   340
Enzyme Assays   341
DNA Studies   342

RADIOLOGY AND NEUROIMAGING   342
Conventional X-rays   342
Ultrasonography   343
Neuroimaging   343

ELECTROPHYSIOLOGICAL METHODS   345

HEMATOLOGIC TESTS   346

EXAMINATION OF BIOPSIED TISSUE   346

PRACTICAL CONSIDERATIONS FOR THE COLLECTION
OF SPECIMENS   350

9   Treatment and Prevention of Neurometabolic Disorders   352

CORRECTION OF THE GENETIC METABOLIC DEFECT   352
Counteracting the Offending Metabolite   352
Acting on the Dysfunctional Enzyme   353
Vitamin Therapy   353
Enzyme Replacement Therapy   359

SYMPTOMATIC TREATMENT   361

PREVENTION   362

Index   365

PREFACE

The hereditary metabolic and degenerative diseases of the nervous system stand alongside the developmental abnormalities, the epilepsies, the cerebral palsies, and the learning disorders as important parts of pediatric neurology. In the past decade, since the publication in 1982 of the first edition of this book, there has been a formidable increase in knowledge about the hereditary metabolic diseases. This came about through new methods of molecular biology, biochemistry, and neuroimaging. New diseases have been discovered, and knowledge of those already known has been greatly expanded. To review these new data comprehensively from the pediatric neurologist's viewpoint has been the motivation for this second edition.

This book is written for clinicians—pediatricians, child neurologists, and adult neurologists. Possibly other specialists, including laboratory scientists, will also find some interest in it. It is our impression that the neurometabolic diseases are now so numerous and diverse in their clinical expressions that the physician needs guidelines. In our work at the E. K. Shriver Center and Kennedy Laboratories of the Massachusetts General Hospital, the Neurology Department of New York University Medical School, and the Child Neurology Service at the University of Louvain (Brussels) we have developed a clinical approach that has been useful to our colleagues and ourselves. A vast number of metabolic diseases of the nervous system have been subdivided in accordance with their age of onset and their predominant neurological syndrome. Not only does this clinical plan facilitate diagnosis, but it also assures that no treatable disease is overlooked.

Knowledge of new technologies for confirmation of diagnosis makes possible the recognition of disease in its preclinical or incipient stage. This has the advantage of enabling the clinician to intercede with any available treatment before the nervous system is irreversibly damaged. But, at the same time, it thrusts the clinician into a new role. Screening procedures of the patient's family and of normal populations of individuals must be devised and applied if they offer reasonable perspectives for prevention and treatment. The results must be evaluated with respect to their reliability, validity, and cost-effectiveness. Families must be educated in the importance of adhering to treatments, some difficult and unpleasant. Parents must be advised and counseled about the risks of bearing other afflicted children. To undertake these new assignments, the neuropediatrician must have knowledge not only of the clinical manifestations of many diseases but also of their biological underpinnings. The latter we have appended to the clinical descriptions.

We are greatly indebted to Dr. Darryl DeVivo for his careful review of our manuscript and for his invaluable critiques and suggestions concerning the paragraphs of this book on mitochondrial disorders. We are also grateful to Dr. Eric Achten, who revised the section on neuroimaging. The authors acknowledge the considerable help received from many colleagues during countless clinical discussions. We are particularly indebted to Joseph Alroy, Rose Mary Boustany, Robert Delong, Elizabeth Dooling, Martin Natowsky, Priscilla Short, Katherine Sims, Philippe Evrard, Gerard Ferriere, Christine Bonnier, Jean-François Gadisseux, Olivier Robain, and Rudy Van Coster. We express our gratitude to Patricia Debluts, Jacqueline Lecuit, Marta Lyon, Jo Serneels, Patricia Stewart, and Ken Wei for their painstaking secretarial work, to Alan Hunt of Keyword Publishing Services Ltd., and to Muza Navrozov, Joseph Hefta, and the staff of McGraw-Hill for their remarkable editorial work.

Gilles Lyon
Raymond D. Adams
Edwin H. Kolodny

NEUROLOGY OF HEREDITARY METABOLIC DISEASES OF CHILDREN

Chapter 1

GENERAL ASPECTS OF HEREDITARY METABOLIC DISEASES OF THE NERVOUS SYSTEM

MATTERS PERTAINING TO ETIOLOGIES

MATTERS PERTAINING TO CLASSIFICATION

CLINICAL CRITERIA OF AN HMD. QUESTIONS OF DEVELOPMENTAL ARREST AND REGRESSION

PLAN OF THIS BOOK

The hereditary metabolic diseases (HMDs) pose a major challenge to neurologists and particularly the neuropediatrician. Most become manifest during childhood and affect the nervous system more often than any other organ system. Clinically, they are difficult to distinguish from one another since the same symptoms and signs occur in many different diseases. Moreover, the same disease may have different presentations, depending in part on the varying age of onset and the stage of development of the child's nervous system. For these reasons, a specific diagnosis often cannot be made on clinical grounds alone.

Reports of new forms of these hereditary metabolic diseases appear regularly in medical journals in an almost bewildering array. New diseases are being discovered and certain well-established hereditary disorders are proving to have a metabolic and/or molecular basis. The details of their biochemistry and molecular genetics may be difficult to comprehend; yet the neuropediatrician must have some familiarity with them in order to make correct diagnoses and rationally direct therapy and prevention. This requires a knowledge of the many laboratory tests that are available and of how to select the ones that are most likely to reveal the exact cause of any given disorder.

Our knowledge of the hereditary metabolic encephalopathies evolved in several overlapping phases. First, the clinical and pathological features were delineated. This allowed for their classification into such categories as neuronal storage diseases, leukodystrophies, poliodystrophies, and subacute necrotizing encephalopathies. In a second phase, the nature of the metabolites accumulating in nerve cells, white matter, visceral organs, and body fluids was identified. In the third phase, the enzymatic defects accounting for the abnormal accumulation (or loss) of the metabolites were discovered. In the fourth phase, genes were mapped to specific chromosomal regions. The most recent phase has involved the cloning of individual genes and the characterization of disease-causing mutations.

The recent advances in molecular biology have had a major impact on neurology. As new diseases were discovered, the extraordinary genetic and clinical heterogeneity of the hereditary metabolic disorders became apparent. The spectrum of their clinical manifestations has proven to be much more diverse than was anticipated a decade ago. A progressive mental regression, a simple mental retardation, an acute life-threatening coma or epileptic status, sudden infant death, or a developmental defect are now all recognized as possible modes of expression. Allelic variants with onset in later years in life, even adulthood, are being observed so that neurologists who see only adult patients must take notice of them. Moreover, by the application of biochemical tests, diagnosis becomes possible before the appearance of the first clinical symptom or sign. Thus, it may be possible to intervene medically before the nervous system suffers serious injury.

Medical progress creates new roles for the child and adult neurologist. The seemingly pointless exercise of affixing a diagnostic label to a rare and untreatable disease now becomes an indispensable step in the planning of a program of treatment and prevention, for which the neurologist must assume responsibility. The neurologist must be prepared to assist in community surveys in a search for heterozygotes; to engage in prenatal and neonatal screening; to serve as a genetic counselor; and to educate patients and their families, as well as physician colleagues, of the need of complying with diets and other treatments even in times of good health.

MATTERS PERTAINING TO ETIOLOGIES

The causes of the disease must always be considered in light of the agency that brings about the abnormal state and without which it cannot occur. The mechanisms of disease refer to the means whereby the causative agency induces tissue change. Terms for the latter are *pathogenesis* and *process*. Both intrinsic and extrinsic factors are involved in pathogenesis.

As the medical model of a disease, the authors accept any maladaptive state of an organ or organism in which there is evidence of a cause and a lesion or a reasonable presumpton of one. The cause initiates a pathogenic process which leads to a change in the function and structure of cells in an organ or organs, and at a certain point gives rise to symptoms and signs recognizable medically. Morphologic changes may be visible to the naked eye or to microscopic examination, and may be only subcellular and inferred from consistency and specificity of clinical manifestations.

The causes of the disease under consideration are genetic. They are attributable to mutations, i.e., alterations of nuclear or mitochondrial DNA. In the case of metabolic diseases of the nervous system, whole populations of neurons or functionally related systems of neurons or some part of their structure is singled out and bears the brunt of the mutation. Thus nerve cells may be affected in their entirety or only some parts of them, such as the axon, myelin sheath, oligodendrocyte, astrocyte, Schwann cell, synaptic connection, neurotransmitters, or neuromodulators. Other organs may be occultly or manifestly affected in some of the disorders, and their dysfunction may, in turn, alter brain function and structure.

In a large number of hereditary metabolic encephalopathies, recent scientific advances have resulted in the discovery of the primary cause (a defective gene), the nature of the gene product (usually an enzyme or an activator protein) and the specific intermediate metabolites (sphingolipids, fatty acids, amino acids, organic acids, or glycogen), which accumulate as a consequence of the enzymatic block.

Technical simplifications now make enzymologic tests available in most hospital laboratories. The possibility of detecting metabolites in body fluids, a clue to the diagnosis of many metabolic disorders, has gained considerably from the use of such methods as gas chromatography/mass spectrometry, thin-layer and liquid chromatography, and mass spectrometry/fast atom bombardment. New or improved techniques in exploring the morphology and function of the brain, such as computed tomography (CT), magnetic resonance imaging (MRI), magnetic resonance spectroscopy (MRS), positron emission tomography (PET), and single proton emission computed tomography (SPECT), are becoming integral parts of the medical examination and provide clues to certain aspects of pathogenesis.

An increasing number of mutant genes causing hereditary metabolic and degenerative diseases affecting the nervous system have been defined and mapped to their chromosomal loci. Detection of their mutations is now possible. This has greatly enhanced diagnostic possibilities, especially when the abnormal protein is difficult to assay, as in dominantly inherited diseases and disorders of mitochondria. The characterization of the specific DNA alteration is also increasingly important for heterozygote detection, prediction of the severity of the disease, presymptomatic diagnosis, and prenatal diagnosis.

Notwithstanding these remarkable advances, we have yet to discover how a primary gene abnormality induces loss of activity of an enzyme or activator protein and in what way the enzyme defect, and particularly the abnormal accumulation of a metabolite, produces brain damage. The filling of this gap of knowledge stands as an important field for future research. Effective therapeutic measures can be achieved only through an understanding of these pathogenic mechanisms. These endeavors offer a prodigious challenge to the neuroscientist. At the present time, it can be said that we do not possess complete knowledge of the pathogenesis of a single hereditary metabolic disease of the nervous system (with the possible exception of pyridoxine dependency). Even in such a well-known disease as phenylketonemia, it is not fully understood how an excess of phenylalanine in brain tissue gradually and irreparably damages nerve cells or myelin; this is also true for all the other amino-acidopathies and organoacidopathies and for all substances accumulating in the nervous system as a result of an enzymatic block. In the sphingolipidoses, it is not known whether the stored lysosomal product damages neurons or is merely an inert by-product of the enzymatic defect. The reasons for the noxious effects of an excess or lack of copper on the brain likewise remain mysterious. Even less do we understand the pathophysiology of disorders in which the normal action of the product of the mutant gene is not known, as is the case in Huntington disease and the spinocerebellar degenerations. The pathogenesis of the brain lesions occurring in Leigh disease and other mitochondrial disorders, or in Zellweger disease and related conditions, remains indeterminate. Nor do we know clearly the basis for the numerous clinical variations (age-related or not) in each disease. Although the mechanisms of neuronal dysfunction and neuronal death are largely unknown, specific neurotoxins appear to play a role in some disorders, for instance, psychosine in Krabbe leukodystrophy; polyglutamine in Huntington disease.

Such insights as have been obtained make us aware of the complex interplay of intrinsic and extrinsic factors during the long maturational period of the human brain. Brain lesions may precede clinical signs. Some disorders strike the fetal nervous system, and children are born with considerable brain damage (as in peroxisomal diseases, disorders of pyruvate metabolism, and some organoacidopathies). In others, such as gangliosidoses, where the disease appears clinically several weeks or months after birth, it has been shown that neuronal lesions are already present in the fetus. From these findings one envisions prospects for fetal therapy. When the disease strikes much later, a combination of different factors might explain the delay and variability of clinical manifestations, which tend to be milder and restricted to certain neuronal systems. Relevant factors may be the degree of residual activity of an enzyme and types of mutations. In disorders related to a defect in mitochondrial DNA (mtDNA), the clinical presentation is probably determined by the proportion of normal to mutated mtDNA in various tissues.

The operation of extrinsic factors is evident in diseases where brain damage is produced or aggravated by seizures, circulatory collapse, acidosis, hyperthermia, or hypoglycemia, or is secondary to the functional decompensation of visceral organs (heart, blood vessels, liver, kidneys, endocrine glands) whose cells may be affected more than or prior to those of the brain.

Episodic neurologic dysfunction may be related to a biochemical abnormality worsened by fasting, excess dietary protein, deficiency of a vitamin, or fever.

Much progress has been made in the treatment of HMDs; however, in many of them, a specific treatment has not been discovered. Apparent obstacles have been (1) occurrence of irrevocable brain damage before birth; (2) the blood-brain barrier, which renders neurons probably inaccessible to enzyme replacement therapies; and (3) our ignorance of the exact pathophysiological mechanisms leading to brain dysfunction.

MATTERS PERTAINING TO CLASSIFICATION

Theoretically, the ideal classification of this group of diseases should be based on cause and pathogenesis. Unfortunately, current knowledge is insufficient to allow their arrangement in such terms. Moreover, their clinical, biochemical, and genetic heterogeneity is so great (for example, more than 50 mutations have been described in Tay-Sachs disease) that no logical order is possible on purely molecular or enzymatic criteria. Therefore, the authors believe that a taxonomy utilizing clinical criteria, i.e., age of onset and syndromes common to groups of diseases, best serves practical medical objectives. This thesis and its potential weaknesses will be elaborated further on.

CLINICAL CRITERIA OF AN HMD. QUESTIONS OF DEVELOPMENTAL ARREST AND REGRESSION

The three main clinical criteria for the determination of a hereditary metabolic and heredodegenerative disease of the nervous system are evidence of *familial coincidence, progressive decline in nervous functioning, and the appearance and progression of unmistakable neurologic signs.* When all these criteria are satisfied by clinical analysis, diagnosis becomes relatively certain. Each criterion has its own fallibilities and may sometimes be difficult to apply.

Hereditary metabolic and degenerative diseases are *transmitted* according to different modes. Knowledge of the type of transmission of each disease is essential for diagnostic purposes.

In *autosomal recessive disorders*, several siblings in a family (boys and girls) may be affected, whereas parents are normal. Twenty-five percent of the children of a carrier-carrier couple are affected, 50 percent are carriers, and 25 percent are without the mutant gene. Each parent has a 50 percent chance of transmitting the gene to his offspring.

In *autosomal dominant* conditions, several generations are affected, females and males equally. Father to son transmission occurs. Children of carriers have a 50 percent risk of being affected. Carrier parents may have various degrees of the disease.

In *X-linked diseases*, only males are affected, and only mothers transmit the disease. Carrier females are usually normal, but a few may manifest some symptoms. Sons of carrier women have a 50 percent risk of having the disease. All daughters of men with the disease are carriers.

In *maternal (mitochondrial) inheritance*, there is a mother to child (boys and girls) transmission, and no transmission from father to child. Female cariers may be affected. (Some mitochondrial disorders have a mendelian, nonmaternal, mode of inheritance.)

Evidence of familial coincidence is frequently lacking and, if present, is not always easy to ascertain. In autosomal recessive disorders, the family may not realize that a previous child has been or is afflicted with the same disease. A sibling may have died of unknown causes or an erroneous diagnosis may have been made; or if the sibling is still living, the clinical picture may be so different that the connection with the other child's condition is not recognized. Also, parents may be ashamed or frightened and therefore deliberately conceal the existence of another affected individual in the family.

Mild degrees of a disease may be overlooked unless other family members (parents, ascendants and collaterals) are carefully examined. For instance, the mother may show subtle but significant evidence of disease in X-linked or mitochondrial disorders of maternal transmission. One of the parents may be affected with a condition which at first may seem to bear no relationship to the child's disorder but which is of major diagnostic importance (for instance, psychological disturbances in a parent of an individual with juvenile Huntington disease).

The ascertainment of a *regression* of neurologic function also may prove to be more difficult than one expects. It is most reliably determined by the juxtaposition of two sets of data; one drawn from the biography of the patient and specifying the level of functioning at different age periods; the other, a developmental scale, drawn from the examination of a large number of sup-

posedly normal infants and children of different ages. Difficulties in the application of this method come from several sources. Information about the patient's developmental status at a succession of age periods usually must come from the parents. If neglectful, unobservant, or themselves mentally impaired, parents cannot supply reliable information. One must then rely upon a series of medical examinations separated by intervals of time (here a succession of photographs and videotapes of the child taken by the parents may prove to be useful). Allowance must be made for the effects of infection, malnutrition, parental neglect, seizures, or drugs, which may in any one examination reduce the patient's capacities in nonspecific ways. And the reliability of a developmental scale depends upon the ages it covers. Early in life, the few reference points are heavily weighted in motor functions, which do not predict more complex behavior and cognitive development. For more complex mental functions, normal individual differences are wider. In early infancy, when many parts of the cerebrum are immature, regression from a higher to a lower level of functioning is more difficult to perceive. Another problem is that in a slowly progressive disease, for a long period, the dysfunction may be indistinguishable from an arrest of development or a nonprogressive disease. In these circumstances, the metabolic nature of the disorder may be missed if sufficient attention is not given to some extraneurologic abnormality or to the results of a few paraclinical investigations, which should systematically be applied to these situations.

The recognition of *newly developing neurologic signs* is an obvious mark of an emerging disease. Here, allowances must be made for the delayed time of appearance and the prominence of signs dependent on the continuously maturing nervous system. For example, a static nonprogressive congenital hemiplegia may not become manifest until the fifth or sixth month of postnatal life, at a time when the corticospinal tract is becoming myelinated. A choreoathetosis from a birth injury may not be evident until the second or third year. A potential epileptic focus acquired at the time of birth or before may not evince a first seizure until childhood; and the form of seizure, whether one of infantile spasms or petit mal is partly conditional upon the level of maturation of the brain. Such a relationship between brain maturation and clinical expression is also possible in the neurometabolic encephalopathies. Moreover there may be particular difficulty when the induction of new neurologic signs is consequent to the use of drug therapy. For example, dystonia or choreoathetotis may be induced by a neurotropic drug in a patient with a chronic or recurrent psychiatric disease (tardive dyskinesia).

To summarize, the neuropediatrician will find that the clinical diagnostic criteria may be difficult to utilize under the following circumstances:

1. When the metabolic disease strikes and terminates life during the first postnatal days or weeks before a significant degree of cerebral function has been attained.

2. When the metabolic disease is of such chronicity that one cannot decide whether there is regression or merely an arrest of function, viz., the regression may have been more or less synchronous with maturation, nullifying the arrest, so to speak.

3. When, on the contrary, the metabolic disorder strikes with such abruptness as to simulate infectious or postinfectious diseases.

4. When the metabolic disease is of such severity and has such widespread destructive effect that few, if any, parts of the nervous system remain sufficiently intact to undergo further derangement.

5. When intercurrent illness, seizures, or drug therapy impair the function of the nervous system to the point that it cannot be properly assessed over brief periods of time.

6. When nutritional abnormalities precede or mask the evidence of neurological dysfunction.

7. When the manifestations of an earlier nonprogressive lesion evolve in relation to the maturational process and simulate an ongoing disease (for instance, hemiplegia, paraparesis, choreoathetosis and secondary microcephaly of perinatal origin).

8. When the loss of some function in fixed cognitive or behavioral disorders, such as echolalic speech, is misinterpreted as evidence of progressive brain damage.

Other special symptoms and signs of metabolic disease are presented in the following chapters under the age period in which they arise.

PLAN OF THIS BOOK

While the age of onset of the hereditary metabolic disorders varies considerably, and for each disorder neurological signs may appear at practically any time between infancy and adolescence or even adulthood, the majority of them have an age of predilection and in each age period different diseases tend to have a common symptomatology, according to the degree of maturation of the brain.

Therefore, our proposed approach to this complex field is to subdivide all the diseases conforming to the diagnostic criteria itemized above into clinical categories according to the predominant age of onset, their principal syndrome(s), and their temporal profile. We believe that the clinician, prepared with such knowledge, can narrow the range of diagnostic possibilities and select more efficiently the appropriate laboratory tests. This approach is a clinical one, and the information elaborated in the chapters that follow is essentially for the clinician. However, it is not possible to strictly separate the clinical and biological aspects of disease, and due importance has been given to biological data of diagnostic importance. We therefore believe that our presentation of the neurometabolic disorders will also be helpful to the laboratory scientist.

Chapter 2

THE NEUROLOGY OF NEONATAL HEREDITARY METABOLIC DISEASES

GENERAL SYMPTOMATOLOGY, CHARACTERISTIC
FEATURES OF NEONATAL HMDs, AND
DIAGNOSTIC TESTS
    General Symptomatology of Neonatal
      Neurologic Disorders
    Clinical and Radiological Characteristics
      of HMDs
    Diagnostic Laboratory Tests

CLASSIFICATION OF HMDs IN THE
NEONATAL PERIOD
    Inherited Disorders of Amino Acid and Organic
      Acid Metabolism
    Neonatal Mitochondrial Encephalopathies
    Disorders of Biotin Metabolism
    Neonatal Peroxisomal Disorders
    Disorders of Carbohydrate Metabolism
    Pyridoxine (Vitamin B_6) Dependency
    Other Metabolic Disorders with a Possible
      Neonatal Onset

CONCLUSIONS

GENERAL SYMPTOMATOLOGY, CHARACTERISTIC FEATURES OF NEONATAL HMDs, AND DIAGNOSTIC TESTS

A number of hereditary metabolic diseases (HMDs) affecting the nervous system manifest themselves immediately after birth. The importance of these diseases outweighs their frequency, because prompt recognition is essential to successful medical intervention. Failure of diagnosis may consign the patient to death or to lifelong impairment of cognition and/or motor development.

Causes of neonatal neurometabolic disorders are numerous. Most of them also occur in infancy, childhood, or adolescence. Some of the aminoacidopathies and disorders of carbohydrate metabolism which reveal themselves at this early period have been among the first recognized inborn errors of metabolism. Some may now be detected by routine neonatal screening. During the last 10 years, improved methods for the detection of metabolites in body fluids have resulted in the description of new inborn errors of organic acid metabolism. Also, new classes of neonatal disorders related to dysfunction of peroxisomes and mitochondria have been brought to light; some of them—such as Zellweger's syndrome and pyruvate de-hydrogenase (PDH) deficiency—seriously affect the brain before birth and are of particular gravity.

The extraordinary progress of biochemistry and molecular biology now allows the prompt recognition and prenatal diagnosis of most neonatal metabolic disorders and their early treatment. However, the new diagnostic procedures would be of no avail if applied indiscriminately. The suspicion of a metabolic encephalopathy rests on clinical examination.

In view of the relative incompetence of the cerebral hemispheres at birth one might wonder whether there is any possibility of achieving reliable diagnoses of neurologic diseases during the neonatal period from clinical observations. The answer is obviously yes, with concessions to reality.

The brain stem, spinal cord, nerves, and muscles are all functioning sufficiently well at this time to sustain muscle tone and body postures, reflex activity, motor automatisms, sucking and swallowing, and such vital functions as respiration, circulation, and temperature control. More complex activities, which probably imply some degree of participation of the cerebral cortex, consist of awareness of surroundings, ocular pursuit, sleep-wake cycles, and crying. They can readily be explored at this age, in addition to the more elementary motor reactions.

As various disorders affecting the immature brain tend to result in similar symptoms and signs, the clinician's role is not an easy one. He must be aware of the general symptomatology of neonatal neurologic disorders, of the clinical elements which allow the suspicion of a hereditary neurometabolic disorder, and of the pertinent laboratory investigations which are indispensable to confirm clinical impressions. These different steps will now be discussed.

General Symptomatology of Neonatal Neurologic Disorders

The functions of the immature nervous system of the neonate which can be assessed as indicators of disease in the neonate are as follows:

1. The state of consciousness: awareness to surroundings, reaction to visual and auditory stimuli.

2. The tone of the limbs and trunk and certain postural mechanisms (as described by André Thomas (1952),[1] Peiper (1963),[2] Prechtl and Beintema (1965),[3] Brazelton (1973),[4] Dubowitz and Dubowitz (1981),[5] and Amiel-Tison and Grenier (1986).[6]

3. Certain motor automatisms (Moro response, supporting, placing and stepping reactions, palmar grasping, tonic neck reflexes).

4. Myotatic and cutaneous reflexes.

5. Spontaneous ocular movements, ocular fixation and pursuit, visual function.

6. Respiration and circulation (partially assessed by the Apgar score).

7. Sucking and swallowing; regulation of appetite.

8. Occurrence of seizures.

Seizures as a Mark of Neonatal Brain Disease
These are among the most frequent expressions of neonatal cerebral disorders.[7,8] A usual feature is their fragmentary nature; seldom are they integrated into a generalized tonic-clonic pattern. Typically they consist of a series of brief jerks or spasms of muscles of some part of the body: the face, mouth, tongue, eyes, respiratory musculature, or limb musculature. There may a brief fixation or tonic turning or rhythmic jerks of the eyes, variations in the pupillary diameter, eyelid flutter; a momentary arrest of respiration, a bout of hyperpnea, sucking movements, drooling; localized rhythmic jerks of the face or hand; or tonic posturing of one limb. These undramatic phenomena may easily be overlooked or attributed to other causes. Sometimes, one must turn to the electroencephalogram (EEG) for assistance. More definite seizure phenomena are multifocal, erratic, clonic jerks, tonic spasms of the four limbs or massive flexion spasms. Rarely seizures may occur in utero. One clinical difficulty is to distinguish some of the brief epileptic movements from jitteriness, a type of rhythmic tremor which is induced and arrested by certain stimuli, and may or may not express a serious medical problem. Although benign familial convulsions are known to occur,[9] persistent neonatal seizures are generally the consequence of a serious brain disorder.

Impaired Alertness, Stupor, and Coma
These states are somewhat difficult to ascertain in the neonate and must be evaluated solely in terms of spontaneous activity and responsivity to stimuli at different times of the day. Levels of alertness vary depending on gestational age, phases of the sleep-wake cycle, and relation to feeding. Periods of alertness are least well defined in the premature infant, but are sufficiently in evidence to be assayed in the full-term infant. When awake and undisturbed in the supine position, the arms and legs are flexed and the limbs intermittently engaged in random, brief, bilateral, usually asymmetrical movements. If asleep, when approached, gentle stimuli will rouse the infant without inducing crying. A moving visual stimulus, particularly a human face, will evoke ocular fixation and pursuit movements. An auditory stimulus will usually arrest motor activity and sucking, and modify the respiratory pattern. Tactile stimuli elicit movements of the limbs; the latter are not stereotyped or obligatory to one pattern and occur after a variable latency. They habituate to repeated stimuli.

Definite and persistent reduction in alertness, as shown by the absence of these responses, signifies an impairment of brain function. Allowance must be made for the time of day, and whether the infant is asleep, hungry, or satiated. Also, assessment within the first 2 or 3 postnatal days must take into account the possible trauma of parturition, the effects of drugs given to the mother, etc.

The language employed in referring to levels of reduced consciousness conforms to that of neurology in general. A term infant who lies with eyes closed most of the time, making few movements, but still briefly arousable is said to be *lethargic*. If arousable responses are extremely difficult to evoke, the state is one of *stupor*. A complete absence of receptivity of stimuli and of responsivity corresponds to *coma*. Degrees of coma (light or deep) are judged by the presence or absence of obligatory reflexive movements of the limbs and presence or absence of brain stem reflexes [pupillary, corneal, vestibular (doll's eye sign); pharyngeal]. Coma may occur in relation to a series of seizures and is then transitory; if persistent and nonepileptic, it must be regarded as a condition of extreme gravity.

Disturbed Vision and Impaired Oculomotor Function Assessment of these functions in the newborn requires some expertise. Normally, by term and in the first week of postnatal life, visual fixation and the following of a bright object or, even better, a human face is demonstrable. These responses are one of the best indications of upper brain stem (and possibly of cortical) function. As remarked above, the impairment of visual fixation and ocular pursuit are often conjoined with lethargy and stupor. In an alert infant, they should call for careful inspection of the lens, retina, optic nerves, retrogeniculate optic pathways, and ocular muscles. If these structures are intact, the possibility of brain dysfunction must be considered. Between the ages of 3 and 6 months, the state of visual attention, discrimination and memory are said to give valuable indications of future intellectual development.[10]

In the stuporous or comatose infant, and also, if necessary, when the child is awake, one can assess the integrity of the oculomotor nuclei and their connections by vestibular stimulation (turning the infant's head or rotation of the whole body when held in a vertical position or irrigating external auditory canals with cold water). Affection of the oculomotor nuclei or nerves abolishes these labyrinthine-ocular reflexes. A unilateral lesion of the brain stem or hemisphere may cause the eyes to deviate contralaterally; only at a later period of life will an acute cerebral lesion cause failure of contralateral gaze.

In general, isolated or multiple palsies of the oculomotor nerves or supranuclear horizontal or vertical gaze palsies are rare in the neonate. Moderate divergence of the eyes in the horizontal plane is usually not abnormal, whereas divergence in the vertical plane is generally indicative of dysfunction. Abnormal movements of the eyes are more frequent. A rapid pendular nystagmus indicates a lesion of the retina or optic nerve, or a congenital nystagmus. In case of visual failure, the optokinetic nystagmus cannot be elicited. During seizures, the eyes may turn or jerk rhythmically in one direction. Ocular flutter (repeated oscillations of the eyes in one plane) and opsoclonus (dancing eyes in all planes) may be taken as a sign of brain stem and cerebellar disorder at any age. A repeated, rapid downward deviation of the eyes and slow return to a central position (ocular bobbing) are indicative of a pontine lesion. Slow "roving" conjugate eye movements in comatose patients assure integrity of brain stem oculomotor mechanisms.

Alterations of pupillary size are not infrequent but are at times difficult to interpret. A slight difference in diameter may be found in normal children. When a markedly dilated pupil is due to a IIId nerve palsy, there is usually a paralysis of some external eye movements and the levator palpebrae muscle as well; pupillary constriction in response to illumination of the contralateral eye is abolished. If not, a lesion of the optic nerve or retina is probable. The slight ptosis and miosis of Claude Bernard-Horner syndrome are easily recognizable. Coma with dilated, fixed pupils is usually irreversible. Bilateral miosis is observed in segmental brain stem lesions affecting the descending hypothalamo-spinal pupillodilator fibers and in various intoxications, but may remain unexplained. Transient changes in the pupillary diameter may be produced by seizures.

Actually, oculomotor responses in the genetic metabolic diseases have not been well studied, but when the above abnormalities appear in a neonate, one should consider a metabolic disease, among others.

Abnormal Postures and Automatisms of the Trunk and Limbs Muscular hypotonia of the limbs and body axis is a common manifestation of neonatal neurometabolic diseases and of many other diseases of the nervous system or musculature as well. If of nervous (or muscular) origin, it is always associated with a marked reduction in overall spontaneous muscular activity. The primary neonatal reactions, such as the Moro response, palmar grasping, supporting reactions, placing and stepping reactions, are enfeebled or abolished. The tonic neck reflexes may be absent or abnormal. Often, the tendon reflexes in hypotonic infants are depressed or absent, and the plantar reflexes absent or clearly extensor in type. Frank paralysis in an alert, responsive infant should direct attention to spinal cord birth injury, motor neuron disease, and severe myopathies, conditions which are usually not attended by evidence of cerebral dysfunction. (Exceptions exist in the congenital myopathies.) In contrast to hypotonia, pertinent hypertonia of limbs and trunk rarely occurs in genetic metabolic diseases of the brain at this age (a notable exception being Krabbe leukodystrophy). When it is observed in the neonatal period, one should first suspect hypoxic-ischemic cerebral damage or brain hemorrhage. Unyielding deformities of the joints at birth (arthrogryposis) are not manifestations of HMDs. (However, deformity of the limbs may be present in a very limited number of disorders, such as glutaric acidemia type II and Zellweger syndrome.)

These clinical disorders, as was remarked, are common to most neonatal diseases. *Severe hypotonia, alterations of consciousness, ocular disorders, feeding difficulties, vomiting,* and *abnormalities of the respiratory rhythm* (apneic and cyanotic attacks), in isolation or in any combination, are present in most neurometabolic conditions.

Clinical and Radiological Characteristics of HMDs (see Table 2-1)

1. Knowledge that a sibling has died from a hereditary metabolic disorder or from some obscure cause in infancy or childhood; neurologic signs in one parent.

2. A free interval of a few days between birth and the first signs of the disorder. (The delay may however be lacking.)

3. Disorder of the respiratory rhythm in the absence of pulmonary and cardiac abnormalities or paralysis of the respiratory muscles. Hyperpnea and apneas may result from metabolic acidosis, brain stem lesions, or the direct action of a metabolite on the respiratory center (and in this case may be associated with respiratory alkalosis as in urea cycle disorders).

4. Peculiar odor of the urine (maple syrup urine disease, isovaleric acidemia, glutaric aciduria type II).

5. Special extraneural abnormalities on clinical or radiologic examination:

   • Unexplained feeding difficulties and vomiting

   • A cardiomyopathy (essentially in the mitochondrial disorders and Pompe disease)

   • A hepatomegaly and splenomegaly

   • Polycystic kidneys by ultrasound

   • Dysmorphic facial features (essentially in peroxisomal, mitochondrial, and organic acid disorders; also lysosomal diseases, such as mucopolysaccharidoses, I-cell disease, and oligosaccharidoses)

   • Skeletal changes (such as patellar calcifications in Zellweger disease)

   • Abnormalities of skin and hair

6. Ocular abnormalities, such as cataracts, corneal opacities, glaucoma, hypoplastic optic nerves, retinal degeneration, which are characteristic of a number of HMDs, but by themselves in no way specific.

7. MRI, CT scans, and ultrasound scanning may occasionally reveal congenital lesions of the white matter, cerebral cortex, basal ganglia, and corpus callosum in some mitochondrial and peroxisomal disorders, which are to be differentiated from the far more frequent ischemic lesions of peri- or prenatal origin.

8. A great majority of children afflicted with HMDs are born at term with normal birth weight and head circumference and no somatic malformations. However, a moderately low birth weight (as for instance in Menkes disease) and a moderate congenital microcephaly are occasionally noted. Macrocephaly is observed in some organoacidopathies and possibly Menkes disease. Congenital defects of limbs, heart, and urinary tract are features of glutaric acidemia type II and, occasionally, of other diseases. Hydrops fetalis occurs occasionally in some of the lysosomal disorders (see Table 7-2).

Diagnostic Laboratory Tests

Once the pediatrician is oriented toward the possibility of an HMD, either because of the presence of one of the elements of suspicion listed above or because of the absence of an evident cause, a few routine tests (Table 2-2) will often provide the necessary confirmation:

1. Standard laboratory tests, essentially measures of the acid-base balance, lactate, glucose, ketone bodies, ammonia and carnitine in blood and/or urine, and protein, glucose and lactate in the CSF, are of importance:

   • Acidosis and ketosis are found in most organic acidurias

   • A major elevation of lactate in blood and CSF immediately suggests a disorder of pyruvate metabolism or of the respiratory chain

   • Hypoglycemia with low ketone bodies (hypoketotic hypoglycemia) is a feature of disorders of mitochondrial fatty acid oxidation

Table 2-1
Distinctive features in the neonatal HMDs

Dysmorphic facial features and other congenital defects	Zellweger syndrome and other peroxisomal disorders Glutaric aciduria type II Pyruvate dehydrogenase deficiency Molybdenum cofactor deficiency Mevalonic aciduria
Polycystic kidneys	Zellweger syndrome Glutaric aciduria type II Carnitine palmitoyltransferase type II deficiency
Characteristic odor of urine	Maple syrup urine disease Isovaleric acidemia Glutaric aciduria type II
Cardiomyopathy or other cardiac defects	Complex I deficiency Complex IV deficiency Disorders of mitochondrial fatty acid β oxidation Glutaric aciduria type II Carnitine palmitoyltransferase type II deficiency Combined deficiency of MMCoA mutase and MHMT Zellweger disease
Abnormality of skin	Holocarboxylase synthetase deficiency
Abnormality of hair	Menkes disease Holocarboxylase synthetase deficiency
Patellar calcifications	Zellweger disease
Adrenocortical insufficiency or adrenocortical lesions	Zellweger disease and other peroxisomal diseases
Hematologic abnormalities	Propionic aciduria Methylmalonic aciduria Isovaleric acidemia Combined deficiency of methylmalonyl-CoA mutase and methyltetrahydrofolate: homocysteine methyltransferase Methyltetrahydrofolate: homocysteine methyltransferase deficiency Galactosemia
Hearing defects	Zellweger disease and other peroxisomal diseases
Ocular abnormalities	Zellweger disease and other peroxisomal diseases Molybdenum cofactor deficiency Mevalonic aciduria Galactosemia Mitochondrial DNA depletion syndrome Maple syrup urine disease Combined MMCoA mutase and MHMT deficiency (Cbl C)
Prenatal cerebral defects	Zellweger and other peroxisomal diseases Pyruvate dehydrogenase complex deficiency Pyruvate carboxylase deficiency Glutaric aciduria type II 3-hydroxyisobutyric aciduria Molybdenum cofactor deficiency

Abbreviations: MMCoA mutase = methylmalonic-CoA mutase; MHMT = methyltetrahydrofolate: homocysteine methyltransferase.

Table 2-2
Plan for the diagnosis of neonatal hereditary HMD:

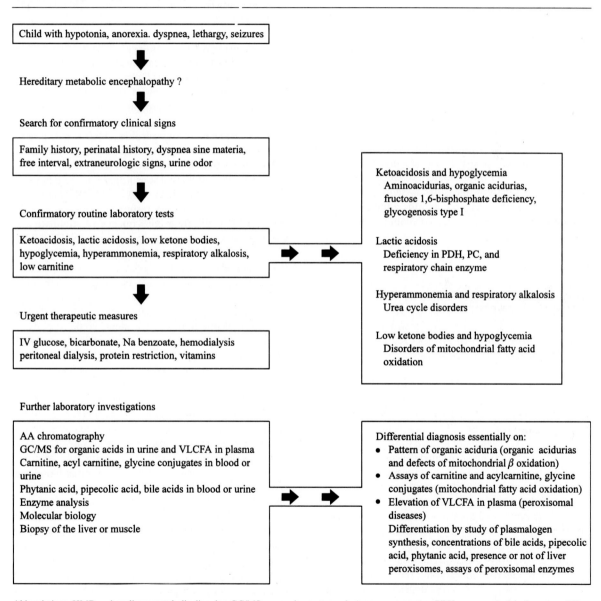

Child with hypotonia, anorexia. dyspnea, lethargy, seizures

↓

Hereditary metabolic encephalopathy ?

↓

Search for confirmatory clinical signs

Family history, perinatal history, dyspnea sine materia, free interval, extraneurologic signs, urine odor

↓

Confirmatory routine laboratory tests

Ketoacidosis, lactic acidosis, low ketone bodies, hypoglycemia, hyperammonemia, respiratory alkalosis, low carnitine

↓

Urgent therapeutic measures

IV glucose, bicarbonate, Na benzoate, hemodialysis peritoneal dialysis, protein restriction, vitamins

Ketoacidosis and hypoglycemia
Aminoacidurias, organic acidurias, fructose 1,6-bisphosphate deficiency, glycogenosis type I

Lactic acidosis
Deficiency in PDH, PC, and respiratory chain enzyme

Hyperammonemia and respiratory alkalosis
Urea cycle disorders

Low ketone bodies and hypoglycemia
Disorders of mitochondrial fatty acid oxidation

Further laboratory investigations

AA chromatography
GC/MS for organic acids in urine and VLCFA in plasma
Carnitine, acyl carnitine, glycine conjugates in blood or urine
Phytanic acid, pipecolic acid, bile acids in blood or urine
Enzyme analysis
Molecular biology
Biopsy of the liver or muscle

Differential diagnosis essentially on:
- Pattern of organic aciduria (organic acidurias and defects of mitochondrial β oxidation)
- Assays of carnitine and acylcarnitine, glycine conjugates (mitochondrial fatty acid oxidation)
- Elevation of VLCFA in plasma (peroxisomal diseases)
  Differentiation by study of plasmalogen synthesis, concentrations of bile acids, pipecolic acid, phytanic acid, presence or not of liver peroxisomes, assays of peroxisomal enzymes

Abbreviations: HMD = hereditary metabolic disorder; GC/MS = gas chromatography/mass spectrometry; PDH = pyruvate dehydrogenase; PC = pyruvate carboxylase; VLCFA = very long chain fatty acids; AA = amino acids.

• Severe hyperammonemia, usually with respiratory alkalosis and without metabolic acidosis, is found in urea cycle disorders

2. Chromatography of blood and urine for amino acids and gas chromatography and mass spectroscopy (GC/MS) for the detection of organic acids in urine and very long chain fatty acids in plasma (elevated in peroxisomal disorders) should be performed whenever a hereditary metabolic disorder is strongly suspected on clinical grounds. These techniques are available in most modern biochemical laboratories.

3. More specialized biochemical enzymatic and molecular procedures are needed for definitive diagnosis, specific treatment, and familial counseling.

4. Whenever a metabolic disorder is suspected, urgent therapeutic measures include intravenous infusion of glucose and bicarbonate, exchange transfusions and peritoneal dialysis, measures to reduce the level of ammonia, protein restriction, and the administration of vitamins [biotin, vitamin B_6, cobalamin, thiamin, or riboflavin (see Table 2-2)].

CLASSIFICATION OF HMDs IN THE NEONATAL PERIOD

Inherited Disorders of Amino Acid and Organic Acid Metabolism

Urea Cycle Disorders The Krebs-Henseleit cycle, by which ammonia is converted to urea, is controlled by six enzymes: N-acetylglutamate synthetase (NAGS), carbamylphosphate synthetase (CPS), and ornithine transcarbamylase (OTC), which are located in the mitochondria of hepatocytes; argininosuccinate synthetase (ASS), argininosuccinate lyase (ASL), and arginase, which are cytosolic enzymes.

Clinical disorders are associated with deficiencies of all six enzymes and are classified as follows: (1) deficient activity of CPS (hyperammonemia type I); (2) of OTC (hyperammonemia type II); (3) of ASS (citrullinemia); (4) of ASL (argininosuccinic acidemia). Each may produce its effect within the neonatal period; (5) several cases of NAGS deficiency have been reported.[11] In all of these conditions, it is the elevation of ammonia levels that gravely endangers the central nervous function and may lead to rapid death if no effective treatment is immediately given. (6) Arginase deficiency, the sixth disorder, has a later onset and a

very different clinical picture. Hyperammonemia is much less marked; only one case has been reported in a newborn, with a rapidly fatal course.[12]

The estimated frequencies of urea cycle enzyme deficiencies are as follows: CPS, 1/1,000,000 to 1/800,000; OTC, 1/80,000; ASS, 1/250,000; ASL, 1/70,000.

Neonatal Symptomatology This is quite uniform and any clinical differences between them are insignificant. Only in X-linked OTC deficiency may the carrier mother present slight signs of neurologic dysfunction after ingestion of excess protein or in conjunction with valproic acid therapy. The patients are born at term and show no evidence of dysmorphia. After a free interval of 1 to 5 days, they begin to feed poorly, to vomit, and to become lethargic, underactive. Irritability, rigidity, opisthotonus, and convulsions appear in some patients. Hyperpnea is generally a striking phenomenon with normal chest x-rays and respiratory alkalosis (overbreathing is probably a consequence of stimulation of the respiratory center by ammonium (NH^{4+}/NH^3)). Hepatomegaly is observed. There may be a bulging of the fontanelle probably related to brain edema. Abnormalities of hair, which occur in the later-onset forms of ASL deficiency, are not present in the neonatal period. Involuntary movements may occur in NAGS deficiency. Without rapid treatment, coma and atonia prevail as the condition worsens, and death results from apnea.

Diagnostic Laboratory Tests There is a considerable elevation of ammonium in plasma (up to 1000 μM and more, instead of 15 to 45 μM in the normal infant) and in the CSF (about 100 μM). Inasmuch as ammonia is a weak organic acid with a pK_a of about 9.3, most of it, at physiological pH values, is in the ionized form, ammonium. The measurement is on venous blood and is determined most commonly by an enzymatic spectrophotometric method.

Hyperammonemia with respiratory alkalosis, absence of ketoacidosis and normal or reduced levels of blood urea, are highly suggestive of a disease of the urea cycle. Other, less important, changes include high levels of glutamine and alanine in blood and CSF, low levels of arginine and ornithine, and normal liver transaminase.

The presence or absence of citrulline and argininosuccinic acid in plasma, and of orotic acid in urine, helps to differentiate between the different disorders (see Table 2-3). Urinary orotic acid is elevated in OTC deficiency and also in ASS and ASL deficiencies and is decreased in CPS deficiency; plasma citrulline levels are very high in ASS deficiency and more moderately elevated in ASL deficiency; and argininosuccinic acid plasma concentrations are high in ASL deficiency. Hyper-ornithinemia has been reported in NAGS deficiency. The final diagnosis rests on enzyme assays and DNA analysis. All enzymes can be measured in liver biopsy specimens. Intestinal mucosa fragments can be used for CPS and OTC, cultured fibroblasts for ASS and ASL, erythrocytes and leukocytes for ASL and arginase; DNA analyses are available for OTC and CPS defects.

Genetics   OTC deficiency is inherited as an X-linked trait. All other urea cycle disorders are autosomal recessive. Allopurinol challenge may be useful for the detection of female heterozygotes for OTC deficiency. The genes for all urea cycle disorders except NAGS have been cloned. Several mutations are responsible for OTC, ALS, and ASS deficiencies.

Prenatal Diagnosis   ASS and ASL deficiencies may be detected in amniocytes but the other enzymes are not expressed in these cells. Fetal liver biopsies were necessary until DNA probes became available. DNA from the chorionic villus can now be used. Prenatal diagnosis is, however, not possible for all families. If the disease mutation is known, direct mutation detection can be done; if not, DNA from other members of the family must be available and informative.

Differential Diagnosis   Hyperammonemia is found in several other conditions, but is less severe than in urea cycle disorders. These include disorders of pyruvate metabolism, glutaric aciduria type II, hydroxymethylglutaryl-CoA lyase deficiency, straight and branched chain organic acidurias, nonketotic hyperglycinemia, and lysinuric protein intolerance. The highest levels ($>400\,\mu$M) occur in propionic acidemia and methylmalonic acidemia. There are lactic acidosis or ketoacidosis, organic aciduria, and high glycine levels in these diseases but these are not found in the urea cycle abnormalities.

There has also been identified a *transient hyperammonemia of the newborn*, a fulminating disorder of unknown origin affecting prematures. It starts on the first day of life with intense respiratory distress, coma, and may be fatal. Some patients recover. Blood ammonia levels may rise above $4000\,\mu$M without any demonstrable enzymatic defect or any other significant biochemical abnormality.

Neuropathology   In most of the infants coming to postmortem examination, the only gross abnormality is swelling of the brain, of both cortex and white matter, with flattening of convolutions, narrowing of sulci, and reduction in size of ventricles. There may be a slight cerebellar pressure cone. Since brain swelling is common to a number of agonal states, particularly if hypoxia and ischemia have intervened, this type of change is difficult to interpret. More significant is a diffuse swelling of protoplasmic astrocytes without obvious change in neurons. One of the authors (RDA) has described a similar condition in liver coma and in experimental hyperammonemia. It is postulated that an accumulation of glutamine in astrocytes exerts an intracellular hyperosmolar state with secondary alteration of the polarization of the cytoplasmic membrane. In the more chronic forms of these diseases in childhood, brain atrophy and neuronal loss has been reported. Periportal fibrosis of the liver is observed in long-term survivors.

Physiopathology   There may be a variety of mechanisms by which ammonia exerts a toxic effect on the brain. An early effect can be an impairment of the conversion of pyruvate to citrate, resulting in the reduced concentration of brain aspartate and glutamate. This could have the clinical consequence of reduced vigilance. More prolonged hyperammonemia could induce an impairment in brain energy production.

Treatment and Course   Blood ammonia concentrations must be reduced to normal as rapidly as possible, to prevent irreversible neurological damage and death. The most effective means is hemodialysis. Other useful methods to promote excretion of ammonia and waste nitrogen through "alternative" metabolic pathways are: intravenous sodium benzoate (250 mg/kg/day) and sodium phenylacetate or phenylbutyrate (250 to 500 mg/kg/day) and citrulline in the case of CPS and OTC deficiencies, and intravenous arginine in the case of ASS and ASL. A high-caloric low-protein diet supplemented with essential amino acids is indispensable.

This treatment may be lifesaving. In surviving children, neurologic sequelae are severe when treatment is not begun before the stage of coma. Even with early treatment, intermittent episodes of hyperammonemia, especially in OTC and CPS deficiencies, marked by vomiting, drowsiness, confusion, and ataxia, may be provoked by excessive protein intake and infection. These may end fatally and leave permanent neurological and mental disorders in survivors.

Table 2-3
Urea cycle disorders[a]

Mode of inheritance	Deficient enzyme	Orotic acid in urine	Plasma citrulline	Plasma argininosuccinic acid
AR	CPS	Low	Low	
X-linked	OTC	High	Low	
AR	ASS	High	Very high ($> 1000\,\mu M$)	
AR	ASL	High	High ($100–300\,\mu M$)	High
AR	Arginase	High	Normal	

[a] The biochemical phenotype of NAGS deficiency is somewhat variable.

Liver transplantation may prove to be another therapeutic option.

Other Phenotypes Intermittent or chronic late-onset forms (Chap. 4).

For a more detailed account of the urea cycle abnormalities, the reader is referred to the chapter by Bruslow and Horwich in *The Metabolic and Molecular Bases of Inherited Diseases*[12] and the review of Batshaw.[13]

Hyperornithinemia-Hyperammonemia-Homocitrullinuria (HHH) Syndrome There are two disorders associated with high concentrations of ornithine in the plasma: gyrate atrophy of the choroid and retina and the hyperornithinemia, hyperammonemia, homocitrullinuria (HHH) syndrome.[14,15]

The HHH syndrome, probably an autosomal recessive disorder, is characterized by the combination of high plasma ornithine concentrations, postprandial hyperammonemia, and homocitrullinuria. Protein intolerance, which is the main feature in this disorder, may be revealed in the first weeks after birth by vomiting, stupor, and seizures. The neonatal course, however, is normal if the infant is breast-fed.

Subsequently, most patients suffer from intermittent episodes of hyperammonemia after ingestion of protein. No ophthalmologic abnormality has been reported. Some patients become mentally retarded and possibly have other neurological signs in late childhood or adolescence. Plasma ornithine concentrations are markedly elevated (mean range, $656\,\mu M$; normal, $10\,\mu M$). Ornithinuria is variable. High levels of homocitrulline are found in the urine. Fasting blood ammonia values are generally normal, but they increase after pro-

tein ingestion. Urinary orotic acid is usually increased. No enzymatic deficiency has been detected. A defect of carrier-mediated transport of orthinine into the mitochondria has been postulated.

Protein restriction and ornithine supplementation (to compensate for a possible defect in ornithine transport into the mitochondria) has resulted in a decrease of hyperammonemia.

Nonketotic Hyperglycinemia Nonketotic hyperglycinemia (NKH) is an inborn error of amino acid metabolism in which large amounts of glycine accumulate in body fluids.[16] Ketosis and abnormal organic acids in blood and urine are not present. The molecular defect is in the glycine cleavage system, a multiple enzyme complex with four protein components, P protein, T protein, H protein, and L protein. Defects in the first three components have been detected in nonketotic hyperglycinemia.

In the majority of cases, NKH is expressed as an extremely severe neonatal disorder, starting usually within the first 2 days of life, but sometimes later. Rapidly increasing stupor, unresponsiveness, marked breathing difficulties, and seizures are the usual manifestations. Within 1 to 3 days, the infant is totally unresponsive and flaccid. Respiratory distress necessitates mechanical ventilation. Seizures are always prominent, usually of the myoclonic type. Hiccuping is frequent. Abnormal ocular jerking may occur. The EEG frequently exhibits a burst-suppression pattern. Brain scans may show defects of the corpus callosum (Fig. 2-1).

Many patients die in the first days or weeks of life. Some survive for a few months without artificial ventilation, but with increasing microcephaly and continuing

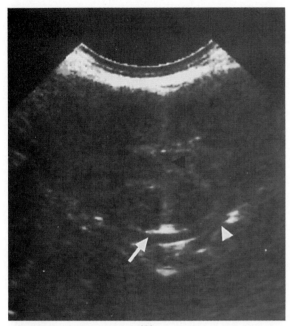
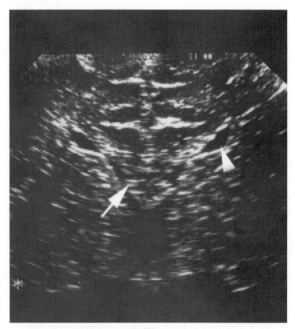

Figure 2-1   **(A)**   **(B)**

Ultrasound scans, coronal plane. (A) Normal neonate. Note corpus callosum (arrow), interhemi-spheric fissure (black arrowhead). Lateral ventricles are virtual (white arrowhead). (Courtesy Dr. M. Ambrosino.) (B) Neonate with nonketotic hyperglycinemia. The corpus callosum is absent. Prolapse of cingulate gyri into third ventricle (arrow). Lateral ventricles displaced laterally (arrowhead).

seizures of various types, including infantile spasms with hypsarrhythmia. There is practically no clinical evidence of brain development.

Biochemical Findings Concentrations of glycine are considerably elevated in plasma, urine, and CSF. Because glycine is normally excreted in the urine, quantitative assays are necessary. Even better for diagnosis is the measurement of glycine in blood. Glycine concentrations in CSF are characteristically elevated. The ratio of CSF glycine to plasma glycine is much higher than in patients with organic acidurias (0.1–0.3; N: 0.01–0.03).

There is no ketosis, acidosis, or abnormal pattern of organic acids in blood or urine.

Diagnosis Measurements of ketone bodies in blood and urine, and gas chromatography/mass spectroscopy for organic acids in urine allows distinction between NKH and some of the conditions causing organic acidemia, especially propionic acidemia and methylmalonic acidemia, which are also associated with hyperglycinemia. Estimation of the CSF/plasma ratio of glycine concentration is very helpful. Differential diagnosis is important as most organic acidurias are treatable. Not to be overlooked is the fact that valproate induces hyperglycinemia.

Neuropathology Various degrees of alteration of the cerebral white matter, including spongy degeneration or cystic degeneration, have been reported in children who have survived for some time. "Agenesis" of the corpus callosum and developmental defects of the cerebral cortex are frequently observed.[17]

Physiopathology The noxious effects of glycine on nerve cells may be related to glycine's role as an inhibitory transmitter in the brain stem and spinal cord, and an excitatory transmitter in the cortex.

Genetics NKH appears to be an autosomal recessive condition. Prevalence has been estimated at 1/250,000. In northern Finland, prevalence is 1/12,000. NKH is probably a genetically heterogeneous disorder.

All patients with the common neonatal type have defects in the P or the T protein. One patient with a different infantile phenotype had a defect in the H protein.

Prenatal diagnosis is not yet possible. However, it might be feasible by the analysis of chorionic villus biopsies.

Treatment No effective treatment of NKH is currently available. Use of dextromethorphan, which blocks NMDA receptor activation by glycine, in association with benzoate, which reduces glycine concentrations, has been tried, apparently with some success. [16,18] Valproate should be avoided.

Other Forms of NKH

- A transient form of neonatal NKH has been described with normal development after treatment with diazepam[19]

- Nonprogressive mental retardation and seizures[20,21]

- Early infantile progressive encephalopathy[22]

- Spinocerebellar degeneration[23]

Maple Syrup Urine Disease

Maple syrup urine disease (MSUD) is caused by defects in the branched chain α keto acid dehydrogenase, a multienzyme complex. This permits accumulation of the branched chain amino acids, leucine, isoleucine and valine, and their keto acids, in body tissues and fluids. Onset of the most common form is in the neonatal period. The less frequent and later-onset varieties with an intermittent or more benign course and a thiamine responsive form are described in Chap. 3.

Clinical Presentation of the Neonatal Type of MSUD Feeding difficulties and a diminished level of responsiveness become apparent between the 4th and 7th day of life, but may occur earlier or as late as the 14th day. In fact, leucine concentrations may rise to abnormal and potentially dangerous concentrations during the first hours of life, prior to evident clinical symptoms. During the following days there develop stupor and abnormalities of the respiratory rhythm, including episodes of apnea, myoclonic jerks, convulsions and opisthotonic spasms. A characteristic odor of urine is an important diagnostic feature, but may pass unnoticed. After several weeks of poor nutritional control the odor becomes most easily detected in earwax. Fluctuating ophthalmoplegia has been observed.[24] The CT scan reveals brain edema, more marked in certain regions such as the centrum semiovale and the cerebellum.

An almost constant feature is a metabolic acidosis, ketonemia, and ketonuria. There may also be hypoglycemia and hypoalaninemia.

If treatment is delayed, death, as well as severe neurological handicaps in survivors, may ensue.

Specific Biochemical Abnormalities A metabolic ketoacidosis makes it necessary for the clinician to consider the possibility of MSUD among other causes. A preliminary screening test for keto acids at the bedside, using a fresh solution of 2N HCl saturated 2,4-dinitrophenylhydrazine may be useful, but diagnosis depends on analysis of urinary organic acids by gas chromatography and mass spectroscopy. The characteristic pattern consists in a marked elevation of branched chain amino acids (BCAAs) and branched chain keto acids (BCKAs) in urine, plasma, and cerebrospinal fluid. The presence of an abnormal metabolite, L-alloisoleucine, is pathognomonic. Plasma leucine is 1000 to 5000 μM. Confirmation is obtained by studying the ability of intact cultured cells to decarboxylate 1-^{14}C-labeled BCAAs or BCKAs; residual activity is less than 2 percent of that in controls.

Genetics MSUD is an autosomal recessive inherited disease. Heterozygotes can be detected by assays on cultured fibroblasts from skin.

Prevalence of the disease is estimated at 1/200,000 live births. In the Mennonite community of North Carolina the rate is 1/176. Branched chain α-keto acid dehydrogenase (BCKD) is a mitochondrial multienzyme complex containing a branched chain keto acid decarboxylase with two α and two β subunits (E1); a dihydrolipoyltransferase (E2); and a dihydrolipoyl dehydrogenase (E3). There are also two regulatory enzymes. MSUD is genetically heterogeneous. The genes encoding BCKD complex are encoded in the nucleus. The E1 α gene is located on chromosome 19, the E1 β gene on chromosome 6, the E2 gene on chromosome 1 and the E3 gene on chromosome 7. The relationship between molecular defect and clinical expression is not clear. The degree of impairment of the BCKD complex does not always correlate with the clinical phenotype. "Environmental" factors such as hypoglycemia, acidosis, anoxia, infection, diet, and the level of maturation of the brain influence the mode of onset and the severity of MSUD.[25]

Neuropathology Brain weight is generally elevated as an indication of edema. Delay in myelination has been reported and chemical analysis is said to reveal a reduction of lipid content, especially of proteolipids and cerebrosides.

There is no evidence of myelin destruction or astrocyte hyperplasia. In one personally observed case which had survived with mental retardation until the age of 3 years, we could detect no nerve cell or myelin alteration using conventional staining techniques.

Pathophysiology: Mechanism of Brain Lesions The mechanism of brain dysfunction is not well understood. However, it appears from clinical experience that very high levels of BCAAs and BCKAs play a major role, especially in the very young infant. Neurological sequelae are a function of the time and efficacy of the dietary control of these metabolites. Experimentally, BCKAs have inhibited adrenergic receptors and may have interfered with energy metabolism (glucose and pyruvate). However, the mechanism of the noxious action of BCKAs on nerve cells remains obscure. Hypoglycemia and cerebral hypoperfusion may also play a role in the pathogenesis of the brain lesions in MSUD as it does in other disorders of amino acid metabolism.

Variants of Neonatal MSUD Three neonates have been reported with ophthalmoplegia and evidence of other cranial nerve palsies (facial diplegia, dysphonia); they were associated with hypotonia and somnolence. The children survived without treatment and several months later had an acute neurological episode with coma. The diagnosis of MSUD was made at that time. With dietary treatment, the ophthalmoplegia disappeared and the neurological status became normal, except for moderate mental deficit. The residual activity of BCKA was 16 percent of controls in one case.[26]

Prenatal Diagnosis Prenatal diagnosis can be made by studying decarboxylation of [1-^{14}C]leucine in amniocytes or, in the first trimester of pregnancy, on chorionic villus biopsies. DNA studies on chorionic villus may be employed for both heterozygote detection and prenatal diagnosis within families with a known mutation.

Treatment and Neonatal Screening It is essential to counteract the effects of hypoglycemia, acidosis, and hypotension. Dialysis or exchange transfusions are rarely necessary. BCAAs should be eliminated from the diet; formulas with no BCAA are available. Protein

should be restricted to approximately 2 g/kg/day and supplemented with a high caloric intake. Nitrogen intake should not be so low as to prevent protein catabolism and the nitrogen/caloric ratio should be controlled. Adjustment to individual needs may be difficult. Thiamine supplementation is recommended in all cases. The urgency of these dietary measures cannot be overemphasized. There may be considerable improvement in neurologic function and even normalization if BCAAs are brought to a normal level in the first weeks of life. Chronic therapy is considered in Chap. 3.

The long-term outcome of neonatal MSUD has much improved in recent years due to early diagnosis and treatment. This is illustrated in series reported by Danner and Elsas.[27] From ten patients seen between 1965 and 1980, only three had their disease recognized before age 1 month. Four died, four were severely impaired, and two were mentally retarded. Of ten other patients seen between 1981 and 1986, all were diagnosed before the age of 1 month. Seven had a normal neurological outcome.

It is clear, therefore, that neonatal screening is important, either on a population basis or by neonatal screening at the bedside, using the current colorimetric methods for the detection of BCKA.

Other Phenotypes The intermittent, chronic form and vitamin A responsive form are described in Chap. 3.

Isovaleric Acidemia: Isovaleryl-CoA Dehydrogenase Deficiency

By 1989, more than 60 patients with this diagnosis had been reported. About half the patients with isovaleric acidemia suffer an acute life-threatening neonatal disorder. The first signs appear usually between the 2d and 5th day of life, but range from the 1st day to the 14th day. At first, the infant refuses food, vomits, and then becomes lethargic and hypotonic. Tremor, myoclonic jerks, or convulsions may occur. An abnormal "sweaty feet," or "cheesy" odor of the urine, due to accumulation of isovaleric acid, is generally present and may suggest the diagnosis. Thrombocytopenia and neutropenia are common, as well as hypocalcemia. If untreated, the child lapses into coma and dies after a few days. Death may result from metabolic acidosis or, occasionally, from hemorrhage or infection.

Routine laboratory tests regularly bring to light a severe metabolic acidosis, ketonemia, and ketonuria. Hyperammonemia is frequently present and may be marked.

Biochemical Abnormalities Isovaleric acid is greatly elevated in the plasma (100 to 500 times normal), and much less so in the urine. Of great diagnostic importance is the attendant elevation of a metabolite of isovaleryl-CoA, isovalerylglycine (2000 to 15,000 μmol/ day; normal $<15\,\mu$mol/day). Isovaleric acidemia is the only disease in which isovalerylglycine can be detected in such amounts. Also large amounts of 3-hydroxyisovaleric acid and numerous other metabolites of isovaleryl-CoA, including isovalerylglucuronide and isovalerylcarnitine, are excreted in the urine. Assay of the activity of isovaleryl-CoA dehydrogenase can be made on fibroblasts by various methods (including the tritium release and fluorometric methods).

Diagnosis This disease must be separated from the several other inherited disorders that give rise to metabolic acidosis in the first days of life. A similar odor of urine can be found in glutaric aciduria II.

The major diagnostic test is the analysis of organic acids in the urine by gas chromatography and mass spectroscopy. A high concentration of isovalerylglycine is characteristic. This metabolite can also be assessed rapidly by proton nuclear magnetic resonance.

A sensitive assay is now available for the detection of the deficient activity of isovaleryl-CoA dehydrogenase in cultured fibroblasts. Heterozygotes can be identified. Several methods permit prenatal diagnosis of the enzyme defect on cultured amniocytes or on the amniotic fluid.

Genetics The disease is inherited as an autosomal recessive trait. Its prevalence has not been established. The gene has been located on the long arm of chromosome 15. Several point mutations have been characterized. Heterogeneity has been shown; to date, six mutant enzymes have been described. Some patients are compound heterozygotes. Intrafamilial variations exist: acute and later-onset disorder have been described in the same sibship.

Treatment Treatment of the acute episode involves control of ketoacidosis and hyperammonemia, and prevention of circulatory crises. Protein restriction is essential. Long-term treatment includes restriction of dietary protein and supplementation with glycine and carnitine. If the children survive, they may display developmental delay and intermittent episodes of acidosis.

Phenotypic Variations The chronic intermittent form is described in Chap. 3. Further details on isovaleric acidemia and other branched chain organic acidurias are given in the literature.[28,29,29a]

Isolated Deficiency of 3-Methylcrotonyl-CoA Carboxylase

This rare disorder, to be distinguished from the biotin-responsive multiple carboxylase deficiency, has been reported in one patient, who became symptomatic at 5 weeks of age with vomiting, lethargy, and convulsions. There was an elevation of 3-hydroxyisovalerate and 3-methylcrotonylglycine in urine. The more common infantile form of this condition is discussed in Chap. 3.

Disorders of Propionate and Methylmalonate Metabolism: Propionic Acidemia and Methylmalonic Acidemia

Propionyl-CoA, formed in the catabolism of several essential amino acids, including leucine, valine, methionine, and threonine, is normally converted to methylmalonyl-CoA which is isomerized to succinyl-CoA. Deficiencies of two enzymes: propionyl-CoA carboxylase, which catalyses the conversion of propionyl-CoA to methylmalonyl-CoA, and methylmalonyl-CoA mutase, which catalyses the conversion of methylmalonyl-CoA to succinyl-CoA, underlie two recessively inherited disorders which begin in the neonatal period. They are called *propionic acidemia* and *methylmalonic acidemia*. Both disorders may also have a later onset (see Chap. 3).

Propionic Acidemia (Propionyl-CoA Carboxylase Deficiency)

Clinical Signs The disease starts one to several days after birth. Anorexia, vomiting, lethargy, hypotonia, poor reactivity, and hyperventilation are the main signs. Seizures occur in some patients. Hepatomegaly may be observed. An erythematous rash may occur. CT scans and MRI show a hypodensity of the cerebral white matter and lesions in the putamen or globus pallidus. Leukocytes and platelets are usually normal at this age. If not treated, the patient usually dies after a few days.

Biochemical Characteristics There is metabolic acidosis and ketosis, hyperglycinemia, and hyperglycinuria; hyperammonemia and hypoglycemia may also occur. Propionic acid is considerably elevated in the blood (as high as 400 mg/dL in some patients) and large quantities are excreted in the urine. The detection of a high level of urinary methylcitrate, 3-hydroxypropionate, propionylglycine, and tiglic acid, which are propionate derivates, is of diagnostic importance. Since propionate and its derivates also accumulate in another disease, methylmalonic acidema, definitive diagnosis requires analysis for propionate-CoA carboxylase in leukocytes and fibroblasts. Activity of this biotin-dependent mitochondrial enzyme is 1 to 5 percent of normal controls.

Prenatal Diagnosis   Propionate-CoA carboxylase activity can be demonstrated in cultured amniotic cells or chorionic villus cells, and methylcitrate by gas chromatography/mass spectrometry analysis of the amniotic fluid.

Enzyme assays in leukocytes taken from umbilical cord blood of newborns allows early preclinical diagnosis in high-risk neonates.

Genetics   Propionic acidemia is transmitted as an autosomal recessive disorder. Two complementation groups have been described due to the presence of two nonidentical subunits, α and β, of the carboxylase molecule. Several mutations are known in the genes for each of these subunits. Heterozygote detection should be possible in families with a known mutation. Intrafamilial variations may occur.

Course and Treatment   Urgent treatment of the neonatal metabolic crisis includes withdrawal of dietary protein and administration of sodium bicarbonate parenterally.

If patients survive, and remain untreated, they may continue to have episodes of metabolic acidosis and neurological dysfunction. Apparently all end up mentally retarded and may have mild chorea or dystonia.[30] Long-term treatment consists mainly of a low-protein diet and possibly biotin and L-carnitine supplementation. Specific antimicrobial therapy (metronidazole) may be of clinical benefit in reducing the amount of propionate in tissues.

Neuropathology   There have been few complete neuropathologic studies. White matter vacuolization or spongiosis has been reported in infants and in those surviving beyond infancy. Focal neuronal loss has been found in the lenticular nuclei. In one case, degeneration of Purkinje and granule cells was found in the cerebellum.

Other Phenotypes
- Late-onset forms will be described in Chap. 3
- Some children with complete deficiency of propionyl-CoA carboxylase have no clinical manifestations

Disorders of Methylmalonate Metabolism   Two disorders of methylmalonic acid that depend on cobalamin coenzymes, adenosylcobalamin (AdoCbl) and methylcobalamin (MeCbl), are described here, as their clinical expression is most frequently in the first weeks or months of life. They will also be referred to in Chap. 3.

Methylmalonic Acidemia (Methylmalonyl-CoA Mutase Deficiency)   Isolated inherited deficiencies of methylmalonyl-CoA mutase are caused by mutations at several different loci. Four distinct defects have been shown: two defects of the mutase apoenzyme: mut^0 (the most frequent) and mut^-; and two defects of adenosylcobalamin (AdoCbl) synthesis: Cbl A and Cbl B.

Clinical Features   Clinical features include lethargy or coma, hypotonia, vomiting, respiratory distress, and failure to thrive. Hepatomegaly and an erythematous rash can occur. Clinical differences between the four groups of methylmalonyl-CoA mutase deficiency are slight. However, patients in the mut^0 class have an earlier onset (80 percent during the first week of life and 7 percent during the first month). In the other group, 30 to 40 percent of patients become ill in the first week and 20 percent or less in the first month.[31]

The mut^0 group has the poorest overall prognosis and Cbl A patients have the best outcome. Some children with methylmalonyl-CoA mutase deficiency have no clinical abnormality.

One patient, a neonate who died at the age of 11 days, initially reported to have methylmalonyl-CoA racemase deficiency,[32] was shown to be a mut^- mutant.

Biochemical Characteristics   There is metabolic acidosis and ketosis. pH may be as low as 6.9 and serum bicarbonate as low as 5 mEq/L. Hyperammonemia is common and hypoglycemia is said to occur in 40 percent of patients. Also, hyperglycinemia is a regular finding. Large amounts of methylmalonic acid accumulate in blood and are excreted in the urine (240 to 5700 mg daily; normal: <5 mg daily). Measurements are made by way of GC/MS. A simple colorimetric assay for methylmalonate may be of an orienting value. Propionate and some of its precursors and metabolites (3-hydroxypropionate, methylcitrate) are also found in excess, but at a lower level than in propionic acidemia. Serum cobalamin levels are normal.

Definitive diagnosis is made by specialized enzymatic assays on cultured fibroblasts or cells from other tissues. Confirmation of the etiological category (mut or Cbl) depends on studies on cultured cells. In the mut^0 type of apomutase deficiency, mutase activity in extracts of cultured fibroblasts is undetectable. In the mut^- type, the mutase apoenzyme is structurally abnormal. Cbl A patients are deficient in a mitochondrial cobalamin reductase whereas the Cbl B individuals are lacking in a mitochondrial adenosyltransferase.

Prenatal Diagnosis Prenatal diagnosis is achieved by assays for methylmalonate and methylcitrate in amniotic fluid. Mutase activity and AdoCbl synthesis are measured in cultured amniotic fluid cells.

Genetics Methylmalonic acidemia is most probably an autosomal recessive disorder. Its prevalence has been estimated in a survey of newborns in Massachusetts at 1 in 48,000 but there are reasons to believe that the disorder is more frequent than this.

Neuropathology One striking feature has been necrosis of the putamen or the globus pallidus. We have observed one case with isolated necrosis of the globus pallidus. The exact mechanism of this lesion is not understood.

Course and Treatment The acidosis, hypoglycemia, hyperammonemia and hypovolemia must be countered by appropriate measures. Dietary protein must at first be withdrawn and later restricted. As soon as a suspicion of methylmalonic acidemia arises, cobalamin supplementation is necessary (1 to 2 mg of cyanocobalamin or hydroxycobalamin intramuscularly daily for several days.) L-Carnitine supplementation and oral antibiotic therapy (metronidazole) may be useful. The response to cobalamin therapy varies with the nature of the defect. It results in a marked decrease in methylmalonate in blood and urine in practically all patients of the Cbl A group and in 40 percent of patients in the Cbl B group. The mut^0 and mut^- classes do not respond.

Combined Deficiency of Methylmalonyl-CoA Mutase and Methyltetrahydrofolate: Homocysteine Methyltransferase Combined deficiency of methylmalonyl-CoA mutase and methyltetrahydrofolate: homocysteine methyltransferase has been related to defects

in the cellular metabolism of cobalamins. These are due to defects in the cytosolic oxidation of Co^{2+} to Co^{3+} (Cbl C and Cbl D mutations) or in the lysosomal pathway affecting the synthesis of both adenylcobalamin and methylcobalamin (Cbl F mutation).

More than 20 children affected with this disorder have been reported. They have been assigned to three biochemically and genetically distinct complementation groups : Cbl C, Cbl D and Cbl F. In Cbl F, cobalamin, after endocytosis, cannot exit from the lysosome, whereas in Cbl C and Cbl D, cobalamin is released from the lysosome but its subsequent reduction is defective. Therefore, in each disorder the production of both MeCbl and AdoCbl is blocked.

In patients belonging to the *Cbl C group*, by far the largest, the disease appears usually in the first days or weeks of life and expresses itself by feeding difficulties, lethargy, hypotonia, and developmental delay. Convulsions may occur. Pigmentary degeneration of the retina, a common finding, is detectable after a few weeks. The majority of these infants have a macrocytic anemia and megaloblastosis. Thrombocytopenia and hypersegmented polymorphonuclear leukocytes are less frequent. Hemolytic episodes and congestive heart failure have been recorded. An erythematous rash may occur. Some children have died in infancy. Most of those who survived were mentally retarded. In a few patients, neurological signs have not developed before childhood or adolescence and this has also been the case of patients in the *Cbl D group* (see Chap. 3). Two patients belonging to the *Cbl F group* had neonatal hypotonia, stomatitis, and minor facial abnormalities.

The diagnosis of the disease is based on the combined finding of methylmalonic aciduria, homocystinuria, and normal serum cobalamin. Homocystinuria is much less marked than in isolated mutase deficiency. Hypomethioninemia and cystathionuria occur in some patients. The association of this combination of biochemical abnormalities makes it possible to eliminate isolated mutase deficiency and other causes of homocystinuria such as cysthationine synthase deficiency, methyltetrahydrofolate:homocysteine methyltransferase deficiency or methylenetetrahydrofolate reductase deficiency, as well as Cbl deficiencies. The disorder is most probably inherited as an autosomal recessive trait.

Treatment Treatment with high doses of hydroxycobalamin, especially by the intramuscular route, has proven useful in some cases. The administration of betaine has been recommended.

Other Phenotypes The infantile phenotype is described in Chap. 3.

Methyltetrahydrofolate: Homocysteine Methyltransferase Deficiency This condition is related to isolated defects of methylcobalamin (MeCbl) synthesis. Two complementation groups have been described, Cbl F and Cbl G. The disease starts usually in the first weeks or months of life with lethargy, poor feeding, vomiting, hypotonia, seizures, and developmental delay. One adult patient presented with gait disturbances and sensory abnormalities.

Megaloblastic anemia, homocystinuria, hypomethioninemia and absence of methylmalonic acidemia are the main biological findings. Serum Cbl and folate concentrations have been normal. Studies of fibroblasts confirm the specific enzymatic defect. Most patients have benefited from hydroxycobalamin therapy.

Sulfite Oxidase Deficiency and Molybdenum Cofactor Deficiency (Combined Deficiency of Sulfite Oxidase, Xanthine Dehydrogenase, and Aldehyde Oxidase)

Clinical Presentation At least 44 patients with combined deficiency of sulfite oxidase, xanthine dehydrogenase, and aldehyde oxidase, an autosomal recessive disorder, have been reported. Children are born at term. The onset is in the first or second week of life. Feeding difficulties, frequent and usually *refractory seizures*, hypomotility, axial hypotonia or limb rigidity, and evidence of pyramidal signs are the usual findings. The head circumference is usually normal at birth, but some patients display various dysmorphic features such as a large head, upturned nose, enophthalmus and telecanthus, a triangular face, a cleft of the soft palate, and a broad nasal bridge. Early microcephaly was present in one child. A characteristic lens dislocation may be present in the neonatal period, but is usually noted only after a few weeks or months of life. Brain neuroradiologic imaging may show multiple cystic cavities in the white matter and various degrees of cortical involvement. It is important to bear this disease in mind when considering the differential diagnosis of ischemic/anoxic perinatal multicystic leukomalacia. The outcome of molybdenum cofactor deficiency is discouraging. Many infants die in the first days or weeks of life. Some survive for several years with severe mental retardation, pyramidal signs, or choreoathetosis.

Patients with isolated sulfite oxidase have been described, with similar clinical and neuropathologic features.

Biochemical Findings Affected individuals excrete large amounts of sulfite, thiosulfate, *S*-sulfocysteine, taurine, xanthine, and hypoxanthine but very low amounts of sulfate, cystine, and uric acid. As a screening procedure, urinary sulfite can be detected with a dipstick test. Deficiency of sulfite oxidase and xanthine dehydrogenase can be verified in cultured fibroblasts and liver tissue.[33] Prenatal diagnosis is possible using chorionic villi.

Neuropathology Severe, diffuse lesions of the brain have been found in all autopsied cases, including cystic necrosis of the cerebral white matter and extensive neuronal loss and gliosis of the cerebral cortex. Lesional asymmetry was marked in one case. The cerebellum was severely involved in one child. There have been no differences between cases of isolated sulfite oxidase deficiency and those of combined sulfite oxidase and xanthine dehydrogenase deficiency.

Pathophysiology The neuropathological findings seem to indicate that the neurologic disease is the consequence of the sulfite oxidase deficiency. Xanthine dehydrogenase deficiency and aldehyde oxidase deficiency do not result in an encephalopathy. Damage to the brain could possibly result from a toxic effect of sulfite accumulation or from deficiency of sulfate.

Treatment Therapeutic measures have not been effective. The use of diets to restrict the intake of precursors of sulfur-containing amino acids and the administration of sulfite-binding substances should be considered.

Clinical Variants One patient with isolated sulfite oxidase deficiency developed normally up to the age of 17 months and then had the sudden onset of hemiplegia followed later by unilateral choreoathetotic movements and seizures.

Mevalonic Aciduria: Mevalonate Kinase Deficiency Up to 1993 only 11 patients had been reported with this multisystem disorder starting usually in infancy or in the neonatal period. A marked delay in neurologic development, seizures, a myopathy, failure to thrive, fever, diarrhea, hepatosplenomegaly, and anemia are the usual manifestations. Cataracts, dysmorphic features

and ataxia have occurred in some patients. Four patients died within the first year of life. There is no metabolic acidosis. Mevalonic acid is elevated in urine. A milder form with mental retardation and ataxia has been reported in one child. Muscle development was poor and levels of creatinine kinase were elevated in late childhood.[34] Clinical symptoms may be related to a defect in cholesterol synthesis, a feature of this disease. A high cholesterol diet has been recommended, with uncertain effects.

Smith-Lemli-Opitz Syndrome Smith-Lemli-Opitz (SLO) syndrome, also caused by a defect in cholesterol synthesis, may manifest itself at birth with hypotonia and dysmorphic features (see Chap. 3).

Neonatal Mitochondrial Encephalopathies

Mitochondrial disorders which produce severe brain dysfunction in the neonatal period belong essentially to one of the following three categories: (1) defects of pyruvate metabolism; (2) defects of the respiratory chain, both of which give rise to a marked hyperlactacidemia (infantile lactic acidosis); and (3) disturbances of fatty acid oxidation comprising defects of the carnitine cycle and defects of β oxidation.[35]

General Clinical Presentation Mitochondrial defects produce multisystem disorders in which the degree of involvement of the brain, muscle, heart, and other organs is variable. Neonates affected with these disorders present a relatively nondescript syndrome of severe hypotonia, lethargy, irritability, abnormal respiratory patterns, convulsions, poor feeding, and vomiting. Hepatomegaly is frequent. Birth weight may be low. Without treatment, most infants die in the first days or weeks of life; others survive for a few months with severe neurological handicaps or, exceptionally, may live longer with minimal sequelae.

Clinical signs which specifically favor mitochondrial disorders in the neonatal period (Table 2-4) include dysmorphic facial features and other congenital abnormalities, a cardiomyopathy, and occasionally renal cysts. Prenatal brain lesions are features of several conditions.

Laboratory investigations which are essential for the verification of mitochondrial diseases include the following:

1. Assays of lactate and pyruvate in blood, CSF, and urine, and analysis of the lactate/pyruvate ratio.

2. Measurement of ketone bodies (hydroxybutyrate and acetoacetate) and glycemia.

3. Measurement of carnitine, and assays of acylcarnitine esters and glycine conjugates in body fluids.

4. Gas chromatography/mass spectrometry for analysis of organic acids, which will serve to differentiate the mitochondrial disorders and to eliminate organic acidemias with lactic acidosis (Table 2-5).

Further characterization of individual diseases requires specific, highly specialized biochemical and molecular techniques.

It should be remembered that some neonatal mitochondrial diseases, especially those with marked lactacidemia, are so rapidly lethal that their cause is difficult to ascertain unless biochemical analysis of postmortem specimens of blood, urine, muscle, and liver are obtained.

Further discussion of the infantile and childhood mitochondrial diseases in this category is to be found in Chaps. 3 and 5

Disorders of Pyruvate Metabolism

Neonatal (and Early Infantile) Pyruvate Dehydrogenase Complex Deficiency Pyruvate dehydrogenase (PDH) is a multienzyme complex located in mitochondria that catalyzes the conversion of pyruvate to acetyl-CoA. It comprises three catalytic enzymes, E_1 (pyruvate dehydrogenase), E_2 (dihydrolipoyl transacetylase), and E_3 (dihydrolipoyl dehydrogenase), plus two regulatory enzymes (pyruvate dehydrogenase kinase and pyruvate dehydrogenase phosphate phosphatase). By far the most common defect is in the $E_{1\alpha}$ component of the pyruvate dehydrogenase (PDH) complex, located on the X chromosome. PDH $E_{1\alpha}$ deficiency is inherited as an X-linked trait. Heterozygous females may be symptomatic.

Clinical Presentation Clinical features are variable.[35–37]

(a) In boys, symptoms usually start in the first days of life and consist of extreme hypotonia, lethargy, weak sucking, and respiratory distress with episodes of apnea. Seizures occur in one third of patients. Birth weight may be low (intrauterine growth retardation). Dysmorphic features and congenital anomalies have been reported in one-fourth of the patients. They include a narrow head, frontal bossing, hydrocephalus, a broad nasal bridge, an upturned nose, micrognathia, low set ears, short fingers and arms, simian hand creases, hypo-

Table 2-4
Distinctive clinical signs of neonatal mitochondrial encephalopathies[a]

Disorders[b]	Facial dysmorphia	Congenital defects[c]	Cardiopathy	Urine odor	Polycystic kidneys	Abnormal muscle biopsy[d]	Congenital brain defects	Other abnormalities
PDH E$_{1\alpha}$ (X-linked)	++	+					+++	Birth weight may be low
PC deficiency							++	
Complex I deficiency			++			++	+	
Complex IV deficiency			++			++ RRF		
Mitochondrial depletion syndrome						++ RRF		External ophthalmoplegia Renal tubular dysfunction
Glutaric aciduria, type II	+++	+++		+	+++		++	Macrocephaly
LCAD deficiency[e]			++					Microvesicular fatty infiltration of liver
SCAD deficiency								Microvesicular fatty infiltration of liver
Carnitine palmitoyltransferase II deficiency			++		++	++		Cardiac arrhythmias Fulminant course
3-hydroxymethylglutaryl-CoA lyase deficiency								

Abbreviations and symbols: PDHC = pyruvate dehydrogenase complex; PC = pyruvate carboxylase; LCAD = long-chain acyl-CoA dehydrogenase; RRF =ragged red fibers; +++ = very frequent or of major diagnostic importance; ++ = frequent; + = not rare. SCAD = short-chain acyl-CoA dehydrogenase.

[a] All patients present with hypotonia, hypomotility, poor reactivity, lethargy or coma, seizures, feeding difficulties, vomiting, abnormal respiratory patterns, and occasionally hepatomegaly.

[b] Autosomal recessive, unless stated otherwise.

[c] Affecting limbs, heart and genitourinary tract.

[d] Include fatty infiltration, mitochondrial abnormalities, ragged red fibers.

[e] VLCAD deficiency has similar features.

Table 2-5
Neonatal mitochondrial encephalopathies: orienting laboratory tests

Deficient enzyme	Lactic acidosis[a]	Organic acidemia	Total carnitine[b]	Acyl carnitine[c]	Ketone bodies	Hypoglycemia	Hyperammonemia	Other abnormalities
PDHC	+ + +							
PC	+ + +				High		+	Hypercitrullinemia Hyperlysinemia
Complex I	+ + +							Hyperalaninemia
Complex IV	+ + +					+		Renal tubular insufficiency
Mitochondrial depletion	+ + +		Low					Metabolic acidosis
Glutaric acidemia II		+ + + DA	Low/normal	Increased	Low	+ + +	+	Metabolic acidosis Hyperaminoaciduria
LCAD[d]		+ + + DA	Low/normal	Increased	Low	+ + +		Metabolic acidosis C^{14}-1-acylcarnitine
SCAD		+ + + DA	Low		Low	+ + +	+	Metabolic acidosis
Carnitine palmitoyltransferase II			Low/normal	Increased		+ + +		Long-chain acylcarnitine in tissues
3-hydroxymethylglutaryl-CoA lyase		+ + +			Low	+ + +	+	Metabolic acidosis

Abbreviations and symbols: PDHC = pyruvate dehydrogenase complex; PC = pyruvate carboxylase; LCAD = long-chain acyl-CoA dehydrogenase; SCAD = short-chain acyl-CoA dehydrogenase; DA = dicarboxylic aciduria; + + + = very frequent or of major diagnostic importance; + + = frequent; + = not rare.

[a] In blood, CSF.

[b] In plasma.

[c] Relative concentration in urine.

[d] VLCAD: acidosis, low carnitine, DA, high creatine kinase.

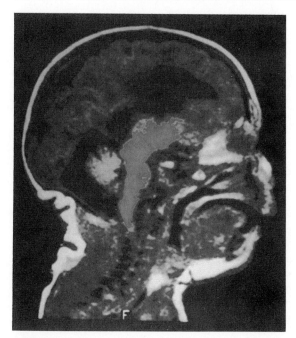

Figure 2-2
Male infant with PDH E_1 deficiency. MRI shows absence of the corpus callosum and severe destructive lesions in white matter and cortex. (Courtesy Dr. Ponsot and Dr. Haengeli.)

spadias, and an anteriorly placed anus. A comparison has been made with the fetal alcohol syndrome, in which acetaldehyde from the maternal circulation is believed to inhibit pyruvate dehydrogenase, presumably causing the somatic malformations. Brain imaging may show a partial or total absence of the corpus callosum, cavitating lesions in the cerebral white matter, severe cortical atrophy, and bilateral low-density lesions in the putamen (25 percent) (Fig. 2-2). There is a marked elevation of lactate in the blood and CSF. The lactate/pyruvate ratio is normal. The residual activity of PDH measured in cultured fibroblasts is low. Many patients die below the age of 6 months.

(b) Some patients have a less dramatic course, including symptomatic heterozygous females. Low birth weight, hypotonia, feeding and swallowing difficulties are usually present in the neonatal period. These children live for several months or even years but make no developmental progress and have hydrocephalus or microcephaly, quadriplegia, optic atrophy, and seizures. There may be abnormal facial features. Neuroradiologic imaging shows severe, evidently prenatal, brain defects. Significant lactate elevation is found in

the CSF, but not always in the blood. The values of residual PDH activity in cultured fibroblasts are variable and are not significantly decreased in some patients.[38,39] If lactic acid is not measured in the CSF, these patients may be thought to have a prenatal nonprogressive encephalopathy of other origin, and the hereditary nature of the disorder may be missed. Definitive proof rests on DNA studies.

Biochemistry. Molecular Biology
● There is an elevation of lactate in blood and CSF, or only in CSF, which constitutes a major element for diagnosis. The lactate accumulation in the CNS may also be shown by proton magnetic resonance spectroscopy of the brain. The lactate/pyruvate ratio is normal (contrary to what is seen in disorders of the respiratory chain).

● Residual PDH activity in cultured fibroblasts is typically low. However, in some patients, particularly heterozygous girls, PDH activity is normal in fibroblasts and decreased in other tissues. In these circumstances the correct diagnosis can only be reached in doing DNA studies.

● Various mutations in the $E_{1\alpha}$ subunit gene of the PDH complex, on the short arm of the X chromosome (Xp22.1) have been characterized. They are mostly sporadic. There is great allelic heterogeneity. Possible explanations for the variability of clinical manifestations include heterogeneity of the underlying mutation and the variable expression of PDH activity in different tissues. For female heterozygotes, the difference of clinical symptomatology could be related to the pattern of X inactivation, which varies from tissue to tissue in the same individual.[40] In some girls, it is believed that PDH deficiency is expressed only in the brain (cerebral lactic acidosis or cerebral PDH deficiency).[38,41] Variability in the expression of PDH deficiency and allelic heterogeneity may complicate the diagnosis and prenatal screening of the disorder. The $E_{1\beta}$ subunit gene is located on chromosome 3.

Neuropathology There is a distinct pattern of obviously prenatal brain defects both in boys and in heterozygous girls with PDH $E_{1\alpha}$ deficiency.[39,42] Lesions consist of atrophy of the cerebral hemispheres, areas of cavitating necrosis in the white matter and basal ganglia, absence (or extreme atrophy) of the corpus callosum, absence of bulbar pyramids, heterotopias of the inferior olives, and in some cases, periventricular heterotopias and fragmentation of the nucleus dentatus. The defect of the corpus callosum is usually not clearly described, but, to our knowledge, classical "agenesis" of the corpus callosum with Probst bundles has not been found. The neuropathological lesions were identical in a boy with a missense mutation and in a girl with a deletion in the PDH $E_{1\alpha}$ gene.[39,43]

Treatment   In certain instances, the systemic lactic acidosis may be reversed or reduced with a high fat/low carbohydrate ketogenic diet or with dichloroacetate, an inhibitor of PDH kinase.

Variants   There is a great variety of clinical expression in PDH complex deficiencies. Other phenotypes of PDH $E_{1\alpha}$ deficiency include the following:

• An early infantile form, generally consistent with Leigh syndrome (Chap. 3).

• A benign late infantile form with fluctuating ataxia (Chap. 3).

• One patient with a deficiency in the E_2 component has been reported.[44] The child presented severe lactic acidosis and hyperammonemia at 2 weeks of age and was later observed to be mentally retarded and microcephalic. The same authors have described two patients with abnormalities of a sixth component of the PDH complex, X protein. Both had chronic lactic acidosis, developmental delay, and poor coordination. One had mental retardation; basal ganglia lucencies on neuroradiologic imaging were present in the other.

• Defects in the E_3 component of the PDH complex located on chromosome 7 are described in Chap. 3 (disorders of the Krebs cycle).

Neonatal Form of Pyruvate Carboxylase Deficiency   Defects of pyruvate carboxylase (PC), an important enzyme in gluconeogenesis, cause two syndromes in the neonate: a severe neonatal disorder (French type) with total lack of enzyme protein, and a more slowly evolving, less dramatic condition (North American type) with some residual enzyme activity (Chap. 3). A late childhood type has also been reported.

The severe neonatal disorder starts at birth with extreme hypotonia, respiratory distress, and lethargy. Convulsions are frequent. Pyramidal signs may become manifest. Paraventricular cavities, ventricular enlargement, and thinning of the corpus callosum may be seen on brain scans. Biochemical abnormalities include major lactic acidosis with increased lactate/pyruvate

ratio, ketosis, citrullinemia, hyperlysinemia, and hyperammonemia.[45]   Citrullinemia, hyperlysinemia, and hyperammonemia reflect aspartate depletion.

Enzyme activity of PC measured in cultured skin fibroblasts is usually absent or extremely low. There are no tissue-specific isoenzymes. Prenatal diagnosis is possible. Most children die within the first four months of life.

Genetics   PC deficiency is an autosomal recessive disease. The gene is located on the long arm of chromosome 11.

Neuropathology and Physiopathology   There is considerable reduction in the number of neurons, "poor myelination," and astrocytic gliosis. Because PC activity is normally high in astrocytes and very low in neurons, it has been suggested that neuronal death is a consequence of the loss of essential metabolites normally provided to neurons by astrocytes. This is purely speculative.

Treatment   Because tissue aspartate levels are low in PC deficiency, aspartic acid supplementation has been advocated with uncertain results. The resultant benefit is only systemic, since aspartate does not cross the blood-brain barrier.

Other Forms of PC Deficiency   Early infantile form (Chap. 3). An intermittent form with repeated episodes of metabolic acidosis and normal neurologic development,[46] or episodic ataxia and mild mental retardation.[46a]

Neonatal Disorders of the Respiratory Chain   Clinical features of the defects of the respiratory chain are varied and may be expressed at different ages. Some of them cause neurologic, muscular, or neuromuscular disturbances, while others primarily affect other organs. Reports made before mitochondrial genetics were understood are difficult to classify. The respiratory chain is influenced by both the nuclear and the mitochondrial genome. In the neonate, deficiency of complex I, complex III and complex IV have been reported (see also Chap. 3).

Isolated Complex I (NADH-Ubiquinone Oxidoreductase) Deficiency   Patients with isolated complex I deficiency may present in the neonatal period with severe respiratory distress and apnea, necessitating artificial ventilation, hypotonia, weakness, cardiac hypertrophy, and hepatomegaly. Biochemical findings consist of elevated blood lactate and pyruvate, marked increase of the lactate/pyruvate ratio, hypoglycemia, and hyperalaninemia. One patient had hypospadias. A CT scan showed decreased density of cerebral white matter.[47] In muscle biopsies, accumulation of very large mitochondria increase in lipids and glycogen have been found. Death occurs in the first weeks of life.

In the brain, a thin corpus callosum, diffuse grayish discoloration of white matter, and "spongiosis" in the cortex, basal ganglia, and brain stem was reported.

Complex I contains at least 25 polypeptides, 7 of which are encoded by the mtDNA. The enzyme defect has been documented in several organs.

Therapeutic trials with riboflavin and sodium succinate have been unsuccessful.

Other forms of complex I deficiency with multisystem involvement are described in Chaps. 3 and 5 (MELAS). Purely myopathic forms develop in childhood or early adult life.

Isolated Complex III (Ubiquinol-Cytochrome-c Oxidoreductase) Deficiency

Complex III deficiency has been reported in one child with neonatal lactic acidosis, hypotonia, seizures, and coma.[47a]

Complex IV (Cytochrome-c Oxidase) Deficiency

As in other deficits of the respiratory chain, patients with cytochrome-c oxidase (COX) deficiency may suffer from a myopathy or a multisystem disorder involving the brain. Patients with a myopathy present at birth with lactic acidosis, hypotonia, and respiratory insufficiency. A cardiopathy[48] and a De Toni-Debré-Fanconi syndrome may be present. Some children die after several months while others recover. There may be ragged red fibers (RRF) in the muscle.

In some patients with overwhelming lactic acidosis, involvement of the brain may be suspected on clinical grounds and because of very high levels of lactic acid in the CSF. The possibility of brain damage has been confirmed recently in a case of neonatal COX deficiency with a cardiomyopathy, hypotonia, lack of neurologic development, athetoid movements of the limbs, and high levels of lactate in the CSF. He died at the age of 4 weeks. At autopsy, one of us found foci of intense gliosis with relative preservation of neurons in the putamen and thalamus.[49]

The most common clinical presentation of COX deficiency is Leigh syndrome (Chap. 3).

The Mitochondrial DNA Depletion Syndrome

In this probably autosomal recessive condition, a primary defect of the nuclear genome is associated with a quantitative reduction of mtDNA. It is an example of "intergenomic signaling defects."[35] This syndrome is probably due to a deficiency of the human mitochondrial transcription factor h-mtTFA,[58] which has recently been described in seven neonates.[59] Marked hypotonia (congenital myopathy) and respiratory abnormalities appeared soon after birth. Seizures occurred in one child and in another there was a severe external ophthalmoplegia. Renal dysfunction with De Toni-Debré-Fanconi syndrome was noted in two of the patients. There was a marked metabolic acidosis with elevation of lactic acid and pyruvate. Total and free carnitine were decreased but esterified carnitine was normal. There were ragged red fibers in the muscle, and liver mitochondria were markedly abnormal (see also Chap. 5).

Defects in Mitochondrial Fatty Acid Oxidation in Neonates

Defects in mitochondrial fatty acid oxidation comprise (a) defects in the carnitine cycle and (b) defects in fatty acid β oxidation. These conditions usually present in infancy or childhood with intermittent episodes of nonketotic hypoglycemia during fasting. They are rare in the neonatal period.

Defects in the Carnitine Cycle

They include primary carnitine deficiency (defect of the carnitine transport system), carnitine palmitoyltransferase type I (CPT I) deficiency, carnitine palmitoyltransferase type II (CPT II) deficiency, and deficiency of carnitine-acylcarnitine translocase. These conditions are rarely expressed in the neonate; they are much more frequent in infancy (Chap. 3). Some have, however, been reported as a cause of a severe neonatal disease.

Neonatal Carnitine Palmitoyltransferase II (CPT II) Deficiency

This rare neonatal type of CPT II deficiency consists of a severe multiorgan disorder which is rapidly lethal. Lethargy, hypotonia, seizures, hyperreflexia, cardiomegaly, hepatomegaly, and renal cysts are the usual clinical features. Cardiac arrhythmia may occur. Blood sugar is low; concentrations of ketone bodies, lactate, pyruvate, and organic acids are normal. Serum carnitine is decreased while the urinary excretion of carnitine is normal. The concentrations of long-chain acyl carnitine are increased in serum and tissue (which could be responsible for the cardiac arrhythmia.[50]) There is an infiltration of cells in muscle (and also heart and most visceral organs) by fine droplets of fat.

In cultured cells, there is a severe reduction in palmitate oxidation and in CPT II activity. The CPT II gene has been assigned to chromosome 1p11-13 and molecular defects have been found in three families. This suggests the possibility of genetic screening for family members.[51] Developmental brain anomalies have been reported in one case.

Deficiency of Carnitine-Acylcarnitine Translocase
This condition has been reported in one newborn infant with seizures, apnea, vomiting, and cardiac dysfunction. Several episodes of lethargy and vomiting upon fasting recurred in the following months. The liver was enlarged. A sibling was also affected. The long-chain acyl carnitine concentrations were elevated and plasma-free carnitine levels were very low. Plasma ammonia levels were high. The enzymatic defect was demonstrated on cultured fibroblasts. The child died of respiratory failure at 32 months of age.[52]

Neonatal Disorders of Fatty Acid β Oxidation (Acyl-CoA Dehydrogenases Deficiencies)
Disorders of mitochondrial fatty acid β oxidation are described in Chap. 3. Very few of them have a neonatal presentation, except glutaric acidemia type II (multiple acyl-CoA dehydrogenase deficiency, MADD). Hypoketonemia, hypoglycemia, carnitine deficiency, and dicarboxylic aciduria are among the most characteristic biochemical findings in this group of diseases. The profiles of urinary acyl carnitines and dicarboxylic acids are important to differentiate between them.

Short-Chain Acyl-CoA Dehydrogenase (SCAD) Deficiency
SCAD deficiency was reported in two neonates[53] with feeding difficulties, vomiting, lethargy, hypertonia, hyperpnea, pale mottled extremities, and hepatomegaly. There was metabolic acidosis, moderate hypoglycemia, hyperammonemia and an increased urinary excretion of dicarboxylic acids, ethylmalonate, methylsuccinate, butyrate, β-hydroxybutyrate, adipate, and lactate. One patient died in the neonatal period; microvesicular hepatic steatosis and brain edema were found. Another patient survived with an apparently normal development to the age of 2 years. SCAD deficiency was documented in skin fibroblasts.

*Long-Chain Acyl-CoA Dehydrogenase (LCAD) Deficiency
Some patients with long-chain acyl-CoA dehydrogenase deficiency can present with major neurological problems in the neonatal period.[54]

Hepatomegaly and hypertrophic cardiomyopathy are usually present. Major biochemical abnormalities include acidosis, hypoglycemia, low levels of ketone bodies in blood and urine, hyperammonemia, low plasma carnitine, and a high concentration of dicarboxylic acids in urine. If the patient survives, episodes of metabolic decompensation during fasting appear in infancy and childhood, and microcephaly becomes evident.

*Very Long Chain Acyl-CoA Dehydrogenase (VLCAD) Deficiency
This recently described disease occurring in neonates has been characterized by ventricular fibrillation, respiratory insufficiency, metabolic acidosis, massive dicarboxylic acidemia, high creatine kinase, and normal plasma carnitine levels. A low-fat diet and carnitine supplements are beneficial.[54a]

The disease is inherited as an autosomal recessive trait. Prenatal diagnosis is possible.

Neonatal Glutaric Aciduria Type II (Multiple Acyl-CoA Dehydrogenase Deficiency)
Glutaric aciduria type II is an autosomal recessive disorder due to a defect of electron transfer of flavoprotein (ETF) or more frequently of ETF dehydrogenase (ETF: ubiquinone oxidoreductase). Both defects lead to "multiple acyl-CoA dehydrogenase deficiency," and to the accumulation and excretion of oxidation products of all substrates normally oxidized by mitochondrial flavin-containing acyl-CoA dehydrogenase.[55]

Newborns, often prematures, present in the first days of life with hypotonia, tachypnea, stupor, vomiting, and occasionally seizures. A "sweaty feet" odor, similar to that of isovaleric aciduria, is often detected. The liver may be enlarged. In most patients, there are remarkable congenital anomalies: macrocephaly, facial dysmorphic features (high forehead, low set ears, hypertelorism), rocker-bottom feet, defects of the anterior abdominal wall, hypospadias and enlarged polycytic kidneys (Fig. 2-3). Metabolic acidosis, marked hypoglycemia, and low ketonuria and ketonemia are characteristic findings and are disclosed by standard laboratory tests. Most patients die in the first few weeks of life. Some survive for a few months and succumb to a cardiomyopathy. A few infants live longer and may develop Reye-like episodes. Severe neurologic sequelae are usual (Chap. 3).

Diagnostic Laboratory Tests
1. Metabolic acidosis; nonketotic hypoglycemia.

*Recent data show that patients reported as having LCAD deficiency have in fact VLCAD deficiency.

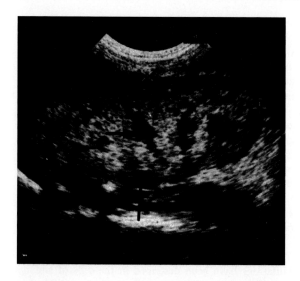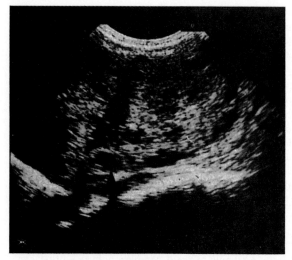

Figure 2-3
Glutaric acidemia type II. Ultrasound scan shows renal cysts (arrows). (Courtesy Dr. Govaerts.)

2. A characteristic organic acid pattern in urine including elevated levels of dicarboxylic acids (adipic, suberic, sebacic, dodecanoic, etc.), glutaric acid, isovaleric acid, isovalerylglycine, isobutyrylglycine and sarcosine.

3. A low or normal concentration of total carnitine in plasma and an increased level of acylated carnitine in urine.

4. Lipid storage of skeletal muscle.

5. The detection of polycystic kidneys by ultrasound.

The catalytic activity of ETF and ETF dehydrogenase is difficult to measure directly. ETF dehydrogenase can be assayed most effectively by electron paramagnetic resonance.

Pathology Lipid storage is found in muscle, liver, renal tubules, and myocardium. Cystic dysplasia of the kidneys is characteristic. In the brain, focal cortical dysplasias (neuronal aggregates in the molecular layer) and other abnormalities of neuronal migration have been reported. Ultrastructural studies have shown moderately electron dense homogeneous membrane-bound cytoplasmic inclusions in neurons and glial cells and kidney epithelial cells.[56]

Treatment Most neonatal patients die within the first few weeks of life. Therapeutic trials with riboflavin and carnitine supplementation have been successful in controlling the disease in some patients with milder forms starting in later life (Chap. 3).

Other Phenotypes Late-onset glutaric aciduria type II (Chap. 3).

Trifunctional Enzyme Deficiency Deficiency of the trifunctional enzyme of mitochondrial β oxidation can give rise to a severe neonatal cardiomyopathy and a state of neonatal neurological distress.[57]

Quantitative analysis revealed a severe depletion of mitochondrial DNA in the affected tissues. Death occurred after a few weeks or months. A late infantile form has been described in three patients.

3-Hydroxy-3-Methylglutaryl-CoA Lyase Deficiency

3-Hydroxy-3-methylglutaryl-CoA lyase (HMG-CoA lyase) is an enzyme located in the mitochondrial matrix that catalyzes the final step in leucine degradation, converting HMG-CoA to acetyl-CoA and acetoacetic acid.

About 30 percent of patients with this autosomal recessive disorder have been symptomatic in the neonatal period.[60] The vomiting, lethargy, respiratory difficulties, and frequently hepatomegaly are associated with metabolic acidosis, absence of ketosis, hypoglycemia, possibly hyperammonemia and elevated serum transaminase. Four organic acids are markedly elevated: 3-hydroxy-3-methylglutaric, 3-methylglutaconic, 3-methylglutaric, and 3-hydroxyisovaleric.

Assays for HMG-CoA lyase may be performed on cultured fibroblasts and leukocytes. Intravenous glucose and bicarbonate are generally effective in alleviating the metabolic abnormalities. Restriction of dietary protein and fat, and supplementation with carnitine are also advised.

Other Types In 70 percent of such patients, the disease starts in the first or second year of life (see Chap. 3).

Disorders of Biotin Metabolism

Biotin, a vitamin of the B complex, acts as a prosthetic group to the four human carboxylases. There are two defects of the biotin cycle, both of which result in multiple carboxylase deficiency and are biotin responsive. (1) *Deficiency in biotinidase* (an enzyme which cleaves biotin from biocytin and biotinyl peptides) usually becomes manifest in early infancy or childhood. A few cases have had a neonatal onset with severe seizures and characteristic cutaneous abnormalities (the same as in holocarboxylase synthetase deficiency). A laryngeal stridor is not uncommon. This disease, also known as late-onset multiple carboxylase deficiency, is described in Chap. 3. (2) *Holocarboxylase synthetase deficiency* (or early-onset multiple carboxylase deficiency) generally becomes clinically apparent soon after birth and is described here.

Holocarboxylase Synthetase Deficiency (Early-Onset Multiple Carboxylase Deficiency) Holocarboxylase links activated biotin to four carboxylases: pyruvate carboxylase, propionyl-CoA carboxylase, 3-methylcrotonyl-CoA carboxylase, which are all located in mitochondria; and acetyl-CoA carboxylase, which is cytosolic. When holocarboxylase synthetase (HS) is deficient, all carboxylases are inactive. HS deficiency is a disorder of "biotinylation."

Little more than 10 patients with (HS) deficiency have been reported in the literature. The disease usually becomes apparent in the first weeks of life or even at birth. Some children have manifested symptoms after several months of life and as late as 15 months in one instance. Most of them exhibit breathing abnormalities such as hyperpnea or apneic spells, hypotonia or hypertonia, lethargy alternating with irritability, anorexia, and vomiting. Seizures also occur. A skin rash appears in more than half of the patients and in some it has been observed before the onset of neurological signs. Rarely there is alopecia. Hypothermia and a special odor of the urine may be noted. CT scans reveal moderate ventricular dilatation and low density changes in the white matter.

All children have metabolic ketoacidosis, organic aciduria, and frequently hyperammonemia during acute episodes. The characteristic pattern of organic aciduria includes an elevated urinary excretion of β-hydroxypropionate, tiglylglycine, methylcitrate, lactate, β-methylcrotonylglycine, and β-hydroxyisovalerate.

Definitive diagnosis requires the demonstration of a deficient activity of holocarboxylase synthetase in peripheral blood leukocytes or cultured skin fibroblasts.

The disease is inherited as an autosomal recessive trait. The gene for HS maps to chromosome 21q2.1. Mutations have been described in the cells of siblings with HS deficiency. Prenatal diagnosis is possible (see Chap. 3 for references).

Treatment with biotin (10 mg/day) usually has a beneficial effect. Clinical symptoms and biochemical abnormalities improve rapidly. Biotin treatment initiated at birth is effective in some patients only. The difference probably has a molecular basis. Prenatal maternal treatment may be useful.

Other phenotypes are mentioned in Chap. 3.

Neonatal Peroxisomal Disorders

A number of disease states are now linked to a dysfunction of peroxisomes. They have their onset in the neonatal period and many pursue a rapidly fatal course. A few evolve more slowly and their full-blown clinical picture emerges only in infancy or in early childhood. X-linked adrenoleukodystrophy is a juvenile peroxisomal disorder (see Chap. 5).

A brief general statement about peroxisomes will be helpful as an introduction to this group of diseases.

Peroxisomes are round cytoplasmic organelles bound by a single membrane, with an average diameter of approximately $0.5 \mu m$. They are found in various amounts in all eukaryotic cells, but are large and more abundant in those of the liver and kidney. They stain with cytochemical reactions for catalase, which is an important means of identification. Among other functions, peroxisomes play an important role in fatty acid oxidation, bile acid synthesis, plasmalogen synthesis, and in the metabolism of pipecolic acid and phytanic acid. In recent years, a number of multisystem diseases with prominent neurologic features have been traced to an impairment of peroxisomal function.[61–64]

In a *first group* there is a virtual absence of peroxisomes and a generalized loss of all peroxisomal functions. Moser[61] terms this "disorders of peroxisome biogenesis" and Wanders[62] "peroxisome deficiency disorders." To this group belong Zellweger disease and a few allied conditions.

In a *second group*, peroxisomes are present but lack a single enzyme of peroxisome β oxidation. This category includes four conditions with a Zellweger-like phenotype and juvenile X-linked adrenoleukodystrophy, as well as two disorders with no involvement of the nervous system (and possibly adult Refsum disease).

In a *third group*, several peroxisomal enzymes are defective. This is the case in the Zellweger-like syndrome and in rhizomelic chondrodysplasia punctata, which is essentially a skeletal disorder, although microcephaly and developmental delay are common (Tables 2-6, 2-7, and 2-8).

Other incompletely characterized forms have been reported. One mimics Leber's *congenital amaurosis*. A benign peroxisomal disorder with ataxia and polyneuropathy has been observed in young children and adolescents. Finally, there are neonates or infants with the Zellweger phenotype but no enzymatic deficit.

In all of these disorders (with two exceptions (Table 2-6)) there is an accumulation of very long chain fatty acids (VLCFAs) in tissues and plasma. The identification of this latter abnormality by gas chromatography stands as a major criterion in the biochemical identification of peroxisomal oxidation disorders. Distinction between various neonatal diseases rests on the combined analysis of intermediate bile products, pipecolic acid, and phytanic acid in plasma, on assessment of plasmalogen synthesis (measurement of dihydroxyacetone phosphate acetyltransferase activity in red blood cells), and on assays of the activity of individual peroxisomal enzymes (Table 2-7). A search for peroxisomes in a liver biopsy or cultured fibroblasts is also useful. Various methods for the prenatal diagnosis of

Table 2-6

Identified types of peroxisomal disorders

	Diseases	Peroxisomes	Peroxisome enzyme defect
Group 1	Generalized loss of peroxisomal function (disorders of peroxisomal biogenesis)		
	Zellweger disease	Absent	Generalized
	Neonatal adrenoleukodystrophy	Absent	Generalized
	Infantile Refsum disease	Absent	Generalized
	Hyperpipecolic acidemia	Absent	Generalized
Group 2	Loss of a single peroxisomal function[a]		
	X-linked adrenoleukodystrophy[b]	Present	VLCFA-CoA synthetase
	Pseudo-neonatal adrenoleukodystrophy	Present	Acyl-CoA oxidase
	Pseudo-Zellweger disease	Present	Peroxisomal thiolase
	Bifunctional protein deficiency	Present	Bifunctional enzyme
	Dihydroxyacetone phosphate acyltransferase deficiency	Present	DHAP-AT
Group 3	Loss of several peroxisomal functions[c]		
	Zellweger-like syndrome	Present	Plasmalogen synthesis and peroxisomal fatty acid β oxidation are deficient

Abbreviations: VLCFA = very long chain fatty acids; DHAP-AT = dihydroxyacetone phosphate acyltransferase.

[a] Also hyperoxaluria type I, acatalasemia.

[b] Described in Chap. 5.

[c] In rhizomelic chondrodysplasia punctata, plasmalogen synthesis and phytanic acid oxidase are defective; peroxisomal thiolase is present in its unprocessed form; VLCFA are normal. (In DHAP-AT, VLCFA are also normal.)

Table 2-7
Main biochemical abnormalities in neonatal peroxisomal disorders

	Group I	Group II				Group III
	ZD-NALD IR-HPA	Pseudo NALD[a]	Pseudo ZD[b]	Bifunctional protein deficiency	DHAP-AT deficiency	Zellweger-like syndrome
Metabolites in body fluids						
VLCFA (plasma)	↑	↑	↑	↑	n	↑
Bile acid intermediates	↑	n	↑	↑	n	↑
Pipecolic acid	↑	n	n	n	n	n
Phytanic acid	↑	n	n	n	n	n
Plasmalogen synthesis	↓	n	n	n	↓	↓
Peroxisomal β oxidation						
Acyl-CoA oxidase	↓	↓	n	n	n	↓
Bifunctional protein	↓	n	n	↓	n	↓
Peroxisomal thiolase	↓	n	↓	n	n	↓
Lignoceroyl-CoA synthetase	↓	n	n	n	n	n
Dihydroxyacetone phosphate acyltransferase	↓	n	n	n	↓	↓
Peroxisomes	0	+	+	+	+	+

ZD = Zellweger disease; NALD = neonatal adrenoleukodystrophy; IR = infantile Refsum disease; HPA = hyperpipecolic acidemia; DHAP-AT = dihydroxyacetone phosphate acyltransferase; ↑ = elevated; ↓ = deficient; + = present; 0 = absent; n = normal.

[a] Oxidase deficiency.

[b] Thiolase deficiency.

most peroxisomal diseases are available. Heterozygote detection is only reliable in X-linked ALD. Therapeutic options are still very limited in the neonatal peroxisomal disorders.

The Clinical Syndromes in the Neonatal Period or Early Infancy Any one or several of the following signs should raise suspicion of a peroxisomal disease in a patient with marked hypotonia and evidence of severe neurological dysfunction:

- *Faciocranial dysmorphic features* including a low and broad nasal bridge, shallow orbital ridges, a high forehead, large fontanelles and an epicanthus.
- *Ocular abnormalities* such as pigmentary degeneration of the retina (confirmed by electroretinogram), cataracts, corneal opacities, and glaucoma.

- *Impaired hearing* established by auditory evoked potentials.
- *Renal cysts* detected with ultrasound and *patellar calcifications*; the latter are practically restricted to Zellweger disease.
- *Hepatomegaly* is common but is not an invariable finding.

The relative frequency of these signs in individual diseases is indicated in Table 2-8. Any one of them, however, may be absent or difficult to detect in the neonate and the clinical picture may initially be uncertain. Therefore, the possibility of a peroxisomal disease in a severely hypotonic neonate, with or without seizures, should prompt the pediatrician to obtain a biochemical test for VLCFAs in plasma. Further biochemical investigations are required to identify the underlying enzymatic defect(s) and to classify the disease.

Table 2-8

Clinical and pathological characteristics of neonatal and early infantile peroxisomal disorders[a]

	ZD	NALD	IR	Pseudo NALD[b]	Pseudo ZD[c]	DHAP-AT def.[d]	Bifunctional protein def.	Z-like syndrome
Onset	Birth	Birth	Birth	Birth	Birth	Birth	Birth	Birth
Course	<1 year	>1 year	>1 year	<1 year	<1 year	<1 year	–	<1 year
Facial dysmorphia	++	+	+	0	+	+	+	+
Ocular abnormalities	++	+	++	+	+	+	+	0
Hearing deficit	+	+	+	+	+	–	–	–
Renal cysts	+	0	0	0	+	0	–	–
Patellar calcifications	+	0	0	0	0	+	+	0
Low adrenocortical reserves or adrenal atrophy	+	+	+	–	+	–	–	–
Neocortical lesions	+	+	+	–	+	–	+	–
Leukodystrophy (astrocytosis in white matter)	+	++	+	–	+	–	–	–
Neuronal migration defects	++	±	–	0	+	–	–	–
Dysplasia of inferior olives	++	0	0	+	0	–	+	–
Purkinje cell heterotopias	++	±	±	+	+	–	+	–

Abbreviations and symbols: ZD = Zellweger's disease; NALD = neonatal ALD; IR = infantile Refsum's disease; Z = Zellweger.

+ = has been reported; – = not known, uncertain; + + = frequent, constant, or marked; ± = slight, inconstant; 0 = absent.

[a] Except for ZD and NALD, pathological reports have been, up to now, very limited.

[b] Oxidase deficiency.

[c] Thiolase deficiency.

[d] In isolated deficiency of DHAP-AT, the phenotype is similar to that of rhizomelic chondrodysplasia punctata.

Classical Zellweger Disease (Cerebrohepatorenal Disease) Zellweger disease (ZD) is a multisystem autosomal recessive disorder associated with a complete absence of peroxisomes in all tissues of the body and a generalized loss of peroxisomal function. Severe hypotonia, absence of psychomotor development, and seizures are apparent from birth or soon after. Signs of major diagnostic importance are the typical craniofacial dysmorphology, ocular abnormalities, renal cysts, and patellar calcifications. Death usually occurs in the first months of life. High levels of very long chain fatty acids in plasma, accumulation of bile acid intermediates, pipecolic acid and phytanic acids in plasma or urine, and evidence of a defective synthesis of plasmalogen are the main biochemical abnormalities. Prenatal diagnosis has been attained. There is no effective treatment. The Zellweger phenotype may be found in other closely related disorders of peroxisomal biogenesis and in other types of peroxisome dysfunction.

Clinical Features Zellweger disease is the most frequent peroxisomal disorder in early infancy. Its incidence has been estimated to be 1 in 50,000 or 1 in 100,000. In a recent series of 235 children with peroxisomal dysfunction (excluding X-linked adrenoleukodystrophy), 101 had ZD.[61]

In the typical patient, soon after birth it becomes apparent that the infant, of generally normal birth weight, is hypotonic and underactive with difficulty in sucking and swallowing, necessitating gavage feeding. In subsequent weeks, the child makes no progress in motor functions and reacts little or not at all to environmental stimuli. This may be due partly to impaired hearing and diminished visual activity, which is frequently revealed by a pendular nystagmus and lack of ocular fixation. Epileptic seizures of various types and severity are common. Tendon reflexes usually cannot be elicited. The head circumference tends to be normal at birth but lags with growth. Failure of growth postnatally becomes evident. The characteristic craniofacial dysmorphic alterations and ocular, visceral, and skeletal abnormalities are key points in diagnosis (Fig. 2-4). Noteworthy are the low and broad nasal bridge, a high forehead, large fontanelles and metopic suture, shallow orbital ridges, epicanthus, a high arched palate, micrognathia, redundant folds of the neck, and external ear deformities constituting a typical constellation. Ocular abnormalities include cataracts and corneal opacities (85 percent), glaucoma (60 percent), optic atrophy, and optic nerve hypoplasia. Retinal degeneration is present in 90 percent of the cases, manifest either as pigmentary degeneration or an extinct electroretinogram. Brushfield spots are frequently observed. Impaired hearing is said to be present in 75 percent of the patients, but is difficult to ascertain. Renal cysts, readily detected by ultrasound, are found in most patients (they may already be present in the fetus). Patellar calcifications and synchondrosis of the acetabulum are present in half the patients. Hepatomegaly is common. Cardiac defects occur (especially ventricular septal and aortic defects). Cryptochidism is frequent. Although clinical evidence of adrenocortical insufficiency has never been mentioned, adrenocortical function is found to be impaired.[65]

Brain stem auditory evoked potentials are usually absent or reduced. The electromyogram (EMG) and nerve conduction velocities are not altered. The CSF is usually normal.

The course of the disease is rapid. Most infants die in the first semester of life. A few have survived somewhat longer. The mean age of death has been 5.7 to 6.8 months in Moser's series.[61]

Biochemical Abnormalities Peroxisomes, when searched for by electron microscopy and cytochemistry for catalase, are virtually absent in liver and kidney cells and cultured fibroblasts. Any catalase activity that is found is localized in the cytosol and is not particle-bound. A few small peroxisomes with electron-dense centers may be found in the liver in some cases. Large, empty vesicles which react with antibodies to the peroxisomal membrane protein (membrane ghosts) have been detected in cultured fibroblasts, but not in the liver.[66] Immunoblotting has shown that all enzymes involved in peroxisomal β oxidation are deficient.

1. A defective synthesis and decreased tissue levels of *plasmalogen* (a variety of ether lipids). Acyl-CoA:dihydroxyacetone phosphate acyltransferase (DHAP-AT) and alkyldihydroxyacetone phosphate synthase catalyze plasmalogen synthesis in the peroxisome. DHAP-AT has been shown to be deficient in various tissues: leukocytes, cultured skin fibroblasts, amniocytes, and chorionic villus cells. Plasmalogen levels are reduced in tissues. In red blood cells, the level varies with age. It is significantly reduced under the age of 20 weeks.[61]

2. Defective peroxisomal β-oxidation and accumulation of VLCFAs in tissues and plasma, notably *hexacosanoic acid* (C26:0) which is increased ninefold over controls in plasma. The C26:0/C22:0 ratio is elevated.

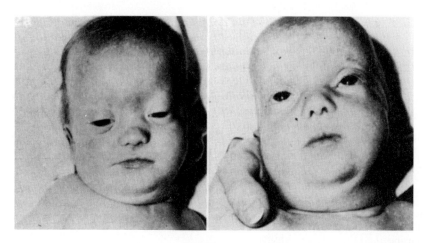

(A)

Figure 2-4
*Zellweger disease. **A**. Typical facial appearance: high forehead; wide set eyes; broad root of nose; shallow supraorbital ridges. **B**. Calcification of patellae. **C**. Ultrasound scan showing cortical cysts in kidney (arrows). (Part **A** courtesy Passarge, I and McAdams, AJ, J Pediatr 71: 69, 1967; part **B** courtesy Dr. Fernand-Alvarez.)*

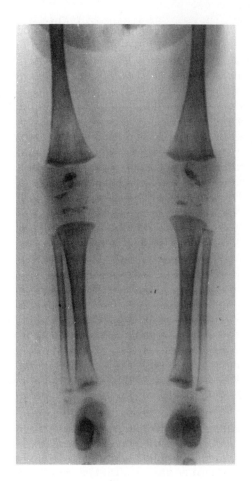

(B)

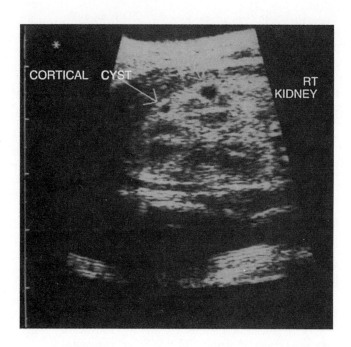

(C)

3. Defects in bile formation resulting in the accumulation of *intermediates of bile acid metabolism.* Levels of trihydrocholestanoic acid (THCA) and dihydrocholestanoic acid (DHCA) are consistently elevated in the plasma.

4. Impaired catabolism and accumulation of *pipecolic acid*, especially the L-isomer in plasma and urine, after the age of 1 month.

5. *Phytanic acid* oxidation in cultured fibroblasts is markedly reduced. Phytanic acid levels in the plasma vary with age. Phytanic acid is exclusively of dietary origin. Concentrations are moderately elevated in ZD after the age of 40 months.

6. Slightly increased amounts of medium-chain dicarboxylic acids are found in the urine.

Molecular Biology and Genetics   ZD is an autosomal recessively inherited disorder. Nine different complementation groups have been found, using cells from patients with defective peroxisomal biogenesis. Genetic mutations have been shown in the genes for two of the peroxisomal integral membrane proteins, peroxisomal assembly factor 1 (PAF 1) coded on chromosome 8q21 and the 70 kd peroxisomal membrane protein (PMP-70), an ATP-binding cassette protein.[67,68]

In two patients, abnormalities in chromosome 7 (7q11.23) have been demonstrated.[69]

Diagnostic Laboratory Tests   Diagnostic laboratory tests include the following:

• Slit-lamp examination of lens and cornea; ultrasonic examination of kidneys and liver and x-rays of lower limbs.
• MRI of the brain showing abnormal convolution pattern and leukodystrophy.
• In biochemical testing, the first step consists in the measurement of plasma VLCFAs by gas chromatography/mass spectrometry. If VLCFAs are elevated, the diagnosis will be confirmed by

1. Analysis of trihydrocholestanoic acid, pipecolic acid, and phytanic acid in plasma or urine, and the assessment of DHAP-AT in red blood cells.

2. Demonstration of a virtual absence of peroxisomes in a liver biopsy (and/or cultured fibroblasts).

3. Measurement of cortisol after stimulation with adrenocorticotropin (ACTH) may also be useful.

Pathological Findings   General pathological findings include fibrosis or nodular cirrhosis of the liver, renal cysts (which may be present in the fetus), various cardiac defects, and adrenocortical lesions similar to those in X-linked adrenoleukodystrophy (ALD). The reticularis and inner fasciculata zone contain striate cells, some of which are ballooned and have lamellar inclusions. These changes may be missed if not specifically sought. Neuropathological findings are unique and are remarkably similar from case to case.[70] They consist of

1. A characteristic pattern of abnormal neuronal migration. Focal areas of microgyria or pachygyria.

2. Pachygyria and disorganization of the inferior olives.

3. Heterotopias of Purkinje cells in the cerebellar white matter.

4. Various degrees of demyelination with astrocytic proliferation in the cerebral hemispheres.

Intracellular lamellar inclusions containing VLCFAs have been demonstrated in gray and white matter.

Differential Diagnosis   The facial appearance and the presence of Brushfield spots may suggest Down's syndrome. Patellar stippling is easily differentiated from the diffuse calcifications of rhizomelic chondrodysplasia punctata, another entirely different peroxisomal disorder. The Zellweger phenotype may occur in a number of other peroxisomal disorders (see below). A correct biochemical diagnosis is important because it permits application of prenatal diagnosis in later pregnancies.

Prenatal Diagnosis   Several methods are available for a reliable prenatal diagnosis in ZD. They consist essentially of assays of VLCFAs and plasmalogen biosynthesis on cultured amniocytes and chorionic villus samples.

Treatment   A dietary regimen to achieve normalization of blood VLCFA levels is currently being tested in the milder forms of the disease.

Other Disorders with the Zellweger Phenotype   A number of other probably recessively inherited peroxisomal disorders have a clinical presentation which is identical or similar to that of Zellweger disease (see Table 2-8). They include three different groups.

A First Group Sharing with ZD a General Loss of All Peroxisomal Enzymes (Group 1, Table 2-6). This group consists of three closely allied conditions which are by order of frequency: neonatal adrenoleukodystrophy, infantile Refsum disease and hyperpipecolic aciduria. Differences between these syndromes and ZD relate to severity of the neurologic abnormality and to the presence of a few clinical and pathological features summarized in Tables 2-7 and 2-8. These conditions, for the most part, were described before our concept of the peroxisomal disorder was formulated. It is not yet known if they represent different entities. Complementation studies have up to now failed to establish a clear relationship between genotype and phenotype. Molecular studies will probably resolve the question.

Neonatal Adrenoleukodystrophy (ALD) The term neonatal ALD was first used by Ulrich et al. in 1978[71] to describe a child with marked hypotonia at birth, severe seizures and absence of psychomotor development, who died at the age of 20 months. Postmortem studies showed demyelination, cerebral "polymicrogyria," and adrenocortical atrophy with ballooned adrenocortical cells containing lamellar cytoplasmic bodies. There was a marked excess of hexacosanoic acid in the brain. Because the pathological and biochemical findings resembled those of X-linked ALD, it was called neonatal ALD, but obviously it is fundamentally different from the juvenile X-linked disorder with that name. It closely resembles ZD but with some differences. In neonatal ALD, facial dysmorphic features are usually less marked or may be absent. The disease is generally less severe and some patients have reached early adolescence. Some of them walk and say a few words but are severely retarded. After a few years, neurological regression becomes evident. A retinopathy with extinction of the electroretinogram (ERG) and deafness are usual. Patellar calcifications and renal cysts are not seen. Clinical signs of adrenal insufficiency are uncommon, but the cortisol response to ACTH is reduced. In one of the Kennedy Institute series, the mean age of death was 36.5 ± 26.4 months compared to 7.0 ± 10.5 months in classical Zellweger disease.[61] At autopsy, disorders of neuronal migration are inconstant and the abnormality of the inferior olive, a striking finding of ZD, is apparently lacking. A sudanophilic leukodystrophy is usually present. In some cases there is perivascular cuffing with lymphocytes. The adrenal pathology may be subtle and not recognized unless specifically sought. Systematic infiltration by lipid-laden macrophages has been reported. The biochemical

abnormalities are similar to those in the Zellweger syndrome. Since they are not observed in the parents of neonatal ALD patients, carrier detection is not possible.

Infantile Refsum Disease In 1982, Scotto[72] and Boltshauser[73] independently described patients with mental retardation, hepatomegaly, sensorineural deafness, pigmentary degeneration of the retina, anosmia, and dysmorphic features. An ultrastructural analysis of a liver biopsy revealed peculiar lamellar structures which led the authors to measure phytanic acid levels in the plasma and to discover that they were markedly elevated. This, together with the sensory disturbances and the hepatomegaly, resembled adult Refsum disease. Subsequent studies demonstrated in all cases of infantile Refsum syndrome the absence of liver peroxisomes and all other biochemical abnormalities found in ZD and neonatal ALD. Levels of phytanic acid in the plasma were found to be equivalent to those seen in patients with ZD and neonatal ALD who survived after the age of 3 months.

The course of the disease is much more prolonged than in ZD and many cases of neonatal ALD.[74] Seizures have not been reported. Most of the affected children are still living and many have reached late childhood or adolescence. All patients are severely retarded and usually able to walk. They have a sensorineural deafness and a pigmentary degeneration of the retina with an extinct ERG, moderately dysmorphic features, essentially a flat bridge of the nose, an epicanthus, and low set ears. Hepatomegaly is usual. Patellar calcifications and renal cysts are absent. Autopsy studies have shown micronodular cirrhosis of the liver, atrophic adrenals, and fat-laden macrophages in multiple organs. There was no evident disorder of neuronal migration in the cortex or abnormality of the inferior olives. A few heterotypic nodules of Purkinje cells were displaced in the molecular layer and aggregates of fat-laden macrophages occurred in the white matter and other organs.[75]

Hyperpipecolic Aciduria There are many similarities between the three patients reported as having hyperpipecolic aciduria and children with neonatal ALD and ZD. All have shown VLCFA abnormalities typical of disorders of peroxisomal biogenesis. The facial dysmorphia in one child was apparently unusual.[61] Peroxisomes were said to be present in one patient, but there are reasons to doubt the validity of this finding,[61] and there is up to now no reason to believe that hyperpipecolic aciduria represents a separate entity. An exception may be three siblings, described by Poll-The et al.,[64] with isolated, increased pipecolic acid, clinical features of a generalized peroxisomal disorder, and of Joubert syndrome.

Other Variants of Disorders of Peroxisomal Biogenesis   In one report[61] the most distinctive finding was a congenital retinopathy with an extinct ERG as in Leber's amaurosis. At 7 months the child was hypotonic and mentally retarded. A hepatomegaly was present, but there were no dysmorphic features and no patellar calcifications. Peroxisomes were absent and the biochemical abnormalities were those of a generalized peroxisomal insufficiency.

Disorders Displaying the Zellweger Phenotype in Which Peroxisomes Are Present and There Is a Deficiency of Only One Enzyme of Peroxisomal β Oxidation (Group 2, Table 2-6)

Peroxisomal Acyl-CoA Oxidase Deficiency (Pseudo-Neonatal ALD)   The first two siblings with this condition have been reported by Poll-The et al.[76]

Hypotonia and seizures were present soon after birth. Subsequently, there was amblyopia due to a pigmentary degeneration of the retina (with an extinct ERG), hearing loss, a delay in psychomotor development, and a latent adrenocortical insufficiency. There was no dysmorphia. Regression in neurological function appeared after the age of 2. Biological abnormalities were confined to an elevation of VLCFAs in the plasma. Plasmalogen, bile acids, and pipecolic acid were normal. Liver peroxisomes were present and appeared even to be enlarged. The activity of peroxisomal acyl-CoA oxidase was deficient due to a large deletion in the gene for this enzyme.[64] Other particulars have since been identified by a complementary analysis. A neuropathological examination made by one of us showed in one patient an olivary pachygyria, as in ZD, and no other abnormality.

Peroxisomal 3-Oxoacyl-CoA Thiolase Deficiency (Pseudo-Zellweger Syndrome)   In 1986, Goldfischer et al.[77] reported a girl with severe neonatal hypotonia and seizures, dysmorphic features of Zellweger syndrome, and no evidence of motor or mental development. She died at the age of 11 months and autopsy showed atrophic adrenals, renal cysts, liver fibrosis, a sudanophilic leukodystrophy, and neuronal heteropia in the cerebral and cerebellar hemispheres. Hepatic peroxisomes were abundant and enlarged. There was an accumulation of VLCFAs and bile acid intermediates in the

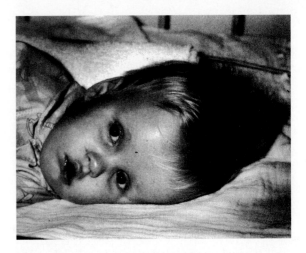

Figure 2-5
Bifunctional enzyme deficiency: facial features. Note the high forehead. (Courtesy Dr. Van Coster.)

plasma. Plasmalogen synthesis was normal. Immunoblotting revealed a deficiency in the peroxisomal 3-oxoacyl-CoA thiolase.[78]

Bifunctional Protein Insufficiency   A bifunctional protein deficiency was found by Watkins et al.[79] in a child presenting with the following clinical picture: severe hypotonia at birth, neonatal seizures, lack of spontaneous movements, depressed deep tendon reflexes, no evidence of mental development, macrocephaly (a high forehead), and large fontanelles (Fig. 2-5). Visual and brain stem auditory evoked responses were delayed. There was no retinopathy, dysmorphia, or renal cysts. A brain biopsy at 6 weeks of age revealed "polymicrogyria." VLCFAs and bile acid intermediates were elevated in plasma. There was no abnormality in the biosynthesis of plasmalogen or in the degradation of pipecolic and phytanic acid. Other patients with isolated bifunctional protein insufficiency have since been identified. Clayton et al.[80] described three children in the same family with severe neonatal hypotonia, refractory seizures, severe retardation, retinopathy, and diminished auditory evoked potentials. Autopsy in one revealed adrenal atrophy and renal cortical cysts. VLCFAs and bile acid intermediates were found to be elevated. Immunoblotting showed that all three peroxisomal β-oxidation enzymes were present, but the bifunctional protein was later shown to be deficient.[81] Autopsy in one case showed a moderate cerebral cortical dysplasia, typical olivary abnormalities, and Purkinje cells heterotopias in the cerebellar white matter.[82]

Dihydroxyacetonephosphate Acyltransferase Deficiency   Two patients with isolated dihydroxyacetonephosphate acyltransferase (DHAP-AT) deficiency have been described. They presented at birth with craniofacial abnormalities, cataracts, pronounced rhizomelic shortening, especially of the upper limbs, and profound hypotonia. These dysmorphic features were similar to those of RCDP. Very long chain fatty acids were normal. But the abnormalities of phytanic acid metabolism and of peroxisomal thiolase typical of RCDP were absent. Only plasmalogen synthesis was deficient, due to the absence of DHAP-AT activity. A milder form of DHAP-AT deficiency has also been described.[83]

A Disorder Displaying the Zellweger Phenotype Characterized by the Loss of Several Enzymes and a Normal Amount of Peroxisomes: The So-Called Zellweger-Like Syndrome (Group 3, Table 2-6)   This condition has been described so far in two unrelated patients.[83a] Their clinical presentation was indistinguishable from that of Zellweger disease. However, peroxisomes were present in normal number and appearance in a liver biopsy. There was an accumulation of VLCFAs and di- and trihydrocholestanoic acids in plasma and evidence of dicarboxylic acids in the urine. Upon immunoblotting the three enzymes involved in peroxisomal β oxidation, as well as the enzyme dihydroxyacetone phosphate acyltransferase (DHAP-AT) involved in plasmalogen synthesis, were deficient.

Disorders of Peroxisomal β Oxidation with a Still Unidentified Enzyme Defect   Several patients have recently been reported with a similar clinical presentation reminiscent of Zellweger disease or neonatal ALD and with evidence of peroxisomal β oxidation defect, but no detectable enzyme deficiency.

A girl with neonatal hypotonia and seizures was reported by Naidu et al.[84] At autopsy, there was a demyelination, adrenal atrophy, hepatic fibrosis and PAS-positive macrophages in several organs. Biochemical abnormalities were confined to an excess of VLCFAs in the plasma. No enzymatic defect could be demonstrated. Mandel et al.[85] have reported two siblings with facial dysmorphism, severe hypotonia, apneic spells, and neonatal seizures. The sole peroxisomal dysfunction consisted of an increase in plasma VLCFAs.

Peroxisomes were present in the liver and all three peroxisomal β-oxidation enzyme proteins were normally present by immunoblotting.

Disorders of Carbohydrate Metabolism

Disorders of Fructose Metabolism   Two disorders of fructose metabolism give rise to severe neurologic dysfunction in the newborn: fructose 1,6-bisphosphatase deficiency and hereditary fructose intolerance.[86]

Fructose 1,6-Bisphosphatase Deficiency   Fructose 1,6-bisphosphatase deficiency is a potentially life-threatening disorder of gluconeogenesis for which an effective treatment exists. Eighty-five cases had been reported up to 1989.[86]

Its mode of inheritance is autosomal recessive. About half the patients have their first symptoms between their 1st and 4th days of life, a period during which young infants are dependent on gluconeogenesis. Hyperventilation and spells of apnea, hypotonia, irritability, convulsions, and lethargy then coma are the usual manifestations. Hepatomegaly may occur. There is marked acidosis, lactacidemia, ketosis, and hypoglycemia. There are also hyperalaninemia and increased concentrations of glycerol.

Diagnosis is established by demonstrating the enzyme deficiency in liver or jejunal biopsies. The acute episodes can be counteracted by the administration of intravenous glucose and sodium bicarbonate which allows further development to be normal. These children are prone to subsequent metabolic attacks during periods of fasting or febrile illness. This can be prevented by a diet limiting fructose and sucrose.

Hereditary Fructose Intolerance (Fructose 1,6-Bisphosphate Aldolase Deficiency)   Hereditary fructose intolerance may manifest itself in newborns who are not breast-fed when they are given fructose or sucrose which induces a profound hypoglycemia, vomiting, convulsions and possibly death. A late-onset, intermittent form occurs in infancy or childhood (see Chap. 3).

Glycogen Storage Diseases   *Type I Glycogen Storage Disease: Von Gierke Disease*   Von Gierke disease is caused by a deficiency of glucose 6-phosphatase in liver, kidney, and intestinal mucosa. It may present in the neonatal period with hypoglycemia and lactic acidosis. *Type II glycogen storage disease* which may be symptomatic soon after birth is discussed in Chap. 3.

An exceptional, rapidly fatal, neonatal form of *glycogenesis type VII* with involvement of muscle and brain has been reported.[87]

Transferase Deficiency Galactosemia

Clinical Features   In this disorder, vomiting and diarrhea appear after birth, a few days after milk ingestion. Failure to thrive, jaundice, hepatomegaly and occasionally hemolysis subsequently occur. Cataracts may be present in the first days of life as demonstrated by slit-lamp examination. High intracranial pressure and a bulging fontanelle have been reported.

If untreated, many children die of overwhelming infection (usually *E. coli*) during the first weeks or from progressive liver failure. In those who survive, mental retardation later becomes evident.

Biochemical Features   Galactosemia and galactosuria are characteristic. Other important biochemical features are proteinuria, generalized aminoaciduria, hyperchloremic acidosis and evidence of liver dysfunction. The specific deficiency in galactose-1-phosphate uridyltransferase (GALT) is revealed in red blood cells. The disease can be detected by population-based neonatal screening tests. The GALT locus has been mapped to chromosome 9p13 and several mutations in the gene have been described.

Treatment and Course   A galactose-free diet (casein hydrolysates and soybean milk) is lifesaving and results in a remarkable cure of the digestive and hepatic symptoms, regression of cataracts, and normal growth. Long-term effects of dietary treatment on intellectual development is usually less than satisfactory (for discussion, see Chap. 3).

Variants   A few patients fail to show a severe neonatal syndrome and are seen in late infancy and childhood with mental retardation, cataracts, and possibly hepatomegaly (see Chap. 3).

Pyridoxine (Vitamin B₆) Dependency

This autosomal recessive hereditary metabolic disorder is characterized by severe neonatal seizures. Convulsions are apparently due to an abnormality of glutamic acid decarboxylase (GAD), for which vitamin B_6 is a cofactor. The result is an insufficient formation of γ-aminobutyric acid (GABA), an inhibitory neurotransmitter. To overcome a defect in the pyridoxal phosphate binding site of GAD, greater than normal doses of pyridoxine (vitamin B_6) are required. Pyridoxine dependency must not be confused with pyridoxine *deficiency* in which the cofactor is missing because of low dietary intake or impaired gastrointestinal absorption. In this instance, the brain is affected and seizures may occur, but other tissues are also deranged.

Clinical Findings   The disease manifests itself during the first few days of life by repeated and prolonged generalized or focal seizures. Convulsions may even start in utero and are perceptible to the mother. Between bouts of seizures, the infant is irritable and jittery, movements may be tremulous, and startle due to auditory stimuli is prominent.

Pyridoxine dependency is demonstrated by the immediate effect of high doses of intravenous pyridoxine (100 to 200 mg). Within a few minutes, seizures disappear and the EEG is normalized. With oral supplementation by 50 mg of pyridoxine daily, seizures do not recur and psychomotor development proceeds normally. High CSF glutamate levels should be normalized.[87a] This treatment must be given indefinitely. If treatment is interrupted, seizures reappear within 2 to 23 days. Without treatment, the seizures persist and are accompanied by severe mental retardation. There is no diagnostic biological test.

In view of the severity of the disease and the extraordinary effect of a specific and innocuous therapy, oral pyridoxine should be systematically tried in all cases of neonatal convulsions.

It has become evident in recent years that the clinical spectrum of pyridoxine dependency is broader than initially described. The onset of seizures may not begin until after several weeks or months and may be severe and prolonged. It is therefore necessary to consider the possibility of pyridoxine dependency in infants with seizures who do not respond to the usual antiepileptic drugs.[88]

Pathological Findings   Only a few patients have come to postmortem examination. One of our patients, a severely retarded, spastic 10-year-old child with pale optic disks was found to have a brain that weighed 350 g less than normal with reduced volume of cerebral white matter. The cerebral cortex appeared normal, but there was depletion of neurons and fibrous gliosis in thalamic nuclei. The cerebellum displayed an abnormal lobular pattern of folia and focal loss of Purkinje cells with microglial clusters in the molecular layer. Glutamate concentrations were elevated and GABA concentrations reduced in the frontal and occipital cortices.[89]

Other Metabolic Disorders with a Possible Neonatal Onset

A few other disorders which may have their first signs in the neonatal period will be considered in the next chapter because the full-blown manifestations of the disease usually do not develop until early infancy or because their neonatal manifestations are relatively rare. They include

- Menkes kinky hair disorder.

- Glycogenesis type II.

- Lysosomal disorders such as Krabbe disease, Niemann-Pick disease, G_{M1} gangliosidosis, Farber disease, Gaucher disease, Sly disease, sialidosis, galactosialidosis, I-cell disease, and sialic acid storage disease. Hydrops fetalis may occur in many of these conditions.

- *Lysinuric protein intolerance.* In this condition, symptoms related to hyperammonemia may occur in neonates who are not breast-fed. They consist of feeding difficulties, vomiting, diarrhea, and poor reactivity. The disorder is usually recognized at a later period (see Chap. 3).

- *β Ketothiolase (mitochondrial 2-methylacetoacetyl-CoA thiolase) deficiency.* One child with this condition has been reported with a neonatal onset. He presented with vomiting, tachypnea, and stupor. All other cases have had a later onset (Chap. 3).

- *5-oxoprolinuria (glutathione synthetase deficiency).* Three children were reported with this disease. In two of them, evidence of severe metabolic acidosis occurred in the first days of life. Considerable quantities of 5-oxoproline were excreted in the urine. Symptomatic treatment of acidosis resulted in a normal development, with moderate mental retardation in one. Both patients showed an increased rate of hemolysis. A third patient had jaundice at birth and subsequently evidence of chronic metabolic acidosis with severe motor and mental handicap. The defect of glutathione synthetase, which causes this disease, is demonstrable in cultured fibroblasts and erythrocytes.

- *2,4-dienoyl-CoA reductase deficiency.* This disorder was detected in one girl who presented in the neonatal period with severe hypotonia, irritability, microcephaly, and feeding problems as well as cardiac hypertrophy. She had a short trunk, arms, fingers, and feet, and a large face. At 2 months of age, she was microcephalic. By ultrasound, the ventricles were enlarged. The patient died at 4 months of age. Metabolic studies revealed hyperlysinemia and carnitine deficiency. Organic acid excretion was normal, but an abnormal acyl carnitine (2-*trans*-4-*cis*-decadienoylcarnitine) was excreted. 2,4-decadienoyl-CoA reductase deficiency was demonstrated postmortem in liver and muscle.

CONCLUSIONS

The reader, after perusing the preceding pages, cannot but be impressed with the commonality of clinical expression of the hereditary neurometabolic diseases in the neonatal period. An identical syndrome—neurological symptoms, dyspnea, vomiting—occurs both in the metabolic diseases and in the far more frequent hypoxic-ischemic encephalopathies, prenatal brain defects, infections, pulmonary disorders, or intoxications.

Nevertheless, a strong suspicion of a metabolic disorder can usually be raised on purely clinical grounds. Typically, such children are born normally at full term and the immediate post-partum responses are normal. There is no microcephaly or developmental defect. Hypotonia, somnolence or stupor, seizures, respiratory dysrhythmias, anorexia, and vomiting appear only after a day or two, or more.

But there are exceptions to this rule. The free interval may be missing, a mild degree of prematurity or intrauterine growth retardation are occasionally noted, and in a few conditions cerebral and somatic development abnormalities are present. Here again, the absence of any perinatal disorder and of radiologic signs of an ischemic encephalopathy are important indications. Also, the presence of nonneurologic abnormalities such as a cardiopathy, a hepatomegaly, renal cysts or skeletal changes, and the existence of a previously affected child in the family, are important clinical clues and lead one to undertake the necessary laboratory investigations. Early detection is essential to prevent further neurologic deterioration by specific therapeutic measures.

Practically all diseases which manifest themselves soon after birth also present later in life.

REFERENCES

1. Andre-Thomas J, Sainte-Anne d'Argassies S: *Etudes Neurologiques sur le Nouveau-né et le Nourrisson.* Paris, Masson, 1952.

2. Peiper A: *Cerebral Function in Infancy and Childhood.* New York, Consultants Bureau, 1963.

3. Prechtl HFR, Beintema D: *The Neurological Examination of the Full Term Newborn Infant.* London, William Heinemann, 1964.

4. Brazelton TB: *Neonatal Behavioral Assessment Scale.* Philadelphia, Lippincott, 1973.

5. Dubowitz L, Dubowitz V: *The Neurological Assessment of the Preterm and Full-Term Newborn Infant.* Philadelphia, Lippincott, 1981.

6. Amiel-Tison C, Grenier A: *Neurological Assessment during the First Year of Life.* New York, Oxford University Press, 1986.

7. Volpe JJ: *Neurology of the Newborn.* 3d ed. Philadelphia, Saunders, 1995.

8. Aicardi J: *Epilepsy in Children*, 2d ed. New York, Raven, 1994.

9. Malafosse A, Beck C, Bellet H, et al.: Benign infantile familial convulsions are not an allelic form of the benign familial neonatal convulsions gene. *Ann Neurol* 35: 479–482, 1994.

10. Miranda SB, Hach M, Fantz RL, et al.: Neonatal pattern vision: a predictor of future mental performance? *J Pediatr* 91: 642–647, 1977.

11. Bachmann C, Colombo JP, Jaggi K: *N*-Acetylglutamate synthetase (NAGS) deficiency: Diagnosis, clinical observations and treatment. *Adv Exp Med Biol* 153: 39–45, 1982.

12. Brusilow SW, Horwich AL: Urea cycle enzymes, in Scriver CR, Beaudet AL, Sly WS, Valle D (eds): *The Metabolic and Molecular Bases of Inherited Disease*, 7th ed. New York, McGraw-Hill, 1995, pp. 1187–1232.

13. Batshaw ML: Inborn errors of urea synthesis. *Ann Neurol* 35: 133–141, 1994.

14. Shih G, Efron ML, Moser HW: Hyperornithinemia, hyperammonemia and homocitrullinuria. A new disorder of aminoacid metabolism associated with myoclonic seizures and mental retardation. *Am J Dis Child* 117: 83–92, 1969.

15. Dionisi Vici C, Bachmann C, Gambarara A, et al.: Hyperornithinemia, hyperammonemia, homocitrullinuria syndrome. Low creatine excretion and effect of citrulline, arginine or ornithine supplementation. *Pediatr Res* 22: 364–367, 1987.

16. Hamos RA, Johnson MV, Valle D: Nonketotic hyperglycinemia, in Scriver CR, Beaudet AL, Sly WS, Valle D (eds): *The Metabolic and Molecular Bases of Inherited Disease*, 7th ed. New York, McGraw-Hill, 1995, pp. 1337–1348.

17. Dobyns WB: Agenesis of the corpus callosum and gyral malformations are frequent manifestations of nonketotic hyperglycinemia. *Neurology*, 39: 817–820, 1989.

18. Hamosh A, McDonald JW, Valle D, et al.: Dextromethorphan and high-dose benzoate therapy for nonketotic hyperglycinemia in an infant. *J Pediatr* 121: 131–135, 1992.

19. Luder AS, Davidson A, Goodman SI, et al.: Transient nonketotic hyperglycinemia in neonates. *J Pediatr* 114: 1013–1015, 1989.

20. Flannery DB, Pellock J, Bonsounis D, et al.: Non-ketotic hyperglycinemia in two retarded adults: a mild form of infantile non-ketotic hyperglycinemia. *Neurology* 33: 1064–1066, 1983.

21. Singer H, Valle D, Hagasaka K, et al.: Non-ketotic hyperglycinemia: studies in an atypical variant. *Neurology* 39: 286–288, 1989.

22. Trauner DA, Page T, Greco C, et al.: Progressive neurodegenerative disorder in a patient with nonketotic hyperglycinemia. *J Pediatr* 98: 272–275, 1981.

23. Bank WJ, Morrow G: A familial spinal cord disorder with hyperglycinemia. *Arch Neurol* 27: 136–144, 1972.

24. Zee DS, Freeman JM, Holtzman NA: Ophthalmoplegia in maple syrup urine disease. *J Pediatr* 84: 113–115, 1974.

25. Peinemann F, Danner DJ: Maple syrup urine disease, 1954 to 1993. *J Inherit Metab Dis* 17: 3–15, 1994.

26. Chhabria S, Tomasi LG, Wong PWK: Ophthalmoplegia and bulbar palsy in variant form of maple syrup urine disease. *Ann Neurol* 6: 71–72, 1979.

27. Danner JD, Elsas LJ: Disorders of branched chain amino acid and keto acid metabolism, in Scriver CR, Beaudet AL, Sly WS, Valle D (eds): *The Metabolic Basis of Inherited Disease*, 6th ed. New York, McGraw-Hill, 1989, pp. 671–692.

28. Sweetman L, Williams JC: Branched chain organic acidurias, in Scriver CR, Beaudet AL, Sly WS, Valle D (eds): *The Metabolic and Molecular Bases of Inherited Disease*, 7th ed. New York, McGraw-Hill, 1995, pp. 1387–1422.

29. Ozand PT, Gascon GG: Organic acidurias: a review. Part 1. *J Child Neurol* 6: 196–219, 1991.

29a. Ozand PT, Gascon GG: Organic acidurias: a review. Part 2. *J Child Neurol* 6: 288–303, 1991.

30. Surtess RA, Matthews EE, Leonard JV: Neurologic outcome of propionic acidemia. *Pediatr Neurol* 8: 333–337, 1992.

31. Fenton WA, Rosenberg LE: Disorders of propionate and methylmalonate metabolism, in Scriver CR, Beaudet AL, Sly WS, Valle D (eds): *The Metabolic and Molecular Bases of Inherited Disease*, 7th ed. New York, McGraw-Hill, 1995, pp. 1423–1449.

32. Kang ES, Snodgrass PJ, Gerald PS: Methylmalonyl coenzyme. A racemase defect: another cause of methylmalonic aciduria. *Pediatr Res* 6: 875–879, 1972.

33. Van Gennip AH, Abeling NGGM, Stroomer AEM, et al.: The detection of molybdenum cofactor deficiency: clinical symptomatology and urinary metabolite profile. *J Inherit Metab Dis* 17: 142–145, 1994.

34. Hoffman GF, Charpentier C, Mayatepek E, et al.: Clinical and biochemical phenotype in 11 patients with mevalonic acidemia. *Pediatrics* 91: 915–921, 1993.

35. De Vivo DC: The expanding clinical spectrum of mitochondrial diseases. *Brain and Development* 15: 1–22, 1993.

36. Robinson BH, MacMillan H, Petrova-Benedict R, et al.: Variable clinical presentation in patients with defective E_1 component of pyruvate dehydrogenase complex. *J Pediatr* 111: 525–533, 1987.

37. Brown GK, Brown RM, Scholem RD, et al.: The clinical and biochemical spectrum of human pyruvate dehydrogenase deficiency. *Ann NY Acad Sci* 573: 360–368, 1989.

38. Brown GK, Haan EA, Kirby DM, et al.: "Cerebral" lactic acidosis: defect in pyruvate metabolism with profound brain damage and minimal systemic acidosis. *Eur J Pediatr* 147: 10–14, 1988.

39. De Meirleer L, Lissens W, Denis R: Pyruvate dehydrogenase deficiency: clinical and biochemical diagnosis. *Pediatr Neurol* 9: 216–220, 1993.

40. Fujii T, Van Coster RN, Old SE et al.: Pyruvate dehydrogenase deficiency: molecular basis for intrafamilial heterogeneity. *Ann Neurol* 36: 83–89, 1994.

41. Prick M, Gabreels F, Renier W, et al.: Pyruvate dehydrogenase deficiency restricted to the brain. *Neurology* 31: 398–404, 1981.

42. Chow CW, Anderson RC, Kenny GC: Neuropathology in cerebral lactic acidosis. *Acta Neuropathol* 74: 393–396, 1987.

43. Dahl HHM, Maragos C, Brown RM, et al.: Pyruvate dehydrogenase deficiency caused by deletion of a 7-p repeat sequence in a $E_{1\alpha}$ gene. *Am J Hum Genet* 47: 286–293, 1990.

44. Robinson BN, MacKay N, Petrova-Benedict R, et al.: Defects in the E_2 lipoyl acetyltransacetylase and X-lipoyl containing component of the pyruvate dehydrogenase complex in patients with lactacidemia. *J Clin Invest* 85: 1821–1824, 1990.

45. Saudubray JM, Marsac C, Cathelineau CL, et al.: Neonatal congenital lactic acidosis with pyruvate carboxylase deficiency in two siblings. *Acta Paediatr Scand* 65: 717–724, 1976.

46. Van Coster RN, Fernhoff PM, De Vivo DC: Pyruvate carboxylate deficiency: a benign variant with normal development. *Pediatr Res* 30: 1–4, 1991.

46a. Stern HJ, Nagar R, DePalma L, et al.: Prolonged survival in pyruvate carboxylase deficiency: lack of correlation with enzyme activity in cultured fibroblasts. *Clin Biochem* 28: 85–89, 1995.

47. Moreadith RW, Batshaw ML, Ohnishi T, et al.: Deficiency of the iron-sulfur clusters of mitochondrial reduced nicotanmimide-adenine dinucleotide ubiquinone oxidoreductase (complex I) in an infant with congenital lactic acidosis. *J Clin Invest* 74: 685–697, 1984.

47a. Birch-Machin MA, Sheperd IM, Watmough NJ, et al.: Fatal lactic acidosis in infancy with a defect of complex III of the respiratory chain. *Pediatr Res* 18: 991–999, 1984.

48. Zeviani M, Van Dyke DH, Servidei S, et al.: Myopathy and fatal cardiomyopathy due to cytochrome oxidase-*c* deficiency. *Arch Neurol* 43: 1198–1202, 1986.

49. Scalais E, Van Coster RN: Personal communications, 1994.

50. Hug G, Bove KE, Soukup S: Lethal neonatal multiorgan deficiency of carnitine palmitoyltransferase II. *New Engl J Med* 325: 1862–1864, 1991.

51. Taroni F, Verderio E, Dworzak F, et al.: Identification of a common mutation in the carnitine palmitoyltransferase II gene in familial recurrent myoglobinuria patients. *Nat Genet* 4: 314–320, 1993.

52. Stanley CA, Hale DE, Gerard TB, et al.: Brief report: a deficiency of carnitine-acylcarnitine translocase in the inner mitochondrial membrane. *New Engl J Med* 327: 19–27, 1992.

53. Aamendt BA, Greene C, Sweetman L: Short-chain acyl-coenzyme A dehydrogenase deficiency: clinical and biochemical study in two patients. *J Clin Invest* 79: 1303–1309, 1987.

54. Hale DE, Batshaw ML, Coates PM, et al.: Long-chain acyl coenzyme A dehydrogenase deficiency: an inherited cause of nonketotic hypoglycemia. *Pediatr Res* 19: 666–671, 1985.

54a. Bertrand C, Langilliera C, Zabot MT, et al.: Very long-chain acyl-CoA dehydrogenase deficiency, etc. *Biochem Biophys Acta* 1180: 327–333, 1993.

55. Loehr JP, Goodman SI, Frerman FF: Glutaric acidemia type II: heterogeneity of clinical and biochemical phenotypes. *Pediatr Res* 27: 311–315, 1990.

56. Harkin JC, Gill WL, Shapiro E: Glutaric acidemia type II: phenotypic findings and ultrastructural studies of brain and kidney. *Arch Pathol Lab Med* 110–399, 1986.

57. Jackson S, Turnbull DM: Other enzyme defects of β-oxidation. Abnormalities of the trifunctional protein, in *Proceedings 2d International Congress on Human Mitochondrial Pathology*, Rome, 1992, 65 (abstract).

58. Poulton J, Morten K, Freeman-Emerson C, et al.: Deficiency of the human mitochondrial transcription factor h-mt TFA in infantile mitochondrial myopathy is associated with mtDNA depletion. *Hum Molecul Genet* 3: 1763–1769, 1994.

59. Moraes CT, Shanke S, Tritschler HJ, et al.: MtDNA depletion with variable tissue expression: a novel genetic abnormality in mitochondrial diseases. *Am J Human Genet* 48: 492–501, 1991.

60. Gibson KM, Breuer J, Kaiser K, et al.: 3-Hydroxy-3-methylglutaryl-coenzyme A lyase deficiency: report of five new patients. *J Inherit Metab Dis* 11: 76–87, 1988.

61. Lazarow PB, Moser HW: Disorders of peroxisome biogenesis, in Scriver CR, Beaudet AL, Sly WS, Valle D (eds): *The Metabolic and Molecular Bases of Inherited Disease*, 7th ed. New York, McGraw-Hill, 1995, pp. 2287–2324.

62. Wanders RJA, Van Roermund CWT, Schutgens RBH, et al.: The inborn errors of peroxisomal beta oxidation: a review. *J Inherit Metab Dis* 13: 4–36, 1990.

63. Moser HW: Peroxisomal disorders, in Rosemberg RN, Prusiner SB, Di Mauro S, Barchi RL, Kunkel LM (eds): *The Molecular and Genetic Basis of Neurological Disease.* Boston, Butterworth-Heinemann, 1993, pp. 351–387.

64. Fournier B, Smeitlink JAM, Dorland L, et al.: Peroxisomal disorders: a review. *J Inherit Metab Dis* 17: 470–486, 1994.

65. Govaerts L, Monnens L, Melis T, et al.: Disturbed adrenocortical function in cerebro-hepato-renal syndrome of Zellweger. *Eur J Pediatr* 143: 10–12, 1984.

66. Hughes JL, Crane D, Robertson E, et al.: Morphometry of peroxisomes and immunolocalisation of peroxisomal proteins in the liver of patients with generalized peroxisomal disorders. *Virchow's Arch A Pathol Anat und Histopathol* 423: 459–468, 1993.

67. Gartner J, Moser H, Valle D: Mutations in the 70K peroxisomal membrane protein gene in Zellweger syndrome. *Nat Genet* 1: 16–23, 1992.

68. Shimozawa N, Suzuki Y, Orri T, et al.: Standardization of complementation grouping of peroxisome-deficient disorders and the second Zellweger patient with peroxisomal assembly factor-I-(PAF-I) defect. *Am J Hum Genet* 52: 843–844, 1993.

69. Naritomi K, Izumikawa Y, Ohshira S, et al.: Gene assignment of Zellweger syndrome to 7q11.23: report of the second case associated with pericentric inversion of chromosome 7. *Hum Genet* 84: 79–80, 1990.

70. Evrard P, Caviness VS, Prats-Vinas J, Lyon G: The mechanism of arrest of neuronal migration in Zellweger malformation. *Acta Neuropathol* 41: 109–117, 1978.

71. Ulrich J, Herschkowitz N, Heitz P, et al.: Adrenoleukodystrophy; preliminary report of a connatal case. Light and electron microscopical, immunohistochemical and biochemical findings. *Acta Neuropathol* 43: 77–83, 1978.

72. Scotto JM, Hadchouel M, Odievre M, et al.: Infantile phytanic acid storage disease, a possible variant of Refsum's disease. Three cases including ultrastructural studies of the liver. *J Inherit Metab Dis* 5: 83–90, 1982.

73. Boltshauser A, Spycher MA, Steinmann B, et al.: Infantile phytanic acid storage disease: a variant of Refsum's disease. *Eur J Pediatr* 139, 317–318, 1982.

74. Poll-The BT, Saudubray JM, Ogier HAM, et al.: Infantile Refsum disease, an inherited peroxisomal disorder. Comparison with Zellweger syndrome and neonatal adrenoleukodystrophy. *Eur J Pediatr* 146: 477–483, 1987.

75. Chow CW, Poulos A, Fellenberg J, et al.: Autopsy findings in two siblings with infantile Refsum disease. *Acta Neuropathol* 83: 190–195, 1992.

76. Poll-The BT, Roels F, Ogier H, et al.: A new peroxisomal disorder with enlarged peroxisomes and a specific deficiency of acyl CoA oxidase (pseudo-neonatal adrenoleukodystrophy). *Am. J. Hum Genet* 42: 422–434, 1988.

77. Goldfischer S, Collins J, Rapin I, et al.: Pseudo-Zellweger syndrome: deficiencies in several peroxisomal oxidative activities. *J Pediatr* 108: 25–32, 1986.

78. Schram AW, Goldfischer S, Van Roermund CWT, et al.: Human peroxisomal 3-oxoacyl-coenzymeA thiolase deficiency. *Proc Natl Acad Sci* 84: 2494–2496, 1987.

79. Watkins PA, Chen WW, Harris CJ, et al.: Peroxisomal bifunctional enzyme deficiency. *J Clin Invest* 83: 771–777, 1989.

80. Clayton PT, Lake BD, Hjelm M, et al.: Bile acid analyses in "pseudo-Zellweger" syndrome: clues to the defect in peroxisomal beta-oxidation. *J Inherit Metab Dis* 11 (suppl 2): 165–168, 1988.

81. Wanders RJA, Van Roermund CWT, Brub S, et al.: Bifunctional enzyme deficiency: identification of a new type of peroxisomal disorder in a patient with an impairment in peroxisomal beta-oxidation of unknown aetiology by means of complementation analysis. *J Inherit Metab Dis* 15: 385–388, 1992.

82. Moser H, Kaufman: Personal communication, 1994.

83. Clayton PT, Eckhardt S, Wilson J, et al.: Isolated dihydroxyacetonephosphate acyltransferase deficiency presenting with developmental delay. *J Inherit Metab Dis* 17: 533–540, 1994.

83a. Suzuki Y, Shimozawa N, Ozii T, et al.: Zellweger-like syndromes with detectable hepatic peroxisomes: a variant form of peroxisomal disorder. *J Pediatr* 113: 841–845, 1988.

84. Naidu S, Hoeffler G, Hoeffler S, et al.: Neonatal seizures and retardation in a female with biochemical changes resembling X-linked adrenoleukodystrophy: a probable new peroxisomal entity. *Neurology* 38: 1100–1107, 1988.

85. Mandel H, Berant M, Aizin A, et al.: Zellweger-like phenotype in two siblings: a defect in peroxisomal β-oxidation with elevated very long-chain fatty acids but normal bile acids. *J Inherit Metab Dis* 15: 381–384, 1992.

86. Gitzelman R, Steinmann B, Vandenberghe G: Disorders of fructose metabolism, in Scriver CR, Beaudet AL, Sly WS, Valle D (eds). *The Metabolic and Molecular Bases of Inherited Disease*, 7th ed. New York, McGraw-Hill, 1995, pp. 905–934.

87. Servidei S, Bonilla E, Diedrich RG, et al.: Fatal infantile form of phosphofructokinase deficiency. *Neurology* 36: 1465–1470, 1986.

87a. Baumeister FAM, Gsell W, Shin YS et al.: Glutamate in pyridoxine-dependent epilepsy: neurotoxic glutamate concentration in the CSF and its normalization by pyridoxine. *Pediatrics* 94: 318–321, 1994.

88. Goutieres F, Aicardi J: Atypical presentations of pyridoxine-dependent seizures: a treatable cause of intractable epilepsy in infants. *Ann Neurol* 17: 117–124, 1985.

89. Lott IT, Coulombe RV, Di Paolo RV, et al.: Vitamin B_6-dependent seizures: pathology and chemical findings in the brain. *Neurology* 28: 47–54, 1978.

Chapter 3

EARLY INFANTILE PROGRESSIVE METABOLIC ENCEPHALOPATHIES: CLINICAL PROBLEMS AND DIAGNOSTIC CONSIDERATIONS

MAIN FEATURES AND DIAGNOSTIC GUIDELINES
    Evidence of Neurological Regression
    Delay in Motor Development
    Neurologic Signs
    Nonneurologic Abnormalities
    Neurologic Disorders in the Family
    The Confirmatory Standard Laboratory Tests
    Neuroradiologic Imaging

EARLY INFANTILE NEUROMETABOLIC DISORDERS WITH A RELENTLESSLY PROGRESSIVE COURSE
    The Sphingolipidoses
    Sialidoses and Sialic Acid Storage Disorders
    Glycogenesis Type II
    The Genetic Early Infantile Leukodystrophies
    Hereditary Metabolic Disorders with Cutaneous Signs
        and Frequent Seizures
    Syndromes with Severe Seizures as a Constant Sign
    An Oculocerebrorenal Syndrome: Lowe Syndrome
    Organoacidopathies with Dystonia or Choreoathetosis
    Disorders of Amino Acids or Organic Acids with Ataxia
    Inborn Errors of Amino Acids, Organic Acids, and
        Carbohydrate Metabolism with Isolated Cognitive
        and Behavioral Abnormalities
    Disorders of Valine Catabolism with Prenatal
        Developmental Defects of the Brain

HMDS WITH ACUTE AND REMITTING NEUROLOGIC DISORDERS
    Disorders with Lactic Acidosis as a Major Metabolic
        Sign
    Disorders with Episodic Nonketotic Hypoglycemia
    Disorders with Intermittent Episodes of Ketoacidosis
    Disorders with Hyperammonemia and Respiratory
        Alkalosis
    Reye-like Syndromes

OTHER DISORDERS WITH CLINICAL EXPRESSION IN THE EARLY INFANTILE PERIOD

CONCLUSIONS

MAIN FEATURES AND DIAGNOSTIC GUIDELINES

The hereditary neurometabolic diseases which become manifest in the first year of life are impressive in their variety and at the same time daunting to the student of children's neurology. It seems to the authors that only by the application of certain clinical principles, which will be enunciated further on in this monograph, is it possible to gain one's bearings in this field of endeavor, i.e., to think of the most likely diagnosis and to select the appropriate laboratory tests after examining the patient.

As a rule, one's suspicion of an HMD at this age of life should be aroused by one or several of the following factual data:

1. Neurologic regression or arrest of development.
2. A delay in development and severe hypotonia, with no evident cause.
3. Presence of a particular neurologic sign.
4. Certain nonneurologic abnormalities.
5. Occurrence of a neurologic disorder of similar or undetermined type in a sibling or other member of the family.

Some of these criteria need further elaboration.

Evidence of Neurological Regression

The types of genetic metabolic disease presenting in the early infantile period of life evince special diagnostic problems not encountered in any other age epoch. Since the disease may begin before significant psychomotor development occurs, the cardinal principle of behavioral regression, enunciated in Chap. 1 is sometimes difficult to apply. The first warning signs may consist of subtle maturational delays rather than obvious loss of recently achieved functions. For parents who have not raised normal children, such slight departures from normality are easily overlooked. Usually the first causes of concern are an observed indifference of the infant to the surroundings, a lack of visual interest evidenced by a failure to fixate on and follow objects with the eyes, poor head control, an inability to roll over and later to sit without support, and an inability to use the hands properly in the prehension of objects and in play. These disorders should serve as warnings of impending disease during the first 6 months of postnatal life.

The uncertainties of neurologic diagnosis may be complicated by the coexistence of certain general difficulties, such as feeding problems (anorexia, vomiting, and intolerance of formula), that result in malnutrition. One may then err by ascribing any delay in neurologic development to nutritional deficiency or merely to being ill, for it is well known that systemic illness may occasion minor delays in psychomotor development.

The diagnosis of a progressive encephalopathy becomes easier when its onset is delayed until the second half of the first year of life, after the infant has attained a higher level of complex behaviors, which are then lost during illness. One may be helped in viewing successive photographs or videotapes of the child taken by the parents. In some patients, regression seems to start abruptly after an infectious illness and the initial diagnosis may then be that of an encephalitis.

Delay in Motor Development

The occurrence of retarded motor development with severe hypotonia and reduced motor activity (with or without loss of tendon reflexes and pyramidal signs) without obvious cause, even when accompanied by feeding difficulties, should always alert the physician as to the possibility of a neurometabolic disorder.

Neurologic Signs

Regarding special neurologic phenomena that provide leads of diagnostic value, the following are of importance: excessive and persistent acousticomotor reactions; marked rigidity and tonic spasms and head retraction; clinical and electrophysiologic evidence of a peripheral neuropathy; choreic movements, choreoathetosis, dystonic postures or ataxia (these towards the end of the first year of life); intermittent respiratory dysrhythmias without pulmonary disease (sine materia) with or without metabolic acidosis; recurrent episodes of acute neurologic distress and coma with vomiting and hyperpnea to be differentiated from infectious or postinfectious encephalopathies (all disorders with acute intermittent metabolic attacks may also produce sudden death).

Ocular abnormalities, present in approximately two-thirds of the neurometabolic disorders, are clearly of great value in diagnosis. Some of them are themselves expressions of the disorders of the nervous system, since the retina and optic nerves are parts of the central nervous system. Other ocular abnormalities are nonneurologic. In the first group are the macular cherry red spot and other types of macular degeneration, chorioretinal degeneration, optic atrophy (all with impaired vision), rapid pendular nystagmus, and other abnormal ocular movements and nuclear and supranuclear ocular palsies. In the second group are cataracts, corneal opacities, and glaucoma. Prenatal ocular defects (coloboma, congenital hypoplasia of optic disks) may also occur. Deafness is less frequent (except in peroxisomal disorders) and may be difficult to detect at this age. Head circumference is usually normal at birth but head growth tends usually to slow after a few months or weeks. Rarely, there is a moderate degree of microcephaly or of macrocephaly at birth; and an early progressive head enlargement is characteristic of a few disorders. Prenatal developmental defects of the brain are present in a limited number of HMDs. These abnormalities are listed in Table 3-5 along with the neurometabolic diseases with which they are most apt to be associated.

An additional remark should be made about seizures. They may occur in many of the diseases under consideration and are frequently of the myoclonic type. In a limited number of neurometabolic disorders, intractable seizures and a status epilepticus constitute a major clinical characteristic (see Table 3-5). In most neurometabolic disorders of this age, seizures are not a dominant manifestation. In any given disease, the frequency and severity of convulsions vary from case to case. It is said that seizures are more frequent when lesions affect the cerebral cortex rather than the white matter, but there are too many exceptions for the rule to be helpful. Moreover, many cerebral diseases involve both gray and white matter, and seizures may develop in diseases of the white matter after axonal loss has resulted in secondary degeneration of cortical neurons.

Nonneurologic Abnormalities

Of the systemic, visceral, and other nonneurologic conditions which suggest a hereditary metabolic disease of the nervous system, the following are ranked in order of their diagnostic importance:

a. Visceromegaly, essentially enlargement of the liver and/or spleen, which may occasionally precede by several weeks or months the appearance of neurologic signs (e.g., in some varieties of Niemann-Pick disease and of Gaucher disease); a cardiomegaly in Pompe disease and some of the mitochondrial diseases and sphingolipidoses; and enlarged polycystic kidneys in glutaric acidemia type II and Zellweger disease.

b. Unexplained malnutrition, poor feeding, vomiting, and diarrhea resulting in failure to thrive.

c. Dysmorphic facial features, characteristic of some of the peroxisomal, mitochondrial and lysosomal disorders and in Lowe syndrome. Some of the gargoyle-like facies of the mucopolysaccharidoses and mucolipidoses can be observed at this age but usually do not become evident before the end of the first year. This abnormality will be discussed in Chap. 4.

d. Skeletal changes and arthropathies ("dysostosis multiplex" and others) which may constitute a crucial diagnostic clue.

e. Various changes of skin and hair.

f. Involvement of the respiratory system: pulmonary infiltrates, chronic rhinitis, stridor, or raucous voice.

g. Disturbances of renal tubular function, liver function (in Alpers syndrome and in the self-limiting episodes of early infantile jaundice in type C Niemann-Pick disease), and adrenocortical insufficiency.

h. Specific or characteristic inclusions in circulating leukocytes and in histiocytes of bone marrow and other organs.

Finally, it should be remembered that a limited number of metabolic disorders affecting the nervous system may give rise to congenital somatic defects of limbs, heart, and the genitourinary system.

Table 3-6 lists the systemic and nonneurologic abnormalities one is likely to find in patients with HMDs of the nervous system and their usual disease linkages.

There are examples of HMDs that cause none of these neurologic or nonneurologic disorders. Inexplicable slowness of development and failure to thrive may be the only indicators of ongoing disease. Under these conditions or because of a family history of mental retardation, seizures or some other obscure disorder, one should be prompted to undertake one or more of the laboratory procedures described below. With the advance of more refined and practical biochemical tests, the screening of all newborn infants will expand or become more widely practiced.

Neurologic Disorders in the Family

A similar, apparently dissimilar, or ill-defined neurologic disease in the family or the unexplained death of a sibling should always alert one to the possible existence of an HMD and should encourage the neuropediatrician to examine other members of the family, looking for subtle forms of disease and to perform appropriate laboratory tests. The pattern of genetic transmission of disease appearing in the early infantile period is autosomal recessive X-linked or maternally inherited. In the latter cases, the carrier mother may be slightly symptomatic. Further discussion of these problems is to be found in Chap. 1 and in conjunction with the description of each disease.

The Confirmatory Standard Laboratory Tests

Although laboratory tests should be selected according to the clinical context, we recommend that the following investigations be performed on any child who is suspected of having an HMD during the first year of life. They include

- Analysis of the blood for glucose, lactic and pyruvic acid, ammonia, ketone bodies, acid-base balance, and carnitine.
- Measurement of the CSF for protein, glucose, and lactate levels.
- X-ray films of chest and skeleton and ultrasound examinations of the heart, kidneys, liver, and spleen.
- A complete ophthalmologic assessment, including slit lamp examination of lens and cornea and if indicated an electroretinogram (ERG).
- Evaluation of nerve conduction velocities and an electromyogram (EMG) is recommended when tendon reflexes are abolished and hypotonia is marked.
- Chromatography of the blood and urine for amino acids, and gas chromatography for detection of organic acids in urine and analysis of fatty acids in blood. These two methods are now available in most biochemical laboratories.
- Neuroradiological imaging.
- In certain circumstances, bone marrow biopsies looking for macrophages with stored products should be undertaken; and also biopsies of conjunctiva, skin, liver, and muscle utilizing electron microscopy (see Chap. 8).

The proper selection and utilization of these tests will be specified in connection with each of the described diseases. More specific identification of the disease in question necessitates the use of enzymatic and molecular techniques, for which one must turn to specialized laboratories.

Neuroradiologic Imaging

Since the first edition of this monograph, computed tomography (CT) scans and, even more, magnetic resonance imaging (MRI) have become virtually indispensable instruments in this field of neurology. While MRI is generally preferred because of its anatomic resolution and freedom from exposure to x-irradiation, CT scanning remains the method of choice to detect cerebral calcifications. It is well known that some lesions of the brain may exist for some time without clinical signs, and certain lesions of the white matter (i.e., leukodystrophies) and basal ganglia necroses may precede the emergence of the characteristic clinical syndrome. Lesions are now being visualized that in times past were known only to pathologists; and in some diseases, still defined mainly

by pathological criteria (as Leigh syndrome and Alpers syndrome), neuroradiologic imaging represents an indispensable step for diagnostic confirmation during life. This statement also applies to metabolic or degenerative disorders starting later in life.

The use of recent techniques, such as MR spectroscopy, MR angiography, positron emission tomography (PET), and single proton emission computed tomography (SPECT), holds promise of advancing knowledge of the functional aspects of brain pathology. These techniques will enable the clinician to utilize a living biopathology in formulations of a disease process. That is not to say that neuroradiologic imaging will ever replace clinical examination; many neurologic problems show no visible changes using MRI or CT. Moreover, some of the changes that are being seen are difficult to interpret. The same neuroradiologic abnormalities may be common to several different disorders (see Chap. 8).

EARLY INFANTILE NEUROMETABOLIC DISORDERS WITH A RELENTLESSLY PROGRESSIVE COURSE

The Sphingolipidoses

General Remarks In this category, there have been identified a number of genetic defects of hydrolytic enzymes. The latter are contained in lysosomes and are necessary for the degradation of sphingolipids. As a result of the deficiency, products of the intermediate metabolism of sphingolipids accumulate in lysosomes (a notable exception being Krabbe disease). Sphingolipidoses (neurolipidoses) are therefore called lysosomal disorders. The concept of inborn lysosomal disorders was created by Hers.[1,2]

The history of neurolipidoses starts in 1881 with the clinical descriptions, by Warren Tay,[3] a British ophthalmologist, and Bernard Sachs,[4] an American neurologist, of an early infantile neurodegeneration with megalocephaly and blindness. They called it *amaurotic idiocy*. For half a century the disease was defined only by its clinical and pathological features. Then, in the early 1960s, the exact nature of the stored material (ganglioside) was finally identified[5] and its ultrastructural characteristics described. Later the enzymatic defect causing the abnormal accumulation of lipids in lysosomes was discovered. Finally, during recent years, cDNAs have been isolated for this and nearly all the other lysosomal enzymes known to be involved in the genesis of the sphingolipidoses. The genes for most have been assigned a chromosomal locus, and a number of them have been cloned. Multiple mutations are now known to be responsible for most of the diseases. Approximately 50 mutations have been described for Tay-Sachs disease alone. Defects in activator protein have also been shown to be involved in certain patients and "pseudo-deficiency" genes have been characterized. These scientific discoveries have informed us that the sphingolipidoses are clinically, enzymologically, and genetically highly heterogeneous, which adds to the difficulty of their classification. It is for this reason that we emphasize the practical advantages of categorizing them by their age-related clinical symptomatology.

We will describe here the early infantile forms of the sphingolipidoses. The late infantile, juvenile, and adult forms will be discussed in Chaps. 4 and 5.

Treatment of the neurolipidoses is still unsatisfactory (see Chap. 8), because brain damage is already present before birth, and the blood-brain barrier constitutes an obstacle to enzyme replacement therapies; and because we are ignorant of most of the pathophysiological mechanisms by which neurons are rendered dysfunctional. Fortunately, heterozygote detection and prenatal diagnosis are possible for most sphingolipidoses, which offers the possibility of genetic counseling.

Neurolipidoses

The Early Infantile G_{M2} Gangliosidoses   The G_{M2} gangliosidoses are a group of autosomal recessive disorders characterized by the accumulation of G_{M2} ganglioside[5] and a few related glycolipids in neurons and to a much lesser extent in other organs. Normally the hydrolysis of gangliosides is accomplished by the action of two structurally related lysosomal enzymes, hexosaminidase A and hexosaminidase B and by the G_{M2} activator protein. Hexosaminidase A is composed of two subunits, α and β ($\alpha\beta$) encoded respectively on chromosome 15 and chromosome 5. Hexosaminidase B has only β subunits ($\beta\beta$). The G_{M2} activator protein, encoded on chromosome 5, is necessary for the degradation of G_{M2} ganglioside by hexosaminidase A. Mutations at any one of these gene loci can result in G_{M2} gangliosidosis. Three enzymatic nonallelic varieties have been described.

1. A defect in the hexosaminidase α subunit that affects the activity of hexosaminidase A and gives rise to Tay-Sachs disease and also to later-onset variants of G_{M2} gangliosidosis.

2. A defect of the β subunit that results in a deficiency of both hexosaminidase A and hexosaminidase B and gives rise to early infantile and juvenile Sandhoff disease.

3. G_{M2} activator protein deficiency (AB variant).

4. In addition, a few patients with a late infantile form of the disease have a hexosaminidase A reacting normally with artificial substrates but inactive with reference to the natural substrate ganglioside G_{M2} or the sulfate derivative of the artificial compound. This latter variety, referred to as variant B1, is allelic with other deficiencies of the hexosaminidase α subunit.

According to Sandhoff and Conzelmann,[6] in vitro studies show a good correlation between the degree of residual activity of hexosaminidase A and the clinical expression of the disease, and the degree and site of neuronal storage. In the early infantile form, the activity of this enzyme is completely absent, while in the late infantile form some degree of residual activity remains (see also Chaps. 4 and 5).

In this chapter, we will describe the early infantile forms of G_{M2} gangliosidosis. Late-onset forms will be described in Chaps. 4 and 5.

Tay-Sachs Disease: Hexosaminidase α Subunit Deficiency (Variant B)   Tay-Sachs disease is an autosomal recessive inherited disorder caused by mutations within the gene encoding for the α subunit of hexosaminidase A. The gene is located on chromosome 15. Deficient activity of hexosaminidase A results in intraneuronal accumulation of G_{M2} ganglioside. The disorder is seen primarily in Jewish children, although this predominance is now much less pronounced as screening and prevention in this group has become widespread.

An abnormal acousticomotor reaction, psychomotor deterioration, together with axial hypotonia and bilateral pyramidal signs, and blindness with macular cherry red spots are the clinical hallmarks of the disease. There is no visceral or skeletal involvement, no abnormalities by electron microscopy of bone marrow and leukocytes, and no abnormal urinary excretion of oligosaccharides. The disease is always fatal, usually between 3 and 5 years of age. There is no known treatment (Fig. 3-1).

Clinical Features   Children with this disease are born at term with a normal weight and head circumference. An exaggerated startle response to sounds, and sometimes to light flashes and tactile stimuli, is usually the first sign of the disease.[7] It may be noted by the

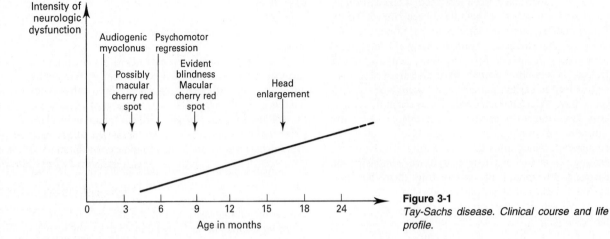

Figure 3-1
Tay-Sachs disease. Clinical course and life profile.

parents in the fourth month and persists throughout the course of the disease. This abnormal acousticomotor response is elicited by sharp, sudden, not necessarily loud, noises and it consists of a brusque extension of the arms and sometimes of the legs, often followed by a few clonic jerks of all the limbs. Blinking, a startled facial appearance, and neck extension are other accompaniments. Repetitive acoustic stimulations, such as hand clapping, will invariably evoke a synchronized recurrence of the response. There appears to be no adaptation to a succession of stimuli. The character of the movement and its pattern and persistence clearly differentiate it from the normal startle reaction of infants, which usually consists of a flexor motor response that undergoes quick adaptation.

Although the acousticomotor response is not restricted to Tay-Sachs disease (and to the Sandhoff variant) but can occasionally be seen in other conditions, such as juvenile G_{M2} gangliosidosis, Krabbe leukodystrophy, or pyridoxine dependency, it does not occur as early or as constantly and persistently in these diseases.

Apart from this sign, which at first can be easily overlooked, the child's development proceeds normally during the first months of life. Not until the fourth to sixth month does psychomotor deterioration become manifest. One of the earliest signs is the inability to maintain the sitting position. As the condition worsens, the infant becomes unable to roll over and loses the first rudiments of both projected and purposeful movements. Spontaneous vocalization ceases, and finally, even head control disappears. Only exceptionally does a child with

Tay-Sachs disease reach the stages of sitting and crawling. The patient's interest in the surroundings vanishes. After a few months, marked axial hypotonia in combination with pyramidal signs is observed, and thereafter the limbs gradually become spastic.

By the end of the eighth month, it has become obvious that the child is blind. Frequently, visual failure is first indicated as early as the fourth month by a pendular nystagmus. Pupillary responses to light can persist long after the infant no longer heeds a visual stimulus. A bilateral macular cherry red spot is found in more than 90 percent of the cases. It consists of a large, conspicuous, whitish gray, circular zone of retinal degeneration in the center of which can be seen the contrasting red macula (Fig. 3-2). The electroretinogram is normal.

In the second year of life, the size of the cranium, which is at first normal, characteristically increases. The enlargement of head circumference often reaches 3 standard deviations above normal, and x-ray films of the skull may reveal separation of sutures. This is due to an enlargement of the brain, not to tension hydrocephalus. However, with the death of neurons and further gliosis, the ventricles may eventually enlarge.

At this stage of the disease, generalized tonic-clonic or minor motor seizures can occur, again often elicited by noise. Laughing spells are another peculiar feature. The EEG, usually normal in the first phases of the disease, undergoes several types of alteration. Paroxysmal slow-wave activity and multiple spike potentials are observed frequently. Hypsarrhythmia may occur. Photic stimulation usually induces no change.[4]

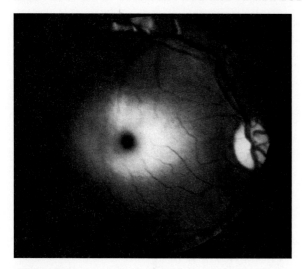

Figure 3-2
Retinal cherry red spot in a patient with Tay-Sachs disease. Note the white ring around the dark macula.

Noteworthy is the fact that there are no signs of peripheral nerve involvement. Nerve conduction velocities remain normal. There are no abnormal facial features. Moreover, the CSF is unremarkable, and there is no evidence of visceral or skeletal involvement. Bone marrow smears are without particularity. Basophilic granulations in leukocytes and vacuolated lymphocytes have only rarely been reported. In the urine there is no increased excretion of oligosaccharides.

By the third year the child has become hopelessly demented, insensate, decerebrate, cachectic, and blind.

Biochemical Diagnosis   Biochemical diagnosis of Tay-Sachs requires the demonstration of an isolated deficiency of hexosaminidase A with normal or elevated activity of hexosaminidase B. Enzymatic studies can be performed on leukocytes using artificial compounds or the natural G_{M2} ganglioside as substrates.

There is an absence or near absence of hexosaminidase A activity. Metabolic studies of cultured skin fibroblasts are needed only when enzyme assays of blood cells are inconclusive.

Genetics   Tay-Sachs disease is inherited as an autosomal recessive trait and is particularly frequent in Ashkenazic Jews of Eastern or Central European descent.[8] The incidence of the disease has been estimated at

1/112,000 of live births in the general population and 1/3900 live births in the Jewish population.

Heterozygotes can be detected by assays of hexosaminidase A in serum, leukocytes, tears, and cultured fibroblasts. Heterozygote frequency is estimated at 1 in 167 in the general population and 1 in 31 in the Jewish population. Systematic carrier detection in populations at risk allows informed genetic counseling and may have an important impact on the increasingly low incidence of the disease in the populations that are screened.

Prenatal Diagnosis   Hexosaminidase A and B can be measured in amniotic fluid, amniocytes, and chorionic villus.

Neuropathology   The brain may be large and heavy (1400 to 2300 g), probably because of an increase in water content and intraneuronal accumulation of gangliosides. Neurons throughout the central nervous system and autonomic ganglia are markedly distended by a fine granular material. Formation of meganeurites is most striking in late infantile or juvenile G_{M2} gangliosidosis (Chap. 4). There is also a loss of neurons. Under the electron microscope the granular material has the appearance of intralysosomal inclusion bodies composed of concentric membranes, hence the name membranous cytoplasmic bodies.[9] The stored substance contains essentially G_{M2} ganglioside. Neurons laden with the material are found throughout the cortex and central nuclear structures and accounts for 12 percent of dry brain weight. Myelin loss and gliosis are observed in the cerebral white matter and seem to be more pronounced than could be expected from simple neuronal loss.

In the retina, the ganglion cells are infiltrated by the same storage material as the neurons in the brain, and it is these distended cells, crowded in the perifoveal regions, that account for the whitish gray appearance of the tissue. The red color of the fovea is given by the choroid shining more brightly through this thinned part of the retina (lacking neurons), according to Greenfield.[10] The pigment epithelial cells, rods, and cones are unaltered, which explains the normal electroretinogram.

A small quantity of lipid-laden cells and an increase of G_{M2} ganglioside have been detected in the liver and spleen of children who have reached the later stages of the disease. To a slight degree the typical ultrastructural inclusions have also been detected in nerve axons of skin and conjunctiva.

Typical neuronal inclusions have been detected in all parts of the central nervous system, especially in the spinal cord and autonomic ganglia of fetuses as early as 12 to 22 weeks gestation. G_{M2} ganglioside has been elevated in the brain of fetuses aged 18 to 20 weeks.

Clinicopathological Correlations It is logical to believe the storage of ganglioside in neurons impairs their function. Although this substance is nontoxic for the cells, its physical accumulation is likely to interfere with intracellular activities, and finally to result in neuronal death. Other mechanisms may also be involved. Gangliosides are implicated in synaptogenesis, and an altered pattern of cellular gangliosides could interfere with synaptic transmission. The pathogenesis of the acousticomotor response is unknown; probably it is due to a disturbance at the level of the brain stem. The increased brain volume is presumably due to the storage material, reactive gliosis, as well as to disturbance of fluid balance between blood and brain.

Differential Diagnosis Tay-Sachs disease is usually easily differentiated from other early infantile HMD without clinically evident extraneurological involvement, such as Krabbe disease and Canavan-Van Bogaert-Bertrand disease.

Treatment Only supportive care can be given. Attempts at enzyme replacement therapies have failed.

Early Infantile Sandhoff Disease (Hexosaminidase β Subunit Deficiency; Variant 0) Sandhoff disease, an autosomal recessive disorder, is caused by mutations of the gene encoding the β subunit of hexosaminidase, on chromosome 5.

Since both hexosaminidase A and hexosaminidase B contain β subunits, the activity of these two enzymes is lacking in this disorder, so G_{M2} ganglioside and other structurally related glycolipids accumulate. There is no ethnic predominance. In fact, no case of Sandhoff disease has up to now been reported in a Jewish child.

Clinical Features In Sandhoff disease, age of onset, duration, and the neurological and ophthalmologic symptomatology are identical to that of Tay-Sachs disease. The distinguishing features, in some patients, are the presence of an enlarged liver and spleen, the occasional presence of skeletal changes similar to those in early infantile G_{M1} gangliosidosis as well as the presence of N-acetylglucosamine-containing oligosaccharides in urine and foam cells in the bone marrow.

Diagnostic Laboratory Tests Demonstration of a lack of activity of both hexosaminidase A and hexosaminidase B in leukocytes, serum, tears, and cultured fibroblasts.

Detection of N-acetylglucosamine-containing oligosaccharides in urine.

Prenatal Diagnosis Prenatal diagnosis is now possible. The existence of Sandhoff disease and a "pseudo-deficiency" (normal individuals with a very low level of hexosaminidase A and B) in the same family has been reported. This may complicate the prenatal diagnosis.

Genetics Sandhoff disease is inherited as an autosomal recessive trait.

Heterozygotes have a reduced level of total serum hexosaminidase (A and B) and a higher than normal percentage of hexosaminidase A.

Pathology and Storage Compounds In the brain, the lesions are similar to those of Tay-Sachs disease, except that under the electron microscope the lamellar intralysosomal inclusions in neurons are more polymorphic hence they are called pleiomorphic cytoplasmic bodies. Evidence of lipid storage in the viscera is more pronounced than in Tay-Sachs disease.

Other differences consist of a marked accumulation of globoside in visceral organs and pronounced storage of G_{A2} glycolipid in the brain.

Differential Diagnosis Tay-Sachs disease and G_{M1} gangliosidosis.

Treatment No specific treatment is available.

G_{M2} Activator Deficiency (AB Variant) The intralysosomal G_{M2} activator, encoded on chromosome 5, is necessary for hydrolysis of G_{M2} ganglioside by hexosaminidase A. Its deficiency leads to accumulation of G_{M2} ganglioside in the α and β subunit deficiencies. But the two hexosaminidases, A and B, are present in normal or elevated amounts in those patients.

This form of G_{M2} gangliosidosis is rare. The clinical phenotype is identical with Tay-Sachs disease.

The diagnosis can be suspected when, in such circumstances, assays for hexosaminidase A and B with artificial substrates are normal.

G_{M2} activator deficiency can be demonstrated in cultured fibroblasts by various highly specialized methods.

Galactosylceramide Lipidosis (Krabbe Leuko-dystrophy)   This type of neurolipidosis is described under genetic leukodystrophies.

Neurovisceral Lipidoses

Early Infantile G$_{M1}$ Gangliosidosis (Type 1)   Infantile G$_{M1}$ gangliosidosis was first recognized as a distinct clinical entity and named "familial neurovisceral lipidosis" by Landing et al. in 1964.[11] An accumulation of G$_{M1}$ ganglioside was documented by O'Brien et al.[12] and by Gonatas and Gonatas in 1965.[13]

Early infantile (type I) G$_{M1}$ gangliosidosis is an autosomal recessive disorder due to a deficiency of the lysosomal enzyme acid, β-galactosidase,[14] resulting in the accumulation of G$_{M1}$ ganglioside in nerve cells and of galactosyl oligosaccharides and keratan sulfate degration products in other tissues. Clinically, the disease is expressed by early psychomotor deterioration, macular cherry red spots, facial dysmorphism, bone deformities, and hepatomegaly. Vacuolated lymphocytes are found in blood and foamy histiocytes in bone marrow smears. Galactose-containing oligosaccharides and keratan sulfate are excreted in the urine[15] (Fig. 3-3).

Clinical Features   Usually, reduced alertness, diminished spontaneous activity, and hypotonia are noted in the first days or weeks of life. Head control may be acquired but sitting posture is never attained. In some instances, the arrest of neurological development becomes evident somewhat later, during the third to sixth month. This is accompanied almost invariably by feeding difficulties and failure to thrive. Many infants have facial and peripheral edema in the first weeks of life.

After a few months, signs of visual failure appear, frequently revealed by a pendular nystagmus. A macular cherry red spot is found in at least 50 percent of the cases but its presence is usually not detected until the sixth month. Seizures may occur, generally during the later stages of the disease. As time passes, hypotonia gives way to spasticity; there are tonic spasms and pyramidal signs. Head size is normal or slightly increased at birth, but later there is secondary microcephaly. Peripheral nerves are spared and the cerebrospinal fluid is normal. Infants surviving beyond 12 months are usually in a state of decerebrate rigidity. They succumb to respiratory failure and bronchopneumonia by the age of 2 years.

The most strongly suggestive signs of the disease are nonneurologic. They consist of special facial features, skeletal changes, hematologic abnormalities, and oligosacchariduria. Hepatomegaly and later splenomegaly are usually present after the sixth month.

Dysmorphic features may be striking. They may be already present at birth but definitely become more apparent with time. They include a wide, depressed nasal bridge, frontal bossing, epicanthal folds, elongate upper lip, gingival hypertrophy or thickened alveolar ridges, puffy eyelids, moderate macroglossia, low-set ears, and a short underslung jaw (chipmunk face) (Fig. 3-4). There is limited mobility, even flexion contractures of the joints, and after a few months, a lumbodorsal kyphoscoliosis may develop. The terminal phalanges tend to be short and stubby.

Laboratory Findings   The most important radiologic signs are in the long bones and spine. They are constant and a clinical diagnosis of early infantile G$_{M1}$ gangliosidosis cannot be made in their absence. Marked subperiosteal bone formation is an early sign; it may be present at birth. Later there is widening of the diaphyses (midshaft) of bones, demineralization, tapering of the extremities, and sloping of the epiphyseal plates. Hypoplasia and beaking of one or more vertebrae at the thoracolumbar junction are characteristic but usually do not become evident before 3–6 months of age. These deformities are similar to those of the mucopolysaccharidoses and frequently are referred to as *dysostosis multiplex*.

Vacuolation is present in 10 to 80 percent of lymphocytes in the blood, and there are finely vacuolated foamy histiocytes in the bone marrow.

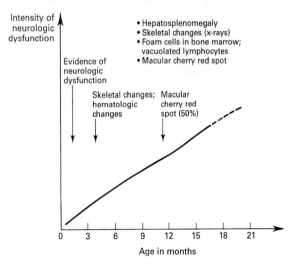

Figure 3-3

G$_{M1}$ gangliosidosis. Clinical course and life profile.

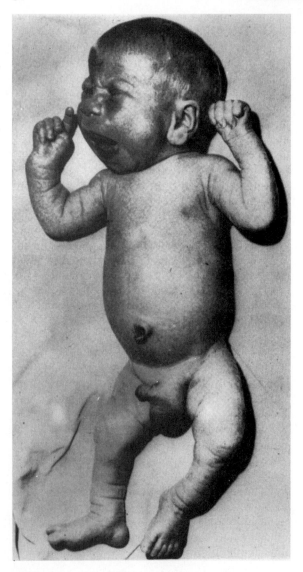

Figure 3-4
Infant with G$_{M1}$ gangliosidosis. Facial dysmorphism: depressed nasal bridge, puffy eyelids, long upper lip, underslung jaw (chipmunk face), hernias, metaphyseal swelling. (Reprinted, by permission, from Metabolic Basis of Hereditary Disease, *1989.)*

Galactose-containing oligosaccharides and a modest increase in keratan sulfate are found in the urine.

Variants and Rare Signs In a few of the proved cases, severe respiratory difficulties have occasionally been an early manifestation. Also the heart may be enlarged, as seen on x-ray films, and cardiac failure has been reported early in the course of the disease due to endocardial fibroelastosis and thickening of the valves. In a few, there has been a paroxysmal atrial tachycardia. Corneal opacities[11] and an exaggerated acousticomotor response have been reported in a few patients.

The late infantile (type 2) and chronic/adult (type 3) forms of G$_{M1}$ gangliosidosis will be described in Chaps. 4 and 5.

Clinical variations in β-galactosidase deficiencies may be caused by differences in residual activity for the different substrates.[15] For instance, patients with higher residual activity for ganglioside G$_{M1}$ than for galactose-containing oligosaccharides and keratan sulfate have severe dysostosis and minimal involvement of the nervous system. This probably explains why a deficiency in β-galactosidase may give rise to the so-called Morquio syndrome type B (MPS IV B) in which there are no neurological signs.

Diagnostic Biochemical Tests There is a complete or nearly complete lack of acid β-galactosidase activity. Assays of this enzyme can be done on leukocytes and cultured fibroblasts. Secondary deficiency of the enzyme exists in I-cell disease and mucolipidosis III. This may raise some diagnostic difficulties. Half-normal enzyme levels of β-galactosidose have been demonstrated in obligate heterozygotes. Urine oligosaccharide analysis is helpful.

Genetics G$_{M1}$ gangliosidosis is transmitted as an autosomal recessive trait. The locus coding for acid β-galactosidase is on chromosome 3 (3p21.33). Detection of heterozygotes and prenatal diagnosis are available.

Pathologic Findings Neurons in the central and autonomic nervous systems are packed with intracytoplasmic granular material, which is shown in electron micrographs to consist mainly of intralysosomal membranous cytoplasmic bodies resembling those seen in Tay-Sachs disease.

Histiocytes in many viscera, hepatocytes, leukocytes, skin fibroblasts, and characteristically, the renal glomeruli are distended with a highly water-soluble substance that is usually dissolved during fixing and embedding, leaving clear vacuoles in the light microscope preparations and a finely fibrillar material on ultrastructural examination. Similar vacuoles are found in cells in the walls of blood vessels within the brain. These vacuoles represent distended lysosomes.

These two types of inclusions reflect the duality of the neurovisceral storage: accumulation of G_{M1} ganglioside in the brain and, to a lesser extent, in the liver and spleen; and galactose-containing oligosaccharides and proteoglycans (keratan sulfate) in the vacuolated cells of liver, spleen, kidney, and cerebral blood vessels.

In an autopsied child with the disease, the accumulation of G_{M1} ganglioside in the cerebral gray matter was greater than normal by a factor of 10, and values in the liver by factors of between 20 and 50.[16] The magnitude of mucopolysaccharide storage is similar to that in Hurler disease and is much higher than that of gangliosides.

In one 17-week-old fetus with G_{M1} gangliosidosis that has been studied in detail, vacuoles and abnormal inclusions were found in the brain, dorsal root ganglia, liver, kidney, lymphocytes, and placenta. β-Galactosidase was absent in amniotic fluid, virtually absent in cultured amniotic cells, and decreased in fetal tissues.

Pathophysiology The mechanisms of neuronal dysfunction in G_{M1} gangliosidosis are unclear. The accumulation of G_{M1} ganglioside in the lysosomes of nerve cells could result in a mechanical disruption of their structure and function and lead finally to cell death. The action of a cytotoxic derivative of glycosphingolipids (lysoderivatives) has been postulated but seems unlikely. Another hypothesis is based on the type of structural changes seen in neurons by Golgi stains, which reveal neoformation of neurites near the cell body and swellings between cell body and axon (meganeurites). These changes could induce profound abnormalities in the interneuronal circuitry. They are, however, found mainly in the later-onset G_{M1} and G_{M2} gangliosidoses. Finally, neuronal membranes, especially the synaptic plasma membrane, contain high proportions of G_{M1} ganglioside, and gangliosides play a role in synaptic transmission. It has been postulated that G_{M1} ganglioside accumulation could affect synaptic transmission. Storage of keratan sulfate is probably responsible for the bone changes.

Differential Diagnosis The following diseases should be considered in differential diagnosis: Niemann-Pick disease (major hepatosplenic storage, no dysmorphia or bone anomalies); Gaucher disease (splenomegaly, Gaucher cells in bone marrow); early-onset mucopolysaccharidosis and mucolipidoses.

Treatment Only symptomatic treatment is available.

Niemann-Pick Disease The first description of this disease in an infant was by Albert Niemann, a German pediatrician, in 1914.[17] In the next 10 years, similar cases were reported, and in 1927 Ludwig Pick was able to identify them as constituting a distinct clinicopathologic entity.[18] The name currently applies to a heterogeneous group of disorders divided by Crocker[19] into four types: A, B, C, and D. Type D was assigned a place in the schema but it probably belongs to or relates to type C.

(1) Types A and B (type I in the classification of Spence and Callahan[20]) are caused by a deficiency in sphingomyelinase, an enzyme first isolated by Brady et al. in 1966. In type A, sphingomyelin accumulates in all tissues, including the brain. This type starts in early infancy, is rapidly progressive, and always causes severe neurologic dysfunction.

In type B, sphingomyelin accumulates essentially in visceral organs and little if at all in the brain. Neurological signs are absent, or limited, or may not become evident until later childhood (see Chap. 4). An adult form of sphingomyelin deficiency has also been reported.

(2) Type C (or type II in the classification of Spence and Callahan) is an entirely different entity with a variety of clinical presentations. There is no consistent defect in sphingomyelinase or, at most, only a partial, secondary defect in cultured fibroblasts can be demonstrated. There is a unique intracellular translocation of exogenous cholesterol with a failure in cholesterol esterification. The defective gene has been mapped to chromosome 18 but the primary defect remains unknown. Although some forms of this condition begin in early infancy, this is a largely juvenile disease which will be described in Chap. 5.

Here we will restrict our description to the early infantile, type A, Niemann-Pick disease.

Early Infantile Niemann-Pick (Type A) This autosomal recessive disorder is characterized by neurovisceral accumulation of sphingomyelin due to a deficit of the enzyme sphingomyelinase.

Early failure to thrive and hepatomegaly usually precede evidence of neurologic regression and appearance of a typical macular cherry red spot. Other important diagnostic data include the presence of foam cells in the bone marrow, vacuolated lymphocytes in the peripheral blood, the absence of significant dysmorphic features and skeletal deformities, and a normal serum level of acid phosphatase (Fig. 3-5).

Clinical Features Feeding difficulties and failure to thrive usually become troublesome in the first weeks of life; hepatomegaly is detectable in the first three months and not infrequently is present even in the neonate. The enlargement of the liver is usually more marked than that of the spleen and precedes the latter. There may be vomiting, diarrhea, and bouts of fever. Jaundice and ascites are present in the advanced stages of the disease. Lymph nodes become palpably enlarged. Respiratory difficulties may be present and x-ray films of the chest often show a fine miliary infiltration of the lungs.

Because of the early appearance and importance of visceral signs and nutritional difficulties, full appreciation of neurologic regression may be overlooked initially, but progressive cerebral deterioration usually becomes unmistakable before the end of the first year and often as early as 6 months of age. The first signs of psychomotor regression are loss of head control, inability to sit and to manipulate objects, reduction in spontaneous movements, and loss of interest in the surroundings. In some instances, the neurologic dysfunction is manifested as delayed development, rather than regression, and one observes only a reduced reactivity to surroundings and a paucity of motor responses.

On examination, a combination of axial hypotonia and bilateral pyramidal signs is usual. Neurogenic impairment of swallowing is another feature and interferes with feeding. Blindness and a coarse amaurotic (pendular nystagmus) have been early signs in a number of patients. The macular cherry red spot is seen in about half of the cases. Seizures may occur, but usually only in the later stages of the disease, and rarely do they constitute a major sign. An exaggerated acousticomotor response cannot be elicited. The head circumference is either normal or moderately reduced. Loss of tendon reflexes and slowed nerve conduction velocity have been reported but this is rare. As the disease progresses, there is increasing tendency to rigidity and opisthotonus. The CSF is normal and the EEG is abnormal but noncharacteristic.

The facial appearance is unremarkable, but a few minor changes such as protruding eyes, epicanthal folds, or mild hypertelorism may occur. Often there is a brownish pigmentation of the skin, especially on the face and extensor surfaces of the limbs. Abnormal pigmentation may also be seen in the oral mucosa. Dysplasia of dental enamel is frequent. There is no clinical or x-ray evidence of deformities of joints or bones.

Of some diagnostic importance is the presence of vacuolated histiocytes (i.e., foam cells) in the bone marrow and vacuolated lymphocytes in the peripheral blood. These findings, however, are not specific. Other relevant routine laboratory findings include normal serum acid phosphatase levels (rarely they are moderately elevated), occasionally a mild anemia and thrombocytopenia and alteration of liver function tests. Enlargement of the placenta has been noted by prenatal ultrasound.

As the disease progresses, cachexia, stunting of growth, respiratory infections, visceromegaly, liver failure, and cerebral deterioration become more advanced. Death occurs in the second or third year of life.

Variants Possible variations in the clinical picture of early infantile Niemann-Pick disease relate essentially to the intensity of visceral signs, the age at onset of the neurologic dysfunction and the absence of a macular cherry red spot.

A note should be included here about *Niemann-Pick disease type B*. This disorder is also due to a lack of activity of sphingomyelinase, leading to an accumulation of sphingomyelin in the viscera, and only to a limited extent in the brain (much less than in Niemann-Pick disease type A). The relative escape of the brain could be due to the presence of a residual activity of sphingomyelinase in this organ.[21] Enlargement of the liver and spleen, and pulmonary infiltration, may be detected in infancy or early childhood. Neurological manifestations are absent at that age, but retinal degeneration, mental retardation, and other neurological signs may appear in childhood, adolescence, or adulthood. This sequence of events is not unlike that which is observed in type III

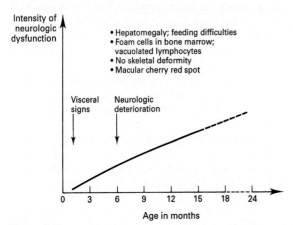

Figure 3-5
Niemann-Pick type A disease. Clinical course and life profile.

Gaucher disease. In the experience of one of us (EHK), in five patients, signs were splenomegaly in two siblings aged 7 and 9, a cherry red macula in an 18-year-old patient, and liver failure in a 43-year-old patient dying of chronic hepatitis. In a 72-year-old patient the disease was recognized only at autopsy. None of these patients had central nervous system manifestations.

Diagnostic Laboratory Tests The activity of sphingomyelinase is less than 5 percent of normal in cell tissue cultures. Leukocytes, fibroblasts, and other tissues can be used for enzymatic assays.

Genetics Infantile Niemann-Pick disease (type A) is inherited as an autosomal recessive trait. Although it is widely distributed, a high proportion of affected children have been Jews of Ashkenazic (eastern European) ancestry (estimated incidence, 1/30,000).

Heterozygotes can be reliably detected by measuring the activity of sphingomyelinase in leukocytes or cultured fibroblasts. The gene for sphingomyelinase has been cloned and mapped to chromosome 11p15. Three mutations account for 95 percent of the mutant Niemann-Pick type A alleles among Ashkenazim, while 50 percent of Niemann-Pick disease type B Ashkenazic patients have one mutation, the delta-R608 lesion.[22]

Prenatal Diagnosis Prenatal diagnosis is possible, by measuring the activity of sphingomyelinase in amniocytes or chorionic villi.

Pathological Findings The bone marrow, spleen, liver, lymphoid system, lungs, and other visceral organs are filled with lipid-laden histiocytes having a foamy appearance. In the normal histologic processing of tissues, the lipid deposits are dissolved by the dehydrating agents, and histiocytes appear to contain multiple translucent vacuoles, hence they are called *foam cells*. In frozen sections the accumulated material is sudanophilic and PAS-negative. Phase microscopy of fresh cells reveals refringent droplets that are partly doubly refractile under polarized light. Under the electron microscope, the cytoplasm is filled with membrane-bound inclusions which are polymorphic and composed of granular bodies with partially membranous inner structures.

Neurons in the central nervous system and autonomic ganglia (mesenteric plexus) are filled with and deformed by the intralysosomal lipid inclusions. Their ultrastructural visualization reveals membranous cytoplasmic bodies similar to those found in Tay-Sachs dis-

ease. Nonspecific lamellar inclusions have been found in Schwann cells.

There is an increase of sphingomyelin in the brain and massive accumulation of this substance in liver and spleen. Sphingomyelin represented 48 percent of total lipids in membranous inclusions in the brain of one patient.[23] Cholesterol is also elevated in visceral tissues and, to a lesser extent, in the brain. However, accumulation of cholesterol is much less than that of sphingomyelin and may be secondary to the primary storage of sphingomyelin. Lipid storage has been found in the brain, liver, and kidney of fetuses and in the placenta.

Differential Diagnosis requires differentiation from type I G_{M1} gangliosidosis, Gaucher disease, sialidosis, sialic acid storage disease, and other disorders causing hepatomegaly, cirrhosis, and jaundice in the newborn and small infant.

Treatment There is no known treatment.

Liver transplants and bone marrow transplants have been attempted without success. Partial correction of the sphingomyelinase deficiency has been achieved in Niemann-Pick type B by repeated subcutaneous implantations of amniotic epithelial cells, but this approach produces only temporary benefits. Therapeutic trials with animal models of Niemann-Pick disease are now feasible and may prove interesting.

Gaucher Disease The disease described in 1882 by Philippe Gaucher[24] as an epithelioma of the spleen without leukemia is now known to be caused by a deficiency in glucocerebrosidase, which allows the accumulation of glucosylceramide in the lysosomes of cells of the reticuloendothelial system. The eponym covers three different disorders: type I, chronic "adult" form, by far the most frequent, is characterized by splenomegaly, hepatomegaly, pancytopenia, and skeletal degeneration. It is of no practical concern to neurologists for it only rarely and secondarily involves the nervous system (and then only by local nerve injury due to hemorrhage or spinal cord compression by collapse of a vertebral body). Type II is the acute neuropathic early infantile form, which is the most dreaded, usually terminating life within a year or two (described below); and type III, a chronic form, which may not affect the nervous system until late childhood or adolescence (see Chap. 5).

Early Infantile Gaucher Disease (Type II Gaucher Disease; Neuropathic Gaucher Disease) Our experience, summarized below, consists of only a few cases. It is a rare, autosomal recessive inherited disease, caused by a deficiency in glucocerebrosidase, which leads to the accumulation of glucosylceramide (glucose-containing cerebroside) in the liver, spleen, and other tissues, and to the destruction of neurons in the brain without intraneuronal lipid storage.

Rapid psychomotor deterioration, spasticity, neck retroflexion, dysphagia, and oculomotor palsies comprise the neurologic syndrome, to which are joined splenomegaly and hepatomegaly. Facial features, skeleton and eyegrounds are normal. Typical histiocytes—Gaucher cells—are present in bone marrow smears, and there is an elevation of acid phosphatase in the serum. Affected children usually die before the age of 2 years (Fig. 3-6).

Clinical Features Neurologic signs in infantile Gaucher disease were first described by Oberling and Woringer.[25] Evidence of neurologic deterioration usually appears before 6 months and frequently before 3 months of age. Approximately 10 percent of patients are obviously abnormal within the first weeks of life. Whatever motor development there may have been up to this age is quickly lost. Occasionally, the disintegration of cerebral functions is more insidious. In all instances neurological signs soon become obvious and constitute a fairly stereotyped picture. Hypotonia invariably gives way to spasticity with bilateral pyramidal signs and there is a persistent and characteristic retroflexion of the neck. Paralytic strabismus with a variety of oculomotor palsies is characteristic; marked dysphagia is another striking feature and a source of feeding problems, leading to aspiration pneumonia. Laryngeal

stridor and trismus (due to bulbar spasticity) are troublesome symptoms in some cases. Awareness of and response to the environment fade rapidly. Seizures are rare and there is no acousticomotor response. Head circumference is usually normal at birth, but head growth rapidly diminishes. The optic fundi are normal. There is no clinical or electrophysiological evidence of peripheral nerve involvement.

Splenomegaly and, to a lesser extent, enlargement of the liver are constant and early findings. Sometimes, it is the enlarged spleen that first attracts medical attention; or the splenomegaly may appear only several months after the onset of neurological signs. Occasionally there is ascites, but jaundice is an exceptional feature of the disease. Hematologic signs of hypersplenism are rare, but late in the disease, anemia, thrombopenia, and leukopenia regularly appear. Recurrent episodes of coughing and respiratory infection are frequent and probably relate to the dysphagia, and to lung infiltration by Gaucher histiocytes. The bone changes that characterize the nonneurologic form of Gaucher disease (type I) are absent.

By the end of life the neurologic functioning has profoundly deteriorated, the face is expressionless, the head and neck are arched backward, the limbs are flexed, and the entire body is rigid. Death occurs usually before the age of 2 years.

Two paraclinical features are essential for the diagnosis of Gaucher disease: the presence of characteristic Gaucher histiocytes in bone marrow smears (see below), and elevation in the serum of tartrate noninhibitable acid phosphatase. Peripheral leukocytes are normal in appearance.

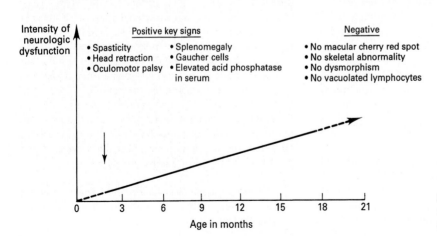

Intensity of neurologic dysfunction

Positive key signs
- Spasticity
- Head retraction
- Oculomotor palsy
- Splenomegaly
- Gaucher cells
- Elevated acid phosphatase in serum

Negative
- No macular cherry red spot
- No skeletal abnormality
- No dysmorphism
- No vacuolated lymphocytes

0   3   6   9   12   15   18   21

Age in months

Figure 3-6
Gaucher type II disease. Clinical course and life profile.

Diagnostic Biochemical Tests The definitive diagnosis is made by assay of glucocerebrosidase in leukocytes or cultured fibroblasts.

Prenatal Diagnosis is based on enzymatic assays of amniocytes or chorionic villus cells and is reliable.

Genetics Gaucher disease type II, like the other types of Gaucher disease, is inherited as an autosomal recessive trait. It is a rare disorder with an incidence that has been estimated at less than 1 in 50,000.[26] There is no ethnic prevalence in contrast with type I Gaucher disease, which is much more common among Ashkenazic Jews. Carrier detection is not reliable because there is some overlap in the level of activity of glucocerebrosidase between heterozygotes and normal controls. Between 5 percent and 20 percent of obligate heterozygotes fall in the normal range. The gene for glucocerebrosidase has been cloned and mapped to chromosome 1. Type II patients have a point mutation at nucleotide base 1448 that causes a substitution of proline for leucine at amino acid 444. Because this acid is immediately adjacent to the active site of the enzyme, its alteration has a particularly severe impact on glucocerebrosidase function.

Pathologic Findings The Gaucher cells that invade the spleen, lymph nodes, liver, capillary alveoli of the lungs, and other organs have a unique appearance (Fig. 3-7). They are 20 to 100 μm in size and their cytoplasm has an irregular wrinkled appearance, because of interwoven fibrils. This feature is visible in ordinary stains and even better in supravital preparations for phase microscopy. Gaucher cells are PAS-positive. Under the electron microscope the storage material is composed of characteristic tubular structures. These Gaucher cells have the same surface markers as histiocytes. Their appearance differs markedly from that of the foam cells seen in the Niemann-Pick lipidoses. The Gaucher cell is not absolutely specific, however, for similar cells have been observed in chronic myelocytic leukemias.

The neuropathological changes are not so easily demonstrated, being of a different nature than those of the other neuroviscera storage disorders. Intraneuronal storage of lipids is not found, even under the electron microscope. A limited number of Gaucher cells are observed around blood vessels or within the parenchyma, and the latter are surrounded by microglial nodules. Multiple areas of neuronal loss and neuronophagic microglial nodules are found in the cortex, tha-lamus, basal ganglia, brain stem, cerebellum, and spinal cord. Glucosylceramide accumulates in the lysosomes of reticuloendothelial cells in the viscera, but little or no increase is detectable in the brain.

Pathophysiology The absence of intraneural lipid storage and the nonspecific neuronal degeneration have prompted the hypothesis that brain lesions in type II Gaucher disease could be the result of some toxic effect of glucosylsphingosine.

The loss of neurons in the brain stem could account for the oculomotor palsies. The dysphagia is attributable to a combination of bulbar and pseudobulbar mechanisms, the latter a reflection of bilateral corticobulbar tract involvement.

Differential Diagnosis The diagnosis of Gaucher disease should be considered in any infant with unexplained splenomegaly, with or without neurological signs. It is very important to point out that splenomegaly may precede neurological signs by several months. In this circumstance, type II Gaucher disease may be difficult to differentiate from types I and III. The diagnosis of type II Gaucher disease cannot be ascertained in the absence of evident neurological deterioration.

Differentiation from G_{M1} gangliosidosis and Niemann-Pick type A is usually easy, because of differences in the involvement of the retina, skeleton, facial features, and hematological signs. Because of the early appearance of spasticity, it may be confused with Krabbe disease unless one detects the splenomegaly.

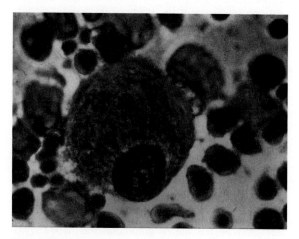

Figure 3-7
Gaucher cell in bone marrow smear.

Treatment   There is no specific treatment for type II Gaucher disease. Organ transplantation and enzyme replacement therapies have proved to be of no real help.

Farber Disease (Lipogranulomatosis); Ceramide Deficiency   This disease was initially reported by Farber, Cohen, and Uzman in 1957.[27] It is a rare autosomal recessive disorder of sphingolipid metabolism due to a deficiency of a lysosomal acid ceramidase, which results in the widespread granulomatous infiltration by ceramide-containing foamy macrophages; the subcutaneous tissues, joints, larynx, and visceral organs are involved, and there is also storage in neurons and glial cells. In its most typical form, it is characterized by painful swelling and deformation of the joints, subcutaneous nodules, dysphonia, dyspnea, and malnutrition. Neurological signs are usually not prominent. Death occurs within the first two years. Patients with a milder form and more prolonged course have been observed. Diagnosis rests on the demonstration of a deficiency of acid ceramidase in fibroblasts or leukocytes. Two other phenotypes have been reported: a neonatal form with marked hepatosphenomegaly and a rapidly progressive neurologic form occurring in early infancy.

Clinical Features   This account is based on approximately 40 cases of Farber disease, which were reported and analyzed by Moser et al. in 1989.[28] There have been no cases in our material at the EK Shriver Center or at the Pediatric Neurology Center of Louvain University. In its most usual form (type 1), the disease starts between birth and 4 months of age. The clinical picture is easily recognizable. The initial signs are swelling and sensitivity of the joints of the hands and feet and a hoarse cry. Subsequently, a severe, progressive generalized arthropathy develops, leading to ankylosis, and there is increasing dysphonia caused by the presence of granulomas on the larynx (visible by laryngoscopy). Characteristic subcutaneous nodules appear on the dorsal surface of the joints, particularly on the fingers, wrists, elbows, and over pressure points on the occiput, spine, and lumbosacral region (Fig. 3-8). Laryngeal and pulmonary infiltrates develop later, resulting in severe dyspnea with an obstructive component. Anorexia, vomiting and swallowing difficulties lead to severe malnutrition. Febrile episodes are frequent. Lymph nodes may be enlarged, hepatomegaly is variable but remains moderate, and the spleen is usually unaffected. The heart may be the site of granulomatous deposits. X-ray films show juxtaarticular bone lesions of destructive type, especially at the incisura ulnaris. Foamy PAS-posi-

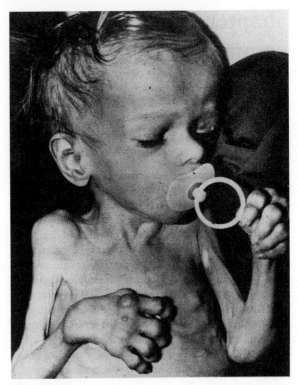

Figure 3-8
Farber disease. Twelve-month-old patient. Note periarticular swelling and subcutaneous nodules, emaciation. (Reprinted, by permission, from Zetterström, Acta Paediatr Scand *47: 501–551, 1958.)*

tive histiocytes may be extracted from the subcutaneous nodules and bone marrow.

Neurologic signs are difficult to detect and interpret in view of the severe degree of articular and cutaneous involvement. The irritability and paucity of movement in these infants may be due to the painful joints, which make the tendon reflexes difficult to elicit. The severe muscle atrophy, which develops rapidly, is surely in part a consequence of the immobilization of the joints and of malnutrition. However, it may also be related to an involvement of the peripheral nervous system. The electromyogram has shown signs of denervation in some patients and peripheral nerve lesions have been reported.[29] Also, lipid storage in the anterior horn cells is important in this disease and might play a role.

There are usually signs of involvement of the pyramidal tract. Blindness and an abnormal grayness of the macula with a red center have been observed. Corneal opacities and lenticular opacities may occur. Infantile spasms and other types of seizures are occasionally seen. Progressive mental deterioration is usual but not constant. The CSF protein level may be markedly elevated. The duration of the disease is short. Death generally occurs within the first two years of life.

Approximately 10 patients have been reported with a longer survival (type 2 and 3). In these cases, onset of the disease was in early infancy or during the second year of life, and death occurred 5 to 18 years later. The lungs were apparently not affected. Two-thirds of the children had a normal intellectual development. Postmortem studies apparently revealed only minimal involvement of the brain.[30]

Clinical Variants   Two additional forms are seen that differ markedly from the common type of Farber disease.

(1) Neonatal onset with hepatosplenomegaly and a fulminating course. In two unrelated children the presenting sign in the first days of life was a marked hepatosplenomegaly with no evidence of involvement of joints, larynx, or skin. Pulmonary infiltrates and fever foreshortened the course of the disease to a few weeks. There was a massive histiocytic infiltration in liver, spleen, and lungs, so malignant histiocytosis was the initial diagnosis. In one child, zebra bodies were found in the anterior horn cells of the spinal cord but the brain was not examined.[31] Interestingly, the sister of this child, who had the same mutant allele, had a more classic form of the disease except that the enlargement of the liver and spleen was more prominent than usual (type 4).

(2) The late infantile neurological form. In three patients belonging to two families, the disease started in the second or third year of life and was essentially characterized by a severe and rapidly progressive mental deterioration, ataxia, pyramidal signs, seizures, polymyoclonia, and cherry red spots (in the two siblings). All had subtle evidence of subcutaneous nodules and arthropathy, but the viscera were spared (type 5).

Pathological Findings   The basic abnormality consists of a granulomatous infiltration by PAS-containing foamy macrophages of joints, subcutaneous tissue, larynx, lungs, and various viscera. The infiltrating macrophages contain both ceramide and glycolipids, namely gangliosides (which are responsible for the PAS-positive staining). They induce a foreign body reaction. In the central nervous system, there is neuronal storage mainly in the anterior horn cells, brain stem nuclei, basal ganglia and ganglion cells of the retina,

and to a lesser degree, in the cerebral cortex. The autonomic nervous system and Schwann cells of peripheral nerves are also involved.[32] Ultrastructural studies have shown special intralysosomal inclusions consisting of comma-shaped curvilinear bodies which are likely to represent ceramide. In neurons and endothelial cells there are also zebra bodies, probably resulting from the presence of gangliosides. High levels of ceramide have been demonstrated in subcutaneous nodules, viscera, and brain. Accumulation of gangliosides and other glycolipids is probably a secondary phenomenon.

Diagnostic Laboratory Tests   The diagnosis of Farber disease rests on the demonstration of a reduced activity of acid ceramidase in cultured fibroblasts, leukocytes, or postmortem tissue. Acid ceramidase activity is usually less than 6 percent of control values.

A useful orienting test consists of the histological examination of a subcutaneous nodule and the detection of foamy macrophages which are PAS-positive (before lipid solvent extraction) and contain the typical inclusions seen under the electron microscope.

Proof of ceramide accumulation in subcutaneous tissue biopsies or postmortem tissue may be obtained by thin-layer chromatography or gas chromatography/mass spectrometry.

Genetics   The mode of inheritance of Farber disease is autosomal recessive. McKusick states that parental consanguinity has not been identified, but consanguinity is described in Tunisian siblings.[32] The prevalence of the disease is unknown, but it is surely quite rare. Obligate heterozygotes have a reduced activity of acid ceramidase in cultured skin fibroblasts and white blood cells.

Prenatal diagnosis by assaying the activity of acid ceramidase on amniocytes or chorionic villus samples is available.

Treatment   There is no specific treatment. Symptomatic therapy includes monitoring of the laryngeal and respiratory function, cosmetic surgery for granulomas, and corticosteroids to relieve pain.

In the future, patients with Farber disease might be good candidates for bone marrow transplantation.

Sialidoses and Sialic Acid Storage Disorders

Sialidoses   Sialidoses are related to a deficiency in acid α-neuraminidase, which results in the excretion of large quantities of sialyl oligosaccharides. Excretion of

these compounds also occurs as a secondary phenomenon in mucolipidoses II and III. Sialidosis type I will be
considered in Chap. 5. Sialidosis type II and galactosialidosis will be described here (and also in Chap. 5).

Sialidosis Type II (Mucolipidosis I) Type II sialidosis is an autosomal recessive disorder characterized
by neurologic, ocular, visceral, skeletal and facial
abnormalities, an excretion of sialylated oligosaccharides and a marked deficiency of the activity of α-neur-
aminidase. The defective gene is encoded on
chromosome 10 (10 pter-q23). Sialidosis type II may
give rise to congenital, infantile, and juvenile disorders.

(1) In the congenital form,[33] infants present at
birth with hydrops fetalis, hepatosplenomegaly, skeletal
dysplasias, ocular abnormalities, and a telangiectasic
skin rash. Infants are either stillborn or live a few
weeks (other metabolic disorders with hydrops fetalis
are indicated in Table 7-2).

(2) In the early infantile form of the disease, hepatosplenomegaly and ascites may be present in the neonate or develop after a few weeks.[34] Dysmorphic
features, such as a puffy facies, a depressed nasal bridge,
and gingival hyperplasia, are noted early. A hepatomegaly may be present. A macular cherry red spot is a
major sign. Punctate lens opacities and deafness may
occur. Neurologic development is severely impaired.
Psychomotor retardation is severe. X-rays disclose periosteal thickening of the long bones, stippling of the
epiphyses, and ovoid vertebral bodies. Foam cells in
bone marrow smears and clear vacuoles in peripheral
lymphocytes can be seen. There may be evidence of a
peripheral neuropathy. On the whole, the phenotype
closely resembles that of infantile G_{M1} gangliosidosis.
The course of the disease is severe and usually leads to
death after a few months or in the second year of life.
Some children live longer with severe mental impairment, intention myoclonus, seizures, and motor difficulties.

Nephrosialidosis A few patients have also had
severe renal dysfunction with proteinuria. They represent a milder form of the disease. They usually come
to attention at age 4 to 6 months with the usual signs
of early infantile type II sialidosis. They may develop
fine corneal opacities. Survival is for several years. At
autopsy one patient had marked storage of inclusion
material in the renal glomeruli and sympathetic ganglia.[35]

(3) Late infantile and juvenile forms exhibit mild
developmental delay, progressively aggravated dys-

morphic facial features, and signs of dysostosis multiplex. Patients eventually become severely disabled.
Death occurs in the second or third decade.

Laboratory Tests
- Thin-layer chromatography of the urine demonstrates a high concentration of sialylated oligosaccharides (several hundred times greater than normal).
- Under the electron microscope, clear membrane-
  bound inclusions are found in biopsies of skin fibroblasts, liver (Kupffer cells), and bone marrow histiocytes.
- There is a marked deficiency of activity of α-neura-
  minidase in cultured fibroblasts, leukocytes, amniocytes, and chorionic villi, and a partial deficiency in
  obligate heterozygotes.
- Prenatal diagnosis can be accomplished.

Pathology Clear vacuoles containing various
lamellar or granular inclusions are found in most
organs, including liver, spleen, lymph nodes, and cerebral neurons.

Galactosialidosis This condition, in which sialyl
oligosaccharides are also excreted in great amounts in
the urine, is characterized by a combined deficiency of α-
neuraminidase and β-galactosidase. It has principally
been reported from Japan[36] but has been seen elsewhere.[37] Its clinical expression is variable and in many
ways resembles sialidosis type II. It presents usually in
late childhood or adolescence, with cerebellar ataxia,
myoclonus, and visual failure. There is a moderate
degree of facial dysmorphism and skeletal changes,
essentially of the spine. A macular cherry red spot and
corneal clouding are usually present; angiokeratomas
have been noted. Vacuolation of peripheral lymphocytes
and foamy cells in bone marrow smears are consistently
present. The progression of the disease is slow.

Early and late infantile forms with visceromegaly
and skeletal dysplasia have also been described.[36] Prenatal diagnosis of the disorder has been achieved.[38]

The primary defect in galactosialidosis is a deficiency of a protective protein encoded on chromosome
20. Serine carboxypeptidase activity is associated with
this protective protein and is markedly reduced.

Sialic Acid Storage Disorders In the sialic acid storage disorders, free sialic acid accumulates in tissue lysosomes and body fluids, possibly as a consequence of a
block in sialic acid egress from the lysosomal compart-
ment of cells. The primary defect is unknown. There are

three clinically distinct conditions: infantile and juvenile sialic acid storage disease and Salla disease. They are allelic variants of a single defect in the lysosomal transport of sialic acid.

Clinical Features   Fifteen cases of the severe infantile form have been reported. Typically, a polyhydramnios, due to a nonimmune hydrops, precedes the premature delivery. At birth, the infant is edematous, pancytopenic and hypoalbuminic. The complexion is usually fair with coarse facies, hepatosplenomegaly, ascites, and inguinal hernias (Fig. 3-9). Cardiomegaly has been reported in 6 of 12 patients and dysostosis multiplex in 5 of 10. One-quarter had a nephrotic syndrome. Death occurred within the first two years.[39]

Morphologic and Biochemical Characteristics Ultrastructural analysis of lymphocytes and skin disclose accumulations of lysosome-bound clear vacuoles containing a small amount of granulofilamentous material. Similar vacuoles are found in bone marrow aspirates. The diagnosis rests on the demonstration of an increased amount of free sialic acid in serum, urine, and cultured skin fibroblasts. Intracellular accumulations of free sialic acid have been found in all organs, including the brain. Urinary excretion of mucopolysaccharides is normal. There is no deficiency in acid α-neuraminidase activity. The defect in this presumably autosomal recessive disease is believed to be in a proton-driven carrier system that transports sialic acid across the lysosomal membrane.

Variants   Increased urinary excretion of free sialic acid without concomitant lysosomal storage has been obtained in a few patients. The defect in these cases appears to be in the feedback inhibition mechanism of the enzyme UDP-*N*-acetylglucosamine-2-epimerase.

The Juvenile Form   Juvenile sialic acid storage disease is rare. It is characterized by developmental delay, mildly coarse facies and hepatomegaly. X-rays disclose mild beaking of the vertebrae. Corneas remain clear. Urine sialic acid levels are elevated.

Salla Disease   Salla disease is named from a region in northern Finland where almost all the cases originated. Many of them had been detected by systematic screening of individuals with mental retardation. Indeed, the clinical picture is not at all characteristic.[40]

Hypotonia and motor retardation are usually evident during the first year of life. Truncal ataxia is generally observed and there may be a nystagmus, which disappears later in life. Exotropia is frequently noted. One-third of patients never walk, or walking is delayed, not being acquired before a mean age of 5 years (2 to 12 years). There are signs of a corticospinal disease and an ataxic gait. Speech is absent or reduced to a few dysarthric words. The mental deficit is profound. The IQ is usually below 20 in adulthood. Patients tend to have a friendly disposition. Seizures are rare. Short stature is usual, and there may be mild coarsening of facial features but no skeletal or ophthalmologic abnormalities. There is no visceromegaly. The life span is nearly normal.

The urinary excretion of sialic acid is increased and abnormal storage of this substance is found within lysosomes. Prenatal diagnosis has been successfully

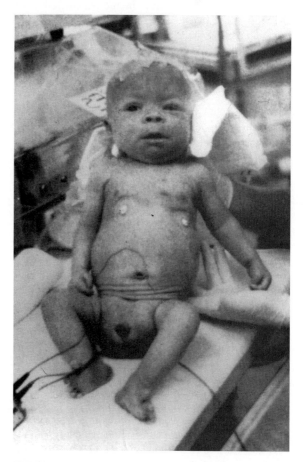

Figure 3-9

Sialic acid storage disease. Seven-week-old infant with broad depressed nasal bridge, puffed eyelids, long upper lip, large forehead, and inguinal hernias.

performed. The genetic locus for Salla disease maps to chromosome 6q14-15.

Glycogenosis Type II (Acid α-Glucosidase Deficiency; Pompe Disease)

This glycogenosis was reported in a Dutch medical journal in 1932 by Pompe.[41] It was classified as type II glycogenosis by Cori.[42] Hers[43,44] demonstrated that it was a lysosomal disorder. In fact, it was the first clearly defined inborn lysosomal disease. It is the only glycogen storage disease in which there is a proven anatomic involvement of the central nervous system.

This condition, inherited as an autosomal recessive trait, is due to a deficiency in a lysosomal acid-1,4-α-glucosidase,[43] which results in the accumulation of glycogen in vacuoles derived from lysosomes in most tissues, including the nervous system.

The disease is characterized by a profound hypotonia and muscle weakness and a cardiomegaly with progressive heart failure.

Clinical Features In its more *common form*, the disease starts during the first weeks or months of life. The most striking manifestation is the reduction of spontaneous motor activity and muscle weakness. Patients lie limply and are unable to hold up their head or will soon lose the ability to do so (Fig. 3-10A); and they are incapable of sitting. Motor reactions of the limbs to stimuli are feeble. There is, however, no muscle wasting and the consistency of muscles is generally firm. Macroglossia is frequent. The deep tendon reflexes are usually depressed or unelicitable. In spite of increasing respiratory failure, the respiratory muscles seem not to be enfeebled as early and severely as in Werdnig-Hoffman disease. Sucking and swallowing are often weakened. The EMG shows a myopathic pattern and striking pseudomyotonic discharges on insertion of the needle electrode (Fig 3-10C). The role played in the clinical picture by glycogen storage in the anterior horn cells is difficult to determine. It may, however, be one element in the mechanism of the progressive muscular weakness and depression of the tendon reflexes. Lingual fasciculations have been reported. Nerve conduction velocities are normal. In contrast to the major motor incapacity, alertness and other mental functions are preserved. When apathy develops later in the disease, it remains difficult to decide whether it is due to the brain lesion or to the cardiomuscular abnormality. Optic fundi and CSF findings are normal.

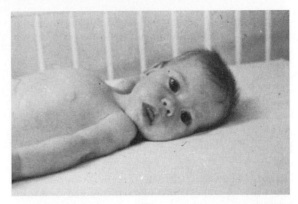

(A)

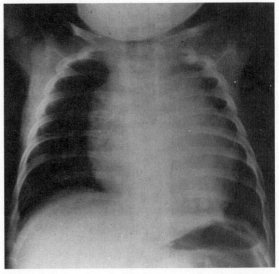

(B)

Figure 3-10
*Pompe disease. **A**. Appearance of infant at 5 months: note protruding tongue. **B**. Chest x-ray film showing marked enlargement of heart. (Part **B** courtesy Dr. de Barsy.)*

The major clinical element for the diagnosis of Pompe disease is a large heart on x-rays of the chest (Fig. 3-10B). There may also be signs of atelectasia of the lungs. The liver enlarges progressively. The electrocardiogram (ECG) is characteristic with a marked shortening of the PR interval and a high amplitude of the QRS complex (Fig. 3-10C). There is no evidence of hypoglycemia or ketosis.

Death results from progressive heart failure and respiratory insufficiency, usually within the first year of

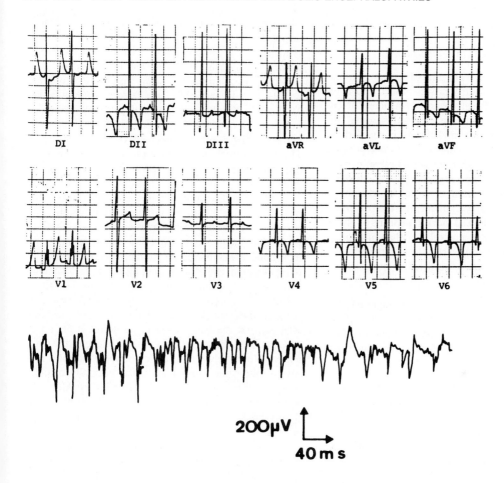

Figure 3-10C
Pompe disease. (Top and middle) ECG shows shortening of PR intervals and large QRS complexes.
(Bottom) EMG: myotonic action potentials. (EMG courtesy Dr. de Barsy and Dr. Knoops.)

life. A few children with less pronounced cardiac involvement have lived longer.

Variants   There are also *late infantile, juvenile, and adult forms* of the disease. Hers et al.[44] have collected 24 patients of both sexes of the late infantile and juvenile types. In these, the disease starts after the child has started to walk, between 1 and 15 years of age. The presenting sign is muscle weakness and the clinical picture resembles that of a myopathy, most particularly Duchenne muscular dystrophy. The consistency of muscles may be rubbery. Initially, heart involvement is minimal or absent. There is no hepatomegaly. An atonic anal sphincter and enlargement of the bladder have been reported. Again, electromyography demonstrates myotonic-like potentials. Some children have been mentally retarded. The disorder is slowly progressive and death occurs often after several years or even in adolescence from cardiorespiratory failure.

In the adult form, there are no complaints before the second or third decade. The condition usually takes the form of a limb-girdle myopathy and coincident involvement of intercostal and diaphragm muscles. Several of our adult patients have died of respiratory insufficiency. The occurrence of the infantile and adult forms in the same family has been reported. This probably indicates the existence of various compound heterozygote states. One family has been reported in which there was pseudo-deficiency of acid α-glucosidase.[45]

Pathologic Findings The ultrastructural examination of all tissues, particularly heart, muscle, and liver, reveals the accumulation of glycogen in lysosomes.[46] Neuropathologic abnormalities consist of intralysosomal storage of glycogen in neuron and glial cells, particularly in the spinal cord, dorsal root ganglia, autonomic ganglia, brain stem nuclei, and dentate nucleus. Lesser involvement of cortical neurons and glia occurs but is inconstant. Glycogen deposits have been described in peripheral nerves. One mentally retarded patient with the late infantile form of the disease showed marked deposits of glycogen in the brain, mainly in glial cells,[47] while in another without mental deficit, glycogen storage in nerve cells was minimal.[48] In the adult cases, no heart or brain lesions have been reported.[49]

Diagnostic Laboratory Tests The diagnosis rests on the determination of acid α-glucosidase mostly in muscle, liver, and lymphocytes. Enzyme assays on chorionic villi and cultured amniocytes have been used for prenatal diagnosis.

Genetics Pompe disease is an autosomal recessive disorder. Heterozygotes can be detected by assays of lymphocytes and other tissues. The locus for acid α-glucosidase has been mapped to chromosome 17q23. The gene is 20 kb long, contains 20 exons and codes for a 105 kD protein. Numerous mutations characteristic of either the infantile or adult form have been described.

Differential Diagnosis In the early infantile form, Werdnig-Hoffman disease and congenital myopathies must be considered. Other early infantile metabolic disorders may give a moderate enlargement of the heart in a different pathologic context (neurovisceral sphingolipidoses, mitochondrial disorders). Exceptionally ethanolaminosis[50] and deficiency of phosphofructokinase and phosphorylase *b* kinase[51] may mimick Pompe disease.

In the juvenile and adult forms, differentiation from muscular dystrophy may be difficult.

The Genetic Early Infantile Leukodystrophies

The term *leukodystrophy* is commonly applied to a group of genetic disorders in which the white matter of the central nervous system is predominantly affected.

The peripheral nerves may also be involved in some of them. Both hypomyelination, due to failure of myelin synthesis, and demyelination, resulting in the breakdown of previously formed myelin, are included.

The recognized types of leukodystrophies are: Krabbe disease, metachromatic leukodystrophy (Chap. 4), juvenile X-linked adrenoleukodystrophy (Chap. 5), Pelizaeus-Merzbacher disease and the sudanophilic leukodystrophies, Canavan disease, and Alexander disease. The pathogenesis of the myelin disorder appears to be different in each disease, and for the most part is not understood.

Krabbe disease and metachromatic leukodystrophy are sphingolipidoses; adrenoleukodystrophy is a peroxisomal disease. Demyelination or dysmyelination is possibly due to a cytotoxic effect on oligodendrocytes in Krabbe disease and to an anomaly in the composition of myelin in metachromatic leukodystrophy. It is related to a defective synthesis of a major myelin protein in Pelizaeus-Merzbacher disease. White matter lesions in adrenoleukodystrophy resemble those of multiple sclerosis, but the basic biochemical defect is unknown. In Canavan disease, the spongiform change in the white matter is probably due to the cytotoxic effect of a neurotransmitter-like compound that is normally confined to the cortex. The specific abnormality in Alexander disease (possibly not a hereditary condition) lies not in dysmyelination but in a generalized abnormality of astrocytes.

Clinically, the leukodystrophies express themselves by evidence of dysfunction of the major cerebrospinal tracts (corticospinal and corticobulbar), cerebellum and cerebellar peduncles, optic nerves, and geniculocalcarine pathways and, possibly, a demyelinating polyneuropathy. Seizures are rare and mental deterioration is not an early sign. There are, however, many exceptions.

Information provided by magnetic resonance imaging (particularly T2-weighted images) is now indispensable for the diagnosis of a leukodystrophy, in the sense that abnormal signals in the white matter are always present. In certain cases, white matter changes on MRI antedate the clinical signs. The topography of the abnormal signals and enhancement with gadolinium may give an indication as to the type of leukodystrophy, but this is not always reliable (see Chap. 8).

For all the major leukodystrophies, the definitive diagnosis rests on enzymatic and molecular studies. Only in Alexander disease does the diagnosis during life depend almost entirely on MRI.

Widespread white matter lesions may be seen also in some patients with Leigh disease, in Zellweger disease, Sjögren-Larsson disease, and a few other metabolic disorders in which there are lesions of both gray and white matter structures. Myelin breakdown also occurs in acquired demyelinating disorders, particularly multiple sclerosis and Schilder disease, and in certain chronic encephalitides (due to HIV or measles virus for instance). Any condition causing widespread neuronal loss may result in some degree of secondary degeneration of myelinated axons in the white matter. Familial cases of white matter and callosal hypoplasia or atrophy of obscure origin have been reported. A transitory delay in myelination may be detected on MRI in infants with a number of different neurologic abnormalities. The significance of this observation remains uncertain.

Krabbe Leukodystrophy; Galactosylceramide Lipidosis (Globoid Cell Leukodystrophy)   Krabbe, a Danish neurologist, reported in 1916 a progressive familial infantile "sclerosis" of the brain.[52] He noted unusual cells in the white matter (which were later termed "globoid cells" by Collier and Greenfield[53]). There had been two earlier descriptions of the same cell type by Bullard and Southard[54] and Beneke.[55]

Krabbe disease is an autosomal recessive disorder known to be caused by a deficiency in galactosylceramidase (galactocerebroside β-galactosidase), a lysosomal enzyme which normally cleaves galactosylceramide to ceramide and galactose. The gene for galactosylceramidase has been mapped to chromosome 14 and has been cloned and sequenced. In the majority of cases the disease starts between 3 and 6 months and has a rapidly fatal outcome. Clinically, it is characterized by generalized rigidity with tonic spasms in association with clinical and electrophysiological evidence of peripheral nerve involvement and a high CSF protein level (Figs. 3-11 and 3-12). There is extensive demyelination in the central and peripheral nervous system. The presence of multinucleated macrophages containing galactocerebroside, the globoid cells, constitutes the pathological hallmark of the disease. The accumulation of psychosine in the central nervous system probably plays a role in the dysmyelinating process. Prenatal diagnosis is available. In about 10 percent of cases, onset is in the late infantile or juvenile period. The juvenile form will be discussed in chapter 5.

Clinical Features   Our clinical analysis is based on 110 recorded cases. In 80 percent of them, the disease began before the age of 6 months and in 25 percent before 3 months (Fig. 3-12).

The usual clinical course is fairly stereotyped. Irritability with bouts of crying, diminished alertness, vomiting, and other feeding problems are usually among the first signs. In many cases, however, the first indisputable and striking abnormality is rigidity. The muscular hypertonia increases progressively, affecting limbs, trunk and neck. Tonic spasms induced by all kinds of stimulation and by feeding lead to opisthotonic recurvation of the trunk and neck. During these spasms, the limbs may undergo clonic movements and there is concomitant crying. Only rarely does auditory stimulation induce a startle response as in Tay-Sachs disease. At first, pyramidal signs (increased tendon reflexes, signs of Babinski and Rossolimo) are quite definite, but later the tendon reflexes become depressed or absent and the spasticity lessens. The peripheral nervous system is affected very early in the disease, so that nerve conduction velocities are markedly reduced. Blindness and optic atrophy appear later along with pendular nystagmus and squints, which are often the earliest signs of visual failure. Rarely, optic atrophy is one of the first signs. Deafness has been observed in a few cases. Episodes of unexplained fever are not uncommon.

Occasionally, the infant has seizures, but seldom do they stand as a major sign. Sometimes they may be difficult to distinguish from muscular spasms and clonic jerks. EEG tracings are altered in nonspecific ways, usually of slow-wave type, but the record may be normal in the early stages of the disease.

The CSF protein level is generally high, ranging from 70 to 450 mg per 100 mL, an abnormality that can

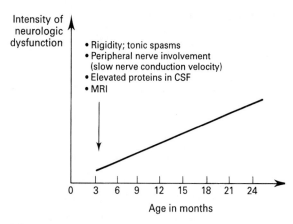

Figure 3-11
Krabbe disease. Clinical course and life profile.

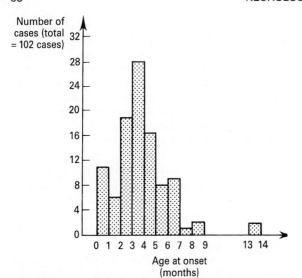

Figure 3-12
Krabbe disease. Clinical course and life profile.

be detected at any time after birth. The electrophoretic pattern is usually normal. An elevation of gamma globulin with an oligoclonal pattern has, however, been reported. In some few instances, the CSF has been normal.

The relative head size is gradually diminished to a moderate degree, usually between 2 and 3 standard deviations from the normal mean. In rare instances, a moderately enlarged head circumference has been reported. Vomiting and anorexia, which tend to occur early, may lead to severe malnutrition, although the birth weight is always normal. Stunting of growth is a prominent finding (up to 10 standard deviations) below normal body length. There seems to be a good correlation between small body size and undernutrition, but not between body size and head circumference. There is no visceromegaly. Finally, the child is blind, spastic and virtually decerebrate.

The course of the disease is relatively brief; in approximately 70 percent of cases the life span does not exceed 1 year and very rarely 2 years. Death is usually due to respiratory difficulties and bronchopneumonia.

Variants   Although the clinical picture of early infantile Krabbe disease is stereotyped in the majority of cases, phenotypic variations are reported more often since the advent of widely available enzymatic testing.

(1) The neonatal variant. The disease may manifest itself in the neonatal period and even at birth. Feeding difficulties, vomiting, and irritability are usually prominent. Soon, body stiffness with clenched fists, twitching, and myoclonic jerks become apparent, especially when the infant is handled. Deep tendon reflexes are usually not depressed, but nerve conduction velocities are already reduced. The interpretation of a high protein content in the CSF may be difficult at that age.

(2) The hypotonic variant.[56,57] In some patients the typical rigidity is absent. Flaccidity, hypomotility, and weakness are the first signs. Deep tendon reflexes are depressed at the initial stage of the disease and nerve conduction velocities are decreased. The weakness and hypotonia of these infants is probably a reflection of the intensity and precocity of peripheral nerve involvement. Differentiation from the congenital hypomyelination neuropathies may be difficult.

(3) In a few patients seizures, in the form of infantile spasms, have been a prominent and early manifestations of the disease.[57]

(4) A fulminating course, leading to death after 3 months has been reported.[58]

(5) The clinical picture may exceptionally consist in uncharacteristic neurological deterioration with seizures and none of the usual signs of classical Krabbe disease.

(6) Late-onset Krabbe disease, which is much rarer, will be discussed in Chap. 5.

Diagnostic Laboratory Tests   Three routine laboratory investigations are essential in seeking support for the diagnosis of Krabbe disease: (1) examination of the CSF, which generally discloses a marked elevation of total proteins; (2) measurement of nerve conduction velocities, which are practically always considerably reduced (nerve conduction velocities may be difficult to measure in the young infant); (3) magnetic resonance imaging, which reveals central white matter demyelination, starting usually in the periventricular regions of the posterior part of the cerebral hemispheres.[60]

The ultrastructural examination of a sural nerve biopsy might be useful in some circumstances, for example, when the enzymatic assay is not readily available (Fig. 8-1) or in case of pseudo-deficiency. In our experience, typical Schwann cell and macrophage inclusions have been detectable at an early stage of the disease, even before the occurrence of typical clinical signs.

The cause of the disease is a deficiency of galactosylceramidase (galactocerebroside β-galactosidase), a lysosomal enzyme which normally cleaves galactosylceramide to ceramide and galactose. Assays of galactosyl-ceramidase are made on leukocytes or cultured fibro-blasts most often using the radiolabeled natural substrate (an artificial substrate can also be used). Residual activities of the enzyme are generally very low.

Assays of glactosylceramidase on leukocytes are used for the detection of heterozygotes. However, carrier detection by this means is not entirely reliable in view of a possible overlap between carriers and normals. This is due, in part, to the presence of a T→C polymorphic base change at nucleotide 1637 of the galactocerebrosidase cDNA, which results in much lower enzyme activity in the presence of homozygosity for C (EK). This difficulty can be circumvented in those families where the base sequence and mutations in the index case have been identified.

Enzymatic assays on chorionic villus or cultured amniotic fluid cells provide the possibility of prenatal diagnosis.

Normal adults with very low levels of galactocer-amidase have been found in one family.[61] The existence of such cases of "pseudo-deficiency" complicates prenatal diagnosis.

Genetics Krabbe leukodystrophy is inherited as an autosomal recessive disorder. The locus for galacto-cylceramidase is on chromosome 14 in the q21-q31 region. The gene encodes a single chain peptide of 669 amino acids. Most Krabbe alleles contain single base substitutions, but a large deletion at the 3' end of the gene, in association with a C $\underline{502}$ T polymorphism, also occurs in genomic DNA of many patients with the early infantile form. The disease is known to occur in most parts of the world but is more prevalent in Sweden in its early infantile form and remarkably infrequent in Finland. In Sweden its incidence has been estimated at 1/25,000.[57] The incidence in the general population is not known.

Pathology The main morphological features of Krabbe leukodystrophy are (1) widespread demyelination (or arrest of myelination) and reactive astrocytic gliosis, usually with sparing of subcortical arcuate fibers. Phylogenetically newer tracts tend to be more severely affected. The number of oligodendrocytes is markedly reduced. Gray matter is spared. (2) The presence, in demyelinated areas, of the characteristic globoid cells, which consist of large PAS-positive[59] mononucleate or multinucleate histiocytes, with a tendency to aggregate around capillaries and venules. Similar cells occur in the peripheral nerves. In electron microscopic preparations,

the cytoplasm of globoid cells and of Schwann cells contain numerous inclusions consisting of straight or curved hollow tubules with longitudinal striation. These inclusions have a crystalloid appearance. A much rarer type of inclusion is the twisted tubule, which resembles that seen in Gaucher disease. Interestingly, although the disease is caused by a defect of a lysosomal enzyme, the tubular inclusions of Krabbe disease are not intralyso-somal.

Chemical Pathology Concentrations of galacto-sylceramide (and sulfatides) are much lower than normal in the whole white matter. Increase of galactosylcera-mide is confined to globoid cells. An important finding is the presence of substantial amounts of galactosyl-sphingosine (psychosine) in the white matter and in other organs. This compound is practically undetectable in normal subjects. The remaining myelin sheaths are ultrastructurally and biochemically normal (this is not the case in metachromatic leukodystrophy, where intact myelin contains an excess of sulfatides).

Fetal Pathology The presence of globoid cells, and a considerable reduction of galactosylceramidase have been observed in 20-week-old fetuses with Krabbe disease.

Mechanism of Deranged Brain Function Formation of specific globoid cells and the lack of total increase of galactosylceramide need to be explained. The following hypothesis is generally accepted.[62] Galac-tosylceramide is an almost exclusive constituent of oli-godendrocytes and myelin. When myelination starts, galactosylceramide is formed which cannot be normally catabolized because of the deficient galactosylcerami-dase. It therefore accumulates in the white matter and stimulates the formation of globoid cells. It has been shown experimentally that galactosylceramide is unique among sphingoglycolipids in inducing the formation of this typical giant cell.

Globoid cells contain galactosylceramide but this substance is not increased in the white matter. Perhaps this is due to the rapid destruction of oligodendrocytes (and probably Schwann cells) and an early arrest of myelination. Destruction of oligodendrocytes has been attributed to an excess of a highly cytotoxic substance, psychosine, which also serves as a substrate for galacto-sylceramidase. Psychosine is almost absent in the normal brain, but forms and accumulates when galactosylcera-midase is deficient.

Differential Diagnosis   The following diseases are to be considered in the differential diagnosis: (1) non-progressive encephalopathies of prenatal origin and fetal encephalitis (when onset is abrupt and gamma globulin and cells are elevated in the CSF); (2) aminoacidopathies in neonates; (3) Leigh disease (a condition in which elevated CSF proteins and a peripheral neuropathy may also occur); (4) G_{M2} gangliosidosis; (5) chronic gastrointestinal disease; and (6) congenital hypomyelination peripheral neuropathies.

Treatment   There is up to now no specific treatment for the early form of Krabbe disease. There are two main obstacles to enzyme replacement therapy by bone marrow transplantation: the difficulty of rapidly delivering the enzyme to the brain across the blood-brain barrier and the fact that important brain damage may already have been present at birth. However, patients with the *later-onset* form of slower progression have benefited from bone marrow transplantation. The theoretical basis for this procedure derives from studies of the twitcher mouse, an enzymatically authentic model of human globoid cell leukodystrophy. After transplantation, the globoid cells gradually disappear, remyelination of the CNS occurs, and survival of the animal is prolonged from between 30 and 40 days to more than 100 days (see Chaps. 5 and 9).

Sudanophilic Leukodystrophies

Introduction   The sudanophilic leukodystrophies constitute a heterogeneous group of genetic disorders that have in common demyelination or defective myelination of the CNS. There are sudanophilic lipids in microglial cells and astrocytes in the affected white matter (from which the diseases obtain their name) but no specific biochemical abnormalities in the brain have been found, except in one variety.

It is noteworthy that myelin degeneration with liberation of sudanophilic lipids as a pathologic criterion lacks the degree of specificity of other myelinopathies, i.e., the globoid cells, metachromatic lipids, astrocytic Rosenthal fibers, spongy degeneration with giant astrocytes that are virtually diagnostic of Krabbe disease, metachromatic leukodystrophy, Alexander disease, and Canavan disease, respectively. Also, any given morphologic variety of sudanophilic breakdown, e.g., patchy demyelination or total absence of myelin, may be associated with several different clinical entities.[62,64,65] It is therefore quite clear that, in the absence of any known biochemical or molecular marker, the genetic and clinical as well as neuropathological data permit only a rough categorization of entities within the group of sudanophilic leukodystrophies, the only exception being Pelizaeus-Merzbacher disease.

A constellation of clinical, genetic, pathologic, and molecular data permits the segregation of two groups of sudanophilic leukodystrophies.

(1) *Pelizaeus-Merzbacher disease* emerges as the only truly distinct entity in this group, a fact confirmed by recent molecular biology studies. The morphological characteristics of this X-linked disorder are mainly the following: (1) the persistence of patches of myelinated fibers in the demyelinated areas, giving a tigroid, patchy, or discontinuous appearance; (2) a paucity of macrophages (scavenger cells); (3) a moderate quantity of sudanophilic lipids localized in astrocytes, and adventitial cells, and (4) a loss of oligodendrocytes. In some cases of Pelizaeus-Merzbacher disease (Seitelberger subtype), there is a total absence of myelin.

(2) *Other unclassified sporadic or familial apparently autosomal recessive leukodystrophies* which differ from adrenoleukodystrophy and Schilder disease. Possibly some of the sporadic cases were examples of Pelizaeus-Merzbacher disease. It is expected that modern techniques of molecular biology will delineate specific disorders within this group.

In this ill-defined and heterogeneous class of diseases, several clinical subtypes may be distinguished.

(1) Early infantile sudanophilic leukodystrophy.[62,66] Anatomically verified cases in this subgroup have been both sporadic and familial and have affected boys as well as girls. The disease starts before the age of 3 months and usually terminates life within 2 years. Any early minor psychomotor achievements are soon erased by rapid deterioration. Neurological signs included spastic paralysis, blindness with optic atrophy, and occasionally, seizures. In some cases, involvement of the peripheral nerves seems probable. The CSF is normal. Marked microcephaly (head circumference 3 standard deviations below mean for age) may be a significant feature.

(2) Late infantile or juvenile sudanophilic leukodystrophy.[63,65,67,68] Occurring either sporadically or in families and in both sexes, the disease usually becomes apparent between 3 and 7 years of age and is of long duration. Neurologic signs are those of a diffuse progressive cerebral disease featuring incoordination, spasticity, occasional involuntary movements, rare seizures, and mental retardation. Nystagmus and optic atrophy are usual. Affected children may live until late adolescence or early adulthood. The neurologic signs and the course of the disease are variable from case to case so

that no clinical picture can be considered typical. In some instances the course is so slow that signs of deterioration are nearly imperceptible over a period of many years, and the diagnosis of nonprogressive, congenital encephalopathy or of cerebral palsy is made erroneously.

(3) Other familial types of leukodystrophy of sudanophilic type:

- Norman et al.[69] have reported two siblings, a boy and a girl, with microcephaly, large ears, nystagmus, and spastic paraplegia. They were both severely retarded. At postmortem examination at 2 and 3 years of age, there was pachygyria and leukodystrophy.

- Congenital, late infantile, juvenile, and adult cases of sudanophilic leukodystrophy with diffuse leptomeningeal angiomatosis have been described by van Bogaert.[70] Seizures, mental retardation, hemiplegia, tremor, dysarthria, and pseudobulbar symptoms were ultimately traced to leptomeningeal angiomatosis, intracortical necrosis, and diffuse demyelination.

- A sudanophilic leukodystrophy with patchy demyelination and striatocerebellar calcifications. This conforms to *Cockayne syndrome* (see Chap. 5).

- Large necrotic lesions of the hemispheric white matter may be seen in Leigh disease, and mistaken for a true leukodystrophy on MRI. We have examined the brains of three patients with these features, two of them in the same sibship, where there were diffuse, irregular cavitary lesions of the white matter and the corpus callosum with sudanophilic lipids in macrophages.

Important to keep in mind, with reference to these classes of diseases, is the fact that sudanophilic lipids in white matter cells are also found in some specific metabolically determined leukodystrophies: X-linked adrenoleukodystrophy, Canavan disease, and Alexander disease.

Very poor myelination in infants, as a part of a generalized encephalopathy, should not be considered as a leukodystrophy.

Pelizaeus-Merzbacher Disease   The name of Pelizaeus-Merzbacher disease[71,72] must be restricted to an X-linked recessive myelin disorder of the central nervous system, caused by a deficiency in *proteolipid protein*, one of the major proteins in myelin.

Clinical Features   Depending on the age of onset and duration, the neurologic symptomatology varies to some extent. Two main patterns have emerged.

In one group, the onset of the disease is in the neonatal period or in the very first months of infancy. The first detectable sign consists in abnormal eye movements and frequently they are accompanied by intermittent shaking movements of the head. The eye movements at first are rapid, irregular oscillations of small amplitude. Some of the movements take the form of a vertical or horizontal (often asymmetric) nystagmus. The ocular abnormality resembles congenital nystagmus or spasms nutans or that of congenital blindness. However, vision at this early stage does not appear to be significantly impaired. The optic fundi are at first normal; optic atrophy, if it is to appear, develops later. Laryngeal stridor is also an early sign in many children.[73,74] In time, different types of abnormal choreiform or athetotic movements of the limbs begin to appear and psychomotor development is by then manifestly slowed. Whatever progress has been made is lost in the third or fourth months of life. Standing and speech are never possible and some infants do not even attain proper head control. Seizures occur occasionally. Pyramidal signs are present in all cases. Marked microcephaly is usual and the body stature is dwarfed. The CSF is normal and the EEG changes noncharacteristic. The natural duration of the disease seldom exceeds 5 to 7 years.

In a second type, the onset is also in the first months of life, or usually somewhat later, and the same peculiar pendular nystagmus and head movements and stridor are again the first signs. Cerebellar ataxia, choreoathetoid movements of the limbs, seizures, pyramidal signs, and spasticity appear later. Pes cavus and kyphoscoliosis become manifest at varying intervals after the onset. Generally the progress of the disease is much slower. Some children are finally able to hold up their heads and sit with support; others never learn to sit.

Curiously, intellectual function in this second type is frequently quite well preserved for a long time, and mental deterioration develops only in the later stage of the disease. Speech is dysarthric and finally becomes incomprehensible. Head circumference is usually reduced. Some of the affected children have survived until the third decade of life.

The results of MRI scans are variable. They may show nonspecific, diffuse and symmetrical abnormalities in the white matter (low intensity on T1-weighted images and high intensity on T2-weighted images).[75] But in certain patients there are no significant changes in the white matter. Brain stem auditory and somatosensory evoked potentials have been consistently abnormal. Visual evoked potentials give variable results and may be normal. An abnormal vestibulo-ocular reflex has been found in affected children and in female carriers, and an apparently unique combination of elliptical pendular and upbeat nystagmus has been reported with high-resolution oculography. But molecular proof of the disease was lacking in these families.

Pathological Findings   These findings were formerly essential for accurate diagnosis. Morphologically, the cerebral and cerebellar atrophy are marked. In most patients there is a characteristic patchy dysmyelination with only small amounts of sudanophilic degradation products. Small islands of preserved myelin are interspersed throughout the demyelinated zones. The number of oligodendrocytes is reduced. In patients with a neonatal onset, myelin has been found to be practically absent in the central nervous system (this picture corresponds to the so-called Seitelberger variant of Pelizaeus-Merzbacher disease). Nerve cells and axons tend to escape damage and peripheral nerves are always normal.

Genetics, Molecular Biology, Pathophysiology
Pelizaeus-Merzbacher disease is inherited as an X-linked trait mapped to Xq22.[76] Carriers are clinically normal, but some have been said to have white matter abnormalities on MRI scanning.[77]

The disease is due to a deficiency in proteolipid protein (PLP) (one of the major myelin proteins). In approximately 30 percent of cases, a variety of point mutations in the PLP gene have been detected, which are frequently specific to a single family. Complete deletion of the PLP gene and duplications have also been found. The consequence of the PLP gene defect is an inability of oligodendrocytes to form normal myelin and the degeneration of many of them. This dichotomy of action may explain the clinical variations of the disease. Mutations in the PLP gene have also been described in two families with X-linked spastic paraparesis.[78,79] One of these mutations, found in the original X-linked recessive spastic paraplegia family reported by Johnston and McKusik in 1962 is identical to the mutation in the rumpshaker mouse, a PLP-deficient animal model.[80]

Diagnosis   Pelizaeus-Merzbacher disease can be considered highly probable in the presence of a typical clinical picture, lack of myelin on MRI scanning, and evidence for an X-linked transmission.

Diagnosis may be difficult in sporadic cases. Brain biopsies have occasionally been used to substantiate diagnosis and facilitate genetic counseling.

A definitive diagnosis can now be established by the demonstration of a defect in the PLP gene. Carrier detection and prenatal diagnosis (on chorionic villi) are possible using molecular biology techniques.

Treatment   There is no known treatment.

Animal Models   The jimpy mouse, which is similar to Pelizaeus-Merzbacher disease, is the result of a mutation that produces a 74-base deletion in the mRNA for PLP. Another mouse model, the rumpshaker, is defective in DM20, an alternatively spliced transcript of the PLP gene. Although myelin deficient, the rumpshaker mouse, surprisingly, has a normal span of life and a full complement of morphologically normal oligodendrocytes. PLP mutations in the rat and dog have also been identified.

Other Leukodystrophies Related to a Defect of a Myelin Protein   A disorder with absence of *myelin basic protein* has been reported in a 25-year-old woman with involuntary movements, ataxia, and mild mental retardation and in her 18-month-old son. There was evidence of defective myelination on MRI. A deletion of the q22.3-qter region of chromosome 18 was demonstrated. The region of this deletion includes the locus for myelin basic protein (MBP).

The 18q-syndrome is now recognized as one of the most common chromosomal deletion syndromes. It is associated with the loss of the distal part of the long arm of chromosome 18, specifically 18q22.3-qter. Affected individuals exhibit growth deficiency, narrow ear canals with hearing impairment, midfacial hypoplasia, carplike mouth, developmental delay, and mental retardation. Brain MRI scans demonstrate a generalized deficiency of central white matter, and molecular studies have shown reduced amounts of genomic DNA coding for MBP.

It is clear from this example that chromosomal studies should be done in cell cases of leukodystrophies of uncertain origin.

Animal Model   A defect of the MBP gene is found in the shiverer mouse.

Spongy Deterioration of the Nervous System; Canavan-Van Bogaert-Bertrand Disease In 1949, Ludo Van Bogaert and Ivan Bertrand[81] described a new familial disease in three Jewish children, which they defined as "amaurotic idiocy with spongy degeneration of the neuraxis." Myrtil Canavan had previously reported, in 1931, as Schilder disease, a case which was retrospectively found to have the same pathological characteristics as the patients described by Van Bogaert and Bertrand.[82]

Spongy degeneration of the nervous system, or Canavan-Van Bogaert-Bertrand disease, as it is now called, is a recessive autosomal disorder characterized by unique pathological changes in the central nervous system. The disease affects mostly infants of Jewish extraction, and its main clinical features are absence of neurologic development or rapid regression, hypotonia with superimposed tonic spasms, gradual enlargement of the head (megalencephaly), and blindness with optic atrophy (Fig. 3-13). There is a high concentration of *N*-acetylaspartic acid in the brain and urine due to a deficiency of *N*-aspartoacylase.

Clinical Features This summary is based on approximately 100 cases of spongy degeneration of the nervous system that have been reported.[83,84] The disease becomes apparent before 6 months (usually around 3 months) and occasionally in the first weeks of life. Lethargy, difficulty in sucking, frequent crying, listlessness, lack of movement, and hypotonia are the usual manifestations. In cases with neonatal onset there is subsequently no sign of psychomotor development.

In most infants, head control and early signs of psychological development are at first delayed, or if attained secondarily lost, between the ages of 3 and 6 months. Motor activity is reduced. As the disease progresses, initial flaccidity is followed by tonic extensor spasms with retraction of the head, spasticity, and bilateral pyramidal signs. The legs become extended and the arms flexed; the neck when not in spasm usually remains hypotonic. Tonic spasms are evoked by handling and sometimes by noise, but the typical repetitive acoustico-motor response of Tay-Sachs disease (with which this disease had been at first confused) is generally not found. Focal or generalized convulsions are not uncommon. The hands and feet are often held in odd postures and movements are suggestive of choreoathetosis.

Of particular importance for the diagnosis are macrocephaly and blindness. A conspicuously large head is usually noted between the third and sixth months of life. Head circumference slowly enlarges with age, usually remaining between 3 and 4 standard deviations above normal. The increase in head size reaches a plateau in some cases after approximately the third year of life. Blindness and optic atrophy without visible change in the retinas become evident between 6 and 18 months. Blindness is frequently preceded by strabismus and pendular nystagmus. MRI reveals nonspecific diffuse abnormalities in the white matter: hypointensity in T1- and hyperintensity in T2-weighted images. The ventricles become somewhat enlarged at an advanced stage of the disease.

The CSF fluid is usually normal, but a slight elevation of protein has been reported in rare instances. The EEG changes are variable. There is no evidence of peripheral nerve involvement.

No visceral, skeletal, cutaneous, or hematologic abnormalities have been noted. Liver function is normal;

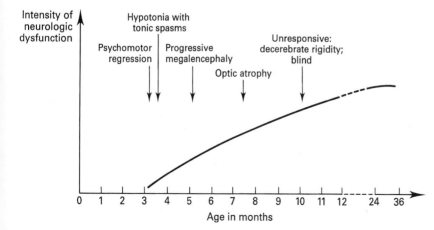

Figure 3-13
Canavan disease. Clinical course and life profile.

fair complexion of the majority of the children has been stressed. In the final stage, children lapse into a state of decerebrate rigidity with pseudobulbar signs. Duration of the disease is usually 1 to 3 years, although survival to 10 or more years has been reported.

Diagnostic   Laboratory   Tests   Considerable amounts of *N*-acetylaspartic acid are excreted in urine, approximately 200 times the amounts found in normal age-matched controls.[85] An elevated level has also been reported in the CSF. *N*-acetylaspartic acid accumulates in the brain, where its signal in early cases can be detected by magnetic resonance spectroscopy.

A profoundly deficient activity of aspartoacylase is found in cultured fibroblasts.

Genetics   Canavan disease is an autosomal recessive disease. The majority of affected children are Jewish, mostly of eastern European origin. The disease has also been observed in natives of Saudi Arabia. Detection of heterozygotes is possible by measuring the activity of aspartoacylase in cultured fibroblasts.

The aspartoacylase gene has been mapped to chromosome 17p13-pter. It spans 29 kb containing 6 exons totaling 1435 base pairs. Among Ashkenazic Jews with Canavan disease, 83 percent of alleles contain the 285Glu→Ala missense mutation and another 13 percent a nonsense mutation at amino acid 231. Nearly 50 percent of alleles in non-Jews with Canavan disease carry a third mutation at amino acid 305, which causes a substitution of glutaric acid for alanine. Testing Ashkenazic Jews for four mutations that account for 99 percent of all the Canavan disease mutations in Ashkenazim has revealed that 1/45 are carriers of the Canavan disease trait.

Prenatal diagnosis is possible by measuring levels of aspartoacylase activity in cultures of chorionic villus or amniocytes, but has proven not to be entirely reliable because of the relatively low levels of the enzyme normally present in these cells. The use of molecular analysis for specific mutations should improve the accuracy of prenatal diagnosis.

Pathologic Findings   The neuropathological features of this disease are unique. They consist of (1) a notable increase in brain weight, which is present in most cases; (2) an absence of myelin, especially in the convolutional white matter; (3) a remarkable spongy change of the lower parts of the cortex, subcortical white matter, and cerebellar cortex; and (4) strikingly enlarged and sometimes monstrous protoplasmic astro-

cytic nuclei (Alzheimer I cells) in most gray matter structures. Ultrastructural morphologic changes in the mitochondria have been observed, without evidence of mitochondrial dysfunction.

Pathophysiology   *N*-acetylaspartic acid is concentrated in brain gray matter and in the white matter, where it is not normally found. *N*-acetylaspartic acid may be toxic to oligodendroglial cells. Since aspartoacylase is primarily a white matter enzyme, it is probable that it acts to protect white matter from *N*-acetylaspartic acid. Its deficiency in Canavan disease could therefore lead to white matter degeneration by the accumulation of *N*-acetylaspartate.

Differential Diagnosis   The following are included in the differential diagnosis: (1) all early infantile encephalopathies with progressive enlargement of the head, essentially Alexander disease, and G_{M2} gangliosidosis, (2) fixed, nonprogressive encephalopathies with megalencephaly, and (3) hydrocephalus, which must be excluded when the ventricles are enlarged.

Treatment   There is no known treatment.

Alexander   Disease   (Leukodystrophy   with Rosenthal Fiber Formation)   This disease, a rare disorder of unproved genetic origin, was first recognized by Alexander in 1949.[86] It is characterized by a unique morphologic change in the astrocytes of the central nervous system, the Rosenthal fibers. A protein, alpha B-crystallin, accumulates in the abnormal astrocytes. In the usual infantile form, megalencephaly psychomotor retardation and seizures are characteristic. In childhood and adulthood, the neurologic symptomatology is variable. Practically all cases of Alexander disease have been sporadic, but there are too few to exclude a genetic origin. Diagnosis is now frequently possible during life by MRI.

Clinical Features   Our experience with this disease consists of four cases. As with most patients, the disease started in early infancy. By 1982, only about a dozen cases had been reported (Table 3-1) mostly in males. A few reports with pathologic confirmation have been published since then, and a number of cases have been recognized during life by typical changes on MRI. A possible familial incidence has been noted in only one case.[88] The first case in our pathologic series had a brother dying at the same age of "encephalitis." Though not absolutely constant, the major sign of the

Table 3-1

Alexander disease: clinical features of infantile cases reported up to 1982

Patient[a]	Sex	Familial	Onset	Death	Head circumference and brain weight	Large head as first sign
86	M		7 months	18 months	50 cm	+
90	M		5 months	7 years	1970 g	+
88	M		4 months	2 years	45 cm (6 months) 53.7 cm (2 years) 1520 g	+
88	M		Birth	31 months	53 cm (5 months) 1690 g	+
88	F		7 years	15 years	990 g	–
91	M		4 months	22 months	1150 g	–
87	M		8 months	15 months	880 g	+
92	F		4 months	8 months	26 cm (birth)[b] 42 cm (4 months) 45.7 cm (8 months) 780 g	+
93	M		4 years	10 years[c]	58 cm (8 years)	–
93	M		2 months	5 months	850 g	–
94	F	+	6 months	19 months	50 cm 1160 g	+
89	F		8 months	4 years[c]	51 cm (2 years) 58 cm (4 years)	+
95	M		9 months	23 months	800 g	–
96	M		9 months	23 months	800 g	+

Symbols: + = markedly enlarged; – = uncertain.   [b] Premature, birth weight 1160 g.

[a] Numbers refer to reference.   [c] Alive at time of report; brain biopsy.

disease is a progressive enlargement of the head, which becomes evident in early infancy and may already be present at birth. Increasing head size is due to megalencephaly, not to hydrocephalus, although the ventricles are somewhat enlarged late in the disease.

In most patients there is arrest of motor and mental development in early infancy, so that the child never achieves head control or the ability to sit. Signs of increased intracranial pressure with bulging fontanelle or papilledema have been noted in two cases in which there was no evidence of hydrocephalus. In other patients, psychomotor development is at first only slightly delayed and neurologic deterioration and mental retardation do not become evident until the second year of life or later. Spasticity and seizures are usual. The optic fundi, CSF, and EEG disclose no significant changes. The course of the disease is variable. Death occurs after a few months or several years.

An important *variant* has been revealed in a few patients with onset of the disease between the ages of 2 and 14 years and without male predominance. The lesions were typical. The clinical picture was that of slowly progressive neurologic deterioration with bulbar and pseudobulbar signs and a bipyramidal syndrome. In some instances, signs of involvement of corticospinal tracts were at first unilateral or intermittent. Mental function was essentially normal. Head size was not reported. Brain weight was low in one autopsied case.

Finally, there is an *adult variant*, which forms a heterogeneous group. To our knowledge, only one of them had the typical diffuse neuropathological features at autopsy. The disease had started at the age of 32 years with a gradual appearance of left hemiplegia. Initially, it was remitting and then progressive. Signs of brain stem, cerebellar and corticospinal involvement developed subsequently. There was no mental deterioration. A tentative diagnosis of multiple sclerosis had been made. There was no information on head size. At autopsy, at age 47, brain weight was 1080 g, there was focal cavitation (but no diffuse demyelination or atrophy of the white matter) and typical Rosenthal fibers, diffusely. Other cases reported as Alexander disease[89] have had clinical and pathologic features resembling multiple sclerosis. Rosenthal fibers were only present in the demyelinated plaques. Since Rosenthal fibers are not specific for Alexander disease, the interpretation of such cases is uncertain.

Neuroimaging   In view of the uncharacteristic and variable picture of Alexander disease, diagnosis during life rests entirely on the results of MRI. Typically, there is an attenuation of hemispheric white matter predominately in the frontal region, with well-defined areas of increased density in the subventricular and subpial regions and in the central white matter (Fig. 3-14). Contrast enhancement may be necessary to reveal this abnormality which is not always discernible.

Pathologic Findings[90-96]   In the early infantile cases, brain weight is usually increased, sometimes markedly so, up to 1600 g. The specific morphologic findings, the so-called Rosenthal fibers, consist of large numbers of rod-shaped or round bodies that stain red with hematoxylin and eosin and black with myelin stains. These are scattered throughout the cerebral cortex and white matter, with a predominance in the subpial, subependymal and perivascular regions. Ultrastructurally Rosenthal fibers consist of masses of granular osmophilic material dispersed among glial fibrils within the cytoplasm of astrocytes. There are also extracellular argentophilic granular deposits, presumably degenerate glial fibers. In addition, the lack or paucity of myelin is usual, with only a few macrophages with sudanophilic lipids. The degree of involvement of white matter is variable from case to case.

It is noteworthy that focal aggregates of these astrocytic fibers were first described by Rosenthal in 1898 in syringomyelia and they have since been reported in many diseases, such as astrocytomas, craniopharyngiomas, chronic inflammatory processes, and multiple sclerosis.

It has been shown that Rosenthal fibers in Alexander disease contain large proportions of alpha-B crystallin.[97] Alpha B-crystallin is one of the major proteins in the lens and in other nonneurologic tissues, but is also expressed in the brain, where it is present in astrocytes and oligodendrocytes. It is not clear if the extraordinary amounts of this compound that accumulate in the brain in Alexander disease are the result of increased synthesis or reduced turnover of the protein. The role of this bio-

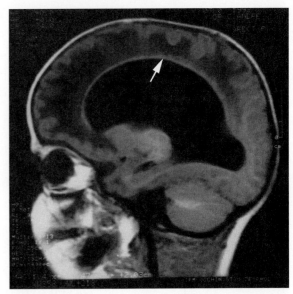

Figure 3-14
Alexander disease. MRI. Attenuation of white matter predominating frontally. Periventricular linear hyperdensification (arrow). (Courtesy Dr. Ponsot.)

chemical finding in the pathogenesis of Alexander disease and the coincident myelin loss remain obscure.

Diagnosis   The diagnosis of Alexander disease should be considered in all infants with signs of neurologic dysfunction of leukoencephalopathic nature and progressive megalencephaly. The results of the CT scan and MRI are of great help and may, when typical, be considered sufficient for the diagnosis. An increase in the CSF level of alpha B-crystallin provides further confirmation of the diagnosis.

In juvenile and adult cases, clinical symptomatology is in no way characteristic, and the possibility of Alexander disease can only be raised in the presence of suggestive neuroradiological findings and proven by way of a brain biopsy.

Treatment   There is no known treatment.

Hereditary Metabolic Disorders with Cutaneous Signs and Frequent Seizures

Disorders of Biotin Metabolism   The four human carboxylases: pyruvate carboxylase, propionyl-CoA carboxylase, β-methylcrotonyl-CoA carboxylase (all located in the mitochondria) and acetyl-CoA carboxylase (in the cytosol), which participate in fatty acid synthesis, amino acid catabolism and gluconeogenesis, are devoid of catalytic activity unless biotin (a B-complex vitamin) is bound to the apoenzymes. There are two defects in the cycle of biotin utilization, which result in multiple carboxylase synthetase deficiencies: biotinidase deficiency and holocarboxylase deficiency. Biotinidase deficiency and some cases of holocarboxylase deficiency are biotin responsive (see also Chap. 2). Isolated deficiencies of one of these carboxylases are not responsive to treatment with biotin.

Biotinidase Deficiency ("Late Onset" Multiple Carboxylase Deficiency)   Biotinidase cleaves biotin from biocytin. Deficiency of biotinidase causes a shortage of free biotin (a vitamin belonging to the B complex), which results in a dysfunction of three mitochondrial carboxylases: propionyl-CoA carboxylase, pyruvate carboxylase, and β-methylcrotonyl-CoA carboxylase.

Clinical Features of Biotinidase Deficiency   Since its first description by Wolf et al. in 1983, sporadic reports of profound biotinidase deficiency have been published. There are also two large series of 31[98] and 68 cases[99] in the literature.

The first symptoms usually appear between 3 and 6 months of age. In some cases, onset is in the neonatal period (Chap. 2) or in the second year of life. Severe and persistent myoclonic seizures in a child with developmental delay and hypotonia are generally the initial neurologic manifestations. Seizures were noted in more than 75 percent of patients and were usually an early symptom. A persistent laryngeal stridor may be another early sign. A major clue to the diagnosis is the presence of cutaneous signs: skin rashes due to a seborrheic or atopic dermatitis and total or partial alopecia, which are present in 70 percent of cases, and less often, a persistent conjunctivitis. The skin rash and alopecia may appear early in the disease. As the child grows, intermittent ataxia, optic atrophy, and sensorineural hearing loss may appear. Most patients present at some time with episodes of metabolic acidosis with hyperlactacidemia, ketosis, possibly hyperammonemia, and also hypoglycinemia. These episodes are characterized clinically by vomiting, lethargy, hyperventilation (Kussmaul breathing) and then apnea. Some children die in a metabolic coma. Over 80 percent of the patients have an organic aciduria, which may be intermittent and is not an early finding. β-Hydroxyisovaleric acid,

β-methylcrotonylglycine, β-hydroxypropionate, and methylcitrate are excreted in abnormal amounts in the urine. In some patients, there has been evidence of an immunological deficiency, which renders the patient susceptible to potentially lethal fungal and bacterial infections.

Laboratory Findings of Diagnostic Value   Two abnormalities are of great diagnostic value: cutaneous signs and an organic aciduria. Organic aciduria is revealed by gas chromatography, a laboratory procedure that should be applied systematically to all children with a progressive neurologic disorder of unknown origin. However, both the cutaneous signs and the organic aciduria may be absent in the initial phase of the disease or even lacking throughout the course of it. It may be useful to measure organic acids in the CSF.[100] We believe, therefore, that biotinidase deficiency should be considered and a therapeutic trial of biotin should be tried in all infants with severe and persistent seizures and developmental delay.

Final diagnosis rests on the demonstration of a deficiency of biotinidase in serum, leukocytes, or cultured fibroblasts. Residual activity is usually very low. Biotinidase activity is also low in the CSF. Heterozygotes can be detected by these methods. Prenatal diagnosis is possible, and a method exists for neonatal screening of biotinidase deficiency.

Variants   These are found among affected individuals, even within a sibship. In infants with a partial deficiency of biotinidase only a seborrheic dermatitis may be present with no neurologic signs.

Genetics   Biotinidase deficiency is an autosomal recessive disorder with an incidence estimated at 1/40,000 births. The gene for biotinidase is on chromosome 3p25. In some patients a major deletion has been identified.

Pathology   Postmortem findings in two children consisted in cerebellar atrophy with loss of Purkinje cells and granule cells; focal areas of necrosis in the cerebrum, cerebellum, and spinal cord; and in one case there was evidence of a "viral encephalitis".

Treatment   Treatment with biotin (5 to 20 mg/day orally) results in a remarkable improvement of cutaneous and neurologic signs. Hearing and visual deficits are more resistant.

Holocarboxylase Synthetase (HS) Deficiency

This disease, which usually starts in the neonatal period, is described in Chap. 2.

In a few patients the disease became manifest in the early or late infantile period with episodes of metabolic acidosis. Developmental delay, seizures, or a skin rash have occasionally preceded an acute metabolic episode. In one child, abnormalities in immunological function were observed.

The human HS gene has been cloned and assigned to chromosome 21q22.1. Several mutations in this gene that have been described are present in the biotin binding domain.[101,102]

Menkes Disease (Steely Hair Disease; Kinky Hair Disease)

Menkes disease is an X-linked hereditary disorder in which insufficient intestinal absorption of copper leads to copper deficiency. Although the primary cellular abnormality remains obscure, defective synthesis of copper enzymes apparently explains most features of the disease. A very early onset of hair abnormalities, abnormal facial appearance, profound neurologic disorder resulting in seizures and rapid neurological deterioration, hypothermia, arterial degeneration, osteoporosis and other skeletal changes, urinary tract abnormalities, and a generally rapidly fatal course constitute the major features of this multisystem disorder. Serum copper and ceruloplasmin levels are very low. In biopsy specimens, copper content is very low in the liver and greatly increased in the intestinal mucosa. Brain copper is reduced. The copper content of cultured fibroblasts is elevated and there is an increased uptake of labeled copper. A truly effective treatment has not yet been devised. A mild form of the disorder has been observed in a few patients.[103] The *occipital horn syndrome* is a closely related disease reported in the literature (Fig. 3-15).

Clinical Features In affected boys, premature delivery, neonatal hypothermia, and hyperbilirubinemia are frequent. Failure to thrive is noted early. Arrest of neurologic development becomes manifest before the third month. Smiling, awareness of surroundings, and head control are either never achieved or are rapidly lost. Lethargy, reduced motility, and spasticity with pyramidal signs appear later. Frequent seizures, whether generalized or focal, are nearly constant manifestations and often occur early in the course of the disease. Multiple asymmetric myoclonic jerks, set off by various types of stimulation, may be elicited. The EEG usually shows multifocal spike and slow-wave activity. The CSF is normal. The optic disks are frequently pale. Retinal degeneration and microcysts of the iris may be found.

The clinical hallmark of the disease is the remarkable appearance of the hair and eyebrows. The hair growth is sparse; hair shafts are poor in pigment and wiry. Many hairs are broken and form a short stubble. Under the microscope the characteristic twisting of the hair shaft, called pili torti, is easily seen (Fig. 3-16). This abnormality becomes more evident after a few weeks of life. The primary hair at birth is usually normal. Seborrheic dermatitis is sometimes present. Nails and teeth are normal but the teeth erupt late. The facial appearance and pallor attract notice—a combination of pudgy cheeks, horizontal and twisted eyebrows, a highly arched palate, and micrognathia. Recurrent episodes of hypothermia and a susceptibility to infections are points of medical interest. Anemia has not been present. Subdural hematomas with skull enlargement are not rare. Otherwise, head growth is at first normal and later tends to be reduced. Skeletal x-rays show a variety of abnormalities, including osteoporosis, metaphyseal spurring with spiky protrusions, diaphyseal periosteal reaction, scalloping of the posterior aspects of the vertebral bodies, and excessive Wormian bone formation (Fig. 3-16). Fractures of the ribs or other bones are frequent. The combination of fractures and a subdural hematoma may lead erroneously to suspicion of child abuse.

Angiography and magnetic resonance techniques reveal remarkable tortuosities, elongations, and variations in caliber of cerebral arteries, and abnormally positioned and supernumerary vessels. Similar changes as well as arterial occlusions are found in the vasculature of limbs, trunk, and viscera. There are diverticuli of bladder and ureters which may rupture and lead to infection; hydronephrosis is another common finding, which may result in serious problems in children who survive for some time. Laxity of skin and joints may be observed. Pulmonary emphysema has been reported. CT scans and MRI may show evidence of cerebral atrophy, focal areas of necrosis, and cerebellar atrophy. Most children die before the age of 18 months, but some have lived with severe neurologic deficits and a variety of medical complications for several years.

Laboratory Findings of Diagnostic Importance In most cases, diagnosis can be made on clinical and radiological grounds. Microscopic examination of the hair is particularly helpful.

Very low levels of serum copper and ceruloplasmin will confirm the clinical impression. As ceruloplasmin and serum copper are normally low in neonates, the

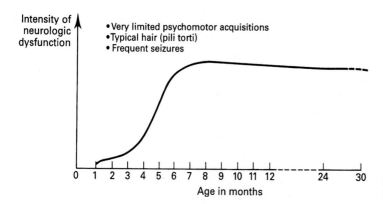

Figure 3-15

Menkes disease. Clinical course and life profile.

significance of this finding cannot be interpreted before the age of 2 to 3 weeks. If doubt persists, assay of copper in liver and intestinal mucosa biopsies and studies of cell cultures can be undertaken. Copper is greatly reduced in the liver and markedly increased in the jejunal mucosa. In cultured fibroblasts copper content is increased. Uptake of administered ^{64}Cu over 24 hours is increased, and its release is reduced. Deficient activity of copper enzymes can be demonstrated in cell cultures, but this test is of little practical use.

The predicted protein encodes a copper-transporting ATPase with similarities to the gene product for Wilson disease. Deletions in the 8.5 kb Menkes transcript have been detected in 13 percent of patients.[104]

Genetics   Menkes disease is inherited as an X-linked trait. The mutant gene is located on the X chromosome in the q13.3 region and has been cloned. Its estimated incidence is 1 to 2 per 100,000 live male births.

About half of the heterozygotes have pili torti. Patchy suntanning in white heterozygotes and mosaic skin depigmentation in black female carriers have been noted.

Full expression of the disease has been reported in three girls.[105] Typical abnormalities in cultured cells are found in some but not all heterozygotes, and this complicates the detection of carriers. Disturbances of copper metabolism in cultured amniocytes or chorionic villi can be used for prenatal diagnosis of Menkes disease in specialized laboratories. In families at risk, mutation analysis may ultimately prove to be the most effective method for heterozygote detection and prenatal analysis.

Pathology   The brain and the cerebellum are atrophic. The cerebral hemispheres exhibit diffuse and focal zones of tissue destruction and gliosis, some of which are clearly the result of vascular occlusion and ischemia. Lesions are particularly severe in the cerebellum. There is also an atrophy of the granular layer and loss of Purkinje cells. The remaining Purkinje cells show abnormal dendritic expansions and processes radiating from the perikaryon, some of which may have occurred prenatally. Abnormal mitochondria have been seen under the electron microscope. In the retina, the ganglion cells are reduced in number and there are microcysts in the pigmentary epithelium. The optic nerve is demyelinated. The arterial changes consist of disruption of the internal elastic lamina and intimal thickening. Such vascular alterations are found in all organs of the body.

The copper content of the brain and liver is markedly reduced and is high in the intestinal mucosa and kidney. The structural abnormality in the hair is due to defective disulfide bonding in keratin.

Pathophysiology and Clinicopathologic Correlations   The basic defect and pathophysiology of Menkes disease remain obscure but a few points have finally been clarified. There is a defective absorption of copper by the intestinal mucosa; copper distributions in the tissues are abnormal (elevated in the intestinal mucosa, kidney, and skin fibroblasts; low in liver and brain); synthesis of copper-containing enzymes is defective (reduced levels of activity of these enzymes have been demonstrated); copper given parenterally does not fully correct the defective synthesis of copper enzymes.

Most of the manifestations of the disease can be explained by a deficiency of the following copper-requiring (linked) enzymes: a deficiency in cytochrome-*c* oxidase and dopamine β-hydroxylase cause the neuronal lesions; deficiency in tyrosinase is responsible for failure of pigmentation, and the deficiency in lysyl oxidase pro-

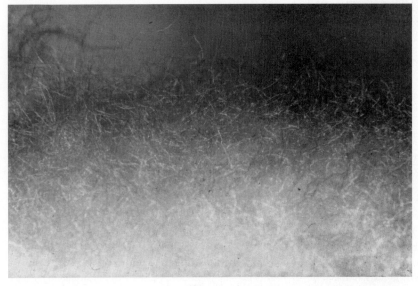

(A)

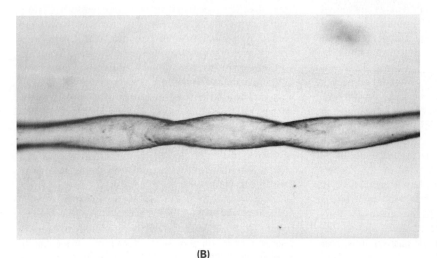

(B)

Figure 3-16
Menkes disease. **A.** *Typical hair: scarce, colorless and friable.* **B.** *Hair shaft as seen under the microscope: pili torti.*

duces a defect in elastin and collagen cross-linking and results in the arterial abnormalities, bladder diverticulae, loose skin and joints, and possibly osteoporosis. Skeletal demineralization would be predicted on the basis of ascorbate oxidase deficiency. Brain lesions are probably the result of both ischemic necrosis and a deficient activity in dopamine β-hydroxylase and cytochrome oxidase. It is probable that many of the effects of the disease begin in utero.

Further research into the pathogenesis and treatment of Menkes disease may be advanced by the study of mottled and brindled mice mutants, which bear a close resemblance to Menkes disease.

Treatment No treatment is fully effective. Copper histidinate, sulfate, glycinate, and other forms of copper have been given parenterally. Daily injections of copper seem to restore normal levels of copper in the serum and liver, but not in the brain. In most cases the treatment has no effect on progressive neurologic deterioration.

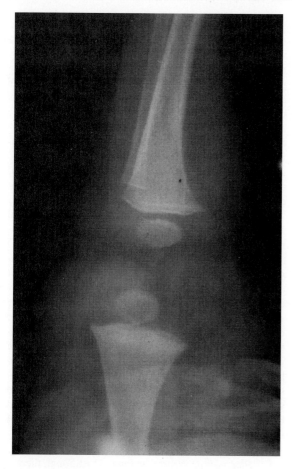

Figure 3-16 (contd.)
C. X-ray film of knee: flaring of metaphyses and bony protrusions.

An exception to this statement may obtain when some children are treated very early. This has led to the suggestion that it might be worthwhile to induce a premature delivery in affected fetuses, or even to start treatment before birth.[105]

Variants

1. *Mild Menkes disease.* In two boys, the disease started after age 2 years. Neurological signs consisted of cerebellar ataxia and mild intellectual deficit. Pili torti, joint laxity, and urinary tract diverticulae were present. Laboratory investigations confirmed the diagnosis.[105]

2. *The occipital horn syndrome.* This disorder, which is now considered as a variety of Menkes disease,

has only been described in a few families. Affected children have only a mild mental deficit or signs of autonomic dysfunction but no other neurological signs. Skin and joint laxity, inguinal hernias, and bladder diverticulae constitute important manifestations of the disease. Chronic diarrhea has been reported. The radiological changes are characteristic. These consist of ossified occipital "horns" and morphological changes in the clavicles and long bones. There may be arterial changes. Laboratory investigations show the same abnormality in copper metabolism as in Menkes disease. Lysyl oxidase levels are low in cultured fibroblasts.

In these milder Menkes phenotypes, mutations have been found in the Menkes disease gene which impair, but do not abolish, mRNA splicing.[106]

Syndromes with Severe Seizures as a Constant Sign

Alpers Syndrome Alpers disease, progressive degeneration of the cerebral gray matter,[107] progressive infantile poliodystrophy,[108] and spongy glioneural dystrophy,[109] are the names given to a clinicopathologic syndrome which probably includes a number of different familial disorders. It can be defined as a rapidly progressive encephalopathy with intractable seizures and diffuse neuronal degeneration.

The lack of specificity of both its clinical and pathologic features has resulted in the application of the term Alpers syndrome to several different conditions, unrelated in terms of genetics and other causal factors. In fact, in many patients reported in the past as having Alpers disease, neurologic signs have followed (or have been aggravated by) such acute accidents as status epilepticus, severe dehydration, hyperthermia, circulatory collapse, inhalation asphyxia, or hypoglycemia.[110] In other children, perinatal brain damage was obviously present.[111] These cases do not belong in the Alpers syndrome category. Another difficulty relates to the interpretation of brain lesions on which the diagnosis of Alpers syndrome heavily relies. It may be difficult to decide if they are the expression of an underlying encephalopathy or are merely secondary to severe and lasting seizures, which may be caused by a variety of disorders.

Nevertheless, a critical review of the literature shows that there is a core group of familial, cryptogenic, rapidly progressive encephalopathies with intractable seizures and widespread neuronal degeneration to which the name of Alpers syndrome can be applied, at least provisionally. It has become increasingly evident that many, but not all, of the patients with Alpers syndrome also have liver disease.[112] This subgroup, which apparently constitutes a coherent entity, has been referred to as the Alpers-Huttenlocher syndrome. We describe here the clinical and pathologic characteristics of Alpers syndrome with and without liver disease.

The Alpers-Huttenlocher Syndrome (Progressive Neuronal Degeneration with Liver Disease; Early Childhood Hepatocerebral Degeneration) Harding has reviewed 32 autopsied cases of this condition.[113] Two siblings were affected in six of the families. In 22 patients the disease started between the ages of 2 and 13 months, 7 in the second year of life, and 3 in late childhood or adolescence. The clinical features were fairly stereotyped. Delivery and the neonatal period were normal. Seizures generally appeared after a period of slow motor and mental development, with failure to thrive and occasional vomiting. Rarely did they constitute the first event. The seizures usually started abruptly, which may be misleading, displayed a variety of clinical expressions, and became intractable with episodes of status epilepticus. Rapid neurological deterioration and blindness ensued. Evidence of overt liver disease (hepatomegaly, jaundice) were occasionally found late in the course of the disease, but biochemical evidence of liver dysfunction and changes in liver biopsies were usually present at or even before the onset of seizures. Characteristic abnormalities in the EEG consisted of very slow waves of high amplitude, mixed with low-amplitude polyspikes. Visual evoked potentials were altered and gradually became extinct. The electroretinogram was normal.

CT scans showed progressive cerebral atrophy with low-density lesions in the medial part of the occipital lobes (Fig. 3-17). Changes in liver biopsy specimens consisted of fatty infiltration, hepatocyte loss, bile duct proliferation, fibrosis, and cirrhosis. In Harding's series, two-thirds of patients died before the age of three. A few had a much more protracted course. At autopsy, the cortical lesions had a diffuse but irregularly patchy distribution, more marked in the calcarine regions. They consisted of severe loss of nerve cells, giving the tissue a loose, spongy appearance and gliosis.

Alpers Syndrome without Liver Disease In a number of typical autopsied cases of Alpers syndrome the liver is apparently normal (see for instance Jellinger[109]). One of us has encountered four such cases, all sporadic, in a period of six years. The clinical

presentation was identical to that described above. Onset of seizures was often abrupt, usually in a child with prior psychomotor delay. Seizures were of many types, generalized, partial or multifocal, with changing patterns in individual patients. A marked myoclonic component was characteristic. Status epilepticus occurred, occasionally followed by prolonged coma or a transient hemiplegia. As myoclonus increased, incoordination of movements became severe. Motor and mental deterioration progressed rapidly. Blindness and optic atrophy were frequent in the latter part of the clinical course. Duration of life from onset of seizures was generally 6 months to 2 years.

In the four cases we have studied, two had cortical and subcortical gray matter lesions consisting of neuronal loss, spongiosis (frequently in a laminar distribution) and marked astrocytosis of the type described by Jellinger as spongy neuroglial dystrophy[109] and similar to that of the Alpers-Huttenlocher syndrome. There was, however, no occipital predominance. In two patients, there was merely widespread, irregularly diffuse, nonspecific neuronal degeneration with mild astrocytosis. The distribution of neuronal loss had none of the characteristic water-shed distribution of lesions seen in the postepileptic or anoxic-ischemic encephalopathies. The relationship between the cases of Alpers disease with and without liver involvement is unclear. It is possible that liver damage could have occurred later in the course of the disease if the child had survived.

Diagnosis of Alpers Syndromes Although there is no specific treatment, it is important to recognize Alpers syndrome during life because of its potentially familial nature. In our opinion the following criteria are required: (1) a rapidly progressive encephalopathy with intractable seizures usually with a myoclonic component and no evidence of retinal degeneration; (2) evidence of progressive brain atrophy with increasing degree of involvement of the cerebral cortex and sparing of white matter in successive CT or MRI scans; (3) absence of an antecedent acute event that could result in cortical destruction (this may be difficult to decide when the disease starts abruptly with status epilepticus); and (4) no evidence of a metabolic disorder, especially that of early infantile lipofuscinosis, which also gives rise to myoclonus and rapid cerebral atrophy with neuronal degeneration (Chap. 4). The problem of a possible mitochondrial dysfunction is discussed below.

In any patient conforming to this description, liver function should be tested and a liver biopsy is justified. If there is unquestionable evidence of a liver

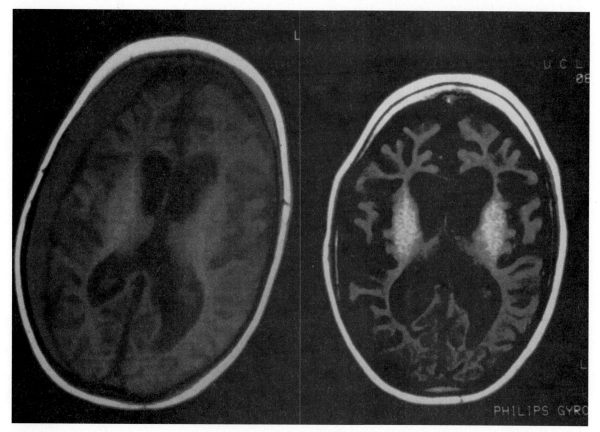

Figure 3-17
Alpers syndrome. Successive brain MR images of infant at 6 months (left) (with extradural blood effusion) and at 14 months to show rapid brain atrophy (striatum is hyperdense) (case with autopsy).

disorder, the diagnosis of Alpers-Huttenlocher syndrome can reasonably be made. If the liver is intact, the diagnosis depends solely on the neuropathological findings (although the comparison of successive MRI films may be very suggestive). A cerebral biopsy can be considered an acceptable procedure in carefully selected cases and with informed consent of the parents, knowing that the biopsy may not be conclusive.

Etiology   The cause (or causes) of Alpers syndrome remain obscure. An autosomal recessive transmission of the disease is a strong possibility in some families, especially those with the Huttenlocher variant.

In several recent reviews, Alpers syndrome is categorized as a mitochondrial disorder because some authors have reported a deficiency in mitochondrial enzymes of the respiratory chain.[114] However, both

the clinical and pathologic characteristics of these patients do not conform strictly to the criteria of Alpers disease, and we believe that evidence is lacking for inclusion of Alpers syndrome in the list of mitochondrial diseases.

Noteworthy is the fact that cortical spongiosis in Alpers syndrome and in Creutzfeld-Jakob disease are in some cases similar. The hypothesis that both disorders could have a similar infectious origin was strengthened when Manuelidis and Rorke[115] recently reported that they were able to induce a spongiform encephalopathy in hamsters injected with brain tissue from a child with Alpers syndrome. This finding has not been confirmed by others.

Clinicopathologic Correlations   Clinical and pathologic evidence are strongly against the brain lesions being secondary to liver dysfunction. Also, it is unlikely that valproate, which may be utilized for seizure control, is responsible for liver lesions. But this medication may possibly aggravate liver lesions.

Treatment There is no specific treatment.

Glucose Transporter Protein Deficiency: DeVivo Disease Ten patients (six boys and four girls) with this condition have been recently reported by DeVivo et al.[116,117] The disease usually starts in infancy with severe seizures. Later, various degrees of mental retardation, motor delay and clumsiness, impaired language, and deceleration of head growth develop. No significant changes were observed in the EEG, and neuroimaging was unremarkable. The hallmark of the disease is a reduced CSF glucose value (30.6 ± 0.32 mg/dL) and a low CSF/blood glucose ratio (0.33 ± 0.07). CSF lactate concentrations are also decreased (0.97 ± 0.03 mM/L). Remarkably, seizures promptly responded to a ketogenic diet (ketone bodies provide energy for brain metabolism and do not depend on the transport of glucose).

There is a reduced uptake of glucose in erythrocytes and reduced immunoreactivity of the human glucose transport protein Glut1. Parents are clinically and biologically normal. It is thought that this condition represents a spontaneous mutation, patients being symptomatic heterozygotes. These observations suggest that in the evaluation of infantile seizures of uncertain origin, CSF glucose should be measured.

Hyper-beta-alalinemia One such patient started at the age of 7 weeks to exhibit lethargy and intractable seizures. The cerebral ventricles were enlarged. Death occurred at the age of 6 months.

An Oculocerebrorenal Syndrome: Lowe Syndrome

Lowe oculocerebrorenal syndrome is an X-linked hereditary disease[118] caused by a deficiency of Golgi phosphatidylinositol 4,5-bisphosphate 5-phosphatase activity.[118a] It is characterized by ocular abnormalities, mainly congenital cataracts and glaucoma, special facial features, marked hypotonia with absent tendon reflexes, severe mental deficiency, and renal tubular disorder with rickets. Glomerular dysfunction appears later, resulting in renal failure in early adolescence. Female carriers can be identified by the detection of lens opacities.

Clinical Features Approximately 100 patients with Lowe syndrome were known to exist in the United States up to 1991. Bilateral nuclear or posterior cataracts are present at birth. The eyes are frequently large with megalocornea and buphthalmos, but they may be of normal size or even small in spite of increased intraocular tension. Glaucoma is present in the majority of cases. Corneal opacities may develop at a later stage. Amblyopia is attended by random oscillatory movements of the eyes. Between 3 and 6 months of age, it becomes apparent that the child suffers a delay in neurologic development and is markedly hypotonic with increased passive mobility of joints. Deep tendon reflexes are usually absent or depressed; they may have been normal initially but disappear after several months. Studies of nerve conduction velocities have been sparse. There is mild slowing and evidence in muscle of denervation in some cases, but not in others. A sural nerve biopsy in a 14-year-old patient showed a decreased number of myelinated fibers, without evidence of demyelination of the remaining axons.[119] There are no pyramidal signs and no paralysis. After the age of 6 months, the infant's hand movements are typical of the blind—slow movements of the hands with extended fingers held before the eyes and rubbing and pressing on the eyes with the fingers. Many of the infants emit a characteristic high-pitched cry. Seizures are rare. Mental retardation becomes more evident as the months pass. The head circumference is normal.

In the second half of the first year of life, growth retardation and the unusual facial features become evident (Fig. 3-18). The facial features comprise a prominent frontal bone, sunken eyes, flaring ears, pale skin, and in some instances, retrognathism. The bone abnormalities take the form of diffuse demineralization and there are typical rachitic deformities consequent upon renal tubular dysfunction.

As the disease progresses, the growth rate slows and renal dysfunction progresses. There is renal tubular acidosis with persistent hyperchloremic acidosis and evidence of progressive glomerular damage resulting in renal failure after the age of 10 years. Late in the disease, arthropathy with noninflammatory joint swellings (of obscure origin) may occur. If responsive to symptomatic treatment, patients may survive into adulthood.

Biochemical Findings Renal tubular dysfunction (Fanconi syndrome) is present in early infancy and persists in later life.[120] It is manifested by proteinuria, which includes both albumin and other proteins of low molecular weight (with a high proportion of β_2-microglobulin); aminoaciduria with a relative sparing of branched

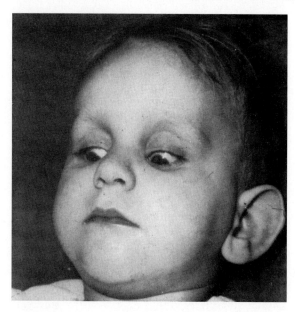

Figure 3-18
Lowe disease. Typical facial appearance: prominent forehead, broad root of nose, large eyes, flaring ears. (Courtesy P. Royer.)

chain amino acids; and phosphaturia with hypophosphatemia. In the serum of many patients there are elevated levels of total protein, increased concentration of α_2-globulin, high concentration of acid phosphatase, elevation of high-density lipoprotein cholesterol, and elevation of creatine kinase. The latter finding suggests involvement of muscle. Blood amino acid concentrations are normal.

Genetics   Lowe syndrome is an X-linked disorder mapped to Xq24-26. Female carriers can be identified by the characteristic lens opacities.[121] Some of them have been fully affected by the disease when they have had an X autosomal translocation. The break point has been placed at Xq25-q26. This information led to the cloning of a gene which encodes a protein with 71 percent homology to human inositol polyphosphate-5-phosphatase, suggesting that Lowe syndrome is an inborn error of inositol phosphate metabolism. This could explain the appearance of cataracts in this disease, since abnormalities in inositol metabolism are believed to be involved in the formation of cataracts in two other diseases, diabetes mellitus

and galactosemia. Assay of phosphatidylinositol 4,5-bisphosphate 5-phosphatase activity has been suggested as a diagnostic test. Mutations in the Lowe syndrome gene have been detected in affected patients.[122]

Neuropathology   Unsettled at this time.

Treatment   Only symptomatic treatment is available. Early phosphate and vitamin D may prevent the development of severe rickets. Glaucoma, when present, must be treated by appropriate medical or surgical means.

Organoacidopathies with Dystonia or Choreoathetosis

Glutaric Aciduria Type I   The clinical presentation of this disease is variable with an acute neurological syndrome in the first weeks or months of life (Chap. 2) or an extrapyramidal disorder in late infancy or early childhood. Progressive dystonia is the most characteristic clinical manifestation. The movement disorder may start out gradually or abruptly, following an infection. Acute episodes of ketoacidosis may occur. On MRI an underdevelopment of the temporal lobes, a "bat-wings" dilation of the Sylvian fissures, and lesions of the lenticular nuclei are characteristic (Fig. 3-19).

This autosomal recessive disease is due to a deficiency of glutaryl-CoA dehydrogenase, a mitochondrial enzyme. It is diagnosed by the detection of glutaric and 3-hydroxyglutaric acids in urine and confirmed by enzyme assays in cultured fibroblasts. Carrier detection has been achieved by measurement of glutaryl-CoA dehydrogenase activity in interleukin-2 dependent cultured lymphocytes.[125]

Glutaric aciduria type I is treated with a special diet in which the intake of lysine and tryptophan are controlled and supplemented with L-carnitine and riboflavin (see also p. 106).

3-Methylglutaconic Acidemia without 3-Methylglutaconyl-CoA Hydrolase Deficiency   Approximately 15 patients have been described with this condition. Neurologic regression starts around 6 months of age. The progressive encephalopathy comprises choreoathetosis, spastic paraplegia, dementia, and later, tapetoretinal degeneration, optic atrophy, and sensorineural deafness.

Levels of 3-methylglutaconate and 3-methylglutarate are elevated in urine. Amniotic fluid levels for these

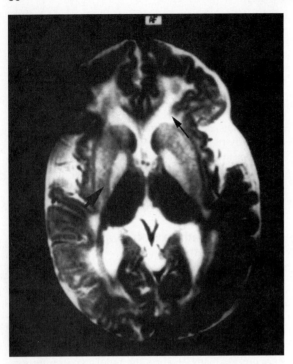

Figure 3-19
Glutaric aciduria type I. MR T2-weighted image. Widening of Sylvian fissures; intense signals from striatum, pallidum, and frontal white matter (arrows). (Courtesy Dr. D'Hooghe.)

metabolites can be measured for prenatal diagnosis of this disorder.[123] Assays for 3-methylglutaconyl-CoA hydrolase are normal.

3-Methylglutaconic Acidemia with 3-Methylglutaconyl-CoA Hydratase Deficiency This condition has been reported in two brothers with speech retardation and fasting hypoglycemia in one of them. 3-Methylglutaconic acid was elevated in the urine. A third patient has been described whose development has been normal.[124]

Disorders of Amino Acids or Organic Acids with Ataxia

One disorder of γ-aminobutyric acid (GABA) metabolism presents with ataxia: succinic semialdehyde dehydrogenase deficiency. Other rare disorders of GABA metabolism have different presentations.

Succinic Semialdehyde Dehydrogenase Deficiency This disorder has been reported in at least 32 children.[126] It is characterized by nonprogressive ataxia, psychomotor retardation, hypotonia, hyporeflexia, aggressive behavior, and occasionally, choreoathetosis and convulsions. Episodic metabolic decompensation or metabolic acidosis have not been observed. Atrophy of the cerebellum may be shown on MRI. The hallmark of the disease is the presence of 4-hydroxybutyric acid in urine, plasma, and CSF, a consequence of the accumulation of succinic semialdehyde. (4-Hydroxybutyric acid is not detectable in normal children.) Free GABA concentrations may be high in the CSF as are those of homocarnosine, a GABA peptide. The enzyme deficiency has been demonstrated in lymphocytes and has been reported in prenatal diagnosis of an affected fetus. Treatment with γ-vinyl GABA, an antiepileptic drug which causes inhibition of GABA transaminase (the enzyme that controls succinic semialdehyde dehydrogenase) has been effective.

Disorders of GABA Metabolism *GABA transaminase deficiency* has been described in two infants of one Flemish family. They presented with profound hypotonia, hyperreflexia, seizures, and neurological delay and died at 1 and 2 years of age, respectively. There was an acceleration of body length.
Other disorders of GABA metabolism probably exist.[126] Measurements of GABA and homocarnosine in the CSF are therefore recommended in all nonprogressive cerebellar ataxias and nonspecific encephalopathies.

L-2-Hydroxyglutaric Acidemia This disorder, which gives rise to cerebellar atrophy and progressive cerebellar ataxia, starts between the ages of 18 months and 10 years. It is described in Chap. 5.

Inborn Errors of Amino Acids, Organic Acids, and Carbohydrate Metabolism with Isolated Cognitive and Behavioral Abnormalities

Practically all amino acidopathies and organoacidopathies may, in addition to their more frequent acute or intermittent forms, manifest themselves by uncharacteristic mental retardation. One example is maple syrup urine disease. Another is nonketotic hyperglycinemia, usually expressed as an extremely severe neurologic disorder in the neonate, but occasionally taking the form of nonprogressive mental retardation, an early infantile progressive encephalopathy, or a complex spinocerebellar or motor neuron disorder. In other aminoacidopathies and in some disorders of carbohydrate metabolism, the only consequence of the accumulation of the offending metabolites in the body is reflected in severe cognitive defects and behavioral disturbances, and occasionally, seizures. Three diseases of this type will be considered here, all of which can be detected by neonatal screening and are relatively frequent:

Phenylketonuria, the prototype of this category of disease, in which normalization of phenylalanine levels in the blood prevents development of mental retardation, although some degree of cognitive deficit usually remains.

Histidinemia, in which the relationship to the accumulation of histidine in the body and the occurrence of mental retardation, if any, remains uncertain.

Galactosemia, a condition in which a galactose-free diet does not effectively prevent the development of intellectual deficits.

Imperfections of our knowledge of the pathogenesis of brain damage in these conditions hampers our ability to devise entirely satisfactory treatments.

Phenylketonuria and the Hyperphenylalaninemias

Phenylketonuria (PKU), one of the most frequent inborn errors of metabolism, is an autosomal recessive disease caused by a deficiency of hepatic phenylalanine hydroxylase (PAH). Evidence of brain damage appears when infants affected with this mutation are exposed to phenylalanine, an essential amino acid that accumulates in the body as a consequence of the metabolic block. In most developed countries, PKU is now detected by routine neonatal screening, and the neurological consequences of the disease can be prevented by early treatment with a phenylalanine-free diet. The main problems that confront the clinician concern the adherence to the diet and monitoring of phenylalanine, the recognition and treatment of maternal PKU, genetic counseling, and the detection of rare, but neurologically severe, forms of hyperphenylalaninemia related to a deficiency of tetrahydrobiopterin.

Clinical Features   The classical clinical picture of PKU can still be encountered in untreated patients who have escaped neonatal screening or who live in countries in which this procedure is not in general use. The mental retardation is always severe. Major behavioral problems are constant and include hyperkinesia, asociality, withdrawal, or elements of a psychotic syndrome. About 25 percent of patients have generalized seizures and the

EEG is abnormal in most cases. Microcephaly is usual after a few years. In older patients, and in rare instances, a pyramidal syndrome or extrapyramidal signs may appear in a few of the patients. Pigment formation is insufficient, leading frequently to a fair skin, blond hair, and blue eyes. Eczema is usual and scleroderma-like changes have been observed. A peculiar, musky body odor may be noted. It is related to the accumulation of phenylacetic acid, a metabolite of phenylalanine. Physical growth is impaired.

Neuropathological studies in older children, who died with PKU, have shown a reduction in brain volume, loss of myelinated fibers, and gliosis in the white matter. Reduction of neuron size and dendritic arborization have also been described, but the consistency of such findings is uncertain.

Pathogenesis of Brain Disorder   All available clinical and experimental data indicate that high levels of phenylalanine, above 1 mM (1000 μmol/L) according to empirical estimates, constitute the main factor in brain dysfunction. Irreversible brain damage occurs essentially during early brain development (neonatal period and the first postnatal weeks of life). However, recent studies indicate that hyperphenylalaninemia may also continue to alter brain function later in life (see below).

The mechanism of brain derangement remains largely unknown despite much experimental work and a number of hypotheses. A better understanding of the pathogenesis of cerebral dysfunction could prove of great therapeutic importance.

Diagnostic Biochemical Findings: Biochemical and Clinical Phenotypes   The upper limit of blood phenylalanine levels in the newborn is 0.15 mM, and in infants 0.12 mM. PKU patients have blood levels above 1.2 mM (1200 μmol/L). Individuals with lower levels (non-PKU hyperphenylalaninemia) have been subdivided into those with levels between 600 and 1200 μmol/L, which are sometimes referred to as "atypical PKU" and those with concentrations of phenylalanine below 600 μmol/L. The latter category, or "mild form," of PAH deficiency is found in not more than 1 to 2 percent of all cases of PAH deficiency. The residual activity of this enzyme is higher than in classical PKU. Mental retardation apparently does not develop in these children.

Phenylalanine is measured by column chromatography or by other methods. High concentrations of phenylpyruvate are found in the urine. This metabolite gives a green color on the addition of $FeCl_3$ in the urine;

the sensitivity of this test is low. The rate of phenylalanine clearance from plasma after an oral or intravenous load of phenylalanine has been used to classify the different phenotypes, but this method is not entirely reliable. Plasma levels and urinary excretion of dopamine are reduced by raised phenylalanine levels. Total values of urinary pterins are elevated. The neopterin/biopterin ratio and concentration of tetrahydrobiopterin are normal.

Enzyme Assay Assay of PAH activity requires a liver biopsy. The residual activity of the enzyme is less than 1 percent in classical PKU, and 5 to 35 percent in the mild form of PAH deficiency.

Neonatal Screening Screening for PKU is simple. At the end of the first week of life, a capillary blood sample is collected on filter paper or in a glass capillary tube and analyzed for phenylalanine. The most widely used method is the semiquantitative microbiologic inhibition assay designed by Guthrie. Column chromatography or fluorometric methods can also be used. Further strict quantitative measurements of phenylalanine are necessary to initiate and monitor the dietary treatment.

Urinary pterins should be systematically analyzed for the detection of tetrahydrobiopterin deficiency, a malignant form of hyperphenylalaninemia. Dried urine samples on filter paper serve for this purpose.

Genetics PKU is an autosomal recessively inherited disorder. Its overall frequency has been estimated between 1/10,000 and 1/15,000 live births. There are wide regional variations. The human gene for hepatic PAH is located on 12q and has been cloned. A number of restriction fragment length polymorphism (RFLP) haplotypes have been identified. More than 60 different point mutations in the PAH gene have been characterized.[127] Most patients with PKU inherit a combination of mutations and are genetic compounds. There is apparently a molecular basis for the phenotypic heterogeneity of the disease.[128] In view of the recent advances in molecular biology, DNA studies are important for carrier screening and prenatal diagnosis, for predicting the clinical phenotypes, and possibly for orienting therapeutic strategies.

Treatment Treatment of PKU is aimed at lowering blood levels of phenylalanine to normal or near normal values by selective restriction of phenylalanine intake. Dietary phenylalanine should be restricted to between 250 and 500 mg/day and plasma phenylalanine maintained well below 1 mM (1000 µmol/L) and above 0.25 mM (250 µmol/L). Excessive restriction impairs growth. If a phenylalanine-restricted diet is given early, ideally before the end of the first month, the adverse consequences of persistent hyperphenylalaninemia are mostly avoided. When treatment is started later, results are much less favorable. Commercial preparations of phenylalanine-free formulas should be adequate in other nutrients to meet anabolic demand and allow normal growth. In older children, elements of the diet are supplied from natural food. Adaptation of the diet in order to maintain the desired levels of phenylalanine is a difficult task, which requires the help of a nutritionist.

Blood phenylalanine levels should initially be measured at frequent intervals. In infants we recommend an assay every week, then every two weeks. Tolerance of phenylalanine varies among patients, and blood levels may be influenced by intercurrent infections and digestive disorders or poor compliance. The diet is unpalatable and strict adherence is difficult for parents, who need prolonged medical help. The effect of early dietary treatment is highly beneficial.[129] Different studies[129] show that the mean IQ of treated children is approximately 93 with higher scores for patients treated before the end of the first month. Late or nontreated individuals have a mean IQ of 45.

It appears that mental development of some of the patients treated early may not be entirely satisfactory. Intelligence quotients remain lower in affected children than in their parents and unaffected sibs.[130] Treated patients with normal or near normal IQs have deficiencies in conceptual skills and visuospatial abilities, attention deficits, and language impairments. Some studies have shown that a discontinuation of the diet even in adolescence was responsible for a decline in cognitive abilities in some patients.[130] Thus, there is growing evidence that "late hyperphenylalaninemia" may also harm the brain and this possibility should be seriously taken into account when discussing the age at which treatment should be stopped. The duration of treatment has been much discussed. Until recently a discontinuance or a major dietary relaxation at the age of 6 to 8 years has been considered safe by most authors. But this policy must now be seriously questioned, and we agree with those who recommend that dietary treatment should be continued throughout adolescence, and perhaps for life.[129] Gene therapy is a consideration in the future for treatment of PKU.

Maternal PKU   A pregnant woman with PKU is at great risk of harming the child she bears, because of her hyperphenylalaninemia. Since effective treatment of children with PKU is now widespread, maternal PKU has become an important problem of health care, and without correct management it could partly overcome the societal benefits of prevention. An intrapartum maternal plasma level of more than 1.1 mM has been given as a threshold value for the estimation of fetal risk, but defects have been observed at much lower concentrations of maternal phenylalanine.

Children from affected mothers are born with severe neurologic defects, microcephaly, intrauterine growth retardation, cardiac malformations, and other anomalies. All cases of maternal hyperphenylalaninemia, even when plasma levels are in the range of "non-PKU" phenylalaninemia should be strictly treated throughout pregnancy, starting ideally before conception. If this is done, prospects for a normal child will be much improved.

Hyperphenylalaninemia due to Tetrahydrobiopterin Deficiency
Deficiency in tetrahydrobiopterin (BH_4)—a cofactor of PAH—impairs the metabolism of phenylalanine, tyrosine, and tryptophan, resulting in hyperphenylalaninemia and a defect of neurotransmitter synthesis. A deficiency in the activity of three different enzymes—dihydropteridine reductase, 6-pyruvoyltetrahydropterin synthase, and guanine triphosphate cyclohydrolase—is a potential cause of this syndrome. PAH activity remains normal.

Although the incidence of BH_4 deficiency is only 1 to 2 per million live births, compared to 150 per million in the hyperphenylalaninemias related to a deficiency in PAH, this condition should be recognized as early as possible because it gives rise to a devastating neurologic illness. In all neonates with hyperphenylalaninemia, pterins should be looked for in the urine. Dried urine samples on filter paper can be used for this purpose.

Clinical Features   Ninety patients with BH_4 deficiency have been collected worldwide by Dhondt up to 1987.[131] In most of them, progressive neurological symptoms appeared between the ages of 2 and 12 months despite excellent dietary control of phenylalanine. The syndrome comprised mental deterioration, intractable seizures, usually with a myoclonic component, arrest in motor development and microcephaly, and occasionally abnormal movements. Unexplained episodes of hyperthermia and of drowsiness or irritability have been observed. There may be progressive calcification of the basal ganglia and other subcortical regions.

Main Biological Features   There are very low levels of the metabolites norepinephrine, serotonin, and dopamine in plasma, urine, and CSF, which are not corrected by lowering phenylalanine blood levels. Values of these metabolites are only moderately depressed in typical PKU, and they are normalized by a phenylalanine-free diet.

The level and/or pattern of pterins in plasma, urine, and CSF are abnormal. Values are usually expressed as levels of total pterins or of BH_4, neopterin/biopterin ratio, and the ratio of oxidized to reduced forms of pterins. Loading tests with BH_4 induce a fall of plasma phenylalanine concentrations, but this procedure is not always reliable. PAH activity is normal.

In dihydropterine reductase (DHPR) deficiency BH_4 levels are greatly reduced; the neopterin/biopterin ratio is low or normal; pterins are essentially in the oxidized form whereas in normal subjects and in PKU patients they are in reduced form. Diagnosis is confirmed by assay of the activity of DHPR in liver biopsy samples, cultured fibroblasts, leukocytes, red blood cells, and dried blood on filter paper.

Measurement of DHPR activity in amniocytes and DNA analysis may serve for prenatal diagnosis. The DHPR locus is on chromosome 4 at p15.31.

In 6-pyruvoyltetrahydropterin synthase (6PTS) deficiency, a disorder of BH_4 synthesis, patients have a greatly increased neopterin/biopterin ratio. The BH_4 loading tests induce a marked reduction in plasma phenylalanine. Low activity of 6PTS is demonstrable in liver and erythrocytes. Prenatal diagnosis has been performed.[132]

In guanine triphosphate cyclohydrolase (GPT-CH) deficiency, a very rare defect, both neopterin and biopterin are low and the neopterin/biopterin ratio is normal. The specific enzyme deficiency is demonstrated in liver biopsy samples and in lymphocytes.

Treatment of BH_4 deficiency   Treatment includes levodopa, carbidopa, and 5-hydroxytryptophan and restriction of phenylalanine intake. Administration of BH_4 has been recommended. Folinic acid has been considered as a reasonable adjunct therapy. Response to this treatment, when started at the latest 2 months after birth, has been beneficial in some children.

Histidinemia
This is one of the most frequent inborn errors of metabolism, but its pathogenicity

remains in question. Its incidence on newborn screening is 1/10,000. It is transmitted as an autosomal recessive trait.

Until 1970, histidinemia was identified essentially by screening children with mental retardation or some other neurologic abnormality. Of those that were positive, about one-third were said to have mental retardation and one-half speech defects, usually associated with mental deficiency. It was then decided that histidinemia might cause specific speech impairment. Other neurologic abnormalities, such as seizures or ataxia, were occasionally mentioned. Siblings of children with histidinemia were frequently found to be normal.

Since then, several surveys in the United States and Japan based on routine neonatal screening failed to find any neurologic abnormality in children with histidinemia. Nevertheless, a Canadian study concluded that 50 percent of siblings with histidinemia had some neurologic impairment of function compared to the 13 percent of neurological abnormalities in nonhistidinemia siblings.

Scriver and Levy[133,134] suggest that histidinemia is an intrinsically benign condition, which may favor the clinical expression of neurologic signs when the brain has been made vulnerable by a previous pre- or perinatal disorder of another type. Thus there could be an entirely benign asymptomatic form as well as another neurological form of the disorder. The offspring of mothers with histidinemia have been normal.

Biochemical Features and Diagnostic Tests The primary defect in histidinemia is a deficiency of the enzyme histidase, which leads to an inability to metabolize histidine to urocanic acid. As a consequence, histidine accumulates in the body. The blood concentration of histidine increases. Other amino acids are normal (except for an occasional elevation of alanine). Urocanic acid, normally present in blood, is not detectable. Oral loading with L-histidine produces a persistent increase of blood histidine. In the urine, there is a striking increase of the level of histidine (3 to 27 nmol/g creatinine, N < 2 nmol/g creatinine) and of the products of histidine transamination (imidazolepyruvic acid). The urinary metabolite imidazolepyruvic acid can usually but not consistently be detected by ferric chloride (upon dipping the phenistic reagent in the urine). Histidine is also increased in the CSF. The deficient activity of histidinase can be demonstrated on the skin. Liver histidase is also low. Chromatographic analysis of the skin shows that urocanic acid is practically absent. The histidase gene has been assigned to chromosome 12q22-q23. It has

been cloned and mutations identified among its 21 exons.

Treatment The biochemical abnormalities are brought under control when children are fed with formulas containing little or no histidine (histidine intake of 20 to 30 mg/kg/day during the first year of life, and thereafter 10 to 20 mg/kg/day). A skin rash may appear when histidine levels are too low. But this diet has no effect on preexisting neurologic abnormalities.

Histidinuria This rare disorder is characterized by increased urinary excretion of histidine and normal levels of histidine in blood. It probably results from a specific defect of intestinal and renal transport. Five children from four families have been reported. All were males. They presented with mental retardation and/or myoclonic seizures.[134]

Urocanic Aciduria In this rare condition, there is a marked excess of urocanic acid in the urine. The activity of urocanase is deficient in the liver. The disorder was first described in four children with mental deficits and growth retardation. Two children identified by neonatal screening were normal.[134] The relationship between urocanic aciduria and nervous system dysfunction is uncertain.

Transferase Deficiency Galactosemia Galactosemia can result from the deficiency of one of three enzymes: galactose-1-phosphate uridyl transferase, galactokinase, and UDP-galactose-4'-epimerase. Classical galactosemia due to a deficiency of galactose-1-phosphate uridyl transferase is an autosomal recessive disorder. It is usually detected by routine newborn screening or, in the neonatal period, by the presence of vomiting, diarrhea, hepatic failure, and hemolysis (Chap. 2). Some children not screened at birth and escaping any neonatal catastrophe may be seen several months or years later because of mental retardation. Some of these patients have a history of vomiting after milk ingestion. Hepatomegaly and cataracts are usual and should always suggest the possibility of a transferase deficiency, namely, galactosemia. The lens findings may be missed if not searched for by slit lamp examination, which reveals punctate lesions of the fetal nucleus or other lenticular abnormalities. Since the association of neurologic deficits and cataracts occurs in many other conditions (see Table 6-11), the diagnosis rests on the demonstration of the enzymatic deficit in erythrocytes. Diagnosis may be indicated by the presence of galactosemia and galactosuria, but the galactosemia may be intermittent. Routine hospital laboratory tests for reducing substances in the urine generally detect only glucose, not galactose.

Treatment   Treatment consists of lifelong elimination of galactose from the diet, which may be difficult to achieve because milk products are in so many foods. Restriction of dietary galactose during pregnancy of women bearing transferase-deficient children seems to have beneficial effects and may be justified as fetal exposure to galactose is probably harmful. The effects of a low-galactose diet on mental development are unfortunately uncertain. Patients diagnosed early and treated well have intelligence below average. There is no clear relationship between the age when therapy is begun and the degree of mental dysfunction. Intelligence quotients vary between 80 and 85. Mental abilities appear to decline progressively with age.[135] Children tend to show abnormalities in visual perception, speech defects, and difficulties with arithmetic. Certain neurological signs have been reported in older patients, including cerebellar ataxia, intention tremor, choreoathetosis, and microcephaly. Many women, even with adequate diets, develop ovarian insufficiency.

From all available data, it appears that mental retardation caused by galactosemia is an irreversible phenomenon. Its mechanism is, however, still unknown, although it has been shown that galactose 1-phosphate and galactitol (the product of an alternate route of galactose metabolism) accumulate in brain and lens more than in other tissues. Pathological findings are of little help for the understanding of the pathogenesis of the disease. They have shown diffuse nonspecific damage, and in some cases, lesions apparently related to liver failure or hyperbilirubinemia. In the lens, the cataract formation clearly seems to be the result of the accumulation of galactitol.

Genetics   Transferase deficiency is an autosomal recessive disorder. Its frequency has been estimated at 1/6200, with great regional variations. The locus for the mutant gene is on chromosome 9p13. Heterozygotes are readily detectable.

Prenatal Diagnosis has been achieved by enzymatic assays on amniocytes or chorionic villus samples.

UDP-Galactose-4-Epimerase Deficiency   In epimerase deficiency galactosemia, a rare disorder, some patients have a symptomatology resembling that of transferase deficiency. In others, the disorder is benign. Epimerase activity is measured in erythrocytes and leukocytes. The gene for this enzyme is coded on chromosome 1.

Galactokinase Deficiency   In galactokinase deficiency the only clinical manifestation consists of cataracts. Galactokinase activity is measured using red blood cells.

Disorders of Valine Catabolism with Prenatal Developmental Defects of the Brain

Rare disorders of valine catabolism are associated with severe neurologic dysfunction and developmental defects of the cerebral cortex.

3-Hydroxyisobutyric Acidemia   Six infants have been reported with 3-hydroxyisobutyric acidemia, a disorder most probably related to a defect of valine metabolism, but for which the primary cause remains unknown. Decreased conversion of ^{14}C-labeled valine and alanine to $^{14}CO_2$ in cultured fibroblasts of one patient has suggested a deficiency of malonic, methylmalonic, and ethylmalonic acid semialdehyde dehydrogenases.[136] Two monozygote twins,[137] with severe intrauterine growth retardation, microcephaly, and very limited neurologic development, exhibited dysmorphic features consisting of a triangular face, a short sloped forehead, hypoplastic orbital ridges, a narrow bitemporal diameter, epicanthus, prominent philtrum, and micrognathia.

The CT scan revealed a lissencephalic or pachygyric cerebrum, agenesis of the corpus callosum and cerebellar hypoplasia. In addition, there were dense calcifications in the frontal lobes and subependymal regions. At autopsy a disorder of cortical migration was confirmed. The biochemical findings consisted of metabolic acidosis and the excretion of large quantities of 3-hydroxyisobutyric acid and other metabolites, indicating a disorder in the metabolism of valine. There were no unusual cysteine conjugates. An excess of 3-hydroxyisobutyric acid was found in the amniotic fluid in an affected fetus. An association between the somatic and the cerebral developmental defect and 3-hydroxyisobutyric acid has been reported in other patients.[137] One 6-year-old boy with the typical picture of an organic aciduria appeared to benefit from treatment with carnitine and a diet restricted in protein.[138]

3-Hydroxyisobutyryl-CoA Deacylase Deficiency A deficiency of 3-hydroxyisobutyryl-CoA deacylase, an enzyme of the catabolic pathway of valine, has been reported in one neonate. There were dysmorphic features, congenital defects of vertebra and heart, agenesis of the corpus callosum and cingulate gyri.[139] Unusual cysteine conjugates were found in the urine.

Other metabolic encephalopathies with brain malformations include Zellweger disease, PDH deficiency (in homozygote males and heterozygote females), glutaric aciduria type II, nonketotic hyperglycinemia, and the Smith-Lemli-Opitz syndrome. They are listed in Table 6-1.

HMDS WITH ACUTE AND REMITTING NEUROLOGIC DISORDERS

A number of different hereditary neurometabolic disorders give rise to acute episodes of drowsiness, stupor, and coma, and neurologic dysfunction. They have a propensity to recur. Between attacks, children may be normal or mildly affected, or display evidence of neurologic or multisystem abnormalities.

Clinically, the acute metabolic attacks consist of vomiting, hypotonia, lethargy, stupor, or coma, respiratory dysrhythmia, and occasionally seizures and ataxia with no significant differences between the syndrome in the various causative diseases.

The type of *metabolic abnormality* detected in routine laboratory screening and the circumstances that precipitate metabolic decompensation are of great diagnostic value. For practical purposes, we will therefore consider successively the intermittent metabolic disorders with:

1. Lactic acidosis
2. Nonketotic hypoglycemia upon fasting
3. Ketoacidosis
4. Hyperammonemia and respiratory alkalosis

Disorders with Lactic Acidosis as a Major Metabolic Sign

These are essentially mitochondrial disorders. They include defects of pyruvate metabolism, of the mitochondrial respiratory chain, and much more rarely, of the Krebs cycle. The most frequent clinical phenotype of this age period is Leigh disease. Since lactic acid elevation occurs in many of the organic acidemias, in some

defects of mitochondrial fatty acid β oxidation, in biotinidase deficiency and other disorders with organic acidemia, these conditions should be ruled out by gas chromatography/mass spectrometry analysis of organic acids in urine. Lactic acidosis is also a feature of fructose 1,6-bisphosphatase deficiency, and of type 1 glycogenosis.

Disorders of Pyruvate Metabolism

Early Infantile Pyruvate Dehydrogenase (PDH) Complex Deficiency Most probably, the great majority of patients with PDH deficiency in early or late infancy conform to the clinicopathologic description of Leigh disease (LD). Most of them have a defect in the E_1 component of the PDH complex. DeVivo and Van Coster[140] have reviewed 65 patients with early infantile PDH deficiency who presented neurologic symptoms between 3 and 6 months of age. Lactate levels were elevated in the CSF and either normal or elevated in the blood, and the activity of PDH was decreased in cultured fibroblasts. At least 85 percent of the autopsied cases had findings that were consistent with Leigh disease (LD). Other children presented with uncharacteristic psychomotor retardation, seizures, pyramidal signs, deceleration of head growth, and mild dysmorphic features. This justifies the undertaking of systematic measurement of lactic acid in blood and CSF in all early-life encephalopathies of uncertain origin.

As indicated in Chap. 2, some patients, frequently heterozygous girls—underdeveloped neurologically from birth and having dysmorphic facial features and severe prenatal brain lesions—may live for several months or years, and the correct diagnosis may only have been reached in the early infantile period or later. *A benign late infantile form*, with episodes of ataxia, postexercise fatigue, transient paraparesis, thiamine responsiveness, and normal mental and motor development, has been described. Several patients with severe, uncharacteristic, and variable neurological signs, including hypotonia, seizures, tachypnea, psychomotor retardation, and lactic acidosis, were found to have a combined deficiency of PDHC and respiratory chain enzymes in muscle biopsies. One child's neuropathology was said to be similar to Leigh disease.[141]

Early Infantile (North American Type) Pyruvate Carboxylase (PC) Deficiency Approximately 18 patients with this condition had been reported by 1992.[140,142] Onset is either in the neonatal period (Chap. 2) or between 2 and 5 months, with severe delay in mental and motor development, hypotonia, pyramidal signs, convulsions, and failure to thrive. Death usually occurs in late infancy and early childhood, frequently during an acute metabolic acidosis.

Serum lactate and pyruvate values are less increased than in the neonatal type, and between the acute episodes, may be only detectable in the CSF. Plasma alanine levels and ketone bodies are also elevated during acute exacerbations. Concentrations of ammonia, citrulline, and lysine, which are elevated in the neonatal form, are usually normal. Episodes of hypoglycemia have been reported.[142] Proximal renal tubular acidosis may be present. The neuropathology has been described in Chap. 2. Therapeutic options are limited. Aspartic acid supplementation may be useful. A low-fat diet is recommended.

Enzyme assays for PC are usually made on cultured fibroblasts. There is no evidence of tissue-specific isoenzymes.

A benign variant with normal neurological development has been reported.[143] This 6-year-old girl had suffered several attacks of metabolic acidosis (elevated lactate, pyruvate, alanine, and ketone bodies), with vomiting; and tachypnea since the age of 7 months, but mental and motor development were normal. A patient with episodic ataxia and mild mental retardation has been reported.[143a]

Previous reports that PC deficiency could cause Leigh syndrome have not been confirmed.[140] Pyruvate carboxylase is also deficient in the biotin-responsive multiple carboxylase deficiency syndromes. The severe "French type" of PC deficiency is described in Chap. 2.

Phosphoenolpyruvate Carboxykinase Deficiency In this rare disease, observed in only five patients, the chemical presentation was associated with hypoglycemia and lactic acidemia. There was hypotonia, underactivity, poor responsivity, and hepatomegaly. One patient had peripheral edema and unexplained episodes of pyrexia. Death occurred in infancy. One patient has survived to age 10 with persistent muscular weakness.[144]

Defects of the Respiratory Chain A defect in complex IV (cytochrome-*c* oxidase) is frequently found in Leigh disease. At least 34 cases have been described. There are numerous other clinical features of respiratory chain defects, some of them presenting as an isolated myopathy or a cardiomyopathy, others as a multisystemic disorder involving the nervous system. Many of the older reports are uninterpretable because the molecular basis of respiratory chain defects was not known at the time.

It appears, however, that an isolated deficiency in complex I (NADH-ubiquinone oxidoreductase), complex II (succinate-ubiquinone oxidoreductase), and complex III (ubiquinol-cytochrome-*c* oxidoreductase) of the respiratory chain may produce in early infancy a syndrome with lactic acidosis, an elevated lactate/pyruvate ratio, weakness, lethargy, myoclonus, arrest of neurologic development, and rapid death from cardiorespiratory failure. Ragged red muscle fibers (RRF) are present in some children with encephalomyopathy, but not in Leigh disease.

The consequences of defects of the respiratory chain in the neonatal period and in the juvenile period are described in Chaps. 2 and 5.

Defects of the Krebs Cycle Three rare congenital defects of the Krebs cycle have been delineated: dihydrolipoyl dehydrogenase (E$_3$) deficiency, fumarase deficiency, and α-ketoglutarate dehydrogenase deficiency.

Dihydrolipoyl Dehydrogenase (E$_3$) Deficiency Infants present a few months after birth with rapid neurological deterioration and persistent lactic acidosis. Symptoms include hypotonia, lethargy and irritability, and respiratory dysrhythmia. Usually there is optic atrophy. The main biological abnormalities consist of high blood concentrations of lactate, pyruvate, and alanine, and elevated levels of α-glutarate and α keto acids. Enzyme assays can be made on cultured fibroblasts. At autopsy, cystic necrosis of the basal ganglia, thalami, and brain stem as well as a loss of myelin are found.

The E$_3$ component is encoded by a gene on chromosome 7q31-q32. The disorder is transmitted as an autosomal recessive trait. A diet restricted in branched chain amino acids has been beneficial.

Fumarase Deficiency At least nine patients have been reported with this condition. Although all patients have had severe neurologic impairment from early infancy, the clinical course was varied with deteriorating neurologic function leading to death by age 8 or 9 months in some, while in others the course was static.[145]

Early-onset cases have had respiratory difficulties, lethargy, anorexia, failure to thrive, and hypothermia. Visual fixation was absent. There was hyperlactacidemia and increased urinary excretion of fumarate, succinate, and citrate were found. A muscle biopsy showed an increased number of subsarcolemmal mitochondria but no typical ragged red fibers. Fumarase activity was low in liver and muscle. One infant died at the age of 8 months. Another exhibited hypotonia, developmental delay and microcephaly during the first year of life. One child was noted to be mentally retarded at the age of 3 years; excessive amounts of fumarate, succinate, and α-ketoglutarate were found in the urine. Fumarase activity was very low in cultured fibroblasts.

We observed two sisters, the offspring of two consanguinous marriages, who presented at 3 weeks of age with repeated vomiting. By age 1 year they had developed severe muscular atrophy, truncal hypotonia, and a pyramidal syndrome. They were also dystonic, had paralysis of upward gaze, generalized seizures, and neutropenia. A CT scan showed ventricular dilatation and mild cortical atrophy. Muscle homogenates were deficient in both cytosolic and mitochondrial fumarase activity. Both activities are coded on the same locus at chromosome 1q. Point mutations have been reported in the fumarase gene.[146]

α-Ketoglutarate Dehydrogenase Deficiency This disorder is essentially characterized by hypotonia, weakness, and failure to thrive, appearing in early infancy. There is hyperlactacidemia, a high lactate/pyruvate ratio, and ketoacidosis.[146a]

Leigh Disease (Subacute Necrotizing Encephalomyelopathy)

Subacute necrotizing encephalomyelopathy was first described as a neuropathological entity by Leigh in 1951.[147] It is characterized by multiple symmetric foci of incomplete necrosis (spongy degeneration) in the brain stem, basal ganglia, thalamus, cerebellum, spinal cord, and optic nerves. The clinical picture reflects both the variability of the lesions and their tendency to predominate in the brain stem, cerebellum, and basal ganglia. In the majority of cases, in addition to pyschomotor retardation and feeding difficulties, the disease expresses itself by intermittent abnormalities of the respiratory rhythm (a most characteristic sign), oculomotor and other cranial nerve palsies, ataxia, a variety of involuntary movements, and optic atrophy. A remitting course with acute exacerbations is frequently observed. In 80 percent of the patients the disease starts before the end of the second year, and death occurs within two years of onset.

Levels of lactate and pyruvate are elevated in the CSF and, less constantly, in blood. The definitive diagnosis of Leigh disease relies on the demonstration of the typical pattern of brain lesions on MRI or at autopsy. Several biochemical and molecular abnormalities have been found to be associated with this disorder, particularly pyruvate dehydrogenase complex (PDHC) deficiency, cytochrome-*c* oxidase (COX) deficiency, and

mitochondrial ATPase 6 gene point mutations. In many cases, a biochemical correlate has not been identified. The disease seems usually to be inherited as an autosomal recessive trait. An X-linked recessive inheritance occurs in some families, and maternal inheritance when the biomolecular defect involves mtDNA. There is no efficient treatment.

Clinical Findings Leigh disease is relatively frequent. More than 200 cases had been published by 1987, and most new cases are no longer being reported. In 55 percent the onset is in the first year, most frequently before the age of 6 months, affecting a previously normal infant. In 25 percent of patients the disease starts between 12 and 14 months. According to DeVivo and Van Coster,[148] patients with PDHC deficiency have an earlier onset (3 to 6 months) than those with COX deficiency (8 to 12 months). A juvenile form and an adult form are known; such cases are described in Chap. 5. There is a predominance in males.

Although we have set the limit of the early infantile period at the age of 12 months, for convenience we will describe here all cases in which the onset is in the first two years of life (Tables 3-2 and 3-3).

In the early infantile period, loss of head control and other motor acquisitions, adynamia, floppiness, and psychic indifference are usually the first parental complaints. Evidence of psychomotor deterioration may appear either insidiously or fairly rapidly, often after a bout of fever or a series of convulsions. Nutritional troubles resulting from poor sucking, anorexia, vomiting, and diarrhea are frequent in the initial stages, and may for some time precede or mask the underlying encephalopathy.

Stunting of body and head growth soon become apparent. When the disease starts in the *second or third year of life* the first neurological complaints are usually difficulty in walking, dystonia, dysarthria, or intellectual regression. Again, nutritional difficulties, vomiting, diarrhea, and failure to thrive, as well as deceleration of head growth, may have preceded the obvious neurological dysfunction.

Unfortunately, some of the signs of infantile Leigh disease, such as axial hypotonia, bilateral, sometimes asymmetrical, pyramidal involvement, seizures, progressive loss of contact with the environment, and irritability, are common to many diffuse, progressive encephalopathies occurring at this age. This adds to the difficulty of diagnosis.

Helpful is the presence of neurologic signs relating to the usual predominance of lesions in the brain stem, basal ganglia, and cerebellum. These occur at variable periods in the course of the disease, sometimes as isolated manifestations and sometimes in many possible combinations. The most important are respiratory disorders, cranial nerve dysfunction, abnormal involuntary movements, and incoordination. These may pursue a remitting course. In the absence of any of these signs the clinical diagnosis of this subacute necrotic encephalomyelopathy is extremely difficult.

(1) Respiratory disorders are fairly constant and highly characteristic. They occur at different periods of the disease; they may be one of the first manifestations. The most frequent are cycles of unexplained hyperventilation lasting a few minutes to several hours, or irregular disturbances of the respiratory rhythm with periods of apnea that may necessitate intubation and respiratory assistance. Also significant, but often overlooked, are minor attacks of dyspnea (air hunger), irregular breathing, gasping, deep sighing respiration, or sobbing without cry. In two of our patients, these breathing difficulties were so prominent and occurred so early that the diagnosis of asthma or some other respiratory disease had been entertained. Respiratory failure is a frequent cause of death. In some instances, major respiratory distress appears to be the consequence of metabolic acidosis, but in most patients no correlation can be established between dyspnea and the lactic acidosis. One patient with Leigh disease due to a deficiency of PDHC was shown to have had the syndrome of central hypoventilation.[149]

(2) Nuclear or supranuclear oculomotor paralyses and other signs of cranial nerve dysfunction are particularly suggestive of the disease. Oculomotor paralyses are usually multiple; there may also be a supranuclear paralysis of lateral or vertical gaze. Total oculomotor paralysis in combination with paralysis of vertical gaze

Table 3-2

Frequency of major signs in subacute necrotizing encephalomyelopathy up to 1982 (85 cases)

Clinical abnormalities	Age at onset				
	1–12 months (48 cases)	12–24 months (22 cases)	2–5 years (8 cases)	5–15 years (7 cases)	Total
Hypotonia	28	17	3	5	53
Pyramidal signs	24	8	6	6	44
Absent tendon reflexes	13	6	2	3	24
Involuntary movements, dystonia	5	1	1	3	10[a]
Cerebellar ataxia	11	8	1	1	21
Seizures	18	2	1	2	23
Myoclonus	3	2			5
Blindness (optic atrophy)	16	5	5	4	30
Oculomotor abnormalities	30	12	7	6	55
Ophthalmoplegia (nuclear and supranuclear)	15	5	5	6	31
Vestibular nystagmus	5	5	2	1	13
Abnormal eye movements	16	8	3	3	30
Paralysis of deglutition	10	1	1	3	15
Paralysis of VIIth cranial nerve	1	1		3	5
Paralysis of XIIth cranial nerve	1				1
Deafness	7		2		9
Mental retardation[b]	27	6	?	?	33
Mental regression[b]	16	9	?	?	25
Respiratory abnormalities	35	16	7	4	62
Lethargy: diminished consciousness	24	19	4	6	53
Feeding problems (and vomiting)	36	11	3	5	55
Failure to thrive	19	9	2		30
Unexplained bouts of fever	13	4	2	1	20
Elevated CSF proteins	10	6	2	1	19

[a]Probably underestimated.

[b]Indications on mental status are often incomplete.

Table 3-3

Age at onset and duration of subacute necrotizing encephalomyelopathy

Age at onset (85 cases)		Duration (84 cases)	
Age	No. cases (%)	Time	No. cases
1–6 months	30 (35.3)	1–6 months	24
6–12 months	16 (18.8)	6–12 months	17
12–24 months	22 (25.8)	12–24 months	15
2–5 years	8 (9.4)	2–5 years	13
5–15 years	7 (8.2)	> 5 years	15
> 15 years	2 (2.3)		

Relation between age at onset and duration (84 cases)

Age at onset	Duration				
	1–6 months	6–12 months	1–2 years	2–5 years	>5 years
1–12 months	14	8	10	7	6
12–24 months	7	9	3	3	
2–5 years	1			3	4
5–15 years	2		1		4
> 15 years			1		1

and retraction of the upper lids have been reported. True vestibular rotary or horizontal nystagmus constitute another sign of involvement of the brain stem. Pendular nystagmus and slow, irregular roving eye movements are more difficult to interpret and may in some cases be due to loss of vision.

Paralysis of deglutition, distinct from the dysphagia of the pseudobulbar syndrome, and other cranial nerve involvement such as facial palsy are observed. Deafness has been reported.

(3) Truncal ataxia, cerebellar intention tremor, and incoordination can in some instances be in evidence at the end of the first year, or later, when the child has started walking. Abnormal movements, of choreiform, dystonic, or athetoid type, can also appear at that age.[149a]

(4) Other important signs are blindness with optic atrophy and pigmentary degeneration of the retina (mtDNA T8993 G mutation), and clinical as well as electrophysiological evidence of peripheral neuropathy. Peripheral neuropathy may eventually cause weakness and atrophy of the limbs. However, the frequency of peripheral nerve involvement is difficult to assess, usually because of incomplete data. In many reports the diagnosis of a peripheral neuropathy is based on

the presence of depressed tendon reflexes. But there are several cases in which there was microscopic evidence of myelin breakdown in a sensory nerve biopsy.

Seizures may occur, especially when the disease starts early and is due to PDHC deficiency or in the NARP T8993 G mutation. Although slow mentation or regression of mental abilities is usual, normal intellectual development is not incompatible with the disease. Secondary microcephaly, after some months, is usual. Unexplained bouts of fever are not rare and profuse sweating may be observed.

(5) Leigh syndrome frequently pursues a remitting course. This characteristic has great diagnostic importance. Fluctuations in the disease may be relatively slight, evidenced only after careful questioning of parents. Or there may be acute exacerbations, induced by an infection consisting of periods of respiratory difficulty, ataxia or involuntary movements, transient nystagmus and cranial nerve paralyses, and vomiting. The neurologic disorders may progress to profound weakness and coma, and metabolic acidosis. Often such an attack is followed by spontaneous improvement that may last for a few weeks to several months.

In rare instances, Leigh disease has an acute, rapidly fatal course. A normal or retarded infant develops convulsions, coma, respiratory dysrhythmia, paralysis of cranial nerves, vomiting, fever, and metabolic acidosis. It may even happen that the duration of the lethal attack is no more than a few days. Obviously, in such circumstances diagnosis is possible only when the typical lesions are found at autopsy.

The duration of the disease is extremely variable. Approximately 80 percent of the patients with infantile subacute necrotizing encephalomyelopathy die within 2 years of onset (in 30 percent death occurs within 6 months). A minority have an acute rapidly lethal course. But others live for more than 5 years, and survival over 10 years has been reported. The relation between age at onset and duration is given in Table 3-3.

Intrafamilial Variations In a survey of 37 families in which several children in the same sibship were affected, the symptomatology tended to be more or less similar, although very rarely absolutely identical, in two successive siblings. In one family, for instance, the age at onset in one sibling was 5 years and 7 months and in another it was 4 years and 10 months. Differences in the duration of the disease among siblings have been found to vary from 2 years to 14 years. When intrafamilial variability is striking, it generally implies a molecular defect involving mtDNA.

Maternally Inherited Leigh Syndrome Maternally inherited Leigh syndrome (MILS) is a rare variety caused by ATP[6] NARP 8993 mutation; retinitis pigmentosa is a major sign that is not found in Leigh syndrome with a Mendelian inheritance. The course is rapidly progressive. There are no RRFs (see also Chap. 5).

Biochemical and Other Laboratory Findings Measurements of lactate and pyruvate are important for the diagnosis of Leigh disease. Lactate and pyruvate are practically always elevated in the CSF. Results in blood are more variable. The lactate/pyruvate ratio also varies. There may be hyperalaninemia. A renal tubular acidosis with generalized nonspecific aminoaciduria has been recorded (de Toni-Debré-Fanconi syndrome). Hyperammonemia, hypoglycemia, and organoaciduria are notably absent.

A deficiency of several mitochondrial enzymes has been demonstrated in patients with Leigh disease: pyruvate dehydrogenase complex (PDHC) deficiency (19 reported cases in 1991 but the frequency is higher)[140,149,150]; cytochrome-*c* oxidase (COX) deficiency (complex IV deficiency) (34 reported cases in 1991)[151]; point mutations in the mitochondrial ATPase 6 gene[153,154]; complex I deficiency (4 cases with late onset reported)[152]; complex II deficiency[152a]; and biotinidase deficiency.[155] Other point mutations in mitochondrial genes have recently been described. In many cases, however, there was no biochemical abnormality. Some patients could possibly have had an enzyme defect restricted to the brain, or some other biochemical abnormality. A deficiency in pyruvate carboxylase, previously reported in Leigh disease, has not been confirmed.

The activity of PDHC and COX can be measured on cultured skin fibroblasts and muscle or liver biopsies. Measurements should be done on two or more tissues because of frequent lack of correspondence between levels of activity in muscle and fibroblasts. For instance, some cases of COX deficiency were only expressed in the muscle.[151] It is possible that in some cases PDHC deficiency is limited to the brain.

Genetics An autosomal recessive mode of inheritance seems probable in many patients. When Leigh disease is related to a mutation in the $E_{1\alpha}$ subunit of PDHC, the disorder is transmitted as an X-linked trait. Female carriers may be variably affected.[156] An unexplained predominance of males is observed in cases of COX deficiency. The mtDNA mutations (in the ATPase 6 gene) are inherited as a maternal, non-Mendelian trait.

Diagnosis In view of the protean nature of the disease and the absence of a unique biochemical or molecular defect, the diagnosis of Leigh syndrome rests on the demonstration of the typical neuropathological lesions. Diagnosis is now possible during life, with a high degree of probability, by MRI. The CT scan is much less reliable. However, other conditions, such as PDH deficiency without Leigh syndrome, glutaric aciduria type I, methylmalonic acidemia, Leber disease, glutaconic acidemia, cryptogenetic familial striatal necrosis, and postinfectious necrosis of the putamen, also cause lesions of the striatum or globus pallidus. Therefore, to be reasonably certain of the diagnosis of Leigh syndrome, one should rely on the combination of the typical pattern of brain lesions on MRI (Figs. 3-20 and 3-21), the demonstration of a high level of lactate in the CSF, and a clinical picture which is consistent with this disorder. Allowance must be made for exceptional cases. In one of our patients, lesions were practically restricted to the spinal cord and optic nerves, and were only minimally present in the brain stem and absent in the basal ganglia. It should be remembered that the

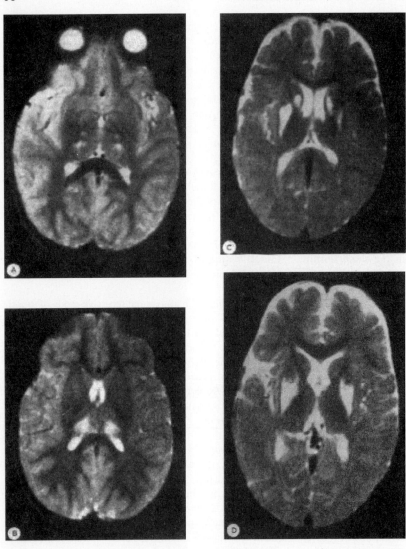

Figure 3-20
*Leigh disease. MRI shows symmetrical lesions in the thalamus and subthalamic nuclei (**A** and **B**) and in the putamen and caudate (**C** and **D**). (Courtesy Dr. Van Coster.)*

lenticular nucleus may be spared, as was the case in Leigh's original description.

As the disorder may be initially quite uncharacteristic, Leigh syndrome should be considered in all cases of early infantile progressive encephalopathy of unknown origin, especially when there is an associated nutritional disorder. In some instances, white matter lesions in the cerebral hemispheres have been so prominent as to mimic a leukodystrophy; we have observed three such patients.

Differential diagnosis includes conditions ranging from active encephalitis and Reye syndrome to many types of slowly progressive encephalopathy. During periods of exacerbation, other mitochondrial disorders and the intermittent types of inherited aminoacidopathies and urea cycle disorders must come under consideration.

Limits of Leigh Syndrome Although the diagnosis of Leigh syndrome, *stricto sensu*, requires the demonstration of the typical brain lesions on neuroimaging, there may not be a fundamental difference between children with the typical clinicopathologic picture, and those with clinical signs of Leigh syndrome, lactic acidosis, and PDHC deficiency, but no evidence of the typical central nervous system lesions. Leigh syndrome is a good example of the problems encountered in defining

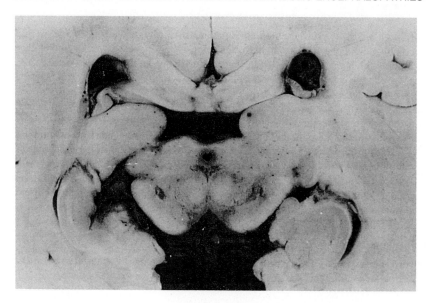

Figure 3-21
Leigh disease. A formalin-fixed brain shows a brain stem with symmetrical necrosis of the third nerve nuclei (arrow) and the substantia nigra (arrowhead).

a disease clinically and pathologically without supportive gene data.

Pathologic Findings The lesions in the nervous system consist of foci of incomplete necrosis with vascular proliferation, spongiform loosening of the neuropil, and relative preservation of neurons, a condition sometimes loosely referred to as spongiosis. The actual proliferation of vessels is not always easy to demonstrate.

These foci, of variable extent and topography, tend to be symmetric and to predominate in the dorsal part of the brain stem, which is only exceptionally spared, and in the lenticular nuclei, thalami, substantia nigra, optic nerves, the dentate nuclei of the cerebellum and spinal cord (Table 3-4, Fig. 3-20). The mammillary bodies are nearly always spared. Involvement of the white matter may occur. Exceptionally, white matter lesions are as prominent as those of a primary leukodystrophy. Cortical lesions are rare; they were not unlike those seen in Mitochondrial Encephalomyopathy, Lactic Acidosis, and Strokelike episodes (MELAS) in one case we studied.

Variations in the intensity of lesions may range from moderate loosening of the neuropil to frank necrosis, probably reflecting degrees of the fundamental biochemical abnormality. Variations in the topography of lesions may be seen in two members of the same family, but striking similarities are more the rule. Segmental

demyelination of peripheral nerves has been observed but is rare. The skeletal muscles are normal.

The lesions in the central nervous system resemble those of Wernicke encephalopathy in adults, a disease due to thiamine deficiency, and are even more like those of thiamine deficiency in the experimental animal (macaque monkey), but their distribution is different.

Clinicopathologic Correlations They are difficult to determine. In most examples, metabolic acidosis cannot account for the respiratory abnormalities. Probably they are related to lesions in the brain stem which are practically constant. Exact topographic correlations prove to be virtually impossible. For example, a typical respiratory disorder may exist in the absence of visible lesions in the tegmentum of the medulla: respiratory dysrhythmia existed in 15 of 84 cases without lesions at that site. When dystonia is present, necrosis of the striatum and thalamus is usually found, but such lesions may exist without involuntary movements.

Treatment There is no specific treatment for Leigh syndrome. Supplementation with B vitamins has had no lasting effect. Recently, the beneficial effects of a ketogenic diet in a patient with PDHC deficiency have been reported.[157]

More research is necessary to explore other therapeutic options, as well as prenatal diagnosis and prevention.

Table 3-4

Neuropathology of subacute necrotizing encephalomyelopathy up to 1982 (80 cases)

Main site of lesions	Age at onset				
	1–12 months (44 cases)	12–24 months (22 cases)	2–5 years (8 cases)	5–15 years (7 cases)	Total
Cerebral cortex	6			1	7
Cerebral white matter	10	5	2		17
Putamen	27	8	3	6	44
Caudate	22	5		6	33
Pallidum	14	1	1	0	16
Thalamus	20	7	1	2	30
Corpus luysi	14	4	5		23
Mammillary bodies	7	2	1		10
Walls of 3d ventricle	5	1	1	1	8
Brain stem	44	20	8	7	79
Mesencephalon					65
Tegmentum	29	13	5	6	53
Periaqueductal gray matter	17	3	5	3	28
Tectum	22	8			30
Locus niger	29	11	5	4	49
Red nucleus	8			1	9
Pons tegmentum	36	18	5	6	65
Medulla oblongata					62
Tegmentum	33	13	3	6	55
Inferior olives	21	9	2	3	35
Cerebellum					43
Dentate nucleus	10	7	2	3	22
White matter	5	5	3	2	15
Superior peduncle	3	1	1		5
Optic chiasmatic nerve or tracts	37	12	2	8	59
Spinal cord					40
Gray matter	11	7	3	1	22
White matter	5	3	10		18
Peripheral nerves[a]	5	3			8

[a] Only a small number have been examined. Lesions are probably more frequent.

Disorders with Episodic Nonketotic Hypoglycemia

Attacks of vomiting, weakness and coma, and respiratory abnormalities are associated with episodes of hypoglycemia and hypoketonemia precipitated by prolonged fasting in disorders of mitochondrial fatty acid oxidation. A cardiopathy, a myopathy, and hepatomegaly may be present. These disorders can be subdivided into defects of the carnitine cycle and defects of β oxidation.[140]

Defects of the Carnitine Cycle There are four of these, involving, respectively, the carnitine transport system, carnitine palmitoyltransferase I, carnitine palmitoyltransferase II, and carnitine-acylcarnitine translocase. These conditions are inherited as autosomal recessive traits.

Defect in the Carnitine Transport System: Primary Generalized Carnitine Deficiency Primary carnitine deficiency is a rare disorder caused by a genetic defect in the carnitine transport system. In addition to episodes of nonketotic hypoglycemia a cardiomyopathy associated with hypotonia and muscular weakness are usually present from infancy or early childhood. The serum and tissue concentrations of carnitine are extremely low. There may be a fatty infiltration of skeletal muscles. Carnitine uptake in cultured skin fibroblasts is negligible and is approximately 50 percent in the heterozygotes. Oral carnitine supplementation is lifesaving.

Carnitine Palmitoyltransferase I (CPT I) Deficiency   This enzyme (CPT I) is located on the inner face of the outer mitochondrial membrane and catalyzes the conversion of long-chain acyl-CoA to long-chain acyl carnitine. There is a marked hepatomegaly. Renal tubular acidosis has been observed. Patients have hypertriglyceridemia, mild hyperammonemia, abnormal liver function, and liver steatosis. Serum carnitine levels are normal or elevated. CK may be elevated. The enzyme is deficient in liver, lymphocytes, and cultured skin fibroblasts. Administration of medium-chain triglycerides may be beneficial.

Carnitine Palmitoyltransferase II (CPT II) Deficiency   This enzyme (CPT II) is located on the inner face of the inner mitochondrial membrane and catalyzes the conversion of long-chain acyl carnitine to long-chain acyl-CoA. The gene has been located on chromosome 1p32.

CPT II deficiency gives rise to a neonatal disorder described in Chap. 2 and a myopathy with myoglobinuria induced by fasting and other provoking factors in later childhood or in the adult. It may also manifest itself in early infancy by abrupt episodes of nonketotic hypoglycemia with coma, liver failure, and cardiomyopathy. Some children have died unexpectedly. The serum carnitine concentrations are decreased in the neonatal and infantile forms, and normal in childhood or adolescence. There may be a fatty infiltration of muscle. The enzyme defect is demonstrated in a muscle biopsy.

Carnitine-Acylcarnitine Translocase Deficiency
This defect has been reported in two infants presenting with seizures, apnea, vomiting, and coma; cardiopathy, hepatomegaly, and myoglobinuria were present. Long-chain acyl carnitine concentrations were elevated. There were very low levels of free carnitine in plasma and a hyperammonemia. Death occurred at the age of 37 months.

Defects in Mitochondrial Fatty Acid β Oxidation (Acyl-CoA Dehydrogenase Deficiencies)   Eight
inherited defects within the mitochondrial β oxidation pathway have been described: medium-chain acyl-CoA dehydrogenase (MCAD) deficiency, long-chain acyl-CoA dehydrogenase (LCAD) deficiency, very long-chain acyl-CoA dehydrogenase (VLCAD) deficiency, short-chain acyl-CoA dehydrogenase (SCAD) deficiency, long-chain 3-hydroxyacyl-CoA dehydrogenase (LCHAD) deficiency, short-chain 3-hydroxyacyl-CoA dehydrogenase (SCHAD) deficiency, electron transfer flavoprotein (ETF) deficiency, and ETF-ubiquinone oxidoreductase (ETF-QO) deficiency (resulting in multiple acyl-CoA dehydrogenase (MADD) deficiency, referred to as glutaric acidemia type II), and trifunctional enzyme deficiency.

Each of these disorders is inherited as an autosomal recessive trait. They present essentially as recurrent episodes of vomiting and coma induced by fasting. Common biochemical features comprise hypoketonemia, hypoglycemia, dicarboxylic aciduria, and carnitine deficiency. The profiles of urinary acyl carnitines and of dicarboxylic acids are important for the differential diagnosis.

Medium-Chain Acyl-CoA Dehydrogenase (MCHD) Deficiency   MCAD is the most common defect of the mitochondrial β oxidation pathway. More than 200 patients have been identified. Its frequency has been estimated between 1 in 10,000 and 1 in 25,000. Estimated heterozygote frequencies are 1 to 2 percent in some populations. Onset is between 5 months and 2 years, with peak incidence between 6 and 18 months.[158]

A significant proportion of children die during the first or a recurrent acute episode (13 percent during the first year and more than 50 percent during the second year of life).[159] For the other patients, if correctly treated, the long-term outlook can be good. Some patients are left with neurological sequelae.

Laboratory Findings   Useful tests are made on urinary organic acids, along with carnitine assays, acyl carnitine identification, and enzyme assays.

In the fasting state, there is an increased urinary excretion of medium-chain (C_6 to C_{12}) fatty acid metabolites and characteristic glycine conjugates (subericglycine and hexanoylglycine). Serum carnitine levels are low and urinary excretion of acyl carnitine is elevated. The ratio of acylated carnitine to total carnitine is increased. There is a highly specific profile of urinary acyl carnitines. Elevated serum transaminases and hyperammonia are usual findings.

The concentration of abnormal urinary metabolites varies greatly and may be detectable only in the fasting state.

Note that the diagnosis can be made postmortem by detection of specific acyl carnitines in the liver using fast atom bombardment mass spectrometry.

Enzyme assays can be done on cultured skin fibroblasts, mononuclear white blood cells, liver, and skeletal muscle. Residual activity of MCAD is usually very low.

Treatment   Treatment with intravenous infusion of 10 percent glucose has proved effective during acute attacks (even in the absence of definite hypoglycemia). Recurrence can be prevented by avoiding prolonged fasting, providing an adequate caloric intake, and reducing fat intake. L-carnitine supplementation may be useful.

Phenotypic Variation: Other Examinations

- In some children during acute episodes, glycemia may be normal (suggesting that the neurological syndrome may not be entirely due to hypoglycemia).
- MCAD may mimic Reye syndrome and may be a cause of sudden infant death.
- Some children have been asymptomatic.

Genetics   MCAD is an autosomal recessive disorder. Healthy heterozygotes are detectable by enzyme assays on cultured skin fibroblasts. Prenatal diagnosis is possible.

The gene has been located on the short arm of chromosome 1. The alteration responsible for the disease in more than 90 percent of cases is an A to G point mutation affecting codon 329, which can be rapidly detected by the polymerase chain reaction (PCR) assay.

Pathology   There is a macrovesicular or microvesicular liver steatosis. Ultrastructural mitochondrial changes seen in Reye syndrome are absent, but some morphological changes in the appearance of mitochondria have been reported. Brain edema is noted in most cases.

Long-Chain Acyl-CoA Dehydrogenase Deficiency (LCAD Deficiency)   LCAD has been identified in 15 patients.[159,160] It shares with MCAD the repeated episodes of vomiting and coma. Once again, hypoglycemia, absence of ketosis, hyperammonemia, secondary carnitine deficiency, and increased urinary excretion of dicarboxylic acids are the characteristic biochemical features.

In contrast with MCAD deficiency, the disease generally starts before 6 months of age, and there may be marked muscular weakness and a hypertrophic cardiomyopathy. Hepatomegaly due to liver steatosis may be present. The course of the disease is variable. Two patients have died, two others are seriously retarded and have severe psychomotor retardation, microcephaly and cerebral atrophy. The other patients had a less devastating course, and experienced muscle cramps and myoglobinuria in adolescence or in adult life.

Laboratory Findings   The main differences from MCAD deficiency are the presence of longer-chain (C_{12} to C_{14}) dicarboxylic acids and acyl carnitines in the urine and the absence of medium-chain glycine conjugates (suberylglycine, phenylpropionylglycine and hexanoylglycine).

Demonstration of the enzyme defect in cultured fibroblasts is necessary for diagnosis.

Treatment   Same as MCAD deficiency.

Short-Chain Acyl-CoA Dehydrogenase (SCAD) Deficiency   SCAD deficiency has been reported in only a few patients with quite variable features, including (1) a lethal neonatal syndrome (see Chap. 2); (2) psychomotor retardation, muscle weakness, microcephaly, poor feeding with low plasma carnitine levels, all appearing during infancy; (3) a myopathy in adulthood.

Muscle and liver tissue are preferable to cultured skin fibroblasts for the enzymatic diagnosis of SCAD, because the deficiency is not always expressed in fibroblasts.[161] Some patients reported as a myopathic form of carnitine deficiency were later found to have muscle-specific SCAD deficiency.

Long-Chain 3-Hydroxyacyl-CoA Dehydrogenase (LCHAD) Deficiency   This apparently autosomal recessive condition has recently been reported in a few patients.[162] The disease appears in early infancy. During acute episodes, hypoglycemia, a low concentration of ketone bodies, lactacidemia, and hyperammonemia are found on routine laboratory screening. The liver is enlarged due to microvesicular or macrovesicular fatty infiltration. A severe myopathy and cardiomyopathy may develop. Death usually occurs in infancy. One patient had a sensorimotor neuropathy, a myopathy with recurrent myoglobinuria, and a pigmentary degeneration of the retina.[163] Some children have had a sibling who died unexpectedly in infancy.

In addition to the C_6 to C_{12} dicarboxylic aciduria seen in almost all patients with β oxidation defects,

---

*See footnote on p. 28.

longer-chain C_{12} to C_{14} dicarboxylic acids are found. A low activity of 3-hydroxyacyl-CoA dehydrogenase is detected in cultured skin fibroblasts. Some patients have a trifunctional enzyme defect. Prenatal diagnosis is possible.[164]

There is no specific treatment.

Short-Chain 3-Hydroxyacyl-CoA Dehydrogenase (SCHAD) Deficiency Only three cases have been described with a phenotype apparently similar to that of LCHAD.[165]

*Very Long Chain Acyl-CoA Dehydrogenase (VLCAD) Deficiency See Chap. 2.

Glutaric Aciduria Type II (Multiple Acyl-CoA Dehydrogenase Deficiency) Patients with glutaric acidemia type II, an autosomal recessive disorder, fall into one of two main groups: a neonatal form, usually with congenital anomalies that was discussed in Chap. 2, and an infantile form which will be described here.

Clinical Features Onset is in the first months of life, sometimes later in the second or third year. Some patients have been asymptomatic until adulthood. The usual clinical manifestations consist in recurrent episodes of vomiting, tachypnea, and lethargy in children with hypotonia and developmental delay. Hepatomegaly and a peculiar odor of urine resembling that of isovaleric acidemia are generally present. Routine laboratory evaluations show metabolic acidosis, hyperlactacidemia, severe hypoglycemia, low ketonemia and ketonuria, and moderate hyperammonemia. Serum transaminases may be elevated. A cardiomyopathy and renal cysts are present in some cases. Association of a nonketotic hypoglycemia and a characteristic organic aciduria is an important diagnostic clue.

Biochemical Findings There is a high urinary excretion of dicarboxylic acids (ethylmalonic, adipic, suberic, dodecanoic, etc.) and of glutaric acid, 2-hydroxyglutaric acid, isovaleric acid, isovalerylglycine, isobutyrilglycine, and sarcosine. The organic aciduria is, however, less pronounced than in the neonatal form of the disease and may be intermittent. The finding of 2-hydroxyglutaric aciduria is important. Lipid storage in muscle and viscera is usually found.

The primary anomaly involves two nuclear encoded proteins: either electron transfer flavoprotein (ETF), or ETF-ubiquinone oxidoreductase (ETF-QO). Both defects affect the electron flux from all mitochon-drial acyl dehydrogenase reactions leading to a *multiple acyl-CoA dehydrogenase deficiency* and consequently to the accumulation and excretion of oxidation products of substrates normally oxidized by the mitochondrial flavin containing acyl-CoA dehydrogenases.

Demonstration of the defective activity of ETF and ETFDH is difficult and necessitates specialized laboratory procedures. The structural gene of ETF is located on 15q23-q25 and has been cloned. Several mutations in this gene have been found in the DNA from patients.

Treatment Oral riboflavin (100 to 300 mg/day), carnitine supplementation, and a diet low in fat and protein have apparently helped some patients.[166]

Other Forms of the Disease

- The neonatal form (see Chap. 2).
- Two patients have been described with only a progressive lipid storage myopathy and carnitine deficiency. Dramatic improvement after riboflavin treatment has been reported in one patient.
- Onset in adulthood with episodic hypoglycemia and limb weakness.

Mitochondrial Trifunctional Enzyme Deficiency The trifunctional enzyme is involved in mitochondrial β oxidation. This enzyme (as well as VLCAD) is bound to the inner mitochondrial membrane, whereas the other enzymes of β oxidation are located in the mitochondrial matrix; it catalyzes the 3-hydroxyacyl-CoA dehydrogenation, 2-enoyl-CoA hydratation and 3-oxoacyl-CoA thiolysis of long-chain CoA esters. Deficiency of the trifunctional enzyme can give rise to neonatal (Chap. 2) or early infantile episodes of drowsiness and coma with nonketotic hypoglycemia. Cardiac failure and hepatic dysfunction are usual. There is an excess of saturated and unsaturated dicarboxylic acids in the urine. Sudden infant death and a rapidly fatal cardiomyopathy have been reported. Some patients have had muscle weakness and myoglobinuria.

A sensorimotor polyneuropathy and a pigmentary degeneration of the retina have been documented in two patients.

All patients had defects of long-chain 3-hydroxyacyl-CoA dehydrogenase, and to a lesser extent long-chain 2-enoyl-CoA hydratase and long-chain 3-oxoacyl-CoA thiolase. There is evidence of biochemical and molecular heterogeneity.[167] Some patients reported to have LCHAD deficiency may, in fact, have had a defect in the trifunctional protein.

Disorders with Intermittent Episodes of Ketoacidosis

Hereditary Disorders of Amino Acid and Organic Acid Metabolism   Most of the inherited disorders of amino acid and organic acid metabolism which become manifest in early (or later) infancy, or which continue their course during this period of life after a neonatal onset, present with intermittent acute, sometimes life-threatening episodes of metabolic acidosis and ketosis promoted by fever, excessive protein intake, or other dietary irregularities. Hypoglycemia, lactacidemia, and hyperammonemia may be associated (ketone bodies are low in β-ketothiolase deficiency). Prompt recognition is essential because rapid initiation of therapy may be lifesaving. The standard treatment of attacks consists of intravenous glucose and bicarbonate, peritoneal dialysis, reduction of protein intake, and vitamin therapy.

The main members of this group of disorders are listed in Table 3-7 and will be described only briefly. Their more common neonatal form is discussed in Chap. 2.

The Intermittent Form of Maple Syrup Urine Disease (MSUD)   The first signs may appear at various ages from infancy to adulthood. During acute episodes of metabolic acidosis, the odor of urine is typical. The level of branched chain amino acids (BCAAs) and branched chain keto acids (BCKAs) is elevated in the urine but returns to normal during vitamin administration and dietary treatment. Death may occur during an acute attack. Leucine decarboxylation by intact cells is 2 to 20 percent of controls.

Treatment   Treatment of the acute attack is directed to normalizing the level of branched chain amino acids (BCAAs) in the blood and counteracting the effects of metabolic acidosis.

Thiamine supplementation should be started immediately (5 to 20 mg/kg/day) as some cases of intermittent MSUD are *thiamine responsive*. Thiamine normalizes the plasma level of leucine, as has also been observed in some cases of neonatal MSUD and can be achieved in more chronic "intermediate" forms of MSUD. It is recommended that this vitamin be given in all forms of the disease. The chronic dietary treatment consists of restricting protein with a reduced level of

BCAAs calculated to be sufficient for the specific needs of patients in accordance with their age, clinical status, and the residual activity of the deficient enzyme. Dietary management has proven to be difficult. A sufficient level of branched chain amino acids needs to be maintained for normal growth.

"Intermediate" Form of MSUD   Clinical symptomatology in this rare form of MSUD, which will require further molecular, enzymatic, and immunologic clarification, is limited to mental retardation and motor delay starting in infancy or early childhood. There is a typical odor of the urine, modest anemia, and occasionally hyperuricemia. A mild metabolic acidosis may be present. The concentration of branched chain amino acids and keto acids in urine is elevated. Leucine decarboxylation is 2 to 40 percent of controls. Restriction of protein results in normal levels of amino acids. Thiamine therapy is recommended.

Propionyl-CoA Carboxylase Deficiency (Propionic Acidemia)   The main biological abnormalities during acute attacks include metabolic acidosis, ketosis, hyperglycinemia, hyperammonemia, and occasionally, hypoglycemia. Lasting neurologic complications may ensue. Thrombopenia and neutropenia are frequent findings. Long-term treatment consists of a low protein diet (0.5 to 1.5 kg/day) or a diet selectively reduced in propionate precursors. Supplementation with biotin and with L-carnitine has been advocated but with uncertain results. Acute attacks of ketoacidosis should be actively treated. The neonatal form of propionic acidemia is described in Chap. 2. The disorder may be asymptomatic.

Methylmalonyl-CoA Mutase Deficiency (Methylmalonic Acidemia)   This essentially neonatal disease may start in early infancy with lethargy, hypotonia, vomiting, failure to thrive, and hepatomegaly. Less frequently there is a late infantile or juvenile onset and a fluctuating course with recurrent episodes of ketoacidosis, hyperammonemia, leukopenia, thrombocytopenia, and anemia.

The proportion of infantile and childhood forms varies strikingly in the different classes of the disease. While in 90 percent of mut^0 patients onset is before the end of the first month (Chap. 2), in an appreciable proportion of the other classes (mut$^-$, Cbl A, Cbl B) the disease starts later. Treatment of methylmalonic acidemia is described in Chap. 2.

Combined Deficiency of Methylmalonyl-CoA Mutase and Methyltetrahydrofolate: Homocysteine Methyltransferase This disorder has its onset mostly in the first two months of life and has been described in Chap. 2. A few patients (in the Cbl C and Cbl D group) have a delayed onset in childhood or adolescence with various neurological symptoms including a myelopathy, dementia, and psychiatric manifestations.

Inherited Disorders of Folate Transport and Metabolism More than 30 cases of *methylenetetrahydrofolate reductase deficiency*, probably an autosomal recessive disorder, have been reported, mostly in females. The initial clinical manifestations have occurred from the first week of life until adolescence or even adulthood. Most patients have been recognized during the first year of life. The usual presentation consisted in nondescript psychomotor retardation, often with microcephaly. Seizures, gait disturbances, and psychiatric manifestations also occurred. In a few patients, recurrent strokes appeared in early adulthood, as a consequence of vascular lesions similar to those seen in classical homocystinuria.[167a]

The deficiency of methylenetetrahydrofolate reductase affects the production of 5-methyltetrahydrofolate, which is needed for remethylation of homocysteine to methionine. Consequently, there is usually a moderate homocystinuria and homocysteinemia with low or normal levels of methionine. Serum folate levels are usually low and cobalamin levels normal. There is no megaloblastic anemia.

In glutamate formiminotransferase deficiency clinical findings have ranged from psychomotor retardation to normal neurological development.

Hereditary folate malabsorption has been described in about 13 patients, 11 of which were girls. The disease is characterized by folate-responsive megaloblastic anemia, mouth ulcers, diarrhea, failure to thrive, and progressive neurologic deterioration. A folinic-responsive peripheral neuropathy has been reported. Treatment consists of large doses of oral or parenteral folates.

All these disorders of folate transport and metabolism are apparently transmitted as an autosomal recessive trait.

Isovaleric Acidemia Isovaleric acidemia is an autosomal recessive disorder due to a deficiency of mitochondrial isovaleryl-CoA dehydrogenase. It is apparently not a rare disease. More than 60 cases had been reported up to 1989. One-half of them presented with an acute neonatal form, which has been described in Chap. 2, and one-half with a chronic intermittent form, which is described here.

The first episode of metabolic decompensation usually occurs in the first year of life, sometimes later. Attacks of ketoacidosis are frequently precipitated by upper respiratory infections or increased intake of protein. The so-called sweaty feet odor of urine is generally present during attacks. Diarrhea, neutropenia, thrombocytopenia, and more rarely, alopecia may occur. Patients have a natural aversion for protein-rich food. The frequency of recurrent episodes of neurologic disorder is variable and tends to diminish with age. Neurological development may or may not be normal. The outcome is much improved by early dietary treatment, consisting of protein restriction and administration of glycine and carnitine.

Diagnostic Biochemical Features During acute episodes, high quantities of isovaleric acid and one of its metabolites, isovalerylglycine, are excreted in the urine. These metabolites are detected by GC/MS or by high-field proton nuclear magnetic resonance. During remissions, levels of isovaleric acid may be low in contrast to isovalerylglycine, which remains high. Determination of the activity of isovaleryl-CoA dehydrogenase can be made on cultured fibroblasts.

Prenatal diagnosis has been achieved.

The gene for isovaleryl-CoA dehydrogenase activity has been localized to the long arm of chromosome 15, q13-q15 and a variety of point mutation have been described in patients. The mechanism of brain damage is not known.

3-Hydroxy-3-Methylglutaric Aciduria (3-Hydroxy-3-Methylglutaryl-CoA Lyase Deficiency) Approximately 20 patients with this disease have been reported. In 30 percent, it began in the neonatal period (see Chap. 2) and in 60 percent between the ages of 3 and 12 months (24 months in one child). Patients with the early infantile form present with recurrent episodes of vomiting, hypotonia, tachypnea, seizures, lethargy or coma, and metabolic acidosis and hypoglycemia. There is no ketosis (a consequence of the role of 3-hydroxy-3-methylglutaryl-CoA lyase in the formation of ketone bodies). Most children have hyperammonemia, elevated serum transaminases, and hepatomegaly. Several patients died during an acute episode. Others remained retarded with microcephaly and evidence of cerebral atrophy on the CT scan. When treated with a diet limited in protein and fat and oral L-carnitine, they may develop normally.

Biochemical Abnormalities Characteristically, there are high levels of 3-hydroxy-3-methylglutaric acid, 3-methylglutaconic acid, 3-hydroxyisovaleric acid, and 3-methylglutaric acid, and a deficient activity of 3-methylglutaryl-CoA lyase in leukocytes and cultured fibroblasts. Heterozygotes can be detected and prenatal diagnosis has been accomplished. The disease is probably inherited as an autosomal recessive trait. The gene for 3-methylglutaryl-CoA lyase has been found on 1pter-p33 and several mutations identified in the coding sequence.

Treatment During the acute episodes, correction of acidosis and hypoglycemia is essential. Chronic treatment consists of a diet restricting protein and fat intake, and avoidance of fasting.

2-Methylacetoacetyl-CoA Thiolase Deficiency (β-Ketothiolase Deficiency)
Severe episodes of ketoacidosis occur in this disorder of isoleucine catabolism; they usually resolve following symptomatic treatment with intravenous glucose and bicarbonate. With protein restriction, the course of the disease is usually benign. Some children have experienced episodic headaches. Motor and mental development are generally normal. The most characteristic metabolite in the urine is 2-methyl-3-hydroxybutyric acid. 2-Methylacetoacetic acid, 2-butanone and tiglylglycine may also be present. The gene for hepatic mitochondrial acetoacetyl-CoA thiolase has been cloned and mapped to 11q22.3-q23.1. Definitive diagnosis of the enzymatic deficit is made on cultured fibroblasts or leukocytes.

This disorder has been reported in approximately 20 patients.

Isolated Deficiency of 3-Methylcrotonyl-CoA Carboxylase
This rare disorder of the leucine degradation pathway is characterized by intermittent attacks of metabolic acidosis and hypoglycemia. Some patients have had alopecia. High concentrations of 3-hydroxyisovaleric acid and of 3-methylcrotonylglycine are found in the urine. The disease can usually be controlled by adequate protein restriction. Enzymatic diagnosis can be made on leukocytes or cultured fibroblasts. Treatment with biotin is without effect, unlike the multiple carboxylase deficiencies.

Glutaric Aciduria Type I
Glutaric aciduria type I is an autosomal recessive disorder of lysine, hydroxylysine, and tryptophan metabolism (see also p. 85). It is characterized clinically by progressive dystonia and acute episodes of ketoacidosis, pathologically by striatal degeneration, and biochemically by a deficiency of glutaryl-CoA dehydrogenase, leading to an accumulation of glutaric acid and 3-hydroxyglutaric acid. Its incidence in Sweden has been estimated at 1 in 30,000. A macrocephaly may be present at birth. Development is normal until the end of the first year of life, or is delayed with manifest hypotonia, beginning in the first months of life. Onset of dystonic postures, grimacing, tongue thrusting and choreoathetotic involuntary movements may appear gradually around the age of 1 to 3 years, or the first manifestations of the extrapyramidal syndrome may be abrupt, following an infection. Episodes of unexplained high fever, possibly related to the extrapyramidal motor activity, are frequent. Intelligence is usually relatively preserved. Acute episodes of ketoacidosis, hypoglycemia, hyperammonemia, and elevation of serum transaminase punctuate the course of the disease. A few patients remain asymptomatic.

Biochemical Findings There is a characteristic organic aciduria having high concentrations of glutaric acid and 3-hydroxyglutaric acid. Urinary excretion of glutaconic acid and of dicarboxylic acids may be very high during acute ketotic episodes. All of these biochemical abnormalities may be absent between acute episodes. Bound glutarate in urine, particularly in the form of glutarylcarnitine, is increased in some cases where the urine organic acid profile is otherwise normal.[168] CT scans and MRI reveal typical atrophy and bilateral necrosis of the caudate nuclei and the putamina, as well as a diffuse brain atrophy predominating in the frontotemporal area with widening of the insular cistern (Fig. 3-19).

Diagnosis rests on the demonstration of a deficient activity of glutaryl-CoA dehydrogenase in leukocytes or fibroblasts. As the typical organoaciduria may not be evident between acute metabolic episodes, the activity of this enzyme should be measured in all children with a progressive dystonic and dyskinetic syndrome. Death usually occurs during the first decade, sometimes after an intercurrent infection or an episode of ketoacidosis.

Genetics Hereditary transmission is autosomal recessive. Most patients have an almost total deficiency of glutaryl-CoA dehydrogenase, while in others the deficiency is partial. The degree of residual enzyme activity correlates apparently with the severity of the disease. There are probably several mutant alleles. The gene has been cloned.[169]

Neuropathology and Physiopathology Cell loss and degeneration of the striatum has been shown to increase with the duration of the disease. Evidence of extrapyramidal symptomatology may antedate the presence of visible striatal lesions in MRI. The cause of striatal dysfunction is unknown. It has been shown that glutaric acid is toxic to striatal cells in culture. The possibility has been raised that glutarate toxicity may be due to repeated depolarization of glutamate receptors, or to an increase in the concentrations of quinolinic acid, a neurotoxin, as a result of the block in glutaryl-CoA dehydrogenase. Also, glutaric, glutaconic, and 3-hydroxyglutaric acids inhibit glutaconic acid decarboxylase in the basal ganglia so that GABA production is profoundly reduced.

Treatment Treatment is generally without great effect, at least in patients in whom damage to the striatum has become irreversible. A low-protein diet, riboflavin, and either baclofen or valproate should be systematically tried, and acute episodes of acidosis and hypoglycemia promptly controlled.

Fructose 1,6-Bisphosphate Deficiency, Late-Onset Intermittent Form

About half the patients with fructose 1,6-bisphosphate deficiency have their first symptoms a few days after birth (see Chap. 2). There is also a late-onset, intermittent form, the disorder starting in early infancy or childhood. Acute episodes are triggered by anorexia, vomiting, or fever. Neurological signs are usually dramatic and may lead to apnea and cardiac arrest. There is a profound acidosis, ketosis, and hypoglycemia, and elevation of lactate and uric acid in blood and urine. Hepatomegaly is often observed. Liver function, renal tubular function, and coagulation are normal. The diagnosis is established by demonstrating the enzyme deficiency in biopsies of liver or jejunum or leukocytes. If treatment is started sufficiently early, neurological and mental development proceed normally. Treatment of acute attacks consists of the correction of acidosis and hypoglycemia. Avoidance of fasting and dietary restriction of fructose and sucrose usually help to prevent further acute episodes. The disorder is inherited as an autosomal recessive trait (see also Chap. 2).

Glycogen Storage Disease Type I (Glucose 6-Phosphatase Deficiency)

This disease may begin in the neonatal period, but more commonly presents at 3 or 4 months of age with hypoglycemic seizures and hepatomegaly. Hypoglycemia and lactic acidosis are triggered by fasting and some infants have died during these episodes. Treatment consists in maintaining normal blood glucose concentrations.

Disorders with Hyperammonemia and Respiratory Alkalosis

Late-Onset Urea Cycle Disorders: the Hyperammonemias

Age of onset varies from early infancy to adolescence and adulthood. There are no major clinical differences between the four major types of late-onset urea cycle disorders: carbamylphosphate synthetase deficiency (CPSD); ornithine transcarbamylase deficiency (OTCD), argininosuccinate synthetase deficiency (ASD), and argininosuccinate lyase deficiency (ALD). There is usually a partial defect of these enzymes, which explains their delayed onset. An abnormality of hair (trichorexis nodosa) is present in ALD and in ASD. In ALD, hepatomegaly is less frequent than in the neonatal form. OTCD is inherited as an X-linked trait and the carrier mother may present with some marks of the disease, such as headaches on protein ingestion. This usually limits her protein intake. The first signs of late-onset urea cycle disorders may coincide with weaning from breast milk, or introduction of cow's milk in the formula. The major biochemical changes during the acute attacks consist of hyperammonemia and respiratory alkalosis. High levels of argininosuccinic acid are characteristic of ALD, and high concentrations of citrulline are found in ASD and to a lesser extent in ALD. Orotic acid levels are elevated in OTCD, ASD, and ALD. Levels of blood glucose, lysine, and glycine are normal. The disease must be differentiated from Reye syndrome, lysinuric protein intolerance and from organic acidemias. The therapeutic recommendations in the late-onset urea cycle defects are identical to those of the neonatal form but with less stringent dietary requirements (see Chap. 2).

Two Disorders with Postprandial Hyperammonemia: Familial Lysinuric Protein Intolerance and the HHH Syndrome

Familial Lysinuric Protein Intolerance Familial lysinuric protein intolerance is an autosomal recessive disorder of dibasic amino acid transport. Approximately 80 patients had been reported up to 1989, half of them in Finland.[170] Evidence of protein intolerance appears after weaning, and is manifested by vomiting, diarrhea, and failure to thrive (see also Chap. 2). In infancy and childhood the patients remain anorectic, and have a marked aversion to proteins. They are underdeveloped and hypotonic with a "loose" skin and prominent abdomen. Growth and skeletal maturation are delayed. Head circumference is normal. Enlarged liver and spleen are usual. In older children, osteoporosis becomes an important complication. Interstitial pneumonia threatens life in some patients. A high-protein diet can produce acute episodes of vomiting, dizziness, lethargy, and coma, related to the hyperammonemia. Increases in protein intake can also lead to psychotic episodes and acute or chronic abdominal pain. Seizures are rare. About one-fifth of the children are moderately retarded mentally.[170]

Biochemical Features A very high level of lysine and a more moderate elevation of arginine and ornithine are found in the urine, resulting in deficiency of these amino acids in plasma. There is a high plasma concentration and urinary excretion of alanine, proline, glutamine, citrulline, glycine, and serine.

Blood ammonia concentration is usually normal during fasting but rises after meals to a degree proportional to protein intake. Blood ammonia is also increased after infections, extensive fasting, or stress. In some patients, there is a moderate persistent hyperammonemia. Urinary orotic acid is increased. Serum urea concentrations are normal during the first months and tend to decrease with time. The exact nature of the amino acid transport defect is not known.

Treatment A diet in which proteins are moderately restricted is the basis of successful treatment and helps to prevent the acute episodes of postprandial hyperammonemia. Citrulline supplementation (300 mg/kg/day) is recommended. The addition of lysine (150 mg/kg/day) aids in growth and development.[171] In acute hyperammonemic crises, intravenous glucose, sodium benzoate, and phenylacetate are usually effective.

Hyperornithinemia-hyperammonemia-homocitrullinuria (HHH syndrome) has been described in Chap. 2.

Reye-like Syndromes

Many hereditary metabolic diseases simulate the condition known in pediatric neurology as *Reye syndrome*. It is described here for the purpose of comparison. Reye syndrome is an acquired condition, which usually occurs a few days after a viral illness (particularly influenza B virus, influenza A, and varicella viruses). The syndrome is comprised of signs of both cerebral and hepatic dysfunction.

The clinical picture includes vomiting, disorientation, loss of consciousness, frequently respiratory abnormalities, possibly seizures, in the absence of focal neurological signs or meningitis. Hepatomegaly develops rapidly but jaundice is not a feature. There is a pronounced microvesicular steatosis of the liver and brain edema. Serum transaminases (SGOT, SGPT) are markedly elevated and there is hyperammonemia and lactic acidosis. Free fatty acids have been found to be elevated in the serum. A transitory generalized decrease of mitochondrial enzyme activities has been demonstrated in the liver and brain, but not in muscle. Statistically, some correlation has been reported between the occurrence of Reye syndrome and aspirin ingestion. The incidence of this syndrome has been steadily declining since 1981.

"Reye-like Syndromes" and Recurrent Comas in the Hereditary Metabolic Disorders The hereditary metabolic disorders that present in this way are listed below. Several biochemical features (such as a marked hypoglycemia, hypoketonemia, an organic aciduria, high levels of NH_3 and a propensity to recur) bear no resemblance to Reye syndrome, which in fact has become a rarity. The distinctive clinical and biochemical characteristics of these disorders, described in this chapter, are given here and listed in Table 3-7.

These conditions include: disorders of mitochondrial fatty acid oxidation; inherited disorders of ammonia metabolism; familial lysinuric protein intolerance; inherited disorders of organic acid metabolism (particularly propionic acidemia and methylmalonic aciduria, isovaleric acidemia, 3-methylcrotonyl-CoA carboxylase deficiency, 2-methylacetoacetyl thiolase deficiency, and 3-hydroxy-3-methylglutaryl-CoA lyase deficiency); and disorders of carbohydrate metabolism (fructose 1,6-bisphosphatase deficiency).

Differential Diagnosis The following disorders, which are not related to a hereditary metabolic defect, may also give rise to recurrent comas and cyclic neurologic dysfunction.

Migraine

Alternating hemiplegia

Some forms of epilepsy (essentially nonconvulsive status epilepticus)

Cyclic vomiting

Adrenocortical insufficiency

Congenital portocaval shunts

Idiopathic recurrent stupor[172]

Munchausen syndrome by proxy

Sudden Infant Death   The sudden infant death syndrome (SIDS), frequent in the first year of life, is defined as the sudden and unexpected death of a previously normal child, which remains unexplained even after autopsy.

All enzymatic defects that may provoke Reye-like syndromes may also cause sudden death in infancy (as, for instance, MCAD deficiency). It is therefore essential to search for an underlying metabolic abnormality in any infant who dies suddenly and unexpectedly. Urine and blood obtained postmortem by bladder or heart puncture and samples of liver and muscle must be submitted to adequate biochemical investigations, based on the knowledge of the type of metabolic disorders that may result in sudden infant death.

Identification of the underlying defect is important for the prevention of such a catastrophe in another sibling.

OTHER DISORDERS WITH CLINICAL EXPRESSION IN THE EARLY INFANTILE PERIOD

Other HMDs which have predominantly a neonatal symptomatology or which become generally manifest in late infancy or early childhood can also, at times, be expressed at age 1 to 12 months. They include essentially the large group of the mucopolysaccharidoses and mucolipidoses, which may already display characteristic facial or skeletal features in early infancy (see Chap. 4), and some of the milder forms of peroxisomal disorders such as infantile Refsum disease and neonatal adrenoleukodystrophy (Chap. 2). Also, the Smith-Lemli-Opitz syndrome belongs to the HMDs. It is briefly described here.

The Smith-Lemli-Optiz Syndrome (SLOS)   One of the most common polymalformative syndromes (with an estimated frequency of 1:20,000), this is now known to be related to a defect in cholesterol biosynthesis. Characteristic facial features and developmental defects (usually evident at birth) include ptosis, low-set and posteriorly rotated ears, broad anteverted nares, micrognathia, hypospadias, and multiple other congenital anomalies of the limbs and visceral organs. Children are microcephalic, mentally retarded, and have serious behavioral problems. They are usually small. Various developmental defects of the brain have been reported. A severe neonatal form (SLOS II) is rapidly lethal.

Plasma cholesterol levels are very low, with an elevation of the cholesterol precursor 7-dehydrocholesterol. The primary defect in SLOS appears to be a deficiency of the enzyme 7-dehydrocholesterol-Δ^7-reductase which catalyzes the conversion of 7-dehydrocholesterol to cholesterol. Recently, marked improvement in neurologic development and behavior has been reported in patients on a high-cholesterol diet.

CONCLUSIONS

There are so many hereditary metabolic diseases which become manifest during infancy that one may wonder whether clinical methodology is really adequate for their recognition and differentiation. To this question the authors would reply in the affirmative, with certain concessions to reality. A variety of discriminatory clues exist to this effect. These are listed in Tables 3-5, 3-6, and 3-7. The reader is reminded that generally the long process of identifying these pleiomorphic conditions begins with the clinical observation of a *gradually emerging neurologic syndrome coincident with psychomotor regression*. It is when the clinical condition deviates from this paradigm that diagnosis proves to be difficult.

In our experience there are five major troublesome areas:

(1) The occurrence of a nonhereditary disease, the course of which is progressive, such as a brain tumor, hydrocephalus, or a chronic encephalitic process. This diagnostic problem is usually resolved by neuroimaging studies, and by appropriate tests in blood and CSF.

(2) When the HMD is merely expressed by a delay in psychomotor development, hypotonia, hypomotility, seizures, and pyramidal signs, with no evidence of progressive deterioration.

This type of apparently static encephalopathy is obviously much more frequently the result of perinatal brain lesions, or of prenatal brain lesions caused by developmental defects, infections, or circulatory disturbances. This large group of brain disorders usually cause characteristic changes, such as congenital microcephaly; chorioretinitis; typical destructive or developmental cerebral lesions or calcifications, which are detected by neuroimaging; and malformations of the face, cranium, eyes, limbs, and other somatic structures.

(text continues on page 118)

Diseases—Heredity	CRS	Blindness early OA	Corneal opacities, cataracts	Oculomotor disturbances	Nystagmus	Auditory myoclonus	Major hypotonia
Tay-Sachs disease—AR	+ + +					+ + +	
Sandhoff disease—AR	+ + +					+ + +	
Krabbe leukodystrophy—AR						±	
Gaucher disease type II—AR				+ +			
G_{M1} gangliosidosis type I—AR	+ +		±co				
Niemann-Pick disease type A—AR	+ +					±	
Farber disease—AR	Macular degeneration						
Defects of pyruvate metabolism (infantile lactic acidosis)—AR, X-linked, maternal inheritance							
Biotinidase deficiency—AR		+					
Alpers syndrome—AR		+ Cortical blindness					
Menkes disease—X-linked							
Pelizaeus-Merzbacher disease—X-linked					+ + +		
Canavan disease—AR		+ + +					
Alexander disease							
Lowe disease—X-linked			c+ + + co+ + +				+ + +
Glycogenesis type II—AR							+ + +
Glutaric aciduria type I—AR							
Methylglutaconic aciduria		+					
3-Hydroxyisobutyric aciduria							

Abbreviations and symbols: AR = autosomal recessive; CRS = cherry red spot; OA = optic atrophy; co = corneal opacities; c = cataract; + + + = very frequent or of major diagnostic importance; + + = frequent (30 to 60 percent of cases); + = not rare; ± = rare.

[a]See also Table 3-6.

Distribution of significant neurological signs and routine paraclinical results in the relentlessly progressive early infantile encephalopathies

Peripheral neuropathy	Dystonia choreo-athetosis	Intractable seizures	Progressive macro-cephaly	High protein in CSF	Other neurologic and extraneurologic characteristics[a]	Typical MRI	Routine biochemical investigations
			+ late				
			+ late				Oligosaccharides in urine
+ + +				+ + +	Rigidity-tonic spasms	+ + +	
					Rigidity splenomegaly		
					Skeletal changes		Elevated serum acid phosphatase Oligosaccharides and keratan sulfate in urine
					Hepatomegaly		
±					Subcutaneous nodules		
					Raucous voice		
	+				Ataxia Dysmorphic facial features Prenatal brain defects	+ + +	Lactate elevated in CSF and blood
		+ + +			Ataxia. Deafness Characteristic skin rash Alopecia Biotin responsive		
		+ + +			Liver disease	+ +	Hepatic insufficiency
		+ + +			Subdural hematoma Brain scan Pathognomonic hair	+ +	Low serum copper
+ + +					Microcephaly	+ + +	
			+ + +				N-acetylaspartic acid elevated in urine
			+ + +			+ + +	
					Glaucoma Cataracts Facial features Large heart Typical EMG		Renal tubular dysfunction + + +
+ + +					Fixed macrocephaly Acute episodes of ketoacidosis Striatal degeneration	+ +	Typical organic aciduria Intermittent ketosis and hypoglycemia
+ + +					Pigmentary degeneration of retina Deafness		Typical organic aciduria
					Prenatal developmental defects of brain Dysmorphic features	+ +	3-Hydroxybutyric aciduria

Table 3-6

Diseases	Hepatomegaly, splenomegaly, hepatic dysfunction	Early anorexia and vomiting	Facial dysmorphism	Skin changes	Hair changes
Gaucher disease type II	+ + +spl				
Niemann-Pick type A disease	+ + +	+ + +		±	
G_{M1} gangliosidosis type I	+ + +	+ + +	+ +		
Farber disease	+			+ + +	
Glycogenesis type 2	+ +				
Menkes disease			+ +	+ +	+ + +
Lowe syndrome			+ + +		
Zellweger disease[a]	+ +		+ + +		
Biotinidase deficiency				+ + +	+
3-Hydroxyisobutyric aciduria		+ + +			
Alpers syndrome	+ + +				

Abbreviations and symbols: + + + = very frequent or of major diagnostic importance; + + = frequent (30 to 60 percent of cases); + = not rare; ± = rare; GC = Gaucher cell; spl = splenomegaly.

[a]Described in Chap. 2.

Distribution of extraneurologic signs in the chronic progressive early infantile encephalopathies

Skeletal and joint lesions	Inclusions in bone marrow histiocytes	Other blood abnormalities	Cardiac abnormalities	Urinary tract and kidney abnormalities	Other nonneurologic clinical abnormalities
	+ + + GC	+			Respiratory infections Hypersplenism (late)
	+ + +	+			Vacuoles in lymphocytes
+ + +		+	±		Oligosaccharides and keratan sulfate in urine Vacuoles in lymphocytes
+ + +	+ + +		+		Raucous voice Dyspnea Malnutrition
			+ + +		
+ + +				+ +	Hypothermia Arterial lesions
+				+ + +	Tubular dysfunction followed by glomerular damage
+ + +				+ + +	Impaired adrenocortical function Biotin responsive

Table 3-7

Disease[b]	Other clinical signs	Attacks mainly triggered by	Metabolic acidosis	Ketone bodies	Hypo-glycemia
MCAD, LCAD deficiencies and other defects of mitochondrial β oxidation	Cardiomyopathy muscle weakness. Liver dysfunction	Fasting		Low	+ + +
Glutaric aciduria type II (multiple acyl-CoA dehydrogenase deficiency)	Cardiomyopathy $\pm$ Renal cysts $\pm$ Hepatomegaly. Odor of urine. (Multiple congenital anomalies in neonatal form.)		+ +	Low	+ + +
Defects of the carnitine cycle					
Primary carnitine deficiency	Cardiomyopathy Muscle weakness	Fasting		Low	+ + +
Carnitine palmitoyl transferase I deficiency	Hepatomegaly	Fasting		Low	+ + +
Carnitine palmitoyl transferase II deficiency	Cardiomyopathy Liver failure Myoglobinuria	Fasting		Low	+ + +
Pyruvate dehydrogenase deficiency (X-linked)	Mostly Leigh syndrome		+ + LA		
Leigh syndrome (AR, X-linked, maternal transmission)	Oculo-motor palsies. Episodic hyperpnea. Ataxia. Choreoathetosis				
Pyruvate carboxylase deficiency			+ +		
3OH-3 Methylglutaric deficiency	Cerebral atrophy	Fasting	+ + LA	Low	+ + +
Biotinidase deficiency	Seizures. Skin rash Alopecia		+ + +	High	
Isovaleric acidemia	Odor of urine Pancytopenia	Protein intake ↑ Fever	+ + +	High	
3-Methyl crotonyl-CoA carboxylase deficiency	Alopecia $\pm$	Protein intake ↑ Fever	+ +		+ +
2-Methylacetoacetyl CoA thiolase deficiency	Diarrhea	Protein intake ↑ Fever	+ + +	High	

Early infantile metabolic encephalopathies with acute, intermittent neurologic episodes[a] and coma

Low serum carnitine	Hyper-ammonemia	Respiratory alkalosis	Distinctive biochemical abnormalities	Treatment[c]	Diagnostic tests
+ +	+ +		Urinary dicarboxylic acids. Acyl-carnitines in urine. Glycine conjugates. Serum transaminase elevated	Avoid fasting. Reduce fat intake. L-carnitine	Enzyme assays on fibroblasts
	+ +		Typical organic aciduria. Serum transaminase ↑	Riboflavin L-Carnitine Low fat diet	Demonstration of defects of ETF or ETF-QO
+ + + extremely low	+ +			Oral carnitine	Carnitine uptake in fibroblasts
	+		Hypertriglyceridemia	Medium-chain triglycerides	Enzyme assay on fibroblasts
					Enzyme assay on muscle
			Lactic acidosis CSF, blood	High fat L-carnitine Thiamine Dichloroacetate	Enzyme assay on fibroblasts and other tissues
			Lactic acidosis CSF		Characteristic MRI. Defects of different mitochondrial enzymes
			Lactic acidosis CSF, blood		Enzyme assay on fibroblasts
	+ +		Typical organic aciduria Serum transaminase ↑	Restriction of fat and protein Avoidance of fasting	Enzyme assay in fibroblasts
	+ +		Typical organic aciduria	Biotin	Enzyme assay on fibroblasts
			Organic aciduria Isovalerylglycine 3-Hydroxyisovalerate	Protein restriction Glycine, carnitine	Enzyme assay on fibroblasts
			Organic aciduria 3-hydroxyisovalerate 3-methylcrotonyl glycine	Protein restriction L-carnitine	Enzyme assay on fibroblasts
			Organic aciduria 2 methyl 3 hydrobutyrate 2 methyl acetoacetate	Protein restriction	Enzyme assay on fibroblasts

Table 3-7 (contd.)

Disease[b]	Other clinical signs	Attacks mainly triggered by	Metabolic acidosis	Ketone bodies	Hypo-glycemia
Glutaric aciduria type I	Dystonia Necrosis of striatum		+ + +	High	+ +
Propionic acidemia	Neutropenia Thrombocytopenia Hepatomegaly Necrosis putamen or globus pallidus	High protein diet Fever	+ + +	High	+ +
Methylmalonic acidemia	Neutropenia Thrombocytopenia Hepatomegaly Necrosis of putamen or globus pallidus	High protein diet Fever	+ + +	High	+ +
Maple syrup urine disease	Odor of urine	High protein diet Fever	+ +		
Carbamyl phosphate synthetase deficiency	Hyperpnea	High protein diet Fever			
Ornithine transcarbamylase deficiency (X-linked)	Hyperpnea Mother symptomatic +	High protein diet Fever			
Argininosuccinate synthetase deficiency	Trichorexis nodosa ±	High protein diet Fever			
Argininosuccinate lyase deficiency	Trichorexis nodosa Hepatomegaly	High protein diet Fever			
Familial lysinuric protein intolerance	Hepatosplenomegaly	High protein diet			
HHH syndrome		Protein ingestion			
Fructose 1,6 bisphosphase deficiency	Hepatomegaly	Fasting Fever	+ + + LA	High	+ + +

[a]In all disorders in this category, acute episodes are characterized by vomiting, irritability, lethargy and coma, respiratory dysrhythmia, occasionally seizures. (All disorders listed in this table may also be responsible for sudden death.)

[b]Inherited as autosomal recessive traits, unless stated otherwise.

[c]In addition to urgent measures to counteract acidosis, hypoglycemia, seizures, circulatory collapse, and hemodialysis.

Symbols: + + + = very frequent or of major diagnostic importance; + + = frequent (30 to 60 percent of cases); + = not rare; ± = rare; LA = lactic acidosis; MCAD = medium-chain acyl-CoA dehydrogenase; LCAD = long-chain acyl-CoA dehydrogenase; ↑ = elevated.

Early infantile metabolic encephalopathies with acute, intermittent neurologic episodes[a] and coma

Low serum camitine	Hyper-ammonemia	Respiratory alkalosis	Distinctive biochemical abnormalities	Treatment[c]	Diagnostic tests
	+ +		Organic aciduria ↑ Glutaric acid and 3 hydroxyglutaric acid ↑ Serum transaminase	Protein restriction L-carnitine Riboflavin Baclofen	Enzyme assays on fibroblasts
			Hyperglycinemia ↑ Propionic acid and derivates	Protein restriction Biotin L-carnitine	Enzyme assay on fibroblasts
	+ +		Hyperglycinemia	Protein restriction Cobalamin L-carnitine	Enzyme assay on fibroblasts
			↑ Branched chain amino acids, and keto acids L. alloisoleucine	Protein restriction Thiamine	Assay on cultured cells
	+ + +	+ +		Sodium benzoate and sodium phenylacetate Low protein diet Citrulline	Enzyme assays on liver and intestinal mucosa
	+ + +	+ +	↑ Orotic acid	Sodium benzoate and sodium phenylacetate Low protein diet Citrulline	Enzyme assays on liver and intestinal mucosa
	+ + +	+ +	↑ Orotic acid ↑ Citrulline + + + ↑ Argininosuccinic acid	Sodium benzoate and sodium phenylacetate Low protein diet Arginine	Enzyme assays on liver and fibroblasts
	+ + +	+ +	↑ Orotic acid ↑ Citrulline + +	Sodium benzoate and sodium phenylacetate Low protein diet Arginine	Enzyme assays on liver and fibroblasts
	+ + +	+ +	↑ Urinary lysine + + + ↑ Orotic acid ↑ Alanine	Low protein diet Citrulline, lysine supplementation	
	+ +		↑ Ornithine in plasma Homocitrullinuria ↑ Orotic acid	Protein restriction Ornithine supplementation	
			↑ Alanine ↑ Uric acid	Avoid fructose, sucrose, fasting	Enzyme assays on liver or jejunal biopsy

Unfortunately, from the clinical standpoint, some of the HMDs also produce prenatal brain defects and somatic malformations. Developmental anomalies of the cerebral cortex, thinning of the corpus callosum, and prenatal destruction of the white matter and lenticular nuclei, occur in some inherited disorders of mitochondria, peroxisomes, amino acids, and organic acids (Table 6-1). Some of these lesions closely resemble those produced by perinatal ischemia. Also, malformations of the face, eyes, limbs, genito-urinary tract, etc., are observed, for instance, in glutaric aciduria type II, the Smith-Lemli-Opitz syndrome, and a limited number of rare aminoacidopathies.

In favour of an HMD, one may be oriented by the presence of neurologic and visceral signs listed in Tables 3-5 and 3-6, but, often, there is no clue. In these circumstances it has been our practice to subject all infants with a nonprogressive neurologic syndrome of obscure origin (excepting those with a very low birth weight, marked congenital microcephaly, and a specific malformative status) to a few systematic paraclinical investigations listed in the first pages of this chapter. Although the results of these investigations are often negative, the importance of early discovery of an HMD outweighs practical and economic objections.

(3) When anorexia, vomiting, diarrhea, or severe liver involvement precedes or masks signs of neurologic dysfunction.

(4) In the presence of acute metabolic episodes with vomiting, hyperpnea, seizures, stupor, and coma, which have propensity to recur. Such symptoms should always suggest an HMD. Some of the biochemical abnormalities detected in routine laboratory screening during these acute attacks are essential for the diagnosis of these conditions. The presence either of lactic acidosis, nonketotic hypoglycemia, ketoacidosis, or hyperammonemia with respiratory alkalosis serve to categorize these diseases and to initiate urgent therapeutic measures. In some patients, clinical features and standard laboratory tests may resemble those produced by Reye syndrome. However, this postviral illness has now become probably less frequent than metabolic disorders.

(5) In case of sudden and unexpected death. Sudden infant death should always raise questions of an HMD. The same diseases which give rise to recurrent episodes of coma can also lead to a sudden death. Except when there is a significant family history, the diagnosis and possibility of prevention rest entirely on biochemical tests performed on blood, urine, muscle, or liver samples collected after the death of the infant. This procedure should be adopted in all instances of sudden, unexplained infantile death.

An accurate diagnosis of most of the early infantile metabolic encephalopathies is now possible, supported by biochemical and molecular methods and modern neuroimaging techniques. Early diagnosis assumes a great importance as an appreciable number of these conditions are amenable to therapeutic intervention. Lifesaving measures and methods to protect the nervous system are now available for many of these diseases.

REFERENCES

1. Hers HG: Inborn lysosomal diseases. *Gastroenterology* 48: 625–633, 1965.
2. Hers HG: The concept of inborn lysosomal disease, in Hers HG, Van Hoof F (eds): *Lysosomes and Storage Diseases*. New York, Academic Press, 1973, pp. 625–633.
3. Tay W: Symmetrical changes in the region of the yellow spot in each eye of an infant. *Trans Ophthalmol Soc UK* 1: 55–57, 1881.
4. Sachs B: On arrested cerebral development with special reference to its cortical pathology. *J Nerv Ment Dis* 14: 541–553, 1887.
5. Svennerholm L: The chemical structure of normal human brain and Tay-Sachs gangliosides. *Biochem Biophys Res Commun* 9: 436–441, 1962.
6. Conzelmann E, Sandhoff K: Biochemical basis of late-onset neurolipidoses. *Dev Neurosci* 13: 197–204, 1991.
7. Schneck L, Maisel J, Volk BW: The startle response and serum enzyme profile in early detection of Tay-Sachs disease. *J Pediatr* 65: 749, 1964.
8. Kolodny EH: Tay-Sachs disease, in Goodman RM, Motulsky AG (eds): *Genetic Diseases Amongst Ashkenazy Jews*. New York, Raven, 1979.
9. Terry RD, Weiss M: Studies in Tay-Sachs disease II. Ultrastructure of the cerebrum. *J Neuropath Exp Neurol* 22: 18–55, 1963.
10. Greenfield JG: The retina in cerebrospinal lipidosis. *Proc Roy Soc Med* 44: 686–689, 1951.
11. Landing BH, Silverman FN, Craig JM, et al.: Familial neurovisceral lipidosis. *Am J Dis Child* 108: 503–522, 1964.
12. O'Brien JS, Stern MB, Landing BH, et al.: Generalized gangliosidosis. *Am J Dis Child* 109: 338–346, 1965.
13. Gonatas NK, Gonatas J: Ultrastructural and biochemical observations on a case of systemic late infantile lipidosis and its relationship to Tay-Sachs disease and gargoylism. *J Neuropathol Exp Neurol* 24: 318–340, 1965.
14. Okada S, O'Brien JS: Generalized gangliosidosis, β-galactosidase deficiency. *Science* 160: 1002–1004, 1968.
15. Suzuki Y, Sakubara H, Oshima A: Beta-galactosidase deficiency, in Scriver CR, Beaudet AL, Sly WS, Valle D (eds): *The Metabolic and Molecular Bases of Inherited Disease*. New York, McGraw-Hill, 1995, pp. 2809–2810.
16. Suzuki K: Cerebral G_{M1} gangliosidosis: chemical pathology of visceral organs. *Science* 159: 1471–1472, 1968.

17. Niemann A: Ein unbekanntes Krankheitsbild. *Jahrb Kinderheilkd* 79: 1–10, 1914.

18. Pick L: Uber die lipoidzellige Splenohepatomegalie typus Niemann-Pick als Stoffwechselerkrankung. *Med Klin* 23: 1483–1488, 1927.

19. Crocker AC, Farber S: Niemann-Pick disease: A review of eighteen patients. *Medicine* 37: 1–95, 1958.

20. Spence MW, Callahan JW: Sphingomyelin-cholesterol lipidoses. The Niemann-Pick group of diseases, in Scriver CR, Beaudet AL, Sly WS, Valle D (eds): *The Metabolic Basis of Inherited Disease*. New York, McGraw-Hill, 1989, pp. 1655–1666.

21. Besley GT, Elleder M: Enzyme activities and phospholipid storage patterns in brain and spleen samples from Niemann-Pick disease variants: A comparison of neuropathic and non-neuropathic forms. *J Inherit Metab Dis* 9: 59–71, 1986.

22. Caggana M, Eng CM, Desnick RJ, et al.: Molecular population studies of Niemann-Pick disease type A. *Am J Hum Genet* 55 (suppl) A: 147, 1994.

23. Kamoshita S, Aron AM, Suzuki K, Suzuki K: Infantile Niemann-Pick disease: A chemical study with isolation and characterization of membranous cytoplasmic bodies and myelin. *Am J Dis Child* 117: 379–394, 1969.

24. Gaucher PCE: *De l'Epithelioma Primitif de la Rate*. Paris, Thèse, 1882.

25. Oberling C, Woringer P: La maladie de Gaucher du nourrisson. *Rev Fr Pediatr* 3: 475–532, 1927.

26. Beutler E, Grabowski GA: Gaucher disease. In Scriver CR, Beaudet AL, Sly WS, Valle D (eds): *The Metabolic and Molecular Bases of Inherited Disease*. New York, McGraw-Hill, 1995, pp. 2641–2670.

27. Farber S, Cohen J, Uzman LL: Lipogranulomatosis. A new lipoglycoprotein "storage" disease. *J Mt Sinai Hosp* 24: 816–837, 1957.

28. Moser HW, Moser AB, Chen WW, et al.: Ceramidase deficiency: Farber lipogranulomatosis, in Scriver CR, Beaudet AL, Sly WS, Valle D (eds): *The Metabolic Basis of Inherited Disease*. New York, McGraw-Hill, 1989, pp. 1645–1654.

29. Vital C, Battin J, Rivel J, et al.: Aspects ultrastructuraux des lésions du nerf périphérique dans un cas de maladie de Farber. *Rev Neurol* 132: 419–427, 1976.

30. Samuelsson K, Zetterstrom R, Ivemark BI: Studies on a case of lipogranulomatosis (Farber's disease) with protracted course, in Volk BW, Aronson SM (eds): *Sphingolipids, Sphingolipidoses and Allied Disorders*. New York, Plenum, 1972, p. 533.

31. Antonarakis SE, Valle D, Moser HW, et al.: Phenotypic variability in siblings with Farber disease. *J Pediatr* 104: 409, 1984.

32. Pellissier JF, Berard-Badier M, Pinsard N: Farber's disease in two siblings, sural nerve and subcutaneous biopsies studied by light and electron microscopy. *Acta Neuropath* 72: 178–188, 1986.

33. Johnson WG, Thomas GH, Miranda AF, et al.: Congenital sialidosis, a new form of alpha-L-neuraminidase deficiency. Its possible relation to hydrops fetalis (abstract). *Neurology* 30: 377, 1980.

34. Aylsworth AS, Thomas GH, Hood JL, et al.: A severe infantile sialidosis: clinical, biochemical and microscopic features. *J Pediatr* 96, 662–668, 1980.

35. Le Sec G, Stanescu R, Lyon G: Un nouveau type de sialidose avec atteinte rénale: la néphrosialidose II. Etude anatomique. *Arch Fr Pediatr* 35: 830–844, 1978.

36. Matsuo T, Egwa I, et al.: Sialidosis type 2 in Japan. *J Neurol Sci* 58: 45–55, 1983.

37. Chitayat D, Applegarth DA, Lewis J, et al.: Juvenile galactosialidosis in a white male. A new variant. *Am J Med Genet* 31: 887–901, 1988.

38. Kleijer WJ, Hoogeveen A, Verheijen FW, et al.: Prenatal diagnosis of sialidosis with combined neuraminidase and beta-galactosidase deficiency. *Clin Genet* 16: 60–61, 1979.

39. Paschke E, Trinkl G, Erwa W, et al.: Infantile type of sialic acid storage disease with sialuria. *Clin Genet* 29: 417–424, 1986.

40. Aula P, Autio S, Raivio KO, et al.: Salla disease: a new lysosomal storage disorder. *Arch Neurol* 36: 88–94, 1979.

41. Pompe JC: Over idiopathische hypertrophie van het hart. *Ned T Genesk* 76: 304, 1932.

42. Cori GT: Glycogen structure and enzyme deficiencies in glycogen storage disease. *Harvey Lect* 48: 145, 1954.

43. Hers HG: Alpha-glucosidase deficiency in generalized glycogen storage disease (Pompe's disease). *Biochem J* 86: 11–16, 1963.

44. Hers HG, Van Hoof F, De Barsy T: Glycogen storage diseases, in Scriver CR, Beaudet AL, Sly WS, Valle D (eds): *The Metabolic Basis of Inherited Disease*. New York, McGraw-Hill, 1989, pp. 437–440.

45. Nishimoto J, Inui K, Okade S, et al.: A family with pseudodeficiency of acid alpha-glucosidose. *Clin Genet* 33: 254–261, 1988.

46. Baudhuin P, Hers HG, Loeb H: An electron microscopic and biochemical study of type II glycogenosis. *Lab Invest* 13: 1139–1152, 1964.

47. Smith HL, Amick LD, Sidbury JB: Type II glycogenosis. Report of a case with four-year survival and absence of acid maltase associated with an abnormal glycogen. *Am J Dis Child* 111: 475, 1966.

48. Smith J, Zellweger H, Afifi AK: Muscular form of glycogenosis type II (Pompe). *Neurology (Minneap)* 17: 537–549, 1967.

49. Martin JJ, de Barsy T, Den Tandt WR: Acid maltase deficiency in non-identical adult twins. *J Neurol* 213: 105–118, 1976.

50. Vietor KW, Havsteen B, Harms B, et al.: Ethanolaminosis: a newly recognized storage disease with cardiomegaly, cerebral dysfunction and early death. *Eur J Pediatr* 126: 61–75, 1977.

51. Danon MJ, Carpenter S, Marrigold JR, et al.: Fatal infantile glycogen storage disease: deficiency of phosphofructo-

kinase and phosphorylase-*b*-kinase. *Neurology* 31: 1303–1307, 1981.

52. Krabbe K: A new familial, infantile form of diffuse brain sclerosis. *Brain* 39: 74, 1916.

53. Collier J, Greenfield JG: The encephalitis periaxialis of Schilder: A clinical and pathological study with an account of two cases, one of which was diagnosed during life. *Brain* 47: 489–519, 1924.

54. Bullard WN, Southard EE: Diffuse gliosis of the cerebral white matter in a child. *J Nerv Ment Dis* 33: 188, 1906.

55. Beneke R: Ein Fall hochgradigster ausgedehnter Sklerose des Centralnervensystems. *Arch Kinderheilkd* 47: 420, 1908.

56. Hagberg B, Kollberg H, Sourander P, et al.: Infantile globoid cell leucodystrophy (Krabbe's disease): A clinical and genetic study of 32 Swedish cases 1953–1967. *Neuropaediatrie* 1: 74–88, 1970.

57. Hagberg B: Krabbe's disease: clinical presentation and neurological variants. *Neuropediatrics* 15 (suppl): 1–15, 1984.

58. Osetowska E, Gail H, Lukasewicz D, et al: Leucodystrophie infantile précoce (type Krabbe): (Remarques sur les proliférations gliales et les atrophies de système qui peuvent s'y observer). *Rev Neurol* 102: 463–477, 1960.

59. Wallace BJ, Aronson SM, Volk BW: Histochemical and biochemical studies of globoid cell leucodystrophy (Krabbe's disease). *J Neurochem* 11: 367–376, 1963.

60. Sasaki M, Sakuragawa N, Takashima S, et al.: MRI and CT findings in Krabbe disease. *Pediatr Neurol* 7(4): 283–288, 1991.

61. Wenger DA, Riccardi VM: Possible misdiagnosis of Krabbe disease. *J Pediatr* 88: 76–79, 1976.

62. Suzuki K, Suzuki Y, Suzuki K: Galactosylceramide lipidosis: globoid-cell leukodystrophy (Krabbe disease). In Scriver CR, Beaudet AL, Sly WS, Valle D (eds): *The Metabolic and Molecular Bases of Inherited Disease*. New York, McGraw-Hill, 1995, pp. 2671–2692.

63. Seitelberger F: Pelizaeus-Merzbacher disease, in Vinken PJ, Bruyn GW (eds): *Handbook of Clinical Neurology*. Amsterdam, North Holland, 1970, vol. 10, p. 151.

64. Merzbacher L: Uber die Pelizaeus-Merzbachersche Krankheit. *Zbl Neur* 32: 202, 1923.

65. Garcin R, Lapresle J, Berger B: Etude anatomoclinique d'un cas de maladie de Pelizaeus-Merzbacher. *Rev Neurol* 112: 449–466, 1965.

66. Diezel PB, Fritzch H, Jakob H: Leukodystrophie mit orthochromatischen Abbaustoffe. Ein Beitrag zur Pelizaeus-Merzbacherschen Krankehit. *Virchows Arch (Pathol Anat)* 338: 371–394, 1965.

67. Seitelberger F: Die Pelizaeus-Merzbacherrsche Krankheit. Klinisch-anatomische untersuchungen zum problem ihrer stellung unter den diffusen sklerosen. *Wien Z Nervenheilk* 9: 228–289, 1954.

68. Jellinger K, Seitelberger F: Pelizaeus-Merzbacher disease. Transitional form between classical and connatal (Seitelberger) type. *Acta Neuropathol (Berl)* 14: 108–117, 1969.

69. Norman RM, Tingey AH.: Sudanophil leukodystrophy and Pelizaeus-Merzbacher disease. In Folch-Pi J, Bauer H (eds): *Brain Lipids and Lipoproteins and Leukodystrophies*. Amsterdam, Elsevier, 1963, pp. 169–186.

70. Van Bogaert L: Familial type of orthochromatic leukodystrophies, in Vinken PJ, Bruyn GW (eds) *Handbook of Clinical Neurology*. Amsterdam, North Holland, 1970, vol. 10, pp. 120–128.

71. Pelizaeus F: Uber eine eigentümliche form spastischer lähmung mit zerebraler scheinungen auf hereditärer grundlage (multiple sklerose). *Arch Psychiatr Nervenkr* 16: 698–710, 1885.

72. Merzbacher L: Eine eigenartige familiäre erkrankungsform (aplasia axialis extra-corticalis congenita). *Z Ges Neurol Psychiatr* 3: 1–138, 1910.

73. Boulloche J, Aicardi J: Pelizaeus-Merzbacher disease: clinical and nosological study. *J Child Neurol* 1: 233–239, 1986.

74. Haenggeli CA, Engel E, Pizzolato GP: Connatal Pelizaeus-Merzbacher disease. *Develop Med and Child Neurol* 31: 803–807, 1989.

75. Van der Knaap MS, Valk J: The reflection of histology on MR imaging of Pelizaeus-Merzbacher disease. *Am J Neuroradiol* 10: 99–103, 1989.

76. Boespflug TO, Mimault C, Melki J, et al.: Genetic homogeneity of Pelizaeus-Merzbacher disease: tight linkage to the proteolipoprotein locus in 16 affected families. PMD Clinical Group. *Am J Hum Genet* 55: 461–467, 1994.

77. Boltshauser E, Schinzel A, Wichmann W, et al.: Pelizaeus-Merzbacher disease: identification of heterozygotes with magnetic resonance imaging? *Helvetica Paediatr Acta* 42: 337–339, 1987.

78. Johnston AW, McKusick VA: A sex-linked recessive form of spastic paraplegia. *Am J Hum Genet* 14: 83–94, 1962.

79. Saugier-Veber P, Munnich A, Bonneau D, et al.: X-linked spastic paraplegia and Pelizaeus-Merzbacher disease are allelic disorders at the proteolipid protein locus. *Nat Genet* 6: 257–262, 1994.

80. Kobayashi H, Marks HG, Matise TC, et al.: The mouse rumpshaker mutation of the proteolipid protein in human X-linked recessive spastic paraplegia. *Am J Hum Genet* 55 (suppl): A5, 1994.

81 Van Bogaert L, Bertrand I: Sur une idiotie familiale avec dégénérescence spongieuse du névraxe. *Acta Neurol Belg* 49: 572–587, 1949.

82. Canavan MM: Schilder's encephalitis periaxialis diffusa. Report of a case in a child aged sixteen and a half months. *Arch Neurol Psychiatr* 25: 299–301, 1931.

83. Banker BQ, Robertson JT, Victor M: Spongy degeneration of the central nervous system in infancy. *Neurology* 14: 981–1001, 1964.

84. Ungar M, Goodman RM: Spongy degeneration of the brain in Israel: A retrospective study. *Clin Genet* 23: 23–29, 1983.

85. Matalon R, Kaul R, Casanova J, et al.: Aspartoacylase deficiency: the enzyme defect in Canavan disease. *J Inherit Metab Dis* 12 (suppl 2): 329–331, 1989.

86. Alexander WS: Progressive fibrinoid degeneration of fibrillary astrocytes associated with mental retardation in a hydrocephalic infant. *Brain* 72: 373–381, 1949.

87. Wohlwill FJ, Bernstein J, Yakovlev PI: Dysmyelinogenic leukodystrophy. *J Neuropathol Exp Neurol* 18: 359–383, 1959.

88. Crome L: Megalencephaly associated with hyaline panneuropathy. *Brain* 76: 215–228, 1953.

89. Russo LS, Aron A, Anderson PJ: Alexander's disease: a report and a reappraisal. *Neurology* 26: 607–614, 1976.

90. Vogel FS, Hallervorden J: Leukodystrophy with diffuse Rosenthal fiber formation. *Acta Neuropathol* 2: 126–143, 1962.

91. Friede RL: Alexander's Disease. *Arch Pathol* 11: 414–422, 1964.

92. Stevenson LD, Vogel FS: A case of macrocephaly associated with feeble-mindedness and encephalopathy with peculiar deposits throughout the brain and spinal cord. *Ciencia* 12: 71–74, 1952.

93. Herndon RM, Rubinstein LJ, Freeman JRM, et al.: Light and electron microscopy observations on Rosenthal fiber in Alexander's disease and in multiple sclerosis. *J Neuropathol Exp Neurol* 29(4): 524–551, 1970.

94. Garret R, Ames RP: Alexander's disease. *Arch Pathol* 38: 379, 1976.

95. Navarro C: Personal communication, 1980.

96. Escourolle R, Baumann N: Etude microscopique, ultra-structurale et neurochimique après biopsie cérébrale et examen post-mortem d'un cas de maladie d'Alexander, in *Proceedings VIII Riunion della sezione di Neuropatologia della Societa Italiana die Neurologia*, Naples, Feb 1972.

97. Goldman JE, Corbin E: Rosenthal fibers contain ubiquitinated alpha-B-crystallin. *Am J Pathol* 139(4): 933–938, 1991.

98. Wolf B, Heard GS, Weissbecker KA, et al.: Biotinidase deficiency: initial clinical features and rapid diagnosis. *Ann Neurol* 18: 614–617, 1985.

99. Hart PS, Hymes J, Wolf B: Biochemical and immunological characterization of serum biotinidase in profound biotinidase deficiency. *Am J Hum Genet* 50: 126–136, 1992.

100. Duran M, Baumgartner ER, Suormala TM, et al.: Cerebrospinal fluid organic acids in biotinidase deficiency. *J Inherit Metab Dis* 16: 513–516, 1993.

101. Suzuki Y, Aoki Y, Ishida Y, et al.: Molecular cloning and chromosomal localization of human holocarboxylase synthetase, a gene responsible for biotin dependency. *Am J Hum Genet* 55 (suppl 3): A244, 1994.

102. Suzuki Y, Aoki Y, Hoshinori I, et al.: Isolation and characterisation of mutations in the human holocarboxylase synthetase cDNA. *Nat Genet* 8: 122–128, 1994.

103. Menkes JH: Kinky hair disease: from bedside to gene therapy. *Int Pediatr* 9 (suppl 2): 55–59, 1994.

104. Tumer Z, Tonnesen T, Horn N: Detection of genetic defects in Menkes disease by direct mutation analysis and its implications in carrier diagnosis. *J Inherit Metab Dis* 17: 267–270, 1994.

105. Danks DM: Disorders of copper transport, in Scriver CR, Beaudet AL, Sly WS, Valle D (eds): *The Metabolic and Molecular Bases of Inherited Disease*. New York, McGraw-Hill, 1995, pp. 2211–2235.

106. Kaler SG, Gallo LK, Proud VK, et al.: Occipital horn syndrome and a mild Menkes phenotype associated with splice site mutations at the MNK locus. *Nat Genet* 8: 195–202, 1994.

107. Alpers BJ: Diffuse progressive degeneration of the gray matter of the cerebrum. *Arch Neurol Psychiatr* 25: 469–505, 1931.

108. Christensen E, Krabbe KH: Poliodystrophia cerebri progressiva (infantilis). Report of a case. *Arch Neurol Psychiatr* 67: 58–73, 1949.

109. Jellinger K, Seitelberger F: Spongy glio-neuronal dystrophy in infancy and childhood. *Acta Neuropathol* 16: 125–140, 1970.

110. Laurence KM, Cavanagh JB: Progressive degeneration of the cerebral cortex in infancy. *Brain* 91: 261–280, 1968.

111. Wolf A, Cowen D: The cerebral atrophies and encephalomalacias of infancy and childhood. *Proc Assoc Nerv Ment Dis* 34: 199–331, 1954.

112. Huttenlocher PR, Solitare GB, Adams G: Infantile diffuse cerebral degeneration with hepatic cirrhosis. *Archiv Neurol* 33: 186–192, 1976.

113. Harding BN: Progressive neuronal degeneration of childhood with liver disease (Alpers-Huttenlocher syndrome). A personal review. *J Child Neurol* 5: 273–287, 1990.

114. Prick MJJ, Gabreels FJM, Renier WO, et al.: Progressive poliodystrophy (Alper's disease) with a defect in cytochrome aa3 in muscle. *Clin Neurol Neurosurg* 85: 57–70, 1983.

115. Manuelidis EE, Rorke LB: Transmission of Alper's disease (chronic progressive encephalopathy), produces experimental Creutzfeld-Jacob disease in hamsters. *Neurology* 39: 615–621, 1989.

116. DeVivo DC, Trifiletti RR, Jacobsen RI, et al.: Defective glucose transport across the blood brain barrier as a cause of persistent hypoglycorrhachia, seizures and developmental delay. *New Engl J Med* 325: 703–709, 1991.

117. DeVivo DC, Garcia-Alvarez M, Ronen G, et al.: Glucose transport protein deficiency: an emerging syndrome with therapeutic implications. *Int Pediatr* 10: 51–56, 1995.

118. Lowe CU, Terrey M, MacLachlan EA: Organic aciduria, decreased renal ammonia production, hydrophthalmos and mental retardation: a clinical entity. *Am J Dis Child* 83: 164–184, 1952.

118a Suchy SF, Olivos-Glander IM, Nussbaum RL: Lowe syndrome gene encodes a phosphatidylinositol 4,5-bisphosphate 5-phosphatase expressed in the Golgi apparatus. *Am J Hum Genet* 57: Suppl. A38, 1995.

119. Charnas L, Bernar J, Pezeshkpour GH, et al.: MRI findings and peripheral neuropathy in Lowe's syndrome. *Neuropediatrics* 19: 7–9, 1988.

120. Charnas RL, Bernardini I, Rader D, et al.: Clinical and laboratory findings in the oculo-cerebrorenal syndrome of Lowe, with special reference to growth and renal function. *New Engl J Med* 324: 1318–1325, 1991.

121. Hittner HM, Carroll AJ, Prchal JT: Linkage studies in carriers of Lowe oculo-cerebro-renal syndrome. *Am J Human Genet* 34: 966–971, 1982.

122. Leahey AM, Charnas LR, Nussbaum RL: Nonsense mutations in the *OCRL-1* gene in patients with the oculo-cerebrorenal syndrome of Lowe. *Hum Mol Genet* 2(4): 461–463, 1993.

123. Chitayat D, Chemke J, Gibson KM, et al.: 3-Methylglutaconic aciduria: a marker for as yet unspecified disorders and the relevance of prenatal diagnosis in a "new" type ("type 4"). *J Inherit Metab Dis* 15: 204–212, 1992.

124. Gibson KM, Lee CF, Wappner RS: 3-Methylglutaconyl-coenzyme-A hydratase deficiency: a new case. *J Inherit Metab Dis* 15: 363–366, 1992.

125. Seargeant LE, Chudley AE, Dilling LA, et al.: Carrier detection in glutaric aciduria type 1 using interleukin-2-dependent cultured lymphocytes. *J Inherit Metab Dis* 15: 733–737, 1992.

126. Jakobs C, Jaeken J, Gibson KM: Inherited disorders of GABA metabolism. *J Inherit Metab Dis* 16: 704–715, 1993.

127. Eisensmith RC, Woo SL: Molecular basis of phenylketonuria and related hyperphenylalaninemias: mutations and polymorphisms in the human phenylalanine hydroxylase gene. *Hum Mutat* 1(1): 13–23, 1992.

128. Okano Y, Eisensmith RC, Guttler F: Molecular basis of phenotypic heterogeneity in phenylketonuria. *New Engl J Med* 324: 1232–1238, 1991.

129. Scriver CR, Kaufman S, Eisensmith RC et al: The hyperphenylalaninemias, in Scriver CR, Beaudet AL, Sly WS, Valle D (eds): *The Metabolic and Molecular Bases of Inherited Disease*. New York, McGraw-Hill, 1995, pp. 1015–1075.

130. Weglage J, Funders B, Wilken B, et al.: Psychological and social findings in adolescents with phenylketonuria. *Eur J Pediatr* 151: 522–525, 1992.

131. Dhondt JL: Les déficits en tetrahydrobioptérine. Enseignements de l'analyse de 90 patients colligés dans le registre international. *Arch Fr Pediatr* 44: 655–659, 1987.

132. Shintaku H, Hsiao KJ, Liu TT, et al.: Prenatal diagnosis of 6-pyruvoyl tetrahydropterin synthase deficiency in seven subjects. *J Inherit Metab Dis* 17(1): 163–166, 1994.

133. Scriver CR, Levy HL: Histidinemia. Part I: Reconciling retrospective and prospective findings. *J Inherit Metab Dis* 6: 51–53, 1983.

134. Levy HL, Taylor RG, McInnes RR: Disorders of histidine metabolism, in Scriver CR, Beaudet AL, Sly WS, Valle D (eds): *The Metabolic and Molecular Bases of Inherited Disease*. New York, McGraw-Hill, 1995, pp. 1107–1124.

135. Schweitzer S, Shin Y, Jacobs C, et al.: Long-term outcome of 134 patients with galactosemia. *Eur J Pediatr* 152: 36–43, 1993.

136. Gibson KM, Lee CF, Bennett MJ, et al.: Combined malonic, methylmalonic and ethylmalonic acid semialdehyde dehydrogenase deficiencies: an inborn error of β-alanine, L-valine and L-alloisoleucine metabolism. *J Inherit Metab Dis* 16: 563–567, 1993.

137. Chitayat D, Meagher-Villemure K, Mamer OA, et al.: Brain dysgenesis and congenital intracerebral calcification associated with 3-hydroxyisobutyric aciduria. *J Pediatr* 121: 86–89, 1992.

138. Ko FJ, Nyhan WL, Wolff J, et al.: 3-Hydroxyisobutyric aciduria: an inborn error of valine metabolism. *Pediatr Res* 30: 322–326, 1991.

139. Brown GK, Hunt SM, Scholem R, et al.: Beta-hydroxyisobutyryl coenzyme A deacylase deficiency: a defect in valine metabolism associated with physical malformations. *Pediatrics* 70(4): 532–538, 1982.

140. DeVivo DC: The expanding spectrum of mitochondrial diseases. *Brain and Development* 15: 1–22, 1993.

141. Sperl W, Ruitenbeek W, Sengers RCA, et al.: Combined deficiencies of the pyruvate complex and enzymes of the respiratory chain in mitochondrial myopathies. *Eur J Pediatr* 151: 192–195, 1992.

142. Robinson BH, Oei J, Sherwood WG, et al.: The molecular basis for the two different clinical presentations of classical pyruvate carboxylase deficiency. *Am J Hum Genet* 36: 283–294, 1984.

143. Van Coster RN, Fernhoff PM, DeVivo DC: Pyruvate carboxylase deficiency: A benign variant with normal development. *Pediatr Res* 30: 1–4, 1991.

143a. Stern HJ, Nagan R, De Palma L, et al.: Prolonged survival in pyruvate carboxylase deficiency: lack of correlation of enzyme activity in cultured fibroblasts. *Clin Biochem* 28: 85–89, 1995.

144. Robinson BH: Lactic acidemia, in Scriver CR, Beaudet AL, Sly WS, Valle D (eds): *The Metabolic and Molecular Bases of Inherited Disease*. New York, McGraw-Hill, 1995, p. 1493.

145. Elpeleg ON, Amir N, Christensen E: Variability of clinical presentation in fumarate hydratase deficiency. *J Pediatr* 121: 752–754, 1992.

146. Coughlin EM, Chalmers RA, Slaugenhaupt SA, et al.: Identification of a molecular defect in a fumarase deficient patient and mapping of the fumarase gene. *Am J Hum Genet* 53: 896 (suppl), 1993.

146a. Guffon N, Lopez-Mediavilla C, Dumoulin PL, et al: 2-Ketoglutarate dehydrogenase deficiency, a rare cause of primary lactacidemia. *J Inherit Metabol Dis* 16: 821–830, 1993.

147. Leigh D: Subacute necrotizing encephalomyelopathy in an infant. *J Neurol Neurosurg Psychiatr* 14: 216–221, 1951.

148. DeVivo DC, Van Coster R: Personal communication, 1993.

149. Kretzmar HA, De Armond SJ, Koch TK, et al.: Pyruvate dehydrogenase complex deficiency as a cause of subacute necrotizing encephalopathy (Leigh disease). *Pediatrics* 79: 370–373, 1987.

149a. Macaya A, Munell F, Burke RE, et al: Disorders of movement in Leigh syndrome. *Neuropediatrics* 24: 60–67, 1993.

150. DeVivo DC, Haymond MW, Obert KA, et al.: Defective activation of the pyruvate dehydrogenase complex in subacute necrotizing encephalomyelopathy (Leigh disease). *Ann Neurol* 6: 483–484, 1979.

151. Van Coster R, Lombes A, DeVivo DC, et al.: Cytochrome-*c* oxidase-associated Leigh syndrome: phenotypic features and pathogenetic speculations. *J Neurol Sci* 104: 97–111, 1991.

152. Fujii T, Ito T, Okuno K, et al.: Complex I (reduced nicotinamide-adenine dinucleotide-coenzyme Q reductase) deficiency in two patients with probable Leigh syndrome. *J Pediatr* 116: 84–87, 1990.

152a. Bourgeois M, Goutières F, Chretien D, et al.: Deficiency in complex II of the respiratory chain presenting as a leukodystrophy in two sisters with Leigh syndrome. *Brain Dev* 14: 404–408, 1992.

153. de Vries DD, van Engelen BGM, Gabreels FJL, et al.: A second missense mutation in the mitochondrial ATPase 6 gene in Leigh's syndrome. *Ann Neurol* 34: 410–412, 1993.

154. Santorelli FM, Shanske S, Macaya A, et al.: The mutation at nt 8993 of mitochondrial DNA is a common cause of Leigh's syndrome. *Ann Neurol* 34: 827–834, 1993.

155. Baumgartner ER, Suormala TM, Wick H, et al.: Biotinidase deficiency: A cause of subacute necrotizing, encephalomyopathy (Leigh syndrome). Report of a case with lethal outcome. *Pediatr Res* 26: 260–266, 1994.

156. Fujii T, Van Coster RN, Old SE, et al.: Pyruvate dehydrogenase deficiency: molecular basis for intrafamilial heterogeneity. *Ann Neurol* 36: 83–89, 1994.

157. Wijburg FA, Barth PG, Bindoff LA, et al.: Leigh syndrome associated with a deficiency of the pyruvate dehydrogenase complex: results of treatment with a ketogenic diet. *Neuropediatrics* 23(3): 147–152, 1992.

158. Stanley CA, Hale DE, Coates PM, et al.: Medium-chain acylCoA dehydrogenase deficiency in children with non-ketotic hypoglycemia and low carnitine levels. *Pediatr Res* 17: 877–884, 1983.

159. Roe CR, Coates PM: Mitochondrial fatty acid oxidation disorders, in Scriver CR, Beaudet AL, Sly WS, Valle D (eds): *The Metabolic and Molecular Bases of Inherited Disease.* New York, McGraw-Hill, 1995, pp. 1501–1533.

160. Treem WR, Stanley CA, Hale DE, et al.: Hypoglycemia, hypotonia and cardiomyopathy: the evolving clinical picture of long-chain acyl-CoA dehydrogenase deficiency. *Pediatrics* 87: 328–333, 1991.

161. Scholte HR, Ross JD, Blom W, et al.: Assessment of deficiencies of fatty acyl-CoA dehydrogenases in fibroblasts, muscle and liver. *J Inherit Metab Dis* 15: 347–352, 1992.

162. Rocchiccioli F, Wanders RJ, Aubourg P., et al.: Deficiency of long-chain 3-hydroxyacyl-CoA dehydrogenase: a cause of lethal myopathy and cardiomyopathy in early childhood. *Pediatr Res* 28: 657–662, 1990.

163. Dioni-Vici C, Burlina AB, Bertini E, et al.: Progressive neuropathy and recurrent myoglobinuria in a child with long-chain 3-hydroxyacyl-coenzyme A dehydrogenase deficiency. *J Pediatr* 118: 744–746, 1991.

164. von Dobeln U, Venizelos N, Westgren M, et al.: Long-chain 3-hydroxyacyl-CoA dehydrogenase in chorionic villi, fetal liver and fibroblasts and prenatal diagnosis of 3-hydroxyacyl-CoA dehydrogenase deficiency. *J Inherit Metab Dis* 17: 185–188, 1994.

165. Tein I, DeVivo DC, Hale DE, et al.: Short-chain L-3-hydroxyacyl-CoA dehydrogenase deficiency in muscle: a new cause for recurrent myoglobinuria and encephalopathy. *Ann Neurol* 30: 415–419, 1991.

166. Peluchetti D, Antozzi C, Roi S, et al.: Riboflavin responsive multiple acyl-CoA dehydrogenase deficiency: functional evaluation of recovery after high dose vitamin supplementation. *J Neurol Sci* 105: 93–98, 1991.

167. Jackson S, Turnbull DM: Other enzyme defects of β-oxidation. Abnormalities of the trifunctional protein, in *Proceedings of the 2nd International Congress on Mitochondrial Pathology*, Rome, 1992, abstract 65.

167a. Rosenblatt DS: Inherited disorders of folate transport and metabolism, in Scriver CR, Beaudet AL, Sly WS, Valle D (eds): *The Metabolic and Molecular Bases of Inherited Disease.* New York, McGraw-Hill, 1995, pp. 311–328.

168. Ribes A, Riudor E, Briones P, et al.: Significance of bound glutarate in the diagnosis of glutaric aciduria type I. *J Inherit Metab Dis* 15(3): 367–370, 1992.

169. Goodman SI, Biery SI, Salazar D, et al.: Production of human GCDH (glutaryl-CoA dehydrogenase) and ETF (electron transfer flavoprotein) in *E Coli. Am J Hum Genet* 55: A173, 1994.

170. Simell O, Rajantie J, Perheentupa J: Lysinuric protein intolerance, in Eriksson AW, Forsins H, Nevanlinna HR, Workman PC, Norio RK (eds): *Population Structure and Genetic Disorders.* London, Academic, p. 633, 1980.

171. de Parscau L, Vianey-Liaud C, Hermier M, et al.: Intolérance aux protéines avec lysinurie. *Arch Fr Pediatr* 45: 809–812, 1988.

172. Tinuper P, Montagna P, Cortelli, et al.: Idiopathic recurrent stupor: A case with possible involvement of the gamma-aminobutyric acid (GABA) ergic system. *Ann Neurol* 31: 503–506, 1992.

Chapter 4

LATE INFANTILE PROGRESSIVE GENETIC ENCEPHALOPATHIES (METABOLIC ENCEPHALOPATHIES OF THE SECOND YEAR OF LIFE)

GENERAL CONSIDERATIONS

PROGRESSIVE WALKING DIFFICULTIES RELATED
TO LESIONS OF THE CENTRAL AND/OR PERIPHERAL
MOTOR NEURONS (SPASTIC PARAPLEGIA AND/OR
PERIPHERAL NEUROPATHY)
    HMDs Which Cause Spastic Paraplegia and/or
      Peripheral Neuropathy
    Spastic Paraplegia, Mental Deterioration,
      and Seizures

UNSTEADY GAIT AND INCOORDINATE
MOVEMENTS RESULTING FROM CEREBELLAR
ATAXIA, DYSTONIA, CHOREOATHETOSIS, OR SOME
COMBINATION THEREOF

INTENTION MYOCLONUS (POLYMYOCLONUS)
VARIABLY ASSOCIATED WITH EPILEPSY AND
CEREBELLAR ATAXIA

INTERMITTENT EPISODES OF ACUTE
NEUROLOGICAL DYSFUNCTION AND COMA

MENTAL RETARDATION AND REGRESSION WITH
PARALLEL DEVELOPMENT OF SKELETAL AND
OTHER SOMATIC ABNORMALITIES
    The Mucopolysaccharidoses
    Disorders with the Hurler Phenotype and no
      Mucopolysacchariduria: Mucolipidoses,

    Disorders of Glycoprotein Degradation
    Concluding Remarks

PSYCHOMOTOR RETARDATION AND ARREST OF
PSYCHIC FUNCTION

GENERAL CONSIDERATIONS

A number of hereditary metabolic encephalopathies become apparent during the second year of life, when children gain motor independence and acquire the first elements of speech.

Loss of motor function is the most frequent and usually the most obvious indication of a progressive metabolic disorder in this age-group. Some children who have started walking, frequently with some delay, have increasing difficulties doing so, while others who have not achieved independent locomotion lose the ability to stand and later to sit. Weakness or unsteady gait and poor coordination, or involuntary movements underlie the difficulty in walking and standing. This may be the consequence of an affliction of both the central corticospinal and peripheral nervous system (as in the leukodystrophies and neuroaxonal degeneration) or it may be due to cerebellar dysfunction or choreoathetosis, dystonia, or a combination of them (as in ataxia telangiectasia). Sometimes the exact classification of the movement disorders may be difficult to specify. Arrest or regression of mental functions and of incipient speech tends either to parallel or to follow motor dysfunction.

In another group of neurologic abnormalities with predominantly gray matter lesions, a combination of intention myoclonus and seizures associated with mental deterioration and retinal degeneration are in the foreground (such is the case of some of the lysosomal storage disease: lipofuscinoses, sphingolipidoses, sialidoses).

In some patients an arrest of intellectual development, mental deterioration, or progressive behavioral abnormalities may stand as the sole or dominant signs of a disease of the nervous system. A large group of such patients may, in addition, display to a varying degree a dysmorphic, skeletal, or visceral abnormality, such as are seen in the mucopolysaccharidoses, mucolipidoses, or disorders of glycoprotein degradation. In a minority, slow mental progress and psychic aberrations constitute the sole expression of the disease. Diagnosis in these latter cases rests on a number of judiciously selected laboratory investigations, listed at the end of this chapter.

Finally, there is a group of patients in this age period who for the first time manifest the effect of diseases due to mitochondrial defects, aminoacidopathies, and organoacidopathies that produce acute remitting, often dramatic neurologic attacks.

In this broad category of diseases, the lesions tend to be diffuse (as they were in the early infantile period), giving rise to a complex symptomatology, expressive of involvement of many different parts of the nervous system—cerebral cortex, retina, cerebellum, basal ganglia, and peripheral nerves. Nevertheless, any given disease in this age period, tends to evince a roughly stereotyped clinical picture. In contrast, in late childhood and adolescence (to be described in the next chapter) lesions tend more often to be restricted to certain well-defined neurological structures, and there is a greater diversity of clinical expression of the same disorder.

While the neurological pictures in some of the late infantile metabolic encephalopathies frequently remain uncharacteristic, there are certain signs or combinations of signs which should alert the clinician to the probability of an HMD.

1. Progressive difficulties in walking related to lesions of the central and/or peripheral motor system.

2. Unsteady gait and ataxia or involuntary movements of the limbs, traceable to lesions of the cerebellum or basal ganglia, singly or in combination.

3. Intention myoclonus (polymyoclonus) often associated with epilepsy and ataxia.

4. Intermittent episodes of acute drowsiness, confusion, stupor, and coma.

5. Mental retardation or regression in combination with skeletal and visceral abnormalities.

6. Delay in psychomotor development.

Here, as in the metabolic encephalopathies of all ages, the ophthalmologic abnormalities—retinal degeneration, corneal opacities, disorders of oculomotricity—assume considerable diagnostic importance.

PROGRESSIVE WALKING DIFFICULTIES RELATED TO LESIONS OF THE CENTRAL AND/OR PERIPHERAL MOTOR NEURONS (SPASTIC PARAPLEGIA AND/OR PERIPHERAL NEUROPATHY)

A disorder of locomotion can be traced to a degeneration of the pyramidal tracts and the sensorimotor nerves in metachromatic leukodystrophy, multiple sulfatase deficiency and neuroaxonal dystrophy.

Motor delay and difficulties in standing and walking may also at that age be due solely to a demyelinating hereditary sensorimotor distal polyneuropathy without central nervous system dysfunction, as in Déjerine-Sottas hypertrophic disease (see Chap. 5).

In Leigh disease, necrotic foci when involving mainly the central motor pathway may result in a spastic paresis; this may be among the first manifestations of the disease; and also there may be a demyelinating peripheral neuropathy. Of diagnostic importance, as pointed out in Chap. 3, are the other more characteristic signs of lesions in the brain stem, basal ganglia, and cerebellum, which appear soon in most cases.

Some of the late infantile neuronal sphingolipidoses may also begin as a progressive spastic paraparesis. Ataxia, polymyoclonus, mental regression, and behavioral abnormalities are other possible manifestations in this group of diseases (Table 4-1). The relatively pure spastic paraplegias, e.g. Strümpell-Lorrain familial spastic paralysis and other "degenerative" forms will be considered in Chap. 5.

When the progression of walking difficulties is slow in young children whose previous motor development has been retarded, one must avoid mistaking these

Table 4-1

	Main characteristic of motor disorder		Peripheral nerve involvement			
	Paraplegia (i.e., weakness or spasticity) as first sign	Ataxia (i.e., incoordination of limbs and trunk)	Absent DTR	Diminished NCV	CSF protein elevated	Retinal abnormalities
Metachromatic leukodystrophy	+		±	+	+	±
Austin disease[b]	+		±	+	+	±
Neuroaxonal degeneration	+		+	0	0	0
Ataxia-telangiectasia		+	±	±	0	0
Late infantile Niemann-Pick disease type C		+	0	0	0	0
Late infantile G_{M1} gangliosidosis (type 2)	+	±	0	0	0	0
Late infantile G_{M2} gangliosidosis		+	0	0	0	±
Late infantile Krabbe disease	+	+	±	±	±	0
Gaucher disease type III	+	+	0	0	0	0
Late infantile Leigh disease	+	+	±	±	±	0

Late infantile metabolic encephalopathies with difficulties in walking and incoordination as the first major neurologic sign[a]

Other neurologic signs important for diagnosis	Enlarged liver or spleen	X-ray skeletal changes	Inclusions in BM and blood leukocytes	Other important clinical features	Specific biological tests
	0	0	0	MRI: white matter lesions	+
	±	+	+	Ichthyosis; MRI as MLD	+
Early intellectual regression; hypotonia	0	0	0	Changes in nerve biopsy; cerebellar atrophy	0
Disorder of oculomotor function; choreoathetosis	0	0	0	Conjunctival telangiectasia; low IgG2 and IgA; high AFP	+
Disorder of oculomotor function; dysarthria; seizures	+	0	+		+
Seizures	0	+	+	Keratan sulfaturia; skeletal changes	+
Seizures, myoclonus	0	0	0		+
Optic atrophy	0	0	0		+
Seizures; disorder of oculomotor function	+	0	+		+
Disorder of oculomotor function; ocular palsies; optic atrophy	0	0	0	Lactic acid ↑ in CSF	±

Abbreviations: DTR = deep tendon reflexes; NCV = nerve conduction velocities; BM = bone marrow; MLD = metachromatic leukodystrophy; AFP = α-fetoprotein; + = constant or very frequent; ± = relatively frequent; 0 = not a feature.

[a] Familial spastic paraplegia, late infantile Krabbe disease and Gaucher disease type III are described in Chap. 5.

[b] Multiple sulfatase deficiency.

metabolic diseases for a fixed spastic diplegia of pre- or perinatal origin. The possibility of the latter disorder becomes more tenable if the child was born prematurely or suffered parturitional asphyxia.

HMDs which Cause Spastic Paraplegia and/or Peripheral Neuropathy

Metachromatic Leukodystrophy (Sulfatidosis)

Introduction Metachromatic leukodystrophy is an autosomal recessive inherited disorder of myelin metabolism, due to a deficiency of arylsulfatase A, or exceptionally, to a defect of a nonenzymatic protein activator, SAP 1 (in which case arylsulfatase levels fall within the normal range). As a result of these defects, galactosyl sulfatide (cerebroside sulfate) accumulates in the white matter of the central and peripheral nervous system; and in addition to the galactosyl sulfatides, small quantities of lactosyl sulfatide are deposited in the kidney, gallbladder and other visceral organs.

The human arylsulfatase gene is located near the end of the long arm of chromosome 22. Its structure has been determined and a number of disease-related mutations identified. The disease occurs most often in the late infantile period usually in the second year of life, but less aggressive forms appear in late childhood or adolescence (between the ages of 3 and 15 years), and in adults. Apparently, differences in the enzymatic defect (reflecting different MLD mutations) account for these variations in clinical expression. MLD-related mutations fall broadly into two groups: group I and group A. The group I patient produces no active enzyme, no immunoreactive protein, and expresses no arylsulfatase A activity in cultured cells. Group A generates small amounts of cross-reactive material and low levels of functional enzyme in cell cultures. Patients homozygous for a group I mutation, or having two different mutations from this group, have the late infantile form of MLD. Most individuals with one type I and one type A mutation develop paraplegia in the juvenile period form, and those with two type A mutations will generally have the adult form. A small number of patients, usually of the juvenile type of MLD, have a deficiency in SAP 1 and normal levels of arylsulfatase A.

To correctly interpret the biochemical data in MLD, it is important to know that extremely low levels of arylsulfatase A may occasionally be found in clinically normal relatives of patients with MLD, and in normal individuals in the general population, or it may occasionally be found in association with a variety of other neurological conditions. These individuals do not have deposits of sulfatides in their viscera and will never develop MLD. In them there is a fairly common polymorphism of the arylsulfatase A gene giving rise to a "pseudo-deficiency". This may interfere with the detection of presymptomatic patients, and heterozygotes, and with prenatal diagnosis.

While the clinical picture of late infantile MLD, the most common form, is fairly stereotyped, features of the juvenile and adult types of the disease are much more varied. We will here describe the early infantile MLD. The late-onset forms of the disease are discussed in Chap. 5.

Late Infantile Metachromatic Leukodystrophy Late infantile MLD is the most frequent form of the disease, representing 60 to 70 percent of all cases. Its incidence has been estimated at 1/40,000 births. We have observed more than 150 cases in a period of 30 years.

Clinical Features The disease starts insidiously in the second year of life (Fig. 4-1). Sometimes, the onset appears to be rather abrupt, as when attention is called to it after an infection. Early development usually proceeds normally and most children will have begun to walk, although often with some delay. About 15 percent do not achieve independent walking. The first clear-cut neurologic signs appear between 14 and 16 months and consist, in most instances, of progressive difficulties in locomotion. The lower limbs become weak with genu recurvatum, and falling is frequent. If walking has not been acquired, the child loses the ability to stand without support. In this initial period, where neurologic findings are restricted to the lower limbs, three different combinations of signs may be found:

1. A flaccid paraparesis with hypotonia, absent tendon reflexes, and normal plantar responses without amyotrophy or deformities. This period of isolated polyneuropathy may last several months, or exceptionally, a year or more before unequivocal pyramidal signs are superimposed.

2. Most frequently, a combination of pyramidal signs (i.e., spasticity, bilateral Babinski and Rossolimo signs) and depressed deep tendon reflexes.

3. A spastic paraplegia with hyperactive reflexes.

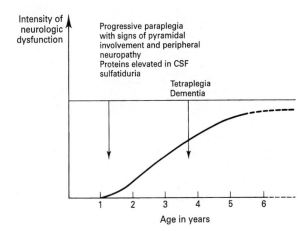

Figure 4-1
Metachromatic leukodystrophy. Clinical course and life profile.

In all three combinations, evidence of peripheral nerve involvement can be obtained by electrophysiologic tests; there is a marked slowing of nerve conduction velocities in motor and sensory nerves. The EMG pattern is initially normal or only slightly altered. Nerve conduction velocities may be reduced also in presymptomatic children.

During the early stages of the disease, the mental status is normal and there is no impairment of vision. However, a nonparalytic squint is not infrequent, and in certain families a pendular nystagmus is one of the first signs to appear.

A high protein content of the CSF is an early and nearly constant finding, and it persists throughout the entire course of the disease. The protein concentration may exceed 100 mg/dL. The electrophoretic pattern of the CSF protein is normal. However, a moderate elevation of the gamma globulins may occur in certain cases (for unclear reasons). MRI reveals a hyperintense signal in the periventricular and central white matter on T2-weighted images. The lesions are not enhanced after gadolinium injection. Initially, the abnormal signals tend to be limited strictly to the periventricular zone of the occipitoparietal regions (Fig. 4-2). They may be missed at that stage in the CT scans.

After a period of 6 to 18 months, as the disease progresses, the child becomes unable to stand and later to sit up. The head is less well controlled and axial hypotonia is increasingly evident. By then the upper limbs are also spastic and weak, and there may be an intention tremor of the arms. Dysarthria, drooling, and dysphagia are conjoined. The tendon reflexes are either hyperactive or impaired. Passive movements of the limbs often seem painful and provoke prolonged crying. By this stage of the disease, other higher cerebral functions have manifestly deteriorated. There may be a failure of vision, and optic atrophy appears in approximately one-third of the patients. The region of the macula may exhibit a peculiar grayish discoloration, and exceptionally, a typical cherry red spot has been reported.

Seizures of various types occur in a small proportion of the patients, but they never constitute a prominent manifestation. EEG abnormalities usually appear late in the disease and are not characteristic. Slight auditory myoclonus has been observed in the advanced stages in rare cases. Head size is usually normal; however, slight enlargement of the skull has rarely been noted.

Although sulfatides accumulate in the kidney, no change in renal function can be detected. The gallbladder fails to fill in cholecystograms as a result of sulfatide deposition in the mucosa. Even in 2-year-old patients, deposition of sulfatides may cause papillomatous transformation of the mucosa of the gallbladder which interferes with its function and causes enlargement (felt as an abdominal mass), or induce cholecystitis.

In the most advanced stages of the disease, the child lies helpless and rigid in decerebrate or decorticate postures, is seized periodically with tonic spasms evoked by stimulation and crying, and exhibits pseudobulbar signs and muscular wasting. Death usually occurs between the ages of 3 and 7 years.

Diagnostic Biochemical Tests and Differential Diagnosis

- Thin-layer chromatography of the urinary sediment will reveal a marked increase of sulfatide level in all patients with MLD. It is unfortunate this test is frequently neglected; it should always be performed when this disease is suspected. In so doing, some errors can be avoided (see "pseudo-deficiency").

- Enzyme assay of arylsulfatase A (ASA) is performed on leukocytes and cultured fibroblasts. When cerebroside sulfate is used as a substrate, almost no enzyme activity is found in patients with MLD. Testing with this natural substrate allows the distinction between MLD patients and a few normal individuals with an unusually low activity of arylsulfatase A.

- In exceptional cases (essentially with the juvenile form), arylsulfatase A activity is normal even when the clinical picture of MLD is fully developed. In this

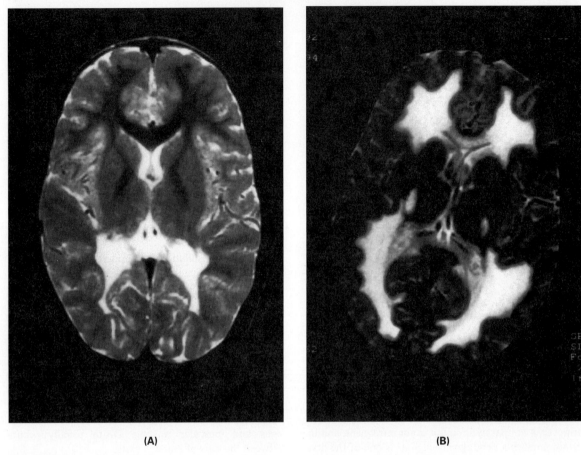

(A)   (B)

Figure 4-2

MLD. MRI shows progressive demyelination of cerebral hemispheres starting posteriorly: **(A)** *at 12 months;* **(B)** *at 18 months.*

instance, the activator protein SAP 1 is deficient, and this can be confirmed by tests using specific antibodies.

• Molecular analysis of DNA is now essential for family screening and prenatal diagnosis, particularly in view of the confusion offered by the pseudo-deficiency allele (see below).

• In rare cases in which there is a discrepancy between clinical and biochemical findings, a sural nerve biopsy or conjunctival biopsy to detect the pathognomonic deposits of sulfatides in Schwann cells and macrophages may be useful (Fig. 8-1).

When the diagnosis of MLD has been made in a child, it is essential to measure the ASA in the other siblings, parents, and relatives to identify heterozygotes and presymptomatic individuals, and to interpret cor-

rectly enzyme assays made on amniocytes or chorionic villi for prenatal diagnosis. It happens that some individuals have a very low ASA activity, approximating 10 to 15 percent of normal (which is much lower than in MLD heterozygotes), with no evidence of MLD (no clinical signs nor sulfatiduria nor metachromatic deposits in peripheral nerves). This state has been termed *ASA pseudo-deficiency*; not to recognize it may lead to major diagnostic errors.

Pseudo-deficiency of ASA Pseudo-deficiency of ASA is caused by a gene (*Pd*), which is allelic with the MLD gene (*MLD*) and is found in about 10 percent of the population. This accounts for its frequent occurrence in MLD obligate heterozygotes, and consequently in siblings of a child with MLD. Homozygosity for the

Family	Arylsulfatase A[a]		Allele status	Comment
	Leukocytes	Fibroblasts		
H-Proband	9.6		MLD/MLD	Affected (LI)
Sibling	11.1		MLD/Pd	Healthy
Father	13.2		MLD/Pd	Healthy
Mother	31.1		MLD/NL	Healthy
G-Proband		11.2	MLD/MLD	Affected (LI)
Sibling		19.7	MLD/Pd	Healthy
Father		17.9	MLD/Pd	Healthy
Mother		99.7	MLD/NL	Healthy
M-Proband	2.7		MLD/MLD	Affected (J)
Mother	8.3		MLD/Pd	Healthy
Father	29.1		MLD/NL	Healthy

Figure 4-3

Arylsulfatase A values and allele status in MLD families with pseudo-deficiency. MLD = metachromatic leukodystrophy; LI = late infantile; J = juvenile; Pd = pseudo-deficiency; NL = normal. (Reprinted from D.A. Wenger and E. Louie, Dev. Neurosci. **13**: 216 *(1991) (ref.1).*

[a]Nanomoles nitrocatechol sulfate hydrolyzed per hour per milligram of protein.

Pd allele or heterozygosity for the *Pd* allele with an allele causing MLD will result in very low levels of ASA. In these circumstances a sibling of an affected child may be misdiagnosed as preclinical MLD (Fig. 4-3).[1,2]

In prenatal diagnosis, it is important to know if either parent carries the *Pd* gene because, if the fetus inherits a *Pd* gene together with an *MLD* allele, this could lead to low levels of ASA and a false diagnosis of MLD. Finally, another source of difficulty occurs when a state of pseudo-deficiency of ASA is associated with a neurological disease which is not MLD.

To summarize, for practical purposes, any individual—parent or sibling of a child with MLD, or a patient with any ongoing neurological disease, or the fetus of parents who have given birth to a child with MLD—with ASA levels at approximately 10 to 15 percent of the normal mean and no sulfatiduria should be suspected of harboring the *Pd* gene. This can be confirmed by special biochemical methods such as the ^{14}C-sulfatide loading tests in cultured skin fibroblasts, amniocytes, or chorionic villi, and with DNA analyses.

In differential diagnosis several conditions must be considered. (1) Early-onset familial sensorimotor polyneuropathy (HMSN type III, Déjerine-Sottas disease), which may be clinically indistinguishable from MLD in its polyneuropathic form or stage. (Note: Extremely low nerve conduction velocities and high protein in the CSF are usually indicative of metachromic leukodystrophy.) It is therefore essential to measure urinary sulfatides and the activity of ASA in any child with a polyneuropathy starting at this age. (2) A congenital or early-onset myo-pathy or motor neuron disease (Wolfhart-Kugelberg disease). (3) Neuroaxonal dystrophy (normal nerve conduction velocities, denervation potentials on EMG, normal CSF, early dementia, cerebellar atrophy). (4) Multiple sulfatase deficiency (additional clinical features are skeletal abnormalities, facial dysmorphia, ichthyosis). (5) Early-onset Strümpell-Lorrain familial spastic paraplegia and other rare forms of familial paraplegias (peripheral nerves and CSF normal). (6) Spastic diplegia of pre- or perinatal origin (in its milder forms and when there is no evidence of prematurity).

Genetics   The pattern of inheritance is autosomal recessive. Heterozygotes can be detected by assay of ASA on leukocytes or cultured fibroblasts. Their level of activity of ASA is usually approximately 50 percent of normal, but there may be some overlap with normal values. When a heterozygote for the MLD gene has also inherited the MLD pseudo-deficiency allele, residual activities of ASA may be much lower. In such circumstances, additional biochemical assays (including sulfatide loading tests in cultured fibroblasts, urine sulfatide analysis, and DNA studies) may be necessary in as many members of the family as possible.

The gene for ASA is located on chromosome 22 in the q13.31-qter region. Several molecular defects in this gene have been identified in MLD patients. One of the alleles (allele I) is associated with the late infantile form of the disease. The gene for the protein activator (SAP 1) has been mapped to chromosome 10.[3]

Pathological and Chemical Findings Sulfatides accumulate in oligodendrocytes and macrophages of the white matter in zones of widespread demyelination in the cerebrum, brain stem, cerebellum, and spinal cord. A small amount may accumulate in some groups of neurons, primarily those of the basal ganglia, brain stem, spinal cord, cerebellum, spinal ganglia, autonomic ganglia, and ganglion cells of the retina. Destruction of the myelin sheaths and, to a lesser extent, axons is widespread. The subcortical fibers and some tracts in the basal ganglia and brain stem are usually partially preserved. In the peripheral nerves, sulfatides accumulate in Schwann cells and in macrophages and there is segmental demyelination. Excessive amounts of sulfatides are found in the renal tubular epithelium and in the epithelium of the gallbladder, where they may induce the formation of large papillomatous formations. In the liver, sulfatides accumulate in hepatocytes, in Kupffer cells, and in the epithelium of bile ducts.

In frozen sections stained by cresyl violet or toluidine blue, sulfatide deposits have a brownish or reddish color (metachromasia), contrasting with the blue cell nuclei of fibroblasts and Schwann cells. Electron microscopic examination localizes the sulfatides to lysosomes; they have a lamellar structure which frequently assumes a prismatic pattern (Fig. 8-1).

Biochemical Analysis Biochemical analysis demonstrates an absolute increase of sulfatides in the white matter. Levels of sphingomyelin, cholesterol, and to an even greater degree, of cerebrosides are decreased. The excess of sulfatide has also been noted in isolated myelin fractions. The concentration of lysosulfatide (a deacylated form of sulfatide) is also increased in cerebral white matter and in peripheral nerves.

An increased concentration of sulfatides has been found in the cerebellum, brain stem, spinal cord, and in isolated myelin sheaths, but not in the still unmyelinated parts of the cerebral hemisphere of a 24-week-old fetus.

Physiopathology The mechanism of myelin breakdown in metachromatic leukodystrophy remains obscure. There is ample morphologic evidence that cellular pathology, particularly intralysosomal accumulations of sulfatides in oligodendrocytes and Schwann cells, precedes demyelination, and there is reason to believe that normal arylsulfatase A activity is necessary for the growth, maintenance, and turnover of the myelin sheaths. It has been suggested that because the composition of myelin is not normal in MLD, it becomes

unstable and breaks down. Another hypothesis favors the idea that myelin breakdown results from the cytotoxic action of lyosulfatide (sulfogalactosylsphingosine) on oligodendrocytes.

Other Forms of MLD MLD may appear at a later period of life from early childhood (3 to 6 years of age) to adolescence and even adulthood (Chap. 5). Although walking difficulties are still a frequent mode of presentation, other neurological features may be seen. Slowing of nerve conduction velocities and protein increase in the CSF are less pronounced; and mental signs and personality changes assume added importance. It is also in this age-group that deficiencies of the protein activator can occur. Studies of substrate turnover in tissue culture suggest that some degree of functional activity persists in patients with late-onset MLD, whereas it is practically absent in the early infantile form.

Treatment and Prevention There is still no effective treatment of MLD. Bone marrow transplantation, when undertaken early, may slow or even halt the progression of the disease. Longer-term follow-up is needed to evaluate the apparent benefits of this mode of therapy (see Chap. 9). When lesions in the nervous system are already well developed, as is usually the case when early infantile MLD is recognized, the risks of the procedure tend to outweigh its potential benefits. Bone marrow transplantation may be a reasonable option in presymptomatic children detected by systematic screening of the siblings of an affected child. In the future, gene replacement therapies will be undertaken.

Genetic counseling for prevention of the disease is based on the detection of heterozygotes and the possibility of prenatal diagnosis. The problems pertaining to these matters have been discussed above.

Multiple Sulfatase Deficiency (Mucosulfatidosis; Austin Disease) Multiple sulfatase deficiency (MSD) is an autosomal recessive hereditary disorder characterized by neurovisceral storage of sulfatides, mucopolysaccharides, and cholesteryl sulfate as a result of the depression of the activity of arylsulfatase A and six other sulfatases. The clinical manifestations present as a neurological syndrome similar to that of early infantile MLD, except that early psychomotor development tends to be more severely retarded. Moreover, there are features reminiscent of the mucopolysaccharidoses, i.e., moderate facial and skeletal deformities, hepatomegaly, deafness, and inclusions in leukocytes. Another impor-

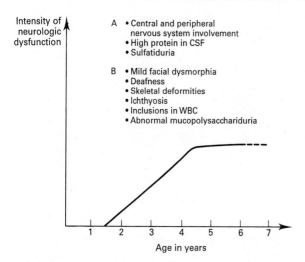

A   • Central and peripheral
         nervous system involvement
     • High protein in CSF
     • Sulfatiduria

B   • Mild facial dysmorphia
     • Deafness
     • Skeletal deformities
     • Ichthyosis
     • Inclusions in WBC
     • Abnormal mucopolysacchariduria

Figure 4-4
Multiple sulfatase deficiency. Clinical course and life profile.

tant feature is ichthyosis. The urine contains excessive quantities of sulfatides as well as heparan sulfate and dermatan sulfate. The genetic mechanism responsible for the multiple sulfatase deficiency appears to involve failure in the posttranslational modification of sulfatases. The details have not been elucidated[3] (Fig. 4-4).

Clinical Features   Approximately 50 cases have been reported from different countries. There have been six in our E.K. Shriver material and three in the Louvain Neuropediatric Center. In about half of the cases the cerebral development during the first year appears to be normal or moderately delayed. Neurologic regression begins between the twelfth and eighteenth month and is manifested by difficulty in walking, weakness of musculature, unsteadiness of movement, and frequent falling. In other patients, early development is markedly retarded and the child may be able to do little more than sit or stand. These latter capacities may not be acquired until the end of the second year and are then lost.

On neurologic examination, there is the characteristic combination of pyramidal signs and peripheral neuropathy, just like that of MLD. The peripheral neuropathy is manifested inconstantly by depressed tendon reflexes, but always by a marked slowing of the conduction velocities of motor and sensory nerves. Nonparalytic squints are frequent. Visual acuity is difficult to assess, and the optic fundi are usually unaltered at this stage. Head circumference is normal or reduced. The

CSF proteins are usually elevated with a normal electrophoretic pattern.

Rapidly, the mental capacities regress. Communicative speech is seldom achieved. Generalized and myoclonic seizures are frequent. Motor deterioration continues, with arm movements becoming awkward and frequently tremulous. By the age of 4 years the child is quadriplegic with pseudobulbar signs and has lost all evidence of meaningful mental activity. There is now an optic atrophy. Other ocular abnormalities include grayish discoloration of the maculas and even cherry red spots and pigmentary degeneration of the retina.[3]

In addition to this neurologic picture, which in many ways is similar to that of MLD, there are a few subtle but significant clinical and paraclinical extraneurologic findings that resemble those of the mucopolysaccharide storage diseases. Facial features are rarely normal: a narrow prominent forehead, depressed nasal bridge, thick eyebrows, and long eyelashes are notable peculiarities. The hands are often stubby and the thumbs are short. The sternum is either prominent or concave. The liver and occasionally the spleen are enlarged. X-ray abnormalities of bone are slight but significant. At the dorsolumbar junction the vertebral bodies are rounded, with slight anterior beaking (marks of hypoplasia). The metacarpal bones are broad and poorly trabeculated, with tapered ends (Fig. 4-5). Other alterations may be found in the pelvis, femoral epiphyses, and ribs. In rare instances these abnormalities are questionable or even absent. In the peripheral blood and bone marrow, metachromatic inclusions similar to those of Hurler disease are seen in lymphoyctes, plasmacytes, and polymorphonuclear leukocytes. As in the mucopolysaccharidoses, deafness is frequent. Corneal opacities are not present (except in an atypical variant described below). A characteristic and nearly constant finding is a diffuse alteration of the skin, usually in the form of a fine ichthyosis (sometimes reported as thick, dry skin) which, unlike ichthyosis vulgaris, is present at birth.

The course of the disease extends over several years and the age at death varies from 3 to 12 years.

Diagnostic Laboratory Findings
• There is an increased urinary excretion of sulfatides, dermatan sulfate, and heparan sulfate.

• Enzyme assays on cultured skin fibroblasts show that, besides the deficiency of arylsulfatase A (found in MLD), there is a loss of activity of arylsulfatase B (*N*-acetylgalactosamine-4-sulfate sulfatase) and arylsulfatase C (steroid sulfatase), and four other sulfa-

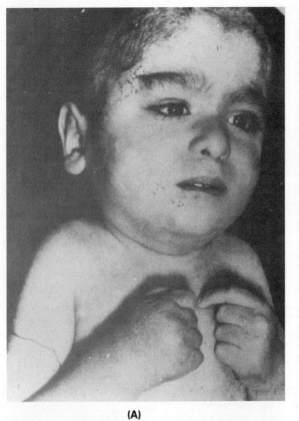

(A)

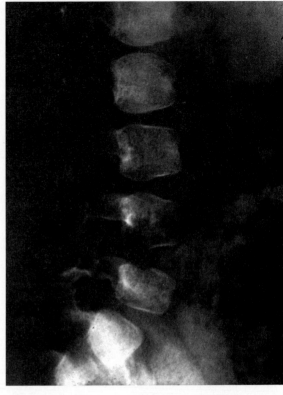

(B)

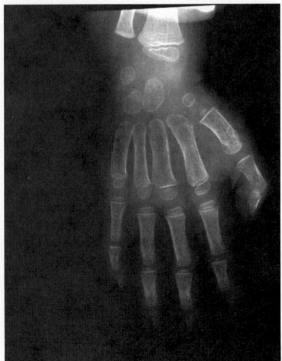

(C)

Figure 4-5

*Multiple sulfatase deficiency. **A**. Boy aged 18 months with slight craniofacial alterations: flat nasal bridge, heavy eyebrows. Note also flexed fingers and ichthyosis. **B**. X-ray film of hand: broad diaphyses and metacarpals with narrow proximal ends. **C**. X-ray of spine of 3-year-old patient; underdeveloped segment of anterior part of vertebral bodies.*

tases that degrade MPS (iduronide-2-sulfate-sulfatase, heparan-*N*-sulfamidase, *N*-acetylgalactosamine-6-sulfate sulfatase, *N*-acetylglucosamine-6-sulfate sulfatase). Deficiency of arylsulfatase C is probably responsible for the ichthyosis.

All of the sulfatases may not be reduced equally. Differences in their activity may be found in different tissues of a given patient, and they vary from patient to patient.

Other important laboratory findings are low nerve conduction velocities; presence of inclusions in peripheral blood and bone marrow leukocytes (Alder-Reilly granules); elevated CSF protein; and intralysosomal inclusions in Schwann cells typical of MLD, in sural nerve biopsy.

Variants

• An early-onset form has been described in two infants with facial dysmorphism, short neck, skeletal deformities (hypoplasia of vertebral bodies and epiphyseal dysplasia), and hepatomegaly, which were present at birth. Both had ichthyosis and corneal clouding before they developed a hydrocephalus. They had a severe deficiency of all the sulfatases.[4]

• Another variant has been reported from Saudi Arabia. Here, there was severe dysostosis multiplex that caused cervical cord compression, macrocephaly, and corneal clouding. Ichthyosis and deafness were absent and mental retardation was mild. Steroid sulfatase was normal in six of the seven patients.

Pathological Findings. Chemical Pathology Neuropathological findings in MSD combine the features of MLD and those of the mucopolysaccharidoses. As in MLD, metachromatic deposits of sulfatides accumulate in glial cells and histiocytes in the demyelinated white matter of the brain, and in Schwann cells and macrophages of peripheral nerves. They accumulate in lysosomes and have the distinctive ultrastructural appearance seen in MLD. In addition, there are clear vacuoles in the vascular pericytes in the brain, and a lamellated storage substance characteristic of ganglioside, in intracortical neurons (as in the MPS).

Biochemical analysis has shown that the stored substances include sulfatides in the brain; mucopolysaccharides (dermatan sulfate and heparan sulfate) in the brain, liver, and kidneys; and cholesteryl sulfate in the liver and kidneys. Gangliosides accumulate in cortical neurons. The ganglioside pattern in these cells (increase in G_{M2} and G_{M3}) resembles that of Hurler disease.

Treatment   No effective treatment is available. We are not aware of any trial of bone marrow transplantation in this disorder.

Neuroaxonal Dystrophy (Seitelberger Disease) This disease was first clearly described in 1963 by Cowen et al.,[5] who coined the term of neuroaxonal dystrophy, and by Lyon and See[6] and Seitelberger et al.[7] Previous reports of this condition had been published by Seitelberger in 1952,[8] and by Rabinowicz and Wildi in 1957.[9] Neuroaxonal dystrophy (NAD) is an autosomal recessive disorder of unknown origin, the most striking features of which are morphologic. Multiple, widespread swellings of axons and presynaptic terminals with typical ultrastructural features, and degeneration of neurons in the pallidum and cerebellum are characteristic. Symptoms usually begin in the second year of life with progressive difficulties in walking, or they may start earlier in the second semester of the first year with psychomotor regression. Hypotonia may be striking. Pyramidal signs, loss of deep tendon reflexes with an EMG showing partial denervation atrophy (but no slowing of nerve conduction velocities), progressive optic atrophy, a normal CSF, and cerebellar atrophy (revealed by MRI) constitute the main symptomatology of the disease (Fig. 4-6).

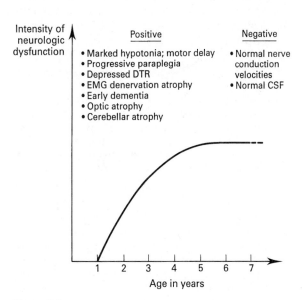

Figure 4-6
Neuroaxonal dystrophy. Clinical course and life profile.

The detection of the typical ultrastructural changes in a peripheral nerve biopsy is necessary for diagnosis.

The distinction between NAD and other disorders with evidence of diffuse axonal dystrophy, namely Hallervorden-Spatz disease and Schindler disease (a recently described metabolic disorder) is not yet clear.

Clinical Features Approximately 40 cases of NAD had been reported by 1982. We have observed seven patients with this condition. The age at onset is usually between 14 and 18 months, rarely up to 3 or 4 years, and sometimes as early as 6 months. A few juvenile cases with seizures and myoclonus have been reported (Chap. 5).

The development of the nervous system is either normal at first or delayed. Most children never achieve a completely independent locomotion, and the first reliable sign is a slowly increasing difficulty in walking. There is a tendency to fall and occasionally unsteadiness of gait. Children in whom the disease starts much earlier (at 6 to 8 months) exhibit a gradual regression of all motor functions, including standing and sitting, and lack of spontaneous activity. Hypotonia in these latter cases is quite marked.

By the time of the first examination, the lower limbs are either spastic or hypotonic, sometimes to such a degree as to suggest a neuromuscular disorder[10]; later, pyramidal signs are indubitable. The deep tendon reflexes may be exaggerated but more frequently they are unobtainable from the start (especially in cases with an early onset) or they become unobtainable as the disease progresses. Diminished sensibility to pain over the lower limbs has been reported.[11] Electromyography usually discloses denervation potentials, especially distally, whereas motor and sensory nerve conduction velocities are relatively normal.

Blindness with optic atrophy is a practically constant finding. The interval between onset of the disease and optic atrophy varies from 10 months to more than 2 years. However, pendular nystagmus and a nonparalytic squint may precede evident failure of vision and can be an early manifestation.

Athetosis and other extrapyramidal signs are not part of the clinical picture, although involuntary movements of face and hands have occasionally been reported late in the course of the disease. Seizures are rare. On EEG tracings, a high-amplitude fast activity is frequently observed. Evidence of progressive mental deterioration coincides with the onset of motor signs. Speech is never attained or is limited. The CSF is normal. The head circumference is normal or moderately reduced after some time. The duration of the disease ranges from 3 to 8 years.

Important Laboratory Tests
● Electrophysiologic data are of diagnostic importance: denervation atrophy on the EMG, normal nerve conduction velocities, abnormal visual and somaesthetic evoked potentials, high-amplitude fast activity in the EEG.

● A normal CSF and cerebellar atrophy on MRI are valuable findings.

● There is no known biochemical abnormality. In particular, both the urinary excretion of oligosaccharides and glycopeptides, and the activity of the enzyme α-*N*-acetylglucosaminidase, are normal (see Schindler disease). The most valuable diagnostic test is the finding of typical ultrastructural axonal alterations in biopsies of skin or conjunctiva (Fig. 4-7). Cerebral biopsies are very rarely needed.

Genetics NAD appears to be inherited as an autosomal recessive trait with no ethnic prevalence. Information concerning transmission of the disease, based on the study of 24 cases in 19 families, reveals that two or more siblings were found to be affected in 6 families. In 2 families the affected children were twins (monozygotic and dizygotic). Girls were more frequently affected than boys (19 girls, 5 boys). The course and symptomatology of the disease was remarkably uniform within a given sibship. Consanguinity in the parents has been noted twice. The parents were unaffected. However, in one family[6] the mother and one of her sisters had what appeared to be a slowly progressive lower motor neuron disease that began at about 20 years of age.

Pathologic Findings The most characteristic pathologic alteration consists of large (50 μm) eosinophilic spheroids, often of a concentric pattern. They are found in all parts of the gray matter but predominate in the posterior horns and Clark columns of the spinal cord, the nuclei gracilis and cuneatus in the medulla, the substantia nigra, the subthalamic nuclei, and the distal parts of peripheral nerves. They represent axonal swellings. Other small (10 μm) perineuronal eosinophilic bodies have been observed in the cortex, the central gray nuclei of the brain, and the anterior horns of the spinal cord.[6] They represent abnormal, enlarged presynaptic endings. Under the electron microscope the

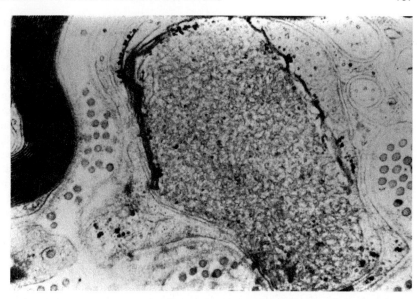

Figure 4-7
NAD. Sural nerve biopsy. Electron microscopy shows typical membrane aggregates in a poorly myelinated axon. (Courtesy Dr. G. Ferrière.)

spheroids and eosinophilic bodies are composed of aggregates of smooth membranes and tubules, which are characteristic.[12]

Other changes include neuron loss and demyelination in the pallidum, with infiltration by fat-laden macrophages and deposition of variable amounts of calcium and iron particles, some of which encrust astrocytes. No significant deposits of iron pigments are seen in the globus pallidus and substantia nigra. There is also an extensive loss of granule and Purkinje cells in the cerebellar cortex and a variable degree of degeneration of ascending and descending fiber tracts in the spinal cord and brain stem.

Diagnosis   NAD should be considered in a child in its second year of life with progressive walking difficulties, or an infant at 6 to 12 months with motor regression and marked hypotonia. In both circumstances tendon reflexes are absent or depressed, with or without pyramidal signs. Blindness with optic atrophy is another important clue. The diagnosis is supported by EMG demonstration of denervation atrophy when the motor and sensory nerve conduction velocities and the CSF are normal. Abnormal visual and somesthetic evoked potentials and cerebellar atrophy on MRI are additional paraclinical abnormalities. The definitive diagnosis of NAD rests on the demonstration in electron micrographs of typical intra-axonal membranous aggregates in the distal part of peripheral nerves or at the neuromuscular junction, in biopsy specimens of the sural nerve (Fig.

4-7). The regular pattern of the membranous aggregates differs from other nonspecific types of intra-axonal inclusions observed in various diseases with axonal degeneration.

The main diagnostic problem is to distinguish NAD from metachromatic leukodystrophy, and neuromuscular disorders. In metachromatic leukodystrophy, nerve conduction velocities are low, the CSF protein is high, and intellectual regression occurs late. NAD can be separated from Schindler disease, a very rare condition where intra-axonal inclusions are also present (see below). The relationship between NAD and Hallervorden-Spatz disease is discussed below. The so-called juvenile NAD is described in Chap. 5.

Nosology and Limits of NAD   Because of the presence of axonal spheroids found in the brain at autopsy, some very atypical cases have been considered as variants of NAD. Brain lesions resembling those of NAD have been found in a 3-year-old child who was demented and blind and who had suffered from frequent seizures from the age of 5 months.[13] A few neonates considered to have a type of NAD have been reported.[14–16] All suffered from a severe early infantile encephalopathy starting in the first days or weeks of life, and fatal outcome within 6 to 18 months. Proof of the diagnosis was based on the demonstration of axonal spheroids and cerebellar atrophy along with other atypical neuropathological features. The nonspecificity of axonal spheroids and one's ignorance of the basic pathogenesis of NAD leaves one uncertain as to whether these cases should be classified as an early infantile form of NAD.

Another small group of cases[7,13] can be set apart by virtue of two sets of data—anatomic and clinical. In addition to otherwise typical brain lesions, there was heavy iron pigmentation of the globus pallidus and substantia nigra. These children died between 7 and 11 years of age with a progressive tremor, rigidity, slowness of movement, and choreoathetosis. Another 9-year-old child presented with progressive optic atrophy, spasticity, and ataxia. At autopsy there were diffuse axonal spheroids, minimal involvement of the cerebellum, and moderate but indisputable evidence of iron deposits (pigmentation) of the pallidum. These cases were considered by their authors either to be examples of an early infantile form of Hallervorden-Spatz disease, a form of NAD, or an "intermediate" form falling between the two.

Some authors have considered NAD as an infantile form of Hallervorden-Spatz disease because of neuropathological similarities. However, differences between the two diseases are more striking than the similarities. The brain in Hallervorden-Spatz disease shows heavy deposits of iron pigment in the globus pallidus and substantia nigra. Moreover, the neuroaxonal swellings are less numerous and less extensive. Also, the cerebellar atrophy is less severe than that in NAD. Of clinical importance is that Hallervorden-Spatz disease has a juvenile onset, a protracted course, and a predominantly extrapyramidal symptomatology, something conspicuously absent in NAD.

While awaiting the results of DNA analysis, the authors advise that NAD and Hallervorden-Spatz disease be treated as separate entities. The relationship of NAD to the so-called juvenile form of NAD and Schindler disease are discussed below.

Mechanisms of the Derangements of Nervous System Function and Clinicopathologic Correlations NAD has been considered by some[12] to be a primary disease of synapses and terminal axons (possibly a disturbance of retrograde axonal transport) with subsequent loss of nerve cells and degeneration of fiber tracts. But its pathogenesis remains unknown. Structurally similar spheroids have been found in the medulla in cases of cystic fibrosis, congenital biliary atresia, and in aging individuals. Experimentally it has been reproduced in rats with vitamin E deficiency and in several types of intoxication.[17] None of these pathogenic factors have been identified in the human disease; that is, no derange-

ment of vitamin E metabolism has been demonstrated in NAD.

Widespread axonal spheroids may also be the consequence of a disorder in glycoprotein metabolism due to a deficiency in α-N-acetylgalactosaminidase (Schindler disease), and this recent discovery may open new avenues to research into the pathogenesis of NAD. However, when specifically looked for, the metabolic abnormality of this disease was not detected in NAD.

Synaptic degeneration in the cerebral cortex would appear to be a logical explanation of the mental deterioration. In this respect, NAD is comparable to the encephalopathy with abnormal presynaptic terminals reported by Gonatas and Goldensohn.[18] The marked hypotonia could be a consequence of axonal disease and cerebellar atrophy. The paucity of extrapyramidal and cerebellar signs is noteworthy.

Schindler Disease (α-N-acetylgalactosaminidase deficiency) Schindler disease is a newly recognized form of infantile neuroaxonal dystrophy resulting from the deficiency of the lysosomal enzyme α-N-acetylgalactosaminidase.[19] The disorder has been described in two brothers. Walking difficulties were noted in one child at the age of 15 months; onset of symptoms in his brother was somewhat earlier. Motor and mental deterioration proceeded at a rapid pace. Myoclonic seizures, pyramidal signs with hyperreflexia and hypotonia, and optic atrophy were additional findings. The CSF was normal. The brain stem auditory, somatosensory, and visual evoked potentials were of low amplitude and delayed. Nerve conduction velocities were normal. The ERG was normal. Atrophy of the cerebrum, cerebellum, and brain stem were observed on MRI scans. The two brothers were bedridden and profoundly retarded by the age of 4 years.

Laboratory Investigations A cortical biopsy showed multiple swellings of terminal or preterminal axons containing sharply demarcated heterogeneous inclusions, comprising dense tubulovesicular and granular structures. Electron microscopy of blood leukocytes, exocrine sweat glands, axons of cutaneous nerves, and cultured fibroblasts showed similar deposits, which were apparently in lysosomes.

An abnormal profile of oligosaccharides and glycopeptides was demonstrated by thin-layer chromatography. The activity of α-N-acetylgalactosaminidase in plasma, leukocytes, cultured lymphoblasts, or cultured fibroblasts was found to be deficient. The α-N-acetylgalactosaminidase gene has been mapped to chromosome

22q13.1→13.2. The cDNA encoding this enzyme has been determined. The disease is inherited as an autosomal recessive trait.

Although a deficiency of α-N-acetylgalactosaminidase has not been found in typical NAD, the discovery of Schindler disease offers new prospects for research into the cause of this disorder. The possibility of another type of abnormality of glycoprotein metabolism should probably be tested.

Clinical Variants   Two additional infants with α-N-acetylgalactosaminidase deficiency have been described. They were the offspring of unrelated Dutch parents. Seizures first appeared in the older child at 11 months and recurred at 28 and 29 months. Psychomotor development was slightly retarded but at 21 months he was able to walk independently and utter simple words. A younger brother, one of twins, aged 9 months, had the same enzyme deficiency. His development seemed normal but was possibly less advanced than his twin sister. The urinary oligosaccharide pattern in the index case was similar but quantitatively much less than that reported for the two Schindler brothers.[20]

An adult Japanese woman with α-N-acetylgalactosaminidase deficiency and urinary glycopeptide excretion similar to the Schindler brothers has also been reported. She had angiokeratoma but was free of neurological signs.

Déjerine-Sottas Disease (HMSN III)   Delay in motor development and difficulties in walking in the second or third year of life may also be caused by Déjerine-Sottas disease, which will be described in Chap. 5.

Late Infantile Leigh Syndrome; Late Infantile PDHC Deficiency   In approximately 25 percent of the cases of Leigh syndrome, the disease starts in the second year of life. This form has been described along with the much more frequent early infantile disease in Chap. 3. The following points will be recalled here: as in many progressive metabolic encephalopathies of this age, the first neurological complaints consist usually of difficulties in walking, dysarthria, and intellectual regression, with evidence of pyramidal tract signs and frequently of cerebellar ataxia.

More characteristic signs relate to the usual predominance of lesions in the brain stem and basal ganglia, the most remarkable of which are nuclear and supranuclear oculomotor paralyses (Fig. 4-8), and unexplained bouts of hyperventilation. Ataxia, dystonia,

optic atrophy, and a peripheral neuropathy may be observed. A remitting course, with periods of dramatic exacerbation of neurologic signs, and even coma are also features of this disease. Another practically constant manifestation consists of nutritional difficulties, vomiting, and failure to thrive, which may precede obvious neurological dysfunction. Lactate levels are usually elevated in the CSF. There is no evidence of a myopathy, and muscle biopsies prove always to be normal.

By definition, diagnosis of Leigh syndrome relies on the demonstration of a typical pattern of symmetrical foci of necrosis in the basal ganglia and brain stem (Fig. 4-8), and occasionally also in the cerebellum and the cerebral white matter. The disease is inherited as an X-linked, an autosomal recessive or a maternal trait. Sev-

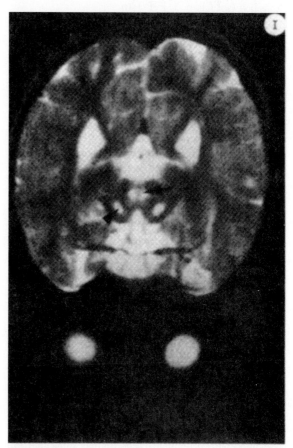

Figure 4-8
Late infantile Leigh disease. First sign in this patient was progressive oculomotor palsies. MRI shows bilateral areas of necrosis in the oculomotor nuclei (arrow) and substantia nigra (arrowhead). (Courtesy Dr. R. Van Coster.)

eral biochemical abnormalities have so far been found to be connected to the syndrome: cytochrome oxidase (COX) deficiency (complex IV), pyruvate dehydrogenase complex (PDHC) deficiency, ATPase 6 gene point mutations, complex I deficiency, and complex II deficiency. A case with a biotinidase deficiency has also been reported (see also Chap. 3). In many cases a biochemical correlate has not been identified.

Some patients with *PDHC deficiency*, but without the typical lesions on the MRI or at autopsy, have had a similar clinical picture. Their exact relationship to Leigh syndrome is uncertain.

Leigh syndrome may also begin in late childhood or adolescence. A benign late infantile or juvenile form with episodes of ataxia, paraparesis, thiamine responsiveness and normal motor development has been described (see Chap. 3, Ref. 140).

Spastic Paraplegia, Mental Deterioration, and Seizures

Late Infantile G_{M1} Gangliosidosis (Type 2)   This is an autosomal recessive disorder due to a deficiency of lysosomal acid β-galactosidase, which results in abnormal accumulation of G_{M1} ganglioside in the nervous system, and of galactose-containing products derived from glycoproteins and keratan-like substances in visceral organs. The β-galactosidase gene is located on chromosome 3.

G_{M1} gangliosidosis usually occurs in early infancy (Chap. 3), but is also seen in late infancy (starting in the second year of life) and with a more chronic course in childhood, adolescence or even in adulthood (Chap. 5).

Described here is the late infantile variety of G_{M1} gangliosidosis: type 2 (Fig. 4-9).

Clinical Features   The disease begins in the second year of life, usually between 12 and 18 months. The first definite sign is difficulty in walking (i.e., disturbance of gait and frequent falling); or if the child has not begun to walk, increasing unsteadiness in sitting and attempting to stand. Purposeful movements of the arms soon become awkward. Speech is rapidly lost. By the time the child has reached the third year, standing and sitting without support are no longer possible and mental regression is severe. A spastic quadriparesis develops, associated with prominent pseudobulbar signs that are responsible for drooling and dysphagia. In some cases, seizures are frequent and may become a major problem. Vision is normal, although nonparalytic squints are frequent. There are no changes in the retina and cornea;

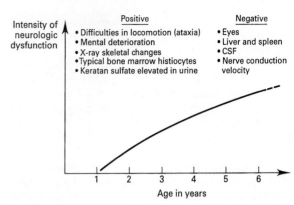

Figure 4-9
G_{M1} *gangliosis type 2. Clinical course and life profile.*

nor any clinical signs of peripheral nerve involvement (nerve conduction velocities are normal). The CSF is unchanged and the EEG is altered but not in any distinctive way. There is usually no significant facial dysmorphism or clinically detectable skeletal deformity; head circumference is normal, and liver and spleen are not enlarged.

On the whole, the clinical picture is quite uncharacteristic. The most helpful aids come from routine laboratory procedures. Skeletal x-ray films, especially of the spine, reveal moderate but distinct and constant changes.[21] The most prominent is a mild anterosuperior hypoplasia of the vertebral bodies at the thoracolumbar junction. Mild hypoplasia of the acetabulae (Fig. 4-10) and proximal deformations of the metacarpal bones are also found. In the bone marrow a few histiocytes show either clear vacuoles or a fibrillary, wrinkled cytoplasm resembling Gaucher cells. Vacuolated lymphocytes have been observed in some cases.[21]

In the final stages of the disease, the patient lapses into a state of decorticate rigidity. Death terminates the illness between the ages of 3 and 10 years, usually from bronchopneumonia.

Diagnostic Laboratory Tests

● The urine contains an elevated quantity of a keratan-like substance and various galactose-containing substances derived from glycoproteins.

● Skin or conjunctival biopsies may reveal clear intracellular vacuoles, like those of the mucopolysaccharidoses.

● Final diagnosis is based on enzymatic assays of leukocytes or cultured fibroblasts. A deficiency of the

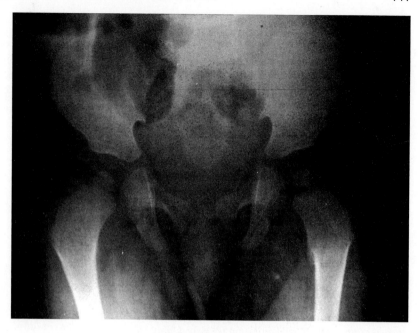

Figure 4-10
Late infantile G_{M1} gangliosidosis type 2. X-ray film of hips. Shallow acetabulae, coxa valga.

lysosomal acid β-galactosidase is readily demonstrated with artificial or the natural substrate G_{M1} ganglioside. Prenatal diagnosis is possible.

Pathological and Biochemical Changes   Pathology of the late infantile (and juvenile) G_{M1} gangliosidosis is qualitatively similar to that of the early infantile form of the disease. It consists of (1) abnormal intralysosomal lamellar cytoplasmic bodies in neurons and glial cells in the central and autonomic nervous system. Cortical neurons are less involved than in the early infantile variety. In juvenile and adult cases storage predominates in the basal ganglia.[22] Intralysosomal inclusions are seen not only in the perikarya but also in the initial segment of the axon (meganeurite).[23] (2) Vacuolization of histiocytes in liver, spleen, lungs, bone marrow and other organs, similar to those found in the mucopolysaccharidoses. (3) Cytoplasmic vacuolization of the renal glomular epithelium.

G_{M1} ganglioside and a lesser amount of asialo G_{M1} ganglioside accumulate in the gray matter of the central nervous system. The main storage substances in the visceral organs consist of galactose-rich products derived from glycoproteins, keratan sulfate, and other carbohydrate-containing materials.[24]

Differential Diagnosis   The clinical picture of the late infantile form of G_{M1} gangliosidosis is not distinc-

tive. Slight changes in the x-rays of the skeleton are most helpful, as are urinary biochemical tests. Metachromatic leukodystrophy and multiple sulfatase deficiency (low nerve conduction velocities, high protein content of CSF), neuroaxonal dystrophy (denervation atrophy with normal nerve conduction velocities), and late infantile Niemann-Pick type C disease (hepatosplenomegaly oculomotor disorder) are among the disorders that must be differentiated from G_{M1} gangliosidosis.

Late Infantile G_{M2} Gangliosidosis   Late-onset G_{M2} gangliosidosis may start in the second year of life with difficulties in walking due to a spastic paraplegia, accompanied by ataxia and polymyoclonus in some patients. But usually this disease starts later in life. It is fully described in Chap. 5.

Late Infantile Niemann-Pick Type C (NPC) Disease   In about a third of the cases, the symptoms of NPC appear during the second year of life (late infancy) with an uncharacteristic neurological picture of a rapidly progressive loss of motor and mental functions and a bipyramidal syndrome. The liver and spleen are generally enlarged and foam cells are found in the bone marrow. Epilepsy is rare. Vision is usually normal, and there is no evidence of a peripheral neuropathy or elevated protein levels in the CSF. Most children with onset of the disease in late infancy die between the ages of 3 and 5 years. (Niemann-Pick type C disease is more fully described in Chap. 5.)

UNSTEADY GAIT AND INCOORDINATE MOVEMENTS RESULTING FROM CEREBELLAR ATAXIA, DYSTONIA, CHOREOATHETOSIS, OR SOME COMBINATION THEREOF

General Features

A typical cerebellar ataxia is practically never an isolated sign in this group of diseases.

In ataxia-telangiectasia, cerebellar signs are eventually accompanied by choreoathetosis, dystonia, and a special disorder of oculomotricity. This full neurologic constellation is quite characteristic. Possible disorders with ataxia in late infancy or early childhood include some of the sphingolipidoses, particularly G_{M2} gangliosidosis, in which gait disturbances and incoordination are accompanied by spastic paralysis, dementia, seizures, often with a polymyoclonus (see Chap. 5). When dystonia and motor retardation appear during the second year of life in a boy, with no history of perinatal damage, Lesch-Nyhan disease (described in Chap. 5) is a prime consideration. Other possible causes are X-linked Pelizaeus-Merzbacher disease (usually recognized earlier, see Chap. 3), Leigh syndrome, the several disorders giving rise to bilateral striatal necrosis (see Chap. 5) and glutaric aciduria type I (Chap. 3).

Some disorders with intermittent cerebellar ataxia, such as PDH deficiency, Leigh disease, MSUD and Hartnup disease, may also manifest themselves in the late infantile period or later. They are listed in Table 6-4.

Ataxia-Telangiectasia Ataxia-telangiectasia was first reported by Syllaba and Henner[25] and by Louis Barr.[26] It is an autosomal recessive disorder of unknown etiology that affects multiple tissues, mainly the thymus and lymphoid tissues, nervous system, skin, conjunctival vessels, and gonads, thus creating a unique clinical syndrome (Fig. 4-11). The neurologic symptomatology is dominated by a complex combination of cerebellar ataxia and choreoathetosis and by a special derangement of oculomotricity. Conjunctival telangiectasias are a pathognomic feature. Recurrent respiratory infections are common and lymphomatous malignancies may occur late in the course of the disease. There are associated disorders of cellular and humoral immunity. The concentrations of IgA, IgG2, and IgE are usually greatly

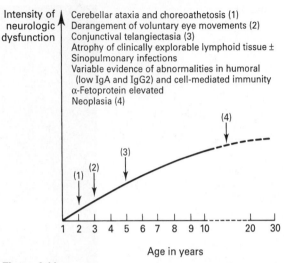

Figure 4-11
Ataxia-telangiectasia. Clinical course and life profile.

reduced. Levels of serum α-fetoprotein are elevated. A sensitivity to ionizing radiation with a tendency to chromosomal aberrations (affecting especially chromosomes 7 and 14) probably plays an important role in the pathogenesis of the disease. The mutant gene for ataxia-telangiectasia (AT) has been mapped to chromosome 11 q22-23 and has recently been cloned.

Clinical Features Our impressions are based on 40 personally observed patients and on a review of the literature. The neurologic disorders are the first clinical manifestations of the disease and usually appear after a period of normal early motor development. As soon as the child walks, between 12 and 18 months (occasionally somewhat later), unsteadiness of gait becomes evident. Also, there is a truncal instability when sitting, which may have been noticed at an earlier date. Initially, the child may exhibit a peculiar gait, walking on tiptoes as if dancing. Gradually the complex disorder of motility unfolds. Although not easy to describe in conventional neurologic terms, it includes elements that may be identified as choreoathetosis as well as cerebellar ataxia in variable proportions from case to case. In a standing position, the child's head and trunk move slowly in undulating side-to-side or in rotational fashion and the body sways in all directions. The head is frequently tilted laterally or thrust forward. The shoulders, upper limbs, and fingers also exhibit motor instability in which slow involuntary movements are combined with incoordination. The involuntary movements persist even when the child lies relaxed in bed. When walking, the gait is wide-based and unsteady, and there is a distressing tendency to fall. Intention tremor and dyssynergia are more variable. In some patients, there is for a period of time relatively pure cerebellar ataxia or choreoathetosis. Rarely, irregular myoclonic jerks of the limbs appear.

In the great majority of patients, usually early in the disease, there is a remarkable derangement of voluntary eye movements (oculomotor apraxia) due to impaired ability to initiate lateral eye movements, and an increased latency and decreased amplitude (hypometria) of voluntary saccades. To look to the side, the patient first makes an abrupt lateral movement of the head, with the eyes turning contralaterally, and then a forced blinking before fixating on the target. The ocular disorder resembles the congenital oculomotor apraxia, described by Cogan.[27] A typical oculocephalic asynergy is demonstrated when the child is asked to look rapidly to the right or the left. The eyes do not follow an abrupt lateral turning of the head; instead they are tonically deviated to the opposite side. When the patient is commanded to look to the side, up, or down, without moving their head, eye movements are slow, grossly saccadic, and frequently incomplete. Sometimes the child will succeed only after a long pause (pseudoparalysis). Pursuit eye movements are easier and fuller than those obtained on command. Nystagmus may be evoked during this procedure. Rapid passive head turns elicit a full (or exaggerated) range of eye movements, demonstrating the absence of oculomotor paralysis. Optokinetic nystagmus is abolished. On labyrinthine stimulation (irrigation of the ears with cold water), there is no nystagmus but instead an obligatory deviation of the eyes to the stimulated side.

Other obvious neurologic signs include dysarthria (speech is slurred, often scanning, and finally, incomprehensible) and drooling. In some patients there is a peripheral neuropathy, indicated by depressed or absent tendon reflexes, distal amyotrophy, deficient proprioceptive sense, and reduced motor fiber conduction velocities. It may be that some of the amyotrophy and depression of tendon reflexes are related to lower motor neuron degeneration and not to a neuropathy. Pyramidal signs and seizures have been recorded but are rare. The CSF is normal. Head circumference can be normal or slightly reduced. The retinas are unaltered.

Mental retardation may be present in the later stages of the disease but the rate of deterioration of intellectual capacities is slow. Children are usually calm and friendly and they exhibit no major behavioral problems. Brain scans may reveal moderate cerebellar atrophy.

The extraneurologic symptomatology is important. In approximately two-thirds of the cases, the children are small and underweight, and their health is plagued by recurrent otitis, sinusitis, and bronchopulmonary infections, most of which seem to be due to common bacteria. Bronchiectasis may develop, as well as clubbing of the fingers. The severity of the respiratory infections has been found by some to correlate well with the magnitude of the immunologic defect.[28] No correlation has been found by others.

Most remarkable are abnormalities of the conjunctivas, skin, and lymphoid tissues. Typical ocular telangiectasias appear usually between the ages of 4 and 7 years, often long after the neurologic changes, although occasionally earlier or much later; and in some cases they never develop. They consist of symmetric, fine, bright red, predominantly arterial, conjunctival vessels that run horizontally at the equator of the ocular bulbs and stop abruptly at the border of the cornea. These features are pathognomonic of AT (Fig. 4-12). In the course of time, cutaneous telangiectasias appear on the ears, nose, cheeks, palate, neck, antecubital and popliteal areas, and the dorsal aspects of the hands and feet. On the nose, cheeks, and limbs, the skin finally becomes atrophic and pigmented, with a senile or poikilodermic appearance. The hair of a number of patients becomes prematurely gray.

Cervical and other lymph nodes, adenoids, and tonsils are generally atrophic, even after repeated upper respiratory tract infections. But there are exceptions to this rule. Lymph nodes may at first be enlarged and later become atrophic.

Among other possible abnormalities are sexual infantilism in older patients, hepatic dysfunction, and derangement of carbohydrate metabolism. Insulin-resistant diabetes can develop in older patients.[28]

The disease progresses slowly, and by age 10–15 years most children are unable to walk, speech becomes incomprehensible, and swallowing is difficult. In some, the disease is milder and its course more chronic. Death usually occurs in the second decade, but some patients do reach adulthood. Pulmonary infections, tumors, or leukemia are frequent causes of death.

Patients with AT have a risk of cancer 60 to 180 times higher than those in the age-matched population. The incidence of malignancies has been estimated at 38 percent.[29,30] The most common ones are lymphoreticular tumors, particularly Hodgkin and non-Hodgkin lymphomas, and acute T-cell leukemias. In older

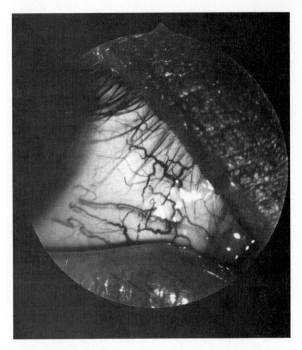

Figure 4-12
Ataxia-telangiectasia. Typical conjunctival telangiectasias.

patients, epithelial tumors of the breast, pancreas, stomach, bladder, ovary, and oral cavity occur with increased frequency. Brain tumors have been reported.[31] There is also an increased incidence of cancer in heterozygotes, particularly breast cancer in women, the risk being possibly increased by diagnostic or occupational exposure to ionizing radiation.[32]

Diagnostic Laboratory Tests   Laboratory tests of major importance for the diagnosis of AT include the demonstration of immunological defects, the detection of chromosomal abnormalities and measurement of serum α-fetoprotein.

Defects of cellular and humoral immunity are not constantly detected, and they vary from case to case even amongst affected siblings and in the same patients at different times in the course of the disease. The most common abnormalities demonstrated by immunoelectrophoresis are the absence or low levels of IgA and IgG$_2$. A deficit of IgG$_4$ and IgE are also frequent, as well as the presence of a low molecular weight form of IgM. Defects of cell-mediated immunity and delayed type of hypersensitivity are revealed by a poor response to common antigens, a decrease of the proliferative

response of T lymphocytes to mitogenic stimulation, and a modest reduction in the number of circulating lymphocytes.

In cell cultures there is an increased sensitivity of the patient's chromosomes to x-radiation, expressed by a fivefold increase in chromosomal breaks as compared to normal. Chromosomal breaks and rearrangements (inversions and translocations) involve more specifically chromosomes 7 and 14. The sites of the breaks include bands 7p14, 7p35, 14q12, 14q32, and 14qter. Recombinations involving 7p14 and 14q32 chromosomal bands are demonstrable. Chromosomes 2 and 22 may be involved and possibly others.

An elevation of the level of serum α-fetoprotein (a fetal protein of hepatic origin) and of the carcinoembryonic antigen are found in most patients.

Genetics   AT is transmitted as an autosomal recessive trait, but many cases have been sporadic. The incidence of the disease is between 1/20,000 and 1/100,000 of the general population. The responsible gene has been mapped on chromosome 11q22-23. Genetic heterogeneity has been suspected on the basis of the existence of several complementation groups.[33] Several mutations have been found within the AT gene which is a multifunctional DNA-activated protein kinase.[33a]

Prenatal Diagnosis   Prenatal diagnosis has been achieved by demonstration of increased chromosomal breaks in cultures of amniocytes from affected fetuses. More secure molecular biological techniques will probably become available in the future.

Pathologic Findings   The most constant and characteristic pathologic finding is the absence or abnormal development of the thymus and all cellular elements of the lymphoid system. Histologically there is a depletion of thymocytes, an absence of Hassall's corpuscles, a lack of corticomedullary demarcation in the thymus, a reduction of lymphocytes, and an absence of germinal follicles in lymph nodes. Dysgenetic abnormalities are found in the ovaries and testicles. Cytomegaly and large dysmorphic nuclei (aneuploidy or polyploidy) are observed in Schwann cells, spinal ganglia, satellite cells, adenohypophysis, liver, and other organs.

Morphologic changes in the central nervous system are remarkably inconspicuous when standard histologic methods are used. Those that are seen do not account for all of the clinical signs. The most definite abnormalities are restricted essentially to the Purkinje and granule cells of the cerebellum, which have degenerated to a varying degree in nonspecific ways. No vascular malformations are seen in the brain. Loss of medullated fibers in peripheral nerves is noted in some cases, and in others there is a disappearance of anterior horn cells in the spinal cord. If there is a neuronal loss of spinal ganglion cells, secondary degeneration occurs in posterior columns. Lesions in the basal ganglia have not been clearly established.

Physiopathology   The physiopathology of this multisystem disorder is still unsolved. One of the basic abnormalities certainly consists of an increased sensitivity of cells to ionizing radiation (not to ultraviolet radiation), probably associated with a defect of DNA repair. Damage to the DNA leads to breaks and rearrangements of chromosomes. Breaks affecting chromosomes 7 and 14 at sites including bands 7p14, 7p35, 14q12, and 14qter are in the vicinity of the IgG genes, T-cell receptor genes and antigen Leu-2/T8 (a T-cell differentiating antigen). A defective regulation of the immunoglobulin gene superfamily (which includes genes for T-cell receptors) has been postulated.[34] There is also evidence of an inability to form mature, normally functioning lymphocytes.[35] These disturbances could favor the emergence of malignancies and recurrent infections. The origin of the nervous system disorder and conjunctival and cutaneous changes, the abnormal development of the thymus and gonads, stunting of body growth, and the persistent production of α-fetoprotein are not explained. Correlation between the neuropathological changes and the neurological syndrome are unsatisfactory. Lesions of the cerebellar cortex (although frequently moderate) could account for the ataxia, but there is no known morphological basis for the choreoathetosis and oculomotor abnormalities.

Diagnosis   The combination of ataxia and/or choreoathetosis, oculomotor apraxia, and typical conjunctival telangiectasias is unique, and the diagnosis is readily confirmed by immunologic and cytogenetic tests and the increase of serum α-fetoprotein, possibly the most constant marker. When conjunctival telangiectasias are not yet present, or if the laboratory tests are inconclusive, the following conditions must be considered in differential diagnosis:

1.   Disorders in which ataxia and/or choreoathetosis are associated with major abnormalities of voluntary eye movements such as juvenile Niemann-Pick type C, juvenile Gaucher disease, some cases of Friedreich ataxia, or the syndrome *ataxia-oculomotor apraxia*.[36] The latter could be a type of spinocerebellar degeneration.

2.   Cogan congenital oculomotor apraxia (in which motor instability is frequent but frank ataxia or athetoid movements and other neurologic abnormalities do not occur).

3.   Some neurological syndromes with immunologic deficiencies. A familial syndrome has been reported with ataxia, spastic diplegia, and a severe deficit of cellular immunity.[37,38] The disease is possibly associated with purine nucleoside phosphorylase deficiency.[39]

Treatment   No specific treatment is available, however, control of infections with antibiotics and their prevention by injections of gamma globulins are important for the comfort of the patients and will prolong their lives. Multiple x-rays should be avoided. Antitumor drugs, rather than radiation therapy, are best used in the treatment of malignancies. However, some authors have recommended the use of low doses of radiotherapy and chemotherapy.[39a] In some cases, tiapride or propanolol have possibly been helpful in controlling incoordination.

INTENTION MYOCLONUS (POLYMYOCLONUS) VARIABLY ASSOCIATED WITH EPILEPSY AND CEREBELLAR ATAXIA

General Features

To an experienced neurologist, intention myoclonus (polymyoclonus) consisting in erratic, arrhythmic, asymmetric, and asynchronous muscular jerks induced or exaggerated by voluntary movement always conveys the idea of a hereditary metabolic or degenerative disorder involving cerebellar nuclei. Myoclonus differs from chorea in the speed of contraction, lasting a fraction of a second only, whereas the choreic movements last a second or more. The polymyoclonus is usually associated with other neurological abnormalities such as seizures and ataxia.

Polymyoclonus occurs in an appreciable number of juvenile metabolic encephalopathies. During the second year of life, it is regularly observed in the lipofuscinoses, some cases of G_{M2} gangliosidosis, of sialidosis type II and in Alpers syndrome (Tables 5-6 and 5-3).

In this section we will present the infantile and late infantile forms of lipofuscinosis and introduce our conception of the lipofuscinoses as a group. Nonmetabolic or degenerative causes of polymyoclonus occurring in the second year of life (e.g. Kinsbourne syndrome) will be discussed in Chap. 6.

The Neuronal Ceroid Lipofuscinoses The neuronal ceroid lipofuscinoses (NCL) are a group of disorders characterized by the intralysosomal aggregation of ceroid and lipofuscin. They constitute a common class of "neurometabolic" disorders of childhood and adolescence. Ceroid and lipofuscin have the unique property of autofluorescence. The nature of the responsible biochemical defect is unknown despite various unconfirmed hypotheses. One idea is that the NCLs are the result of lipid peroxidation. Other proposals are that they represent a deficiency in proteases or protease inhibitors, or an abnormal metabolism of dolichols. But it is now believed that elevated levels of dolichols in urine and brain are a secondary phenomenon. Recently it has been shown that mitochondrial ATP synthase C protein is also stored in neurons, but the meaning of this is not yet known.[40]

Four major forms of NCL have been described. They differ with respect to age of onset, clinical symptomatology, neurophysiologic abnormalities, and pathological findings. Dyken[41] describes six other atypical categories of ceroid lipofuscinoses. The ones most clearly defined are: infantile (INCL, NCL₁, Santavuori-Haltia disease); late infantile (LINCL, NCL₂, Jansky-Bielschowsky disease); juvenile (JNCL, NCL₃, Spielmeyer-Vogt disease); and adult (NCL₄ or Kufs disease). LINCL and JNCL, which are also referred to as Batten disease, are by far the most frequent varieties in most countries, whereas INCL has most often been observed in Finland. In a series of 319 patients with NCL, JNCL represented 51 percent, LINCL 36.3 percent, INCL 11.3 percent and Kufs disease 1.3 percent.[42] There are other reviews in the literature.[43–45]

Neuronal ceroid lipofuscinoses are autosomal recessive disorders except for some families of the adult form in which the mode of inheritance seems to be autosomal dominant. The genes for infantile and juvenile forms are localized to the short arms of chromosome 1 and chromosome 16, respectively. The abnormal protein synthesized by these genes has not yet been identified. A recent study has revealed that LINCL is not an allelic form of the juvenile or infantile subtypes.[46]

The clinical features of NCL consist of various combinations of seizures, myoclonus, ataxia, mental symptoms, and retinal degeneration. Ophthalmologic and electrophysiologic studies, neuroradiologic ima-

ging, and above all, ultrastructural analysis of skin or conjunctiva are essential to differentiate NCL from other neurometabolic disorders, such as the sphingolipidoses, which may have a similar neurologic symptomatology.

The specificity of the various intralysosomal inclusions (osmiophilic granular deposits, curvilinear bodies, and fingerprint deposits) has been the subject of much discussion, particularly the justification of using them as markers of the different NCL. Although the intralysosomal inclusions are somewhat pleiomorphic, especially in older patients, one type of deposit predominates in each form of NCL in biopsy specimens of skin cells (skin cells grown in culture appear normal and lose their distinctive ultrastructure).

Within brain homogenates from the late infantile and juvenile NLC there are specific accumulations of subunit C of mitochondrial ATP synthase. Storage of this material also occurs in cultured cells and urine of patients with LINCL.[47,48]

NCLs are incurable disorders, but therapies for symptoms may be helpful. Prenatal diagnosis may be considered in INCL and JNCL, where the mutant gene has been mapped. Early infantile and late infantile NCL will be described in this chapter, juvenile and adult forms in the next chapter.

Infantile Neuronal Ceroid Lipofuscinosis (INCL; NCL₁; Santavuori-Haltia-Hagberg Disease) Infantile neuronal ceroid lipofuscinosis is a rare autosomal recessive disorder, which has a widespread geographical distribution but appears to be strongly centered in Finland, where its incidence is 1/20,000. It was described by Santavuori et al. in 1974.[49] Its most striking feature is the rapidity with which it leads to a widespread destruction of neurons to a degree unknown in all metabolic encephalopathies except for Alpers syndrome. The neurologic deterioration results in myoclonus, ataxia, visual failure, progressive brain atrophy, and early loss of electrocortical activity. Before the end of the third year, the child becomes completely unresponsive (Fig. 4-13). The gene for NCL₁ has been mapped to chromosome 1p by linkage analysis.

Clinical Features The onset is between 12 and 18 months, with arrest and then regression of all psychomotor acquisitions. However, some indication of retarded development may have already become apparent by 8 months.

Apathy, mental dullness, and diminished activity are frequently the first marks of the disease to be noticed

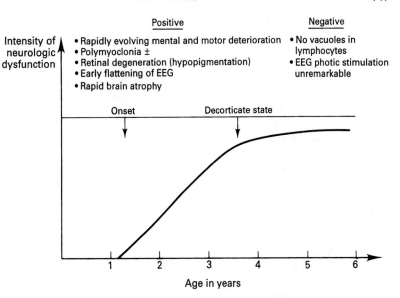

Figure 4-13
NCL₁. Clinical course and life profile.

by parents and may antedate other neurologic signs. Some children display an "autistic" type of behavior,[49] seemingly with complete loss of contact with surroundings but maintaining gestural stereotypes, particularly "knitting movements." Simultaneously, or somewhat later, other neurologic signs rapidly appear and progress. Incoordination of the limbs makes it impossible for patients to walk or to stand, abilities acquired by most of the children before onset of the disease. Marked generalized hypotonia with normal or exaggerated tendon reflexes is frequently noted at this stage. Myoclonic jerks appear soon and are a constant feature, if not early in the illness, by the end of the second year. Atonic, astatic, or generalized seizures are rarer. Failure of vision comes on rapidly. Abnormalities of the retina are seen early in the disease. They consist of hypopigmentation, narrowing of the vessels, brownish discoloration of the macular region, and later, optic atrophy. There is no aggregation of pigment deposits. The ERG is always abolished, even in patients with an apparently normal fundus.

Head circumference is normal at birth, but microcephaly becomes evident in the second year. Brain growth seems to stall after the first year of life, and thereafter the head rarely grows beyond 45 to 47 cm. Successive CT or MR scans reveal a very rapidly progressive cerebral and cerebellar atrophy, the major feature of the disease. MRI may show hypointense areas in the thalami and questionable hyperintense signals in the periventricular white matter.[50]

In the EEG, there is characteristically an early, generalized diminution of wave amplitudes progressing rapidly to an almost isoelectric flattening of the tracings within 1–2 years. EEG photic stimulation responses are unremarkable. Absence of spindles during sleep and flat cortical somesthetic evoked potentials are early electrophysiologic signs.[50] The CSF is normal on routine examination, but there may be an oligoclonal type of gamma globulin on agar electrophoresis and a progressive decrease of the tau fraction. In the peripheral blood, azurophilic hypergranulation of neutrophils is present in many of the patients, but there are no vacuolated lymphocytes. The bone marrow is normal. The EMG and nerve conduction velocities are normal.

By the third year of life, the children have usually become completely vegetative, unable to make interpretable responses or movements. Spasticity with exaggerated tendon reflexes and tonic spasms are prominent by then. The mean age at death has been 7 years.

Diagnostic Laboratory Tests   Three laboratory tests are essential: (1) rapidly progressive flattening of the EEG; (2) neuroradiologic imaging which exposes the progressive brain atrophy; (3) ultrastructural analysis of biopsy samples of skin or conjunctiva (or rectal myenteric plexuses) to reveal the typical finely granular osmiophilic lysosomal bodies in mesenchymal cells (or autonomic ganglia); (4) DNA studies.

Linkage analyses have shown the INCL gene to be located on the short arm of chromosome 1. This finding makes *prenatal diagnosis* possible.[51] Inclusions are present in chorionic villus cells.

Pathologic Findings Macroscopically, cerebral and cerebellar atrophy is the important finding. The brain weight is markedly diminished. Cerebral and cerebellar cortices as well as central gray structures are nearly completely devoid of neurons and are massively invaded by histiocyte-microgliocytes and astrocytes. Persisting neurons, mainly in the thalami and basal ganglia, brain stem structures, and spinal cord, as well as microgliocytes are filled with autofluorescent granular material readily stained by PAS and Sudan black. Similar granules are found in the spleen, pancreas, and lymph nodes. There is no spongiosis or marked astrocytic hyperplasia, as in Alpers syndrome, a condition also characterized by rapid cortical destruction. Photoreceptor cells and ganglion cells of the retina are destroyed.

Under the electron microscope, the inclusions in persisting cortical neurons, astrocytes, and microglia and in neurons of the autonomic ganglia (myenteric plexus) appear as dense, membrane-limited spherical bodies of finely granular structure.

Differential Diagnosis Late infantile G_{M2} gangliosidosis and Alpers syndrome may come under consideration.

Treatment There is no known treatment.

Late Infantile Neuronal Ceroid Lipofuscinosis (LINCL; NCL_2; Jansky-Bielschowsky Disease; Early-Onset Batten Disease) Jansky-Bielschowsky disease is an autosomal recessive hereditary disorder characterized by a dramatic neurologic symptomatology, including numerous generalized seizures, myoclonic jerks, ataxia, mental deterioration, and visual failure, appearing over a period of months. Characteristically, slow photic stimulation induces occipital spikes on the EEG, and visual as well as somatosensory evoked potentials are very large. Typical intralysosomal inclusions with *curvilinear bodies* can be detected in skin biopsies. There is no ethnic or geographic predominance for the disease (Fig. 4-14).

Clinical Features The disease usually starts between the ages of 2 and 4 years, after a period of normal or moderately retarded early psychomotor development. Nocturnal restlessness with a markedly reduced desire for sleep may be an early sign. The first manifestation of the disease is usually seizures, which rapidly increase in frequency and tend to be intractable. They assume several forms, even in the same individual: generalized tonicoclonic convulsions, myoclonic or atonic seizures, staring spells. They are soon accompanied by irregular asynchronous, asymmetric myoclonic jerks (polymyoclonia), which usually become more severe as the disease progresses. The myoclonus is evoked by proprioceptive stimuli, voluntary movement, or emotional excitement. Ataxia ensues, a combination of action myoclonus and cerebellar incoordination. Signs of involvement of corticospinal tracts are usually present. The

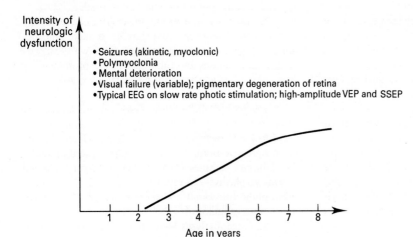

Figure 4-14
NCL_2. Clinical course and life profile.

child's motor disability soon becomes quite marked. Mental faculties deteriorate and speech becomes thick and slurred. Vision fails with time and most children are blind by the age of 6 years. The optic fundi are abnormal except in the early phase of the disease. There is macular degeneration with varying types of discoloration and hyperpigmentation, or a diffuse pigmentary degeneration. Optic atrophy follows. The ERG becomes extinct and may be abnormal even before any clear evidence of visual loss and ophthalmoscopic change.

Electrophysiologic findings are of great diagnostic importance. In the EEG, a low rate of photic stimulation (1 to 2 per second) elicits the characteristic high-amplitude occipital spikes (Fig. 4-15). Giant visual evoked potentials and high somatosensory evoked potentials are typical. CT scans and MRI reveal brain atrophy, which predominates in the cerebellum. Hypointense areas may be seen in the thalami and putamina and hyperintense areas in the periventricular white matter. The CSF is normal. Unlike the juvenile form of ceroid lipofuscinosis, there are no vacuolated lymphocytes. Death usually occurs before the end of the first decade.

Variants   There is some degree of variability in the expression of late infantile lipofuscinosis, as noted by Santavuori, who described some of the cases she observed as *"variant of Jansky-Bielschowsky disease."*[52] This variant, sometimes designated NCL5, is frequent in the genetically isolated population of Finland. Its gene locus has been mapped to 13q31-32.[53]

The clinical and neurophysiological features of this condition overlap both LINCL and JNCL. The disease starts at age 4 to 7 years with such uncharacteristic signs as mental regression and motor clumsiness. Epilepsy, myoclonus, ataxia, and frank mental deterioration do not develop until age 7 to 10 years. Macular degeneration, an extinct ERG, and the aforementioned electrophysiologic triad are observed at age 8 to 10 years. Vacuolated lymphocytes are absent.

Diagnostic Laboratory Tests   Paraclinical tests useful for diagnosis include:

- Ophthalmoscopy and ERG.

- Electrophysiologic studies: EEG with low photic stimulation, and visual evoked and somatosensory evoked potentials.

- Brain MRI.

- Ultrastructural study of skin or conjunctival biopsy reveal the typical intralysosomal inclusions in mesenchymal cells. These consist of multiple small, arciform, lamellar structures called curvilinear bodies (Fig. 8-1).

- The gene locus for LINCL has not been identified, but it has been shown that the disease is not an allelic form of the infantile or juvenile type of neuronal ceroid lipofuscinosis.[46]

Pathologic Findings   The brain, especially the cerebellum, is in most cases grossly atrophic with severe loss of cortical neurons in the cerebellum and less severe

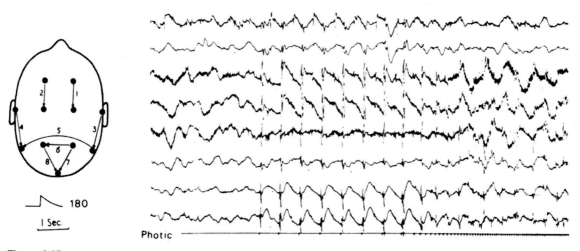

Figure 4-15
NCL2. EEG shows typical high-amplitude occipital spikes induced by low-frequency photic stimulations.

loss in the cerebral cortex, basal ganglia, and thalamus. Surviving neurons of the central nervous system and the peripheral autonomic system (myenteric plexuses) are moderately distended by granules that stain with Sudan black, are PAS-positive, and autofluoresce in ultraviolet light. The deposits in the perikaryon extend into an enlarged axon hillock (meganeurite).

In practically all of the published ultrastructural studies, and this accords with our experience, the neuronal inclusions have the form of curvilinear bodies (or multilamellar cytosomes). Fingerprint-like lamellar structures may also be found in some cells, especially endothelial cells. There are similar structures in peripheral nerves and in many other tissues, including histiocytes in skin, conjunctiva, muscle, and spleen.

In the retina, several reports have specified degeneration of the rods and cones as well as pigment neuroepithelium.

Differential Diagnosis   Diagnosis may be difficult early in the disease. In any previously normal child, aged 2 to 6 years, who displays arrest or regression of mental abilities, increasing clumsiness, action myoclonus and seizures, LINCL should be considered as one of the possibilities.

LINCL may masquerade as severe idiopathic epilepsy, Lennox-Gastaut syndrome, late infantile G_{M2} gangliosidosis, and other progressive disorders with seizures, myoclonus, and ataxia but without extraneurologic involvement.

Treatment   There is no specific treatment.

• Other rare forms of ceroid lipofuscinosis are to be found in the literature.[41,42,54]

• Juvenile and adult NCL are described in Chap. 5.

INTERMITTENT EPISODES OF ACUTE NEUROLOGICAL DYSFUNCTION AND COMA

Diseases with intermittent neurologic signs in early infancy (Chap. 3 and Table 3-7) may continue into late infancy or even into childhood and adolescence. In the second year of life, the causes of this category of disorders are *defects of mitochondrial β oxidation, defects of the carnitine cycle, maple syrup urine disease, urea cycle disorders, propionic acidemia, methylmalonic acidemia, other organic acidemias, familial lysinuric protein intolerance, fructose 1,6-bisphosphate deficiency, some cases of Leigh syndrome and PDH deficiency*. The

acute episodes take the form of derangement of consciousness (irritability, lethargy, mental confusion, or coma); cerebellar ataxia, tachypnea, and occasionally seizures may be conjoined. Frequently they are accompanied by anorexia and vomiting.

The cerebellar symptomatology may be relatively pure and at other times the movement disorder is difficult to distinguish from choreoathetosis. In some instances, the neurological symptomatology consists only of an acute loss of consciousness, or seizures and coma followed by ataxia during recovery. Such attacks are frequently elicited by fasting, excessive protein intake, or infections. It is important to know about triggering factors, which vary according to the nature of the metabolic defect, because they help to indicate measures for treatment and prevention of acute episodes.

Self-limited neurologic attacks last a few days or weeks and may recur for months or years. Pronounced attacks may be fatal. Such an outcome can generally be prevented by the rapid correction of obvious and potentially dangerous metabolic changes, such as hypoglycemia, hyperammonemia, and acidosis.

Further treatment and prevention is based on the precise diagnosis of the underlying metabolic disease. For many of these disorders strict dietary measures and vitamin therapy are essential (see Chaps. 3 and 9 and Table 9-1). Juvenile diseases with intermittent, acute episodes of neurological dysfunction are described in Chap. 5 and listed in Table 6-4.

MENTAL RETARDATION AND REGRESSION WITH PARALLEL DEVELOPMENT OF SKELETAL AND OTHER SOMATIC ABNORMALITIES

Beginning in the second and third year of life, several diseases may be found to underlie mental retardation, slow intellectual deterioration, behavioral abnormalities, and frequently auditory and visual impairment in association with striking somatic abnormalities. Either the systemic or the cognitive disturbances may be the first to attract attention. Included in this group of disorders are the mucopolysaccharidoses, the mucolipidoses, G_{M1} gangliosidosis, multiple sulfatase deficiency, the disorders of glycoprotein degradation (fucosidosis, mannosidosis, aspartylglucosaminuria, and sialidosis), and sialic acid storage disorders.

These conditions have in common a number of progressive nonneurologic abnormalities. The two most distinctive are coarse facial features and characteristic skeletal changes called *dysostosis multiplex*. The degree of these abnormalities varies greatly in the different diseases and may not be obvious before several years. Other abnormalities of diagnostic importance are corneal opacities, deafness, recurrent respiratory infections from infancy, hepatosplenomegaly, and hernias. Cognitive deficits are present in most but not all of these conditions.

The Mucopolysaccharidoses

The mucopolysaccharidoses (MPSs)[55–58] are a group of inherited diseases caused by a deficiency of lysosomal enzymes needed for the degradation of mucopolysaccharides (glycosaminoglycans). As a result, there is an accumulation of undegraded or partially degraded mucopolysaccharides in the tissues and an excretion in the urine. Glycosaminoglycans consist of polysaccharide chains attached to a polypeptide core through a xylose link. Each of the polysaccharides contains as many as 100 or more sugar residues joined together in repeating disaccharide units of uronic acid and sulfated hexosamine. Each MPS is the result of a defect in the degradation of the sugar derivatives or their sulfated residues. The mucopolysaccharides that are stored in the body and excreted in the urine are dermatan sulfate, heparan sulfate, keratan sulfate and chondroitin sulfate. The defective enzyme, the type of mucopolysaccharide stored in the body and excreted in the urine, and the diseases to which they correspond are listed in Table 4-2.

Mental deterioration is a feature of Hurler disease (MPS I H), the severe form or Hunter disease (MPS II), and all subtypes of Sanfilippo disease (MPS III). It is less conspicuous in the Hurler-Scheie syndrome (MPS I H/S) and the mild form of MPS II, but rare in the other MPSs. The degree of mental dysfunction is particularly marked in MPS III, in which mental signs are in the foreground and the systemic abnormalities are slight and subtle. Other possible neurological and sensory signs include deafness, common to all the MPSs (especially marked in MPS II), corneal opacities, retinal degeneration, tension hydrocephalus, and compression of the cervical spinal cord, peripheral nerves or roots by skeletal abnormalities. The two latter complications (and deafness) may also occur in forms of MPS with no cerebral dysfunction, especially Maroteaux-Lamy disease (MPS VI).

Common to the MPSs are various degrees of dysostosis multiplex, "gargoyle-like" facial features and recurrent respiratory infections dating from infancy. Hepatosplenomegaly and hernias are prominent in some varieties.

The probable anatomic basis for cerebral dysfunction is the accumulation of gangliosides in neurons, and in some patients there is an added tension hydrocephalus due to mucopolysaccharide deposition, histiocytic infiltration, and collagen proliferation in the meninges. In addition to direct involvement of the nervous system, the child's motor performance may be greatly hampered by the existence of skeletal deformities, and social communication may be made difficult by the deafness and amblyopia.

Under the light microscope there is a combination of diffuse storage of a lipid substance in neurons, enlargement of perivascular spaces, adventitial thickening of small vessels in cerebral white matter, and an infiltration of the meninges by fibroblasts and collagen.

Under the electron microscope the accumulated substance in neurons appears to consist of different types of intralysosomal cytoplasmic inclusions, the most characteristic of which have been designated zebra bodies. In our experience, neuronal storage tends to be most marked in MPS III. Clear vacuoles containing a finely granular filamentous material are also visible in adventitial cells and in the pericytes of brain capillaries. They are similar to the substance contained in vacuoles in the liver and other organs and probably contain mucopolysaccharides.

Biochemical analysis has shown the accumulation of gangliosides to be relatively slight (in contrast to the gangliosidoses) with a fairly characteristic increase of the monosialogangliosides, G_{M1}, G_{M2} and G_{M3}. The exact mechanism of intraneuronal ganglioside storage is not clear. It is known that mucopolysaccharides can inhibit the action of the β-galactosidase that acts on G_{M1} ganglioside. Therefore, accumulation of MPS might be expected to interfere with the normal turnover in situ of G_{M1} ganglioside. However, the mucopolysaccharide content of the brain is not demonstrably elevated. Mucopolysaccharides are stored in the liver, spleen, bone marrow chondrocytes, white blood cells, and other tissues. The stored substances under the electron microscope have the appearance of clear intralysosomal vacuoles which are empty or contain only small amounts of a finely granular material. Deposition of mucopolysaccharides in connective tissue leads to the marked thickening of skin and mucosae. In the heart there is thickening of the endocardium and valves, and narrowing of the coronary arteries.

Hurler Disease (MPS I H) Hurler disease (MPS I H) is an autosomal recessive disorder caused by a deficiency of α-L-iduronidase (a deficiency which is also the

Table 4-2

Type	Inheritance	MPS in urine	Enzyme defect
Hurler MPS I H	AR	DS HS	α-L-Iduronidase
Hurler-Scheie MPS I H/S	AR	DS HS	α-L-Iduronidase
Scheie MPS I S	AR	DS HS	α-L-Iduronidase
Hunter MPS II, severe form	X-linked	DS HS	Iduronate sulfatase
Hunter MPS, II, mild form	X-linked	DS HS	Iduronate sulfatase
Sanfilippo MPS III	AR	HS	A: Heparan N-sulfamidase B: α-N-acetylglucosaminidase C: acetyl-CoA: α-glucosaminide N-acetyltransferase D: N-acetylgalactosamine-6-sulfatase
Morquio MPS IV, types A and B	AR	A: KS C-6-S B: KS	A: N-acetylglucosamine-6-sulfatase B: β-galactosidase
Maroteaux-Lamy MPS VI	AR	DS	Arylsulfatase B
Sly MPS VII	AR	DS HS C4,6S	β-glucuronidase

Classification and main characteristics of the mucopolysaccharidosis

Gene locus	Nonneurologic signs	Neurologic signs
4p16.3	Distinct facial features Dysostosis multiplex Dwarfism Hepatosplenomegaly Heart disease Obstructive respiratory insufficiency Respiratory infections Corneal clouding	Severe mental deficiency Deafness Pigmentary degeneration of retina Hydrocephalus
4p16.3	Hurler phenotype, milder Micrognathism	Mild mental deficiency Deafness Compression of cervical cord (rare)
4p16.3	Corneal opacities Stiff joints, claw hands Long survival	Normal intelligence Carpal tunnel syndrome Cervical cord compression (rare)
Xq28	Hurler phenotype but no corneal opacities Skin lesions	Mental retardation Pigmentary degeneration of retina Hydrocephalus
Xq28	Hurler phenotype, slower course Longer survival. No corneal opacities	Intelligence normal
17q11-21 12q14	Abnormal facial features, and bone changes mild, initially absent. Corneal opacities nearly always absent.	Severe mental deteriorations Behavioral abnormalities Seizures and pyramidal signs
16q24.3	Distinctive bone changes Hypoplasia of odontoid Corneal clouding	Normal intelligence Compression of cervical spine and spinal roots
5q13-q14	Dysostosis multiplex Corneal clouding	Normal intelligence, usually Carpal tunnel syndrome Spinal cord compression Hydrocephalus (rare)
7q21.1-q22	Variable Hurler phenotype Corneal clouding Inclusions in leucocytes Severe neonatal form	Mental retardation in some cases

Abbreviations: AR = autosomal recessive; DS = dermatan sulfate; HS = heparan sulfate; KS = keratan sulfate; C-6-S = chondroitin 6-sulfate; C4,6S = chondroitin 4,6 sulfate.

The term MPS V is no longer used.

cause of Scheie disease and Hurler-Scheie disease). Dermatan sulfate and heparan sulfate accumulate in the tissues and are excreted in the urine. Gangliosides are stored in neurons.

In a sense, Hurler disease stands as the prototype of all MPSs. The patients are clinically normal at birth and up to the first or second year of life, although mild facial changes, chronic rhinorrhea, hernias, hirsutism, and periostal changes on x-rays of the long bones may have been noted at an earlier date. When the child sits, mild kyphosis may be evident. From the second year of life, the facial dysmorphism and skeletal deformities become increasingly conspicuous. Coarsening of the facial features, a depressed nasal bridge, frontal bossing, a large tongue protruding from an open mouth, coarse hair and skin, thick eyebrows, and a large scaphocephalic head constitute a characteristic and easily recognizable physiognomy. It is sometimes referred to as gargoylism (Fig. 4-16). There are also dwarfism, dorsolumbar kyphosis and lumbar lordosis, claw hands with stubby digits, and limited joint motility.

The combination of bony abnormalities seen clinically and in x-ray films (cf. description by McKusick[58]) are referred to as *dysostosis multiplex* and are present to some degree and with minor variations in the other mucopolysaccharidoses, in the mucolipidoses, multiple sulfate deficiency, glycoprotein storage diseases, sialidoses, and G_{M1} gangliosidosis. The skull is dolicocephalic with synostosis of the longitudinal suture, and the calvarium is thickened. The sella turcica is enlarged and J- or omega-shaped. The dorsolumbar vertebral bodies are rounded and one or two are smaller and recessed. A broad hook develops at the apex of the hypoplastic vertebrae, owing to the fact that the anterosuperior part of the body is rudimentary. The ribs tend to widen distally and are broader than the intercostal spaces. The pelvis flares and the tibias are small. The acetabulae are shallow and their roof is oblique. Coxa valga is present. The diaphyses of metacarpal bones and the shafts of the long bones are wider than the epiphyses. There is tapering of the proximal ends of the metacarpal bones. The humerus is angulated and the glenoid fossa shallow (Fig. 4-17). All these abnormalities are detectable by the second year of life and become progressively more evident.

Other virtually constant findings are enlargement of liver and spleen, chronic rhinitis, repeated respiratory infections and breathing difficulties due to obstruction of the airway by enlargement of the tonsils and adenoids, thickening of the mucosa of the respiratory tract, and narrowing of the trachea. Cardiac abnormal-

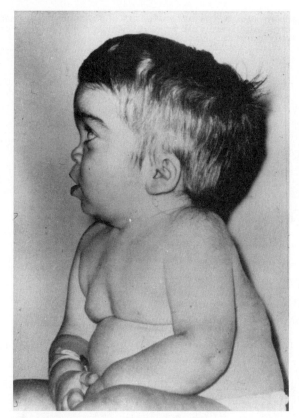

Figure 4-16
Hurler disease. An 18-month-old child with typical profile: large scaphocephalic head, short neck, kyphosis.

ities are frequent, including myocardial thickening, pulmonary hypertension, valvular dysfunction, angina pectoris, and myocardial infarction due to coronary artery stenosis.

Leukocytic inclusions are found in the blood and bone marrow. In the peripheral blood, lymphocytes contain intracytoplasmic vacuoles in the center of which are dark granules in Giemsa-stained preparations (Gasser type I cells). Polymorphonuclear cells may contain abnormal black granules (Alder-Reilly bodies). In bone marrow smears, round or curvilinear inclusions are visible within the intracytoplasmic vacuoles of plasmacytes. In monocytes there are coarse abundant basophilic granules (Gasser type II cells). Nearly all cases exhibit neurosensory and conductive hearing difficulties; conductive difficulties are due to middle ear infections and deformity of the ossicles. Corneal opacities are con-

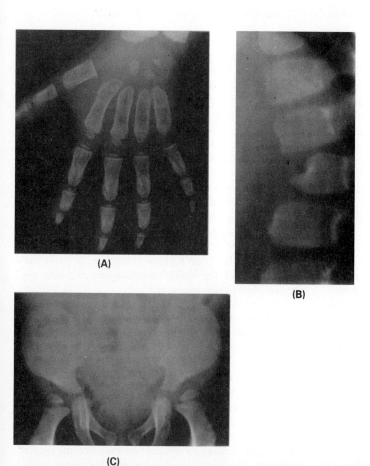

(A)

(B)

(C)

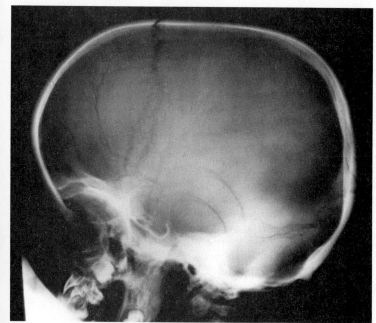

(D)

Figure 4-17
*Hurler disease. X-ray films of skeleton. **A**. Lack of diaphyseal constriction of metacarpals, pointed proximal ends. **B**. First lumbar vertebra is hypoplastic, beaked, and posteriorly displaced, causing gibbus. **C**. Flaring iliac wings, shallow acetabula with oblique roof, coxa valga. **D**. Large dolicephalic skull with diastasis of coronal suture and omega-shaped sella turcica due to raised intracranial pressure.*

stant, but early in the disease they can only be detected with the slit-lamp.

Neurologic development is normal or moderately retarded until the end of the first year; it then becomes arrested. Mental decline and motor dysfunction proceed at a slow pace. Social behavior is usually relatively well preserved, but in some patients agitation and aggressivity are troublesome. Correct evaluation of the status of the motor system is rendered difficult because of the ankylosis of the joints. After some time, signs of a corticospinal tract disorder are usual and there is occasionally evidence of lower motor neuron involvement and even of peripheral neuropathy. Defective hearing and corneal clouding add to the child's difficulties. There may be clinical and radiologic evidence of raised intracranial pressure with papilledema and progressive enlargement of the head, which may contribute to the mental regression (Fig. 4-17). In addition to corneal opacities, pigmentary degeneration of the retina and, not infrequently, optic atrophy are conjoined, contributing to the visual impairment. The optic atrophy is probably a consequence of meningeal lesions or of raised intracranial pressure. In CT scans and MRI, various degrees of ventricular dilation and white matter hypodensities may be found. Death usually occurs in the first decade of life from obstructive airway disease, respiratory infections, or cardiac complications.

Diagnostic Laboratory Tests Excessive amounts of heparan sulfate and dermatan sulfate are found in the urine. Enzyme assays on leukocytes and cultured fibroblasts are the definitive diagnostic procedure, reflecting the deficiency of α-L-iduronidase.

Detection of heterozygotes is possible and *prenatal diagnosis* has been successfully performed.

A deficiency in α-iduronidase is also found in the Hurler-Scheie syndrome and in Scheie disease (see below). Pseudo-deficiency of α-iduronidase has been reported.[59]

The iduronidase gene has been localized on chromosome 4p16.3. The structure and sequence of the gene are now known and more than 30 different mutations have been described. These account for at least 90 percent of the genotypes, including some Hurler–Scheie and Scheie phenotypes.[60–62]

Pathology As described in the introduction to the mucopolysaccharidoses.

Treatment of Hurler Disease Symptomatic treatment is important. Removal of tonsils and adenoids,

measures to alleviate airway obstruction (including the use of continuous positive airway pressure during sleep), correction of hernias, shunting of hydrocephalus, and treatment of heart failure are obvious measures to be undertaken under appropriate circumstances. General anesthesia should be administered with caution.

Bone marrow transplantations have been effective in some cases, leading to improvement of airway obstruction and other somatic abnormalities as well as the clouding of the corneas. Its efficacy for reversing neurological signs has not been proven. The advantages versus the potential risk of bone marrow transplantation should be weighed in any given case before the procedure is recommended (for details see Chap. 9). The degree of response depends not only on early institution of the bone marrow transplant, prior to the development of the major complications, but also on the α-L-iduronidase genotype.[63]

Hurler-Scheie Syndrome (MPS I H/S) Patients with this autosomal recessive disease have the features of Hurler disease but normal or near normal intellectual development. The disease usually manifests itself later than MPS I H, between 3 and 8 years. The skeletal and other systemic abnormalities tend to progress at a slower rate. Some patients have a micrognathia, which is part of the characteristic facies. When the patients reach adolescence, valvular heart disease, myocardial insufficiency, and respiratory obstruction may become major problems. The use of continuous positive airway pressure during sleep may alleviate breathing difficulties. Compression of the spinal cord by cervical pachymeningitis has been observed. Some patients reach early adulthood.

Hunter Disease (MPS II) Hunter disease, the only X-linked disorder among the mucopolysaccharidoses, is caused by a deficiency of iduronate sulfate that results in storage and excretion of excessive quantities of dermatan sulfate and heparan sulfate. There is an increase of gangliosides in neurons. The clinical picture is similar to that of Hurler disease except for the absence of corneal opacities. The presence in some patients of macular whitish skin lesions over the back, shoulders, and thighs is a distinctive feature. Two clinical entities with identical biochemical abnormalities have been described.

(1) In the *severe form of MPS II*, the phenotype is that of MPS I with marked dysmorphic facial features, skeletal dysplasia, short stature, hepatosplenomegaly, hernias, cardiac abnormalities, infections and obstruc-

tive respiratory complications, chronic diarrhea, severe hearing loss, and the development of communicating hydrocephalus. Corneal opacities are conspicuously absent, but a retinal degeneration may develop, leading to amblyopia. Mental retardation and neurologic involvement are similar to those of Hurler disease. Death from obstructive respiratory insufficiency or cardiac dysfunction occurs usually between the ages of 10 and 15 years.

(2) In the *mild form of MPS II*, somatic features are generally similar to those of the severe form but develop much more slowly (Fig. 4-18). Intelligence is preserved, normal social development is usually achieved. Survival is possible into late adult life (fifth to sixth decade and more). Hearing impairment is probably constant, and retinal degeneration may occur. A carpal tunnel syndrome is common. Chronic papilledema has been reported without clear evidence of raised intracranial pressure.

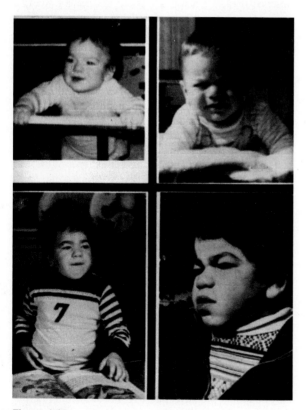

Figure 4-18
Mild form of Hunter disease. Successive facial features of a child at 1, 2, 4, and 6 years of age.

Laboratory Findings   In both clinical forms of the disease, heparan and dermatan sulfate are excreted in large amounts in the urine. The demonstration of a deficiency of iduronate-2-sulfatase in leukocytes or cultured fibroblasts is required for a firm diagnosis of MPS II. The gene for iduronate-2-sulfatase has been localized to the Xq28 region, and its sequence determined. Large deletions in the gene, found in some patients, tend to correlate with more severe degrees of mental retardation.[64-66]

Carrier detection is difficult. An enzyme activity of less than 50 percent of normal is required. Normal levels in a female relative of a patient with Hunter disease does not rule out heterozygosity. Enzyme analysis of single hair bulbs has been used. The availability of iduronate-2-sulfatase cDNA should improve carrier detection for females at risk, especially in those families where the mutation has been observed. The Hunter syndrome has been reported in girls, possibly as a result of the inactivation of the nonmutant maternal chromosome, or by other mechanisms. It is likely that some females previously thought to have MPS II did in fact have multiple sulfatase deficiency. Prenatal diagnosis is available.

Pathology of the Severe Form of MPS II   As described in the introduction to the mucopolysaccharidoses.

Treatment   See Hurler disease.

Sanfilippo Disease (MPS III)   Sanfilippo disease presents as a distinctive clinical syndrome caused by the deficiency of four different enzymes required for the degradation of heparan sulfate. As a result, heparan sulfate accumulates in the body and is excreted in the urine. Gangliosides are stored in neurons. The mode of inheritance is autosomal recessive.

Unlike the other mucopolysaccharidoses, Sanfilippo disease is primarily a neurologic disorder. The neurologic symptoms appear early and are marked, whereas craniofacial, skeletal, and other somatic abnormalities are mild.

Four phenotypically similar genetic variants of this disease have been recognized, each related to a defect of one of the following enzymes: heparan-*N*-sulfatase (sulfamidase) (type A), α-*N*-acetylglucosaminidase (type B), acetyl-CoA: α-glucosaminide-*N*-acetyltransferase (type C), and *N*-acetylglucosamine-6-sulfatase (type D). The genes for type B and type D have been mapped to chromosome 17q11-21 and 12q14, respectively, and their cDNAs have been cloned.

Neurologic Signs Mental deterioration is the dominant sign of this condition. Early mental and motor development are normal or somewhat retarded. Evidence of intellectual arrest and speech delay, and frequently hyperkinesia and aggressive behavior become manifest between the ages of 2 and 6 years. Mental deterioration and loss of speech soon follow and within a few years the patients have become severely demented. Because of marked aggressivity the children may be difficult to manage. Others become withdrawn and seemingly out of contact with their environment. Insomnia is frequent. Deafness occurs but is often difficult to corroborate because of the mental status. Seizures are not rare and may be an inaugural manifestation. Corneal opacities, even when searched for with the slit-lamp are almost always absent, but pigmentary degeneration of the retina and optic atrophy have been described. Signs of motor impairment usually become evident somewhat later. At first, walking becomes unsteady and use of the hands clumsy. Before the end of the first decade, locomotion is no longer possible and the patient remains confined to bed.

The neurologic examination, in addition to revealing signs of bilateral corticospinal tract involvement, may disclose marked amyotrophy, depressed tendon reflexes, and EMG signs of denervation atrophy. Nerve conduction velocities have usually been normal, pointing to the possibility of anatomic involvement of the anterior horn cells. In some cases, conduction velocities have been slowed.

There is to our knowledge no clear report of raised intracranial pressure such as may develop in Hurler disease. However, since the anatomic conditions responsible for communicating hydrocephalus are the same in both conditions, this complication certainly is a possibility and should be kept in mind in searching for a cause of the cerebral disorder. MRI may show marked cerebral atrophy.

Nonneurologic Signs Mild hepatosplenomegaly may be detected in young patients but is unusual in older children and adolescents.

Dysmorphic facial features, which are slight or even unnoticeable in the first years, tend to be more evident as time passes, but they always remain quite moderate (Fig. 4-19). The first years of growth may be accelerated, but usually the child becomes stunted after the age of 10 years. Joint stiffness is slight, and kyphosis

is absent or minimal. The skin is often thick. The teeth are usually carious. Chronic rhinitis and repeated respiratory infections and chronic diarrhea may complicate the disease. Cardiopathy is absent or mild.

X-ray changes in the skeleton consist essentially of a thickened calvarium with underpneumatization of the paranasal sinuses and mastoids, ovoid dorsal and lumbar vertebral bodies with occasional slight anterior beaking (Fig. 4-19), a reduction in the height of the iliac wings, and an abnormal formation of the acetabula with underdevelopment of femoral heads. The long bones are less affected.

Leukocytic inclusions in the blood and bone marrow are identical to those seen in Hunter disease and Hurler disease.

The average duration of the disease is 8 to 10 years. There are few patients who live beyond their twentieth year.

Subtypes of Sanfilippo Disease In view of the absence of any consistent clinical differences, specific enzyme assays must be performed to determine the subtype of the disease. However, statistically, some differences have been observed. *Sanfilippo A* disease is the most common variety and apparently the most severe. In a study in the Netherlands,[67] dementia was noticed before the age of 6 in 83 percent of cases, and this variety seems to have a more rapid progression and a shorter survival than *Sanfilippo B* and *Sanfilippo C* syndromes. Unusually mild cases of Sanfilippo B disease have been noted in the Netherlands series; the patients developed dementia only in the third and fourth decades of life. We have observed a mildly affected adolescent with Sanfilippo C disease.

Diagnosis Excessive amounts of heparan sulfate are excreted in the urine in all the varieties of MPS III. Sanfilippo D patients excrete also *N*-acetylglucosamine-6-sulfate. Definitive diagnosis is achieved by specific enzyme assays of cultured fibroblasts or leukocytes. *Prenatal diagnosis* is also possible by enzyme assays on chorionic villi. Carrier detection is feasible.

Because dysmorphic facial features and other somatic abnormalities characteristic of the MPS are usually slight and may be altogether absent, and the neurologic signs are rather nonspecific, the diagnosis of MPS III may be difficult. Patients with this disease may be thought to have undifferentiated mental retardation or psychiatric disorders, or even primary epilepsy.

An additional difficulty lies in the fact that spot tests, which are used routinely for the detection of

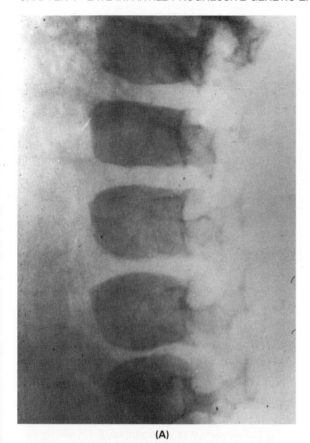

(A)

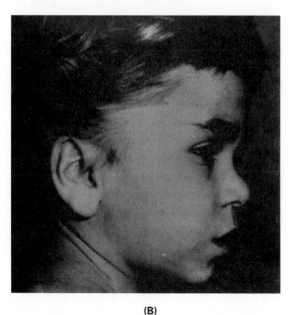

(B)

mucopolysaccharides in the urine, are frequently negative in MPS III. If MPS III is suspected, one is well advised to proceed directly to the enzyme assays, which are reliable and specific.

Pathology Neuropathological abnormalities are identical to those of Hurler disease and Hunter disease, although in our experience intraneuronal storage is much more severe.

Treatment Treatment has been purely symptomatic. Bone marrow transplantations have been performed in a few cases with questionable results (see also Chap. 9).[68]

Other Mucopolysaccharidoses

Mental retardation is usually not a feature of the other mucopolysaccharidoses, but neurological complications may occur occasionally.[67]

Scheie Disease (MPS I S) As in Hurler disease (MPS I H) and Hurler-Scheie disease (MPS I H/S), Scheie disease (MPS I S) is characterized by a deficiency in α-L-iduronidase. This leads to the accumulation in the body and excessive urinary excretion of dermatan sulfate and heparan sulfate. The clinical phenotype is, however, completely different. In Scheie disease, short neck, stiff joints, cloudy corneas, and aortic valve disease are the main clinical features. There is no craniofacial dysmorphia and the dysostosis multiplex is very mild. Intelligence is normal and life span is not shortened. Onset of significant symptoms, such as joint stiffness in the hands or corneal opacities, occur after the age of 5, and diagnosis is seldom made before late childhood.

Neurological complications include the carpal tunnel syndrome (Fig. 4-20), and much more rarely a myelopathy probably consequent to compression of the spinal cord by thickened cervical dura. Retinal degeneration and glaucoma may occur, and with corneal opacities, contribute to visual impairment. Hearing loss has been reported.

Figure 4-19
*Sanfilippo disease. **A.** Lateral view of dorsolumbar spine. Poor development of anterior parts of vertebral bodies, and ovoid dysplasia. **B.** Profile of a 6-year-old boy: low nasal bridge, thick lips, heavy eyebrows, and hirsute forehead. (Part **B** courtesy Dr. Maroteaux.)*

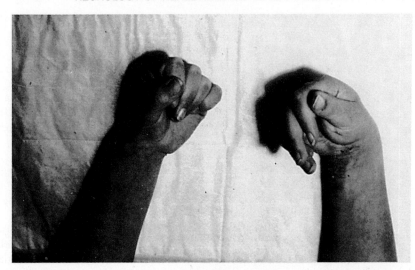

Figure 4-20
Scheie disease. Deformation of hands in an adult patient. Scar of surgical operation for carpal tunnel syndrome on the right.

Morquio Disease (MPS IV) Morquio disease (MPS IV) exists in two genetically different but phenotypically similar forms, A and B. Neurologic signs are related to the skeletal abnormalities. There is a potential danger of high cervical cord compression because of a constant and severe hypoplasia of the odontoid process and ligament laxity; consequently, there is a threat to life by atlantoaxial subluxation. Surgery to stabilize the upper cervical spine may be a necessary preventive measure. Lesions of the spinal cord or spinal roots may also arise as a result of the diminished anteroposterior diameter of the spinal canal. The vertical dimension of the spine is shortened and the spinal cord may descend too low in the lumbar spine.

Here, the accumulation of an oligosaccharide derived from keratan sulfate is the result of a deficiency of *N*-acetylgalactosamine-6-sulfatase in Morquio type A and β-galactosidase in Morquio type B. The gene for *N*-acetylgalactosamine-6-sulfatase has been mapped to 16q24.3, cloned and sequenced. The β-galactosidase deficiency in Morquio type B patients is the same as that which accounts for G_{M1} gangliosidosis. A variety of different mutations in the genes for these two enzymes have been described in Morquio disease.

Maroteaux-Lamy Disease (MPS VI) Maroteaux-Lamy disease (MPS VI) is an autosomal recessive disorder that produces a deficiency of *N*-acetylgalactosamine-4-sulfatase (arylsulfatase B). It has many of the features of Hurler syndrome, but mental development is usually normal. However, the affected children are handicapped by the severity of the skeletal abnormalities

and the visual impairment due to corneal clouding. Exceptionally, the children may be slightly retarded, a condition that may be overlooked because of an excellent social adjustment. The vertebral changes may lead to cervical or thoracolumbar spinal cord compression. The carpal tunnel may be constricted. Hydrocephalus has been reported. Respiratory insufficiency may develop secondary to severe scoliosis and to narrowing of the airway by accumulation of mucopolysaccharide.

The deficiency of arylsulfatase B (*N*-acetylgalactosamine-4-sulfatase) in this autosomal recessive disease results in the accumulation of dermatan sulfate. Several mutations in the gene for this enzyme, located on chromosome 5q13-q14, have been described. An adult-onset form of Maroteaux-Lamy disease is believed to be caused by mutations with a less severe effect, permitting the expression of greater residual enzyme activity.

Sly Disease (MPS VII) Sly disease (MPS VII) is caused by a deficiency of β-glucuronidase. The clinical presentation may be very similar to that of Hurler disease, but milder forms exist. Coarse metachromatic inclusions in granulocytes constitute a characteristic feature. Moderate mental retardation may exist. A severe *neonatal form* of β-glucuronidase deficiency has been reported in two infants with hydrops fetalis, dysostosis multiplex, and evidence of a lysosomal storage disease. The locus for the β-glucuronidase gene has been assigned to 7q21.1-q22 and several mutations have been found in patient DNA. The course of the illness in a patient followed by one of us has been modified by simultaneous transplantation of the liver and bone marrow.

Multiple Sulfatase Deficiency (Mucosulfatidosis)
This disorder was discussed under the spastic paraplegias and/or peripheral neuropathies towards the beginning of this chapter.

Mucopolysaccharidosis with Athetosis and Keratan Sulfaturia   This disorder is described in Chap. 5.

Disorders with the Hurler Phenotype and no Mucopolysacchariduria: Mucolipidoses, Disorders of Glycoprotein Degradation

In the late 1960s, Van Hoof and Hers[69] and Spranger and Wiedemann[70] drew attention to a group of patients with a phenotype resembling that of the mucopolysaccharidoses who did not excrete excessive amounts of mucopolysaccharides in the urine. These disorders have been called *mucolipidoses (MLs)* because lipids as well as polysaccharides were found in the tissues and cells of the patients.

Four types of ML have been described: ML type I or sialidosis, ML type II or I-cell disease, ML type III or pseudo-Hurler polydystrophy, and ML type IV. This classification is not ideal because there are considerable biochemical and clinical differences between the four disorders. ML II and ML III are to be set apart because their pathogenesis differs fundamentally from that of the other lysosomal diseases. The Hurler phenotype is not present in ML IV, and sialidosis type I. Three other diseases with the Hurler phenotype and no mucopolysacchariduria, mannosidosis, fucosidosis, and aspartylglycosaminuria, as well as the sialidoses are now usually classified as *disorders of glycoprotein degradation*. The urine of these patients contains large amounts of oligosaccharides (sialyloligosaccharides in sialidoses and neutral oligosaccharides in the other diseases). They are readily detected by thin-layer chromatography.

The diseases with a more or less severe Hurler phenotype and no mucopolysacchariduria are listed in Table 4-3.

The Mucolipidoses   We will describe under this heading MLs II, III, and IV. Mucolipidosis I refers to the sialidoses. Sialidosis type II is described in this chapter and in Chaps. 3 and 5, and sialidosis type I in Chap. 5.

Mucolipidosis II (I-Cell Disease)   The pathogenic mechanism of mucolipidosis II (ML II) is funda-

mentally different from that of the other lysosomal storage disorders. An abnormality of lysosomal enzyme transport has been demonstrated in cells of mesenchymal origin. The lysosomal enzymes are synthesized normally but lack a recognition marker that targets them to lysosomes.[71] Therefore, newly synthetized enzymes are secreted into body fluids. The recognition marker that targets lysosomal enzymes to lysosomes is mannose-6-phosphate, and in ML II an enzyme which catalyzes the synthesis of mannose-6-phosphate is deficient. Knowledge of this pathogenic mechanism is essential to understanding the basis of the biochemical tests necessary for the diagnosis of the disease.

In cultured fibroblasts from patients, dense inclusions accumulate in the cytoplasm, justifying the name of I-cell disease (inclusion cell disease) coined by Leroy and Demars[72,73] and used as a synonym for ML II. I-cell disease is inherited as an autosomal recessive trait. Mucolipidosis III has the same biochemical abnormalities as ML II.

Clinical Features   The disease has an early onset and a rapid course. Neonates tend to be "small for date." Motor retardation is evinced early; by the second year, mental retardation has become obvious. Speech is not attained and most children do not walk.

At birth the gums are hyperplastic, and within the first months of life, abnormal facial features, limitation of joint movement, thick skin, hirsutism, and radiologic changes of the long bones begin to appear. Changes in long bones are reminiscent of infantile osteomalacia (rickets) and consist of generalized demineralization, periosteal new bone formation, coarse trabeculation, and broad irregular metaphyseal lines. Similar changes may be seen in type I G_{M1} gangliosidosis, fucosidosis, mannosidosis and mucopolysaccharidoses.

Hydrops fetalis has been reported. Fetal ultrasounds have shown short femurs and intrauterine growth retardation.

In the second and third year, facial dysmorphism and skeletal dysplasia, similar to the changes seen in cases of Hurler disease, are obvious, but there is no scaphocephalic deformation of the skull (Fig. 4-21). Instead, the head tends to be brachycephalic and there may be frank synostosis of the coronal sutures. Gingival hyperplasia is particularly prominent. Hepatosplenomegaly is present but not marked. Hernias are common. Cardiomegaly and heart murmurs are frequent, with aortic insufficiency. Corneal opacities are usual. The optic fundi are normal. Hearing is impaired in some patients. Lymphocytes in blood and bone

Table 4-3

Disease[a]	Clinical features	
ML II, I-cell disease	Hypertrophy of gums osteomalacia from infancy; Hurler phenotype; brachycephaly; cardiopathy; corneal opacities; rapid deterioration	Severe mental deficit and motor delay; deafness (inconstant)
ML III, pseudo-Hurler, polydystrophy	Dwarfism; skeletal changes similar to those of Morquio disease; corneal opacities; aortic insufficiency	Moderate mental retardation in 50 percent; carpal tunnel syndrome; retinal degeneration
ML IV	Corneal clouding; face, bones, and viscera are normal; protracted course	Severe psychomotor retardation; retinal degeneration
α-Mannosidosis	Hurler phenotype marked to mild; corneal and lens opacities	Severe to moderate mental deficit; deafness; hydrocephalus
β-Mannosidosis	No facial, skeletal, or hematological abnormalities; angiokeratoma	Mental retardation; hearing loss
Fucosidosis	More or less severe Hurler phenotype; cardiopathy; enlarged salivary glands; angiokeratoma (type III)	Severe to moderate mental deterioration; severe neurologic signs (type I)
Aspartylglucosaminuria	Short stature; joint laxity; mild Hurler phenotype	Various degrees of mental retardation; behavioral and psychiatric manifestations
Sialidosis type II (ML I)[b]	Hurler phenotype	Intention myclonus; mental and motor deficit; cherry red spot; possibly angiokeratoma; renal dysfunction

Abbreviations: ML = mucolipidosis; MPS = mucopolysaccharidosis/mucopolysaccharides; OS = oligosaccharides.

[a] All diseases are autosomal recessive.

[b] Infantile and juvenile sialidosis type II and galactosialidosis are also discussed in Chaps. 3 and 5, and sialidosis type I is described in Chap. 5.

Disorders with the Hurler phenotype and no mucopolysacchariduria: mucolipidoses, disorders of glycoprotein degradation

Diagnostic laboratory tests	Deficient enzyme	Mutant gene
No excess of MPS or OS in urine; increase in serum levels of lysosomal enzymes; low levels of lysosomal enzymes in cultured fibroblasts but high levels in extracellular medium; characteristic inclusions in cultured skin fibroblasts	*N*-acetylglucosaminyl-l-phosphotransferase	4q21-q23
No excess of MPS or OS in urine; lysosomal enzymes as in ML II	*N*-acetylglucosaminyl-l-phosphotransferase	4q21-q23
MPS and OS normal in urine; typical lysosome inclusions in skin biopsies and other tissues		
Mannose-containing oligosaccharides in urine; no mucopolysacchariduria	α-Mannosidase	19p13.2-q12
Oligosacchariduria (mannosyl-1,4-glucosamine)	β-Mannosidase	Chromosome 4
High levels of fucose-containing oligosaccharides in urine; no MPS in urine; NA and Cl content of sweat increased	α-L-Fucosidase	1p34.1-p.36.1
High concentration of aspartylglycosamine in urine	Aspartylglucosaminidase	4q32-q33
Excess sialic acid-containing oligosaccharides in urine; no MPS in urine	α-Neuraminidase	10p ter $\rightarrow$ q23

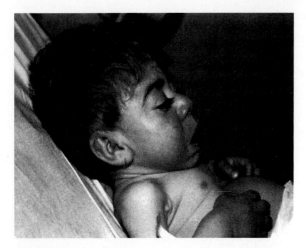

Figure 4-21
I-cell disease in a 2-year-old girl. Facial features similar to those of Hurler disease except for brachycephaly. Deformation of hands, protruding abdomen.

marrow contain cytoplasmic vacuoles, most of which are empty or very rarely contain a dark granule. Persistent nasal discharge and repeated respiratory infections are part of the disease. Urinary excretion of mucopolysaccharides is normal.

The full-blown picture of I-cell disease resembles that of Hurler disease, but there are the following differences: the disease starts earlier and has a more rapid course; neurologic dysfunction is more severe; there is a striking gingival hypertrophy; the head is not scaphocephalic; the hematologic findings are different; and there is no mucopolysacchariduria. Death occurs in most instances between the ages of 5 and 8 years, usually because of congestive heart failure or pulmonary infection.

Diagnostic Laboratory Tests   (1) The diagnosis of I-cell disease can be confirmed biochemically by measuring the activity of lysosomal enzymes in serum and cultured fibroblasts. There is a 10 to 20-fold increase in serum β-hexosaminidase, iduronate sulfatase, and arylsulfatase A. If cultured fibroblasts are available, the characteristic pattern of low levels of lysosomal enzymes in fibroblasts and a high concentration of these enzymes in the extracellular medium can be demonstrated. (2) A deficiency in the activity of N-acetylglucosaminyl-1-phosphotransferase in cultured fibroblasts or leukocytes will serve as the final proof of the diagnosis. Levels of activity of this enzyme are very low or undetectable.

Prenatal Diagnosis   Prenatal diagnosis of I-cell disease can be made by testing for the elevated lysosomal enzyme activity in amniotic fluid and the decreased activity of these enzymes in cultured amniotic cells, and by measuring the activity of the phosphotransferase in these cells. Cultured cells from chorionic villi have also been used.[74]

Carrier detection is possible. Heterozygotes have intermediate levels of activity of phosphotransferase in leukocytes and cultured fibroblasts and may have somewhat elevated levels of serum β-hexosaminidase.

The phosphotransferase gene has been mapped to 4q21-q23, but reports of its structure and sequence have not yet appeared.

Pathologic Findings.   Cultured skin fibroblasts contain coarse, refractile, cytoplasmic granules when observed with phase microscopy. These inclusions are thought to be characteristic of this condition and, as was stated, have given it the name of I-cell (inclusion cell) disease. Under the electron microscope the granules appear as dense intralysosomal inclusions. There are also vacuoles, the contents of which have not been ascertained, but they probably include oligosaccharides, mucopolysaccharides, and lipids.

Ultrastructural studies of the hepatocytes have disclosed no clear vacuoles but instead a small number of dense bodies. However, clear vacuoles do exist in the Kupffer cells and fibroblasts in the periportal spaces. These vacuoles have also been seen in the glomerular epithelium of the kidney and in pericytes in the brain. There are dense lamellar inclusions in neurons and astrocytes.

Cardiac enlargement with endocardial and myocardial fibrosis has been prominent in some cases.

No storage of mucopolysaccharide has been detected in the liver.

Treatment   Bone marrow transplantation has been carried out, to our knowledge, in three patients.[75,76] The result was favorable both on the biochemical defects and on some of the somatic abnormalities, but the neurological status was not improved.

Mucolipidosis Type III (Pseudo-Hurler Polydystrophy)   This rare autosomal recessive condition shares the same pathogenic mechanisms with ML II, but the clinical picture is much milder, and survival into adulthood is not unusual. ML III is characterized by dwarfism, skeletal abnormalities reminiscent of Morquio disease with severe involvement of bones of the pelvis, scapula, and hands, a moderately dysmorphic appearance, corneal opacities and in some patients retinal degeneration and aortic insufficiency. There are multiple-flexion ankyloses of the fingers and reduced mobility of other joints. No urinary excretion of MPS is detectable. The level of lysosomal hydrolases in the serum is elevated. Approximately half of the patients have some degree of learning disability or moderate mental retardation. A carpal tunnel syndrome may occur. The activity of *N*-acetylphotransferase in leukocytes and cultured fibroblasts is less severely depressed than in ML II.

Mucolipidosis IV   Mucolipidosis IV has been reported in approximately 20 patients, most of them of Ashkenazi Jewish parentage. The authors (EHK) have observed 15 additional patients. Corneal clouding, retinal degeneration, and profound motor and mental retardation are present, but facial features are unaltered and there are no skeletal changes or visceromegaly.[77]

Arrest of neurologic development and visual impairment usually become evident between 3 and 8 months of age. Corneal opacity, the most characteristic feature of mucolipidosis IV, is generally observable in early infancy but may not be detected until the second year of life or even later. In one 5-year-old child no corneal opacities could be found. Retinal degeneration with evident amblyopia are generally found and the ERG is extinct. Motor development is severely impaired. While some affected children have been able to sit or stand with support, none of them were able to walk without assistance. Hand play and other manual activities are grossly impaired. Mental development is very poor. Some children have acquired a few words, but speech is lacking in the majority of them. Frank psychomotor regression is usually not observed. Most children are of short stature and have a small head circumference (frequently below the 3d percentile). Facial dysmorphism, skeletal abnormalities, and organomegaly are conspicuously absent. There is no excess of mucopolysaccharides or oligosaccharides in the urine. The disease has a protracted course, which extends well into adolescence and early adulthood.

The diagnosis is based on the demonstration of lysosomal inclusions in conjunctival and skin biopsies. Under the electron microscope, the lysosomal deposits seen in conjunctival and dermal fibroblasts consist of concentric membranous bodies similar to those of the gangliosidoses, and of granulofibrillar material (Fig. 4-22). Clear vacuoles are also observed. Similar deposits exist in leukocytes and the cells of biopsy specimens of

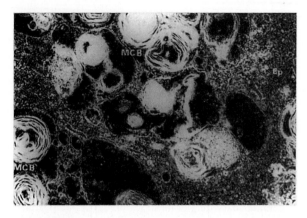

Figure 4-22
Mucolipidosis IV. Conjunctival biopsy. Electron microscopy shows concentric membranous bodies (MCB) in mesenchymal cells (not seen in Tay-Sachs disease).

the liver, spleen, and brain. They are present in neurons. In the liver multilamellar cytosomes are visible in hepatocytes and clear vacuoles in Kupffer cells. Biochemical analysis of cultured fibroblasts and brain biopsy material have shown an accumulation of gangliosides, mainly G_{M3} and G_{D3}, and also phospholipids and mucopolysaccharides (probably as a secondary phenomenon). The enzyme defect leading to the storage of these substances is unknown. Suggestion of a neuraminidase deficiency as the basis of the disease has not been confirmed. The characteristic ultrastructural changes have been found in cultured amniotic cells and chorionic cells, and this has been used for prenatal diagnosis.

Treatment   The corneal clouding can be prevented and also reversed by protecting the cornea with regular use of artificial tears or with contact lenses.

Disorders of Glycoprotein Degradation   Glycoproteins consist of oligosaccharide chains attached to a protein core. The proteins are synthesized on polysomes in the rough endoplasmic reticulum and the oligosaccharides are added as the polypeptides pass through the smooth endoplasmic reticulum to the Golgi apparatus. Oligosaccharides are degraded in the lysosomes. Two types of oligosaccharide chains are formed, one of which, the *N*-glycosidic asparagine-linked type, serves as substrate to the lysosomal enzymes which are deficient in the diseases discussed here.[78]

Disorders of glycoprotein degradation are α-mannosidosis, β-mannosidosis, fucosidosis, aspartylglucosaminuria, and the sialidoses. Another disorder of glyco-protein metabolism, still of unknown cause, is the carbohydrate-deficient glycoprotein syndrome.

α-Mannosidosis α-Mannosidosis is an autosomal recessive inherited disease related to a deficiency in the lysosomal enzyme α-mannosidase, which results in the accumulation of mannose-containing oligosaccharides in tissues and body fluids. Approximately 70 patients have been reported, but this does not reflect the relative frequency of the disorder. Affected patients have mild to moderate coarsening of facial features (Fig. 4-23), some

degree of dysostosis multiplex, mental retardation, and vacuolated lymphocytes. Deafness, lenticular and corneal opacities, hepatomegaly, and repeated respiratory infections are other prominent parts of the disorder. Large amounts of mannose-rich oligosaccharides are excreted in the urine.

Two forms of α-mannosidosis have been distinguished, but more likely there is a continuum of clinical expression rather than a clear separation into two phenotypes. In the infantile variety (type I) mental deterioration is severe; facial dysmorphism, dysostosis multiplex, and hepatomegaly are obvious. The course of the disease is brief, with death occurring usually between 3 and 10 years of age.

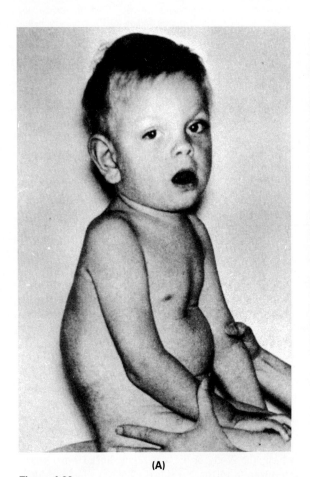
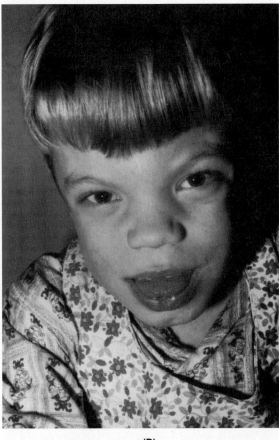

(A)   (B)

Figure 4-23

α-Mannosidosis. **A.** General aspect of a $2\frac{1}{2}$-year-old boy with open mouth (upper respiratory difficulties) and thoracic kyphosis. The child was deaf. **B.** Facial appearance of a 5-year-old girl: broad nose with depressed bridge, thick lips, and protruding tongue. (Part **A** courtesy B. Kjellman et al., J. Pediatr. 75: 366, 1969.)

In the milder juvenile form (type II), the clinical picture may be at first quite uncharacteristic. During the first year of life, motor development is normal or somewhat retarded. Later, speech is delayed and remains imperfect. In the second and third years, mental retardation becomes evident but is of variable degree. Motor performance is poor and movements are clumsy. Progression of the neurologic abnormality is hardly noticeable, at least for many years. Consequently, the diagnosis of developmental mental retardation or cerebral palsy would be tenable were it not for one or several of the following features: deafness, ocular findings, subtle facial dysmorphism, skeletal abnormalities in x-rays, recurrent respiratory infections, hematologic findings, and possibly hepatomegaly.

Hearing loss is usual and has been noted as an early sign. Spokelike posterior lens opacities and superficial corneal opacities are distinctive findings. Slight to moderate dysmorphic features comprise prominent forehead, large jaw, depressed nasal bridge, coarse features, and hyperplasia of the gums (Fig. 4-23). Vertebral bodies are ovoid, flattened, or with a beak-like deformity like that of the mucopolysaccharidoses. A kyphoscoliosis may be present. Poor trabeculation of the long bones, a thick cranial calvarium, and synostosis of the longitudinal suture are important radiological findings. A destructive synovitis may occur in older patients. Susceptibility to multiple upper respiratory tract infections with copious nasal discharge appears in infancy and may persist throughout the disease. The liver may be enlarged and hernias are often present. Between 20 and 90 percent of the lymphocytes in the peripheral blood contain translucent vacuoles, and a proportion of polymorphonuclear leukocytes are coarsely granulated. Foamy histiocytes have occasionally been found in the bone marrow. The disease has a protracted course extending well into adulthood. Late in the disease, hydrocephalus (as in the mucopolysaccharidoses) and a spastic paraplegia may occur.

Diagnostic Laboratory Tests   Excessive amounts of mannose-containing oligosaccharides are excreted in the urine. Thin-layer chromatography will easily disclose the particular pattern of oligosacchariduria which is characteristic of this disease. There is no mucopolysacchariduria.

The deficient enzyme, lysosomal acid α-mannosidase, may be detected in leukocytes and cultured fibroblasts, but not reliably in the plasma. The neutral, Golgi-associated mannosidase is not affected. Thin-layer chromatography of urinary oligosaccharides reveals a ladderlike series of orcinol-stained bands of increasing molecular weight. Heterozygote detection is possible and prenatal diagnosis has been achieved. The persistence of a high residual activity of α-mannosidase in some patients must be taken into account. The acid α-mannosidase gene has been mapped to 19p13.2-q12 and cloned.

Pathology   In the central nervous system, there is a marked and widespread distention of neurons, which, under the electron microscope, are seen to contain multiple clear membrane-bound vacuoles with fine reticulogranular inclusions and other types of deposits. Similar lysosomal vacuoles are found in the liver and other organs.

Treatment   The residual activity of α-mannosidase can be stimulated by zinc ions, but oral therapy with zinc sulfate has not been beneficial. In one patient, who died 18 months after successful bone marrow transplantation, the somatic effects of the disease were reversed, but storage within the brain was not affected.

β-Mannosidosis   Eleven patients with β-mannosidosis have been reported.[79] Mental retardation, hearing loss, and possibly seizures occur without hepatomegaly, facial dysmorphism, skeletal changes, or leukocyte inclusions. Angiokeratomas and tortuosity of retinal vessels have been observed. Other signs have included aggressive behavior, severe epilepsy, spastic quadriplegia, and a peripheral neuropathy. There is excessive urinary excretion and tissue accumulation of oligosaccharides, particularly mannosyl β-1,4-glucosamine. The specific deficiency of β-mannosidase can be demonstrated in leukocytes, cultured fibroblasts, and plasma. The gene encoding betamannosidosis has been localized to chromosome 4.

In one patient with dysostosis multiplex and dysmorphic features, a combined deficiency of β-mannosidase and sulfamidase was found.

Fucosidosis (Alpha-L-Fucosidosis)   Fucosidosis is an autosomal recessive inherited disorder caused by the deficient activity of the enzyme α-L-fucosidase leading to the accumulation of fucose-containing oligosaccharides, glycopeptides, and glycolipids in the tissues and urine.[80,81] Only oligosaccharides are stored in the brain.

Clinical Features.   At least 80 patients with fucosidosis have been reported.[82] The severity of the disease and its clinical expression vary, but in the majority of patients neurological dysfunction is prominent.

In about 60 percent of patients with type I fucosidosis signs of neurologic deterioration appear early, between 6 and 18 months and progress rapidly to a state of decerebrate rigidity and abolition of all mental activity. In other children (type II) neurological regression is only evident in the second or third years of life and proceeds at a somewhat slower pace. There are no corneal opacities and the optic fundi are normal.

Gargoyle-like facial features are more or less pronounced, but they may be very mild in infants. Skeletal abnormalities are slight and essentially restricted to the dorsolumbar spine; they consist of anterior beaking of the vertebrae. In the infant there may be rickets-like changes (Fig. 4-24). Other findings include hepatomegaly, cardiomegaly with ECG changes, nonfunctioning gallbladder, enlarged salivary glands, thickened skin with excessive sweating, and a marked susceptibility to upper respiratory tract infections.

Peripheral lymphocytes contain vacuoles and granular inclusions. Histiocytes with inclusions surrounded by vacuoles have been reported in bone marrow smears. The sodium and chloride content of sweat and saliva may be increased. Urinary mucopolysaccharides are not elevated.

In the early and late infantile form of fucosidosis, death usually occurs between the fourth and sixth year.

In another form of the disease (type III), neurologic signs are noted in the first few years of life but progress slowly to a state of severe mental and motor deterioration by adolescence or adulthood. Coarse facial features, skeletal deformities, or dwarfism become progressively evident. The main distinguishing feature is the presence of angiokeratoma of the same type and distribution as in Fabry disease. The skin lesion is essentially distributed on the external genitalia, abdomen, buttocks, and thighs. (Angiokeratomas also occur in sialidosis and β-mannosidosis.) There are telangiectasic lesions in the mouth. Tortuosity of conjunctival vessels and a pigmentary degeneration of the retina have been reported. These patients may survive for many years.

A clear distinction between the three forms of the disease is somewhat artificial, there is a virtual continuum of clinical expression. "Type I" and "type II" may appear in the same family.[83]

Diagnostic Laboratory Tests On thin-layer chromatography of urine an excessive amount of fucose-containing oligosaccharides and glycolipids can be demonstrated.

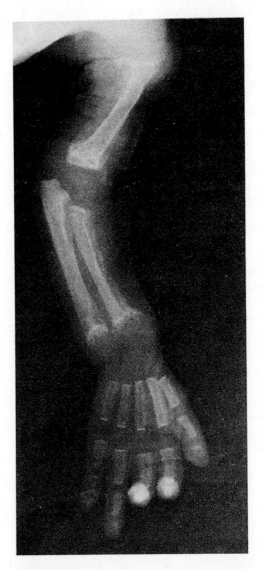

Figure 4-24
Fucosidosis. X-ray appearance of arm of a 7-month-old patient. Note rickets-like epiphyseal skeletal changes. (Courtesy Dr. Dupont and Dr. Maroteaux.)

The finding of marked deficiency of the lysosomal enzyme α-L-fucosidase in serum, leukocytes, and cultured fibroblasts provides the final proof of diagnosis. As the residual activity of this enzyme may exceptionally be relatively high, it is always necessary to carry out thin-layer chromatography for oligosaccharides. Between 6 and 11 percent of the normal population have markedly depressed α-L-fucosidase activity in the serum, but not in leukocytes. Therefore serum and plasma are not suitable for enzymatic diagnosis of fucosidosis.

In conjunctival biopsies, clear vacuoles are seen in epithelial and mesenchymal cells. Carrier testing is possible and *prenatal diagnosis* has been successfully performed. The gene has been mapped to the short arm of chromosome 1 at position 1p34.1-p36.1. As of this writing, 15 mutations in the α-L-fucosidase gene have been described.

Pathologic Findings and Biochemical Pathology The most striking microscopic features are clear vacuoles in the cells of most tissues including neurons, hepatocytes and Kupffer cells, and cells of the spleen, lung, kidney, heart, and skin.

There were unique ultrastructural changes in the neurons of one case. Two types of vacuoles were found in the perikaryon: clear vacuoles and vacuoles filled with a fine granulofilamentous material, a picture different from that of Hurler disease. In the liver, hepatocytes and Kupffer cells contain clear vacuoles, as in gargoylism, in addition to multilamellar membrane-bound inclusions, as in the sphingolipidoses.

Clear vacuoles have been reported in dermal capillaries, epithelial cells of sweat glands, and in cells in conjunctival biopsies.

Fucose-containing oligosaccharides, glycoproteins, and glycosphingolipids are stored in the tissues. In the brain there appears to be only an excess of fucose-containing oligosaccharides, whereas in the liver there is a major accumulation of glycolipids.

Treatment Bone marrow engraftment in canine fucosidosis has been followed by improvements in the peripheral and visceral lesions and in a more gradual improvement in the central nervous system pathology.[84] Both human and canine fibroblasts in fucosidase deficiency can be corrected by retroviral-mediated gene transfer.[85] However, we are not aware of any attempt at enzyme replacement therapy in patients with fucosidosis.

Aspartylglucosaminuria Aspartylglucosaminuria is an autosomal recessive inborn error of metabolism caused by a deficiency of the lysosomal enzyme aspartylglucosaminidase (N-aspartyl-β-glucosaminidase) that cleaves the bond between asparagine and N-acetylglucosamine during the lysosomal degradation of N-linked glycoproteins. As a result, aspartylglucosamine is stored in body tissues and excreted in the urine. The majority of patients have been found in Finland. The aspartylglucosaminidase gene has been localized to the long arm of chromosome 4 at the position of 4q32-q33 and has been cloned and sequenced. Two point mutations responsible for aspartylglucosaminuria have been identified in Finnish patients and a total of at least 11 mutations worldwide have been detected.

Clinical Features In 1993 over 200 cases had been diagnosed in Finland. The disorder has also been seen in several other European countries, in America, and in Japan, accounting for an additional 40 or more cases.[86]

Affected children are more or less mentally retarded from early childhood. Speech is delayed and remains poor or is never acquired. Severe behavioral abnormalities, with alternate periods of hyperactivity and apathy, have been recounted. Psychotic manifestations are possible. A gradual regression of mental function develops insidiously between the ages of 6 and 15 years. Motor deterioration is usually mild; the movements are clumsy and slight signs of corticospinal tract disorder may be evident. Some patients have seizures. Other findings include a short stature, joint laxity, brachycephaly, abnormality of the skin (photosensitivity, large nevi, angiokeratoma in one patient), and neutropenia. The course of the disease is protracted. Many patients reach adulthood. The CSF is normal or shows a low albumin content. The EEG is nonspecific. Corneal clouding and retinal abnormalities have not been reported, but crystal-like lens opacities are observed in some patients.

The differentiation of this condition from a nonprogressive congenital encephalopathy may prove difficult, especially in young children. Of great importance for diagnosis are subtle nonneurologic signs, such as a coarse facies with a broad nasal bridge, anteverted nostrils, a large nose, thick lips, sagging cheeks, and epicanthal folds. Often these changes are slight or absent before the age of 10 years. The liver may be enlarged and abdominal hernias are common. Cardiac valvular insufficiency is not frequent, but cardiac murmurs may be heard. X-ray investigation reveals minimal skeletal changes, but most particularly there are Hurler-like deformities of the thoracolumbar vertebral bodies, subperiosteal thickening, and thickening of the calvarium with underdeveloped cranial sinuses. Vacuolated lymphocytes are found in the blood. None of these signs is specific, but together they serve to orient the clinician toward this group of diseases.

Diagnostic Laboratory Tests Firm diagnosis of aspartylglucosaminuria rests on biochemical data. As the few clinical signs which are in favor of this diagnosis are frequently lacking in the first decade, it might not be illogical to include biochemical screening for this disease among the laboratory investigations performed systematically in young children with mental retardation of unknown origin, despite its rarity outside Finland.

Patients with aspartylglucosaminuria excrete large amounts of aspartylglucosamine in the urine. Increased concentrations of this compound can be detected by chromatography or by a quantitative test based on the enzymatic determination of aspartylglucosamine. (When chromatography is performed, heating of the paper or plate at 100°C for a few minutes is important when a ninhydrin reagent is employed.)

The final diagnosis rests on the demonstration of a marked deficiency of aspartylglucosaminidase in plasma, leukocytes, or cultured skin fibroblasts. *Prenatal diagnosis* has been achieved and heterozygotes can be detected using enzyme assays in fibroblasts or lymphocytes.[87]

Late Infantile Type II Sialidosis and Galactosialidosis Type II sialidosis and galactosialidosis may be recognized in some patients during the second year of life. Progressive difficulties in walking, seizures, myoclonus, mental retardation, macular cherry red spots, and Hurler-like dysmorphic and skeletal features are characteristic. These disorders and sialic acid storage diseases are described in Chap. 3.

Late infantile and juvenile type II sialidosis, galactosialidosis, and sialic acid storage disorders are described in Chap. 5.

The Carbohydrate-Deficient Glycoprotein Syndrome The carbohydrate-deficient glycoprotein (CDG) syndrome was described in 1984 by Jaeken and Van den Bergh. Approximately 70 patients with this disorder have been reported, mostly in the Scandinavian countries, but also in Belgium, Great Britain, and Japan.[88–90]

The CDG syndrome is characterized by the presence of abnormal, carbohydrate-deficient glyco-

proteins, particularly transferrin. (Transferrin is a glycoprotein with a polypeptide chain and carbohydrate chains terminating in sialic acid.) An abnormality in dolichol-linked oligosaccharide synthesis has been described.[91] The gene for this autosomal recessive multisystem disease has been linked to the short arm of chromosome 16.

Clinical Features The disease usually manifests itself during the first year of life by a marked delay in psychomotor development, hypotonia, feeding problems, and failure to thrive.

Ocular fixation is absent or poor. Nonparalytic strabismus is frequent. The deep tendon reflexes may be depressed. Unexplained episodes of stupor may occur, sometimes preceded by fever. Rhythmic head movements and respiratory difficulties have been reported. Very characteristic dermatologic findings are the presence of fat pads and areas of atrophic skin on the buttocks and arms, and inverted nipples, but they are not present in every patient. There is frequently some evidence of hepatic involvement (elevated serum transaminase and occasionally moderate hepatomegaly). Cardiac insufficiency with pericardial effusions have been reported.

While a few patients die in infancy, most survive and become able to stand, but usually they remain incapable of walking by the time they reach childhood and adolescence. There are atrophy and weakness of the lower limbs with evidence of either a peripheral neuropathy or lower motor neuron impairment (absent tendon reflexes and moderately low nerve conduction velocities); cerebellar ataxia; pigmentary degeneration of the retina; severe mental retardation (IQ 40 to 60) with no clear evidence of progressive intellectual deterioration and no behavioral problems. Growth is stunted and kyphoscoliosis and thoracic deformities develop. There may be a peculiar facies with a prominent nose and large ears. "Stroke-like" episodes are reported[92] but poorly described. Hypogonadism is evident when the patients reach adulthood.

On MRI, cerebellar atrophy is a striking finding, usually with atrophy of the pons. This has led some authors to consider CDS syndrome as a cause of *olivopontocerebellar atrophy*. This terminology may not be entirely justified (see Chap. 6).

Diagnostic Laboratory Tests
• A useful screening test is a measurement of the thyroxine-binding protein, which is significantly below normal.

• The critical diagnostic test rests on the demonstration by electrofocusing of an abnormal proportion of disialotransferrin and asialotransferrin, replacing the normal tetrasialotransferrin in serum and CSF.

• A decrease in sialic acid, galactose, and N-acetylglucosamine has also been shown in measurements of total serum glycoproteins and also of purified transferrin. Transferrin, α-1-antitrypsin and probably other glycoproteins consist of both normal and carbohydrate-deficient fractions. This suggests a defect in the incorporation of carbohydrate moieties in transferrin and other glycoprotein molecules. Current techniques, including analyses of the isoforms of transferrin, α-antitrypsin, and α_1-fetoprotein in chorionic villus biopsies and amniotic fluid, do not permit prenatal diagnosis of the carbohydrate-deficient glycoprotein syndrome.[93]

Concluding Remarks

In the mucopolysaccharidoses, mucolipidoses, and disorders of glycoprotein degradation, with very few exceptions, the common clinical denominator is a constellation of progressive nonneurologic changes which constitute the "Hurler phenotype": characteristic facial features, dysostosis multiplex, respiratory insufficiency and respiratory infections, cardiopathy, hepatosplenomegaly, deafness, and frequently corneal opacities. Involvement of the brain may be severe, moderate, or absent.

In some disorders in which mental retardation is present, the Hurler phenotype becomes evident in late infancy, progresses rapidly, dominates the clinical picture, and rapidly orients the neuropediatrician toward this category of disorders. This is particularly the case in Hurler disease, the severe form of Hunter disease, I-cell disease, some patients with sialidosis, fucosidosis, and α-mannosidosis. Marked craniofacial, skeletal, and visceral abnormalities are also prominent in MPS IV, MPS VI, MPS VII and mucolipidosis III, in which intelligence is normal or only moderately affected.

In the presence of a Hurler-like syndrome in a young child, some clinical differences may be distinctive: corneal opacities are lacking in the X-linked Hunter disease and there may be typical skin lesions; in I-cell disease there is a severe early-onset neurological deterioration, and the head is brachycephalic instead of being scaphocephalic as in Hurler disease; angiokeratoma may be a feature of fucosidosis.

In other diseases the facial and skeletal abnormalities are mild and may not be apparent in young children. They become progressively more obvious with age. Here, patients come to medical attention because of poor intellectual performances, language disorders; or mental deterioration, behavioral problems, such as aggressivity and hyperkinesia, seizures, and poor motor performance. This constellation of findings is peculiar to Sanfilippo disease, in which mental deterioration and behavioral problems are prominent, aspartylglucosaminuria, some cases of mannosidosis and fucosidosis.

These children may be mistakenly thought to have congenital nonprogressive mental retardation or a psychiatric disease of nonmetabolic origin, or a progressive encephalopathy of other cause, if sufficient attention is not given to subtle clinical clues, such as changes in facial appearance, thick hair and eyebrows, a tight skin, hirsutism, a slight lumbar kyphosis, progressive hearing loss, recurrent rhinitis and respiratory infections since infancy (which are rarely lacking), umbilical and inguinal hernias, moderate enlargement of liver or spleen, and vacuoles in leukocytes. Additional diagnostic help can be obtained by the demonstration of slight but characteristic and practically constant changes on x-ray films of the thoracolumbar spine, hips, and metacarpals, and in some disorders by the discovery of corneal opacities on slit-lamp examination.

Finally, in a few disorders in which neurologic signs are in the foreground, dysmorphic facial features and dysostosis multiplex are totally absent; this is the case of type I sialidosis, which gives rise to epilepsy, myoclonus, and macular cherry red spots (see Chap. 5); and of mucolipidosis IV, characterized by profound mental retardation and marked corneal opacities.

In any patient in which a suspicion of mucopolysaccharidosis or "mucolipidosis" is raised on clinical grounds, a number of biochemical tests will furnish the answer. As some of the young patients with these diseases lack all stigmata of Hurler syndrome, we believe that certain easily performed screening tests for these relatively frequent diseases should be systematically undertaken in all children with mental retardation or mental deterioration of uncertain origin.

As a first step, mucopolysaccharides and oligosaccharides should be sought in the urine and lysosomal enzymes (which are markedly elevated in I-cell disease and mucolipidosis III) looked for in the plasma. For the detection of oligosaccharides in the urine, thin-layer chromatography is widely available. Spot tests, which constitute quick and inexpensive methods for the preliminary evaluation of the mucopolysaccharides, may give false positive and false negative results (especially in MPS III).[67] Therefore, chromatography and the demonstration of the specific enzyme defects in leukocytes or cultured fibroblasts is needed to firmly establish the diagnosis. As for mucolipidosis IV, there are no specific biochemical abnormalities, and an ultrastructural study of skin or conjunctival biopsy is necessary for diagnosis.

Other neurological disorders may occur in the mucopolysaccharidoses irrespective of the presence of mental dysfunction. They are caused by thickening of the intracranial or intraspinal meninges or bony abnormalities in the spine and limbs, and some of them may necessitate urgent surgical intervention. Tension hydrocephalus is relatively common and may play a role in the mental impairment. In the more slowly evolving diseases, compression of the spinal cord, usually in its cervical segment, is not rare and may be particularly dramatic in Morquio disease, as a consequence of atrophy of the odontoid and atlantoaxial instability, and in Maroteaux-Lamy disease. Peripheral nerve entrapment and particularly the carpal tunnel syndrome are relatively common. Claw hands is an early and striking phenomenon in Scheie disease.

Bone marrow transplantations in the mucopolysaccharidoses and mucolipidoses have led to significant improvement of somatic abnormalities and of corneal deposits, but their effect on cerebral function is much less obvious (see Chap. 9).

PSYCHOMOTOR RETARDATION AND ARREST OF PSYCHIC FUNCTION

With reference to the conditions described in this chapter, it should be kept in mind that some diseases may not at first cause an actual regression but merely a delay in motor and/or intellectual development, or problems in behavior (this last point will be discussed in Chap. 5). Only by a succession of spaced neurologic examinations will neurologic deterioration eventually emerge.

This is true of some of the mucopolysaccharidoses, mucolipidoses, and disorders of glycoprotein degradation before obvious skeletal and visceral signs are present; some sphingolipidoses such as metachromatic leukodystrophy and G_{M1} gangliosidosis; neuroaxonal dystrophy; inherited disorders of amino acids and organoacids; transferase deficiency galactosemia; mitochondrial and peroxisomal disorders.

Where the clinical examination offers no clue, the diagnosis eventually rests on the result of a limited number of radiological, biological, neurophysiological, and histological tests, which we believe are justified in the diagnosis of apparently nonprogressive neurologic conditions of uncertain origin. (This problem will be taken up again in Chap. 5 and has been considered in the conclusion of Chap. 3.)

Our approach is summarized below:

When any one or a group of the following clinical signs are present, the possibility of an HMD should be considered

Nonneurologic signs

Subtle dysmorphic facial features (check siblings)

Kyphosis, diminished joint mobility, claw hands

Growth failure

Feeding difficulties, vomiting

Recurrent respiratory infections

Abnormalities of skin and hair

A cardiopathy

Mild enlargement of liver or spleen

Family history: evidence for a hereditary disorder and its type of transmission.

Neurologic signs

Pyramidal signs with no perinatal antecedent

Depressed tendon reflexes

Dystonia, choreoathetosis, ataxia, action myoclonus

Cataracts; retinal or macular degeneration; optic atrophy; disorders of oculomotricity

Hearing loss

A previous self-limiting episode of lethargy or ataxia

When any of these signs is present, and in any child with unexplained psychomotor retardation or behavioral abnormality of uncertain origin, we recommend the following laboratory investigations to detect a possible HMD

In all cases

Slit-lamp examination of cornea and lens

X-ray films of skeleton (spine, hips, hands)

Measurement of protein, lactic acid and glucose in the CSF

Search for inclusions in peripheral blood leukocytes

Chromatography of urine for amino acids, organic acids, mucopolysaccharides, oligosaccharides

GC/MS of plasma for very long chain fatty acids

Ultrasound scanning of heart, liver, spleen, and kidneys

Magnetic resonance imaging of brain

Karyotyping

According to clinical context

ERG

Nerve conduction velocities, somatosensory evoked potentials

Brain stem auditory evoked potential

GABA and organic acid measurement in CSF

Measurement of uric acid in urine

Measurement of adenylosuccinyl lyase in urine

Serum electrophoresis for transferrin isoforms

Bone marrow aspiration if facial dysmorphia, skeletal or visceral changes

Lysosomal enzymes determination; skin, muscle or nerve biopsies

REFERENCES

1. Wenger AD, Louie E: Pseudodeficiency of arylsulfatase A and galactocerebrosidase activities. *Dev Neurosci* 13: 216–221, 1991.
2. Francis GS, Bonni A, Shen N, et al.: Metachromatic leukodystrophy: multiple non-functional and pseudo-deficiency alleles in a pedigree. Problems with diagnosis and counselling. *Ann Neurol* 34: 212–218, 1993.
3. Kolodny EH, Fluharty AL: Metachromic leukodystrophy and multiple sulfatase deficiency, in Scriver CR, Beaudet AL, Sly WS, Valle D (eds): *The Metabolic and Molecular Bases of Inherited Disease.* New York, McGraw-Hill, 1995, pp. 2693–2739.
4. Vamos E, Liebaers I, Bousard N, et al.: Multiple sulphatase deficiency with early onset. *J Inherit Metab Dis* 4: 103–104, 1981.
5. Cowen D, Olmstead EV: Infantile neuroaxonal dystrophy. *J Neuropathol Exp Neurol* 22: 175–236, 1963.
6. Lyon G, See G: La dégénérescence neuro-axonale infantile (maladie de Seitelberger). Etude anatomique d'une observation. *Rev Neurol* 109: 133–155, 1963.
7. Seitelberger F, Gootz P, Gros H: Beitrag zur spatinfantilen Hallervorden-Spatzche, Krankheit. *Acta Neuropathol* 3: 16–28, 1963.
8. Seitelberger F: Eine unbekannte form von infantilen Lipoidspeicher krakheit des gehirns, in *Proceedings 1st International Congress on Neuropathology*, Rome, 1952, vol. 3, p. 323.
9. Rabinowicz T, Wildi E: Spastic amaurotic axonal idiocy, in Cumings JN (ed): *Cerebral Lipidoses.* Oxford, Blackwell, 1957, pp. 34–47.
10. Aicardi J, Castelein P: Infantile neuroaxonal dystrophy. *Brain* 102: 727–748, 1979.
11. Huttenlocher PR, Gilles FH: Infantile neuroaxonal dystrophy; clinical pathological and histochemical findings in a family with 3 affected siblings. *Neurology* 17: 1174–1184, 1967.
12. Hedley-Whyte ET, Floyd MB, Gilles H, Uzman BG: Infantile neuroaxonal dystrophy. A disease characterized by altered terminal axons and synaptic endings. *Neurology* 18: 891–906, 1968.
13. Indravasu S, Dexter RA: Infantile neuroaxonal dystrophy and its relationship to Hallervorden-Spatz disease. *Neurology* 18: 693–699, 1968.
14. Crome L, Weller SDV: Infantile neuroaxonal dystrophy. *Arch Dis Child* 40: 502–507, 1965.
15. Jellinger K: Neuroaxonale dystrophie. *Ver Dtsch Ges Pathol* 52: 92–126, 1968.
16. Kamoshita S, Neustein HB, Landing BH: Infantile neuroaxonal dystrophy with neonatal onset. *J Neuropathol Exp Neurol* 27: 300–323, 1968.
17. Toga P, Berard-Badier M, Gambarelli-Dubois D: La dystrophie neuroaxonale infantile ou maladie de Seitelberger. Etude clinique, histologique et ultrastructurale de deux observations. *Acta Neuropathol (Berl)* 15: 327–350, 1970.
18. Gonatas NK, Goldensohn ES: Unusual neocortical presynaptic terminals in a patient with convulsions, mental retardation and cortical blindness. An electron microscopic study. *J Neuropathol Exp Neurol* 24: 539–562, 1965.
19. Schindler D, Bishop DF, Wolfe DE, et al.: Neuroaxonal dystrophy due to lysosomal α-N-acetylgalactosaminidase deficiency. *New Engl J Med* 320: 1735–1740, 1989.
20. De Jong J, van den Berg C, Wijburg H, et al.: Alpha-N-acetylgalactosaminidase deficiency with mild clinical manifestations and difficult biochemical diagnosis. *J Pediatr* 125: 385–391, 1994.
21. O'Brioen JS, Ho MW, Veath ML, et al.: Juvenile G_{M1} gangliosidosis: clinical pathological, chemical and enzymatic studies. *Clin Genet* 3: 411–434, 1972.
22. Suzuki K: Neuropathology of late onset gangliosidoses. A review. *Dev Neurosci* 13: 205–210, 1991.

23. Purpura DP, Suzuki K: Distortion of neuronal geometry and formation of aberrant synapses in neuronal storage disease. *Brain Res* 116: 1–21, 1976.

24. Suzuki K: Cerebral G_{M1} gangliosidosis: chemical pathology of visceral organs. *Science* 159: 1471–1472, 1968.

25. Syllaba L, Henner K: Contribution à l'indépendance de l'athetose double idiopathique et congénitale. *Rev Neurol* 1: 541–562, 1926.

26. Louis Barr M: Sur un syndrome progressif comprenant des télangiectasies cutanées et conjonctivales symétriques à disposition naevoide et des troubles cérébelleux. *Confin Neurol* 4: 32–42, 1941.

27. Zee DS, Yee RD, Singer HS: Congenital ocular motor apraxia. *Brain* 100: 581–599, 1977.

28. Sedgwick RP, Boder E: Ataxia telangiectasia, in Vinken PJ, Bruyn GW (eds): *Handbook of Clinical Neurology, vol. 14: The Phakomatoses.* Amsterdam, North Holland, 1972, pp. 267–339.

29. Gatti RA, Good RA: Occurrence of malignancy in immunodeficiency diseases. *Cancer* 28: 89–98, 1971.

30. Gatti RA: Localizing the genes for ataxia-telangiectasia: a human model for inherited cancer susceptibility. *Adv Cancer Res* 56: 77–104, 1991.

31. Schuster J, Hart Z, Stimson CW, et al.: Ataxia telangiectasia with cerebellar tumor. *Pediatrics* 37: 776–781, 1966.

32. Swift M, Reitnauer P, Morell D, et al.: Breast and other cancers in families with ataxia-telangiectasia. *New Engl J Med* 316: 1289–1294, 1987.

33. Jaspers NG, Gatti RA, Boan C, et al.: Genetic complementation analysis of ataxia-telangiectasia and Nijmegen breakage syndrome in a survey of 50 patients. *Cytogen Cell Genet* 49: 259–263, 1988.

33a. Savitsky K, Bar-Shira A, Gilad S, et al.: A single ataxia telangiectasia gene with a product similar to PL-3 kinase. *Science* 268: 1749–1753, 1995.

34. Peterson RDA, Funkhouser JD: Speculations on ataxia-telangiectasia: defective regulation of the immunoglobulin gene superfamily. *Immunology Today* 10: 313–315, 1989.

35. Carbonari M, Cherchi M, Paganelli R, et al.: Relative increase of T-cells expressing the gamma/delta rather than the alpha/beta receptors in ataxia telangiectasia. *New Engl J Med* 332: 73–76, 1990.

36. Aicardi J, Barbosa C, Anderman E, et al.: Ataxia-oculomotor apraxia: a syndrome mimicking ataxia telangiectasia. *Ann Neurol* 24: 497–502, 1988.

37. Hagberg B, Hansson O, Liden S, et al.: Familial ataxic diplegia with deficient cellular immunity. A new clinical entity. *Acta Paediatr Scand* 59: 545–550, 1970.

38. Graham-Pole J, Ferguson A, Gibson AAM, et al.: Familial dysequilibrium-diplegia with T lymphocyte deficiency. *Arch Dis Child* 50: 927–933, 1975.

39. Duy R, Stephenson JBP, Gibson B, et al.: Neurology of purine nucleoside phosphorylase deficiency. Paper presented at the meeting of the European Federation of Child Neurology Societies, Paris, Feb 1991.

39a. Abadir R, Hakami N: Ataxia-telangiectasia with cancer: an indication for reduced radiotherapy and chemotherapy doses. *Br J Radiol* 56: 343–345, 1983.

40. Rider AJ, Dawson G, Siakotos AN: Perspective of biochemical research in the neuronal ceroid-lipofuscinosis. *Am J Med Genet* 42: 519–524, 1992.

41. Dyken PR: Reconsideration of the classification of the neuronal ceroid lipofuscinoses. *Am J Med Genet Suppl* 5: 69–84, 1988.

42. Wisniewski KE, Kida E, Paxtot OF, et al.: Variability in the clinical and pathological findings in the neuronal lipofuscinoses. *Am J Med Genet* 42: 525–532, 1992.

43. Santavuori P: Neuronal ceroid lipofuscinosis in childhood. *Brain Dev* 10: 80–83, 1988.

44. Boustany RM, Abroy J, Kolodny EN: Clinical classification of neuronal ceroid-lipofuscinosis subtypes. *Am J Med Genet Suppl* 5: 47–58, 1988.

45. Goebel HH: Neuronal ceroid-lipofuscinoses: the current status. *Brain Dev* 14: 203–211, 1992.

46. Williams R, Vesa J, Jarvela I, et al.: Genetic heterogeneity in neuronal ceroid lipofuscinosis. *Am J Hum Genet* 53: 931–935, 1993.

47. Kominami E, Ezaki J, Muno D, et al.: Specific storage of subunit c of mitochondrial ATP synthase in lysosomes of neuronal ceroid lipofusinosis (Batten's disease). *J Biochem* 111: 278–282, 1992.

48. Wisniewski KE, Golabek AA, Kida E.: Increased urine concentration of subunit c of mitochondrial ATP synthase in neuronal ceroid lipofusccinoses patients. *J Inherit Metab Dis* 17: 205–210, 1994.

49. Santavuori P, Haltia M, Rapola J: Infantile so-called neuronal ceroid-lipofuscinosis. *Dev Med Child Neurol* 16: 644–653, 1974.

50. Santavuori P, Raininko R, Vanhanen SL, et al.: MRI of the brain, EEG sleep spindles and SPECT in the early diagnosis of infantile ceroid lipofuscinosis. *Dev Med Child Neurol* 34: 61–65, 1992.

51. Vesa J, Hellsten E, Makela TP, et al.: A single PCR marker in strong allelic association with the infantile form of neuronal ceroid lipofuscinosis facilitates reliable prenatal diagnostics and disease carrier identification. *Eur J Hum Genet* 1: 125–132, 1993.

52. Santavuori P, Rapola J, Nuutila A: The spectrum of Jansky-Bielschowsky disease. *Neuropediatrics* 22: 92–96, 1991.

53. Savukoski M, Kestila M, Williams R, et al.: Defined chromosomal assignment of *CLN5* demonstrates that at least four genetic loci are involved in the pathogenesis of human ceroid lipofuscinoses. *Am J Hum Genet* 55: 695–701, 1994.

54. Aicardi J: *Diseases of the Nervous System.* New York, Cambridge University Press, 1992, p. 402.

55. Sly WS: The mucopolysaccharidoses, in Bondy PD, Rosenberg LE (eds): *Metabolic Control and Disease.* Saunders, Philadelphia, 1980, p. 545.

56. Spranger J: The systemic mucopolysaccharidoses. *Ergeb Inn Med Kinderheilkd* 32: 165–178, 1972.

57. Neufeld EF: Lessons from genetic disorders of lysosomes. *Harvey Lect* 75: 41–60, 1981.

58. McKusick VA: The genetic mucopolysaccharidoses. *Medicine* 44: 445–470, 1965.

59. Taylor HA, Thomas GH: Pseudodeficiency of α-L-iduronidase. *J Inherit Metab Dis* 16: 1058–1059, 1993.

60. Scott HS, Guo XH, Hopwood JJ, et al.: Structure and sequence of the human alpha-L-iduronidase gene. *Genomics* 13: 1311–1313, 1992.

61. Bach G, Moskowitz SM, Tieu PT, et al.: Molecular analysis of Hurler syndrome in Druze and Muslim Arab patients in Israel: multiple allelic mutations of the *IDUA* gene in a small geographic area. *Am J Hum Genet* 53: 330–338, 1993.

62. Bunge S, Steglich C, Kleijer WJ: Mucopolysaccharidosis type I. Identification of 93% of mutant alleles in a group of 70 patients. *Am J Hum Genet* 55: A214, 1994.

63. Hopwood JJ, Vellodi A, Scott HS, et al.: Long-term clinical progress in bone marrow transplanted mucopolysaccharidosis type I patients with a defined genotype. *J Inherit Metab Dis* 16: 1024–1033, 1993.

64. Adinolfi M: Hunter syndrome: cloning of the gene, mutations and carrier detection. *Dev Med and Child Neurol* 35: 79–85, 1993.

65. Whitley CB, Jonsson JJ, Aronovich EL: Automated direct sequencing of the iduronate-2-sulfatase gene reveals a vast spectrum of mutations causing Hunter syndrome (mucopolysaccharidosis type II) and a "hot spot" at R468. *Am J Genet* 55: A249, 1994.

66. Yamada Y, Tomatsu S, Sukegawa K, et al.: Mucopolysaccharidosis type II (Hunter disease): 13 gene mutations in 52 Japanese patients and carrier detection in four families. *Hum Genet* 92(2): 110–114, 1993.

67. Neufeld EF, Muenzer J: The mucopolysaccharidoses, in Scriver CR, Beaudet AL, Sly WS, Valle D (eds): *The Metabolic and Molecular Bases of Inherited Disease*. New York, McGraw-Hill, 1995, pp. 2465–2494.

68. Vellodi A, Young E, New M, et al.: Bone marrow transplantation for San Filippo disease type B. *J Inherit Metab Dis* 15: 911–918, 1992.

69. Van Hoof F, Hers HG: The abnormalities of lysosomal enzymes in mucopolysaccharidoses. *Eur J Biochem* 7: 34–44, 1968.

70. Spranger JW, Wiedemann HR: The genetic mucolipidoses. Diagnosis and differential diagnosis. *Human Genetik* 9: 113–139, 1970.

71. Hickman S, Neufeld EF: Hypothesis for I cell disease: defective hydrolases that do not enter lysosomes. *Biochem Biophys Res Commun* 49: 992–999, 1972.

72. Leroy JG, De Mars RI: Mutant enzymatic and cytological phenotype in cultured human fibroblasts. *Science* 157: 804–806, 1967.

73. Leroy JG, Spranger JW, Feingold M, et al.: I-cell disease. A new clinical picture. *J Pediatr* 79: 360–365, 1971.

74. Parvathy MR, Mitchell D, Ben-Yoseph Y: Prenatal diagnosis of I-cell disease in the first and second trimester. *Am J Med Sci* 297: 361–364, 1989.

75. Kurobane I, Aikawa J, et al.: Bone marrow transplantation in I-cell disease, in Hobbs JR (ed): *Correction of Certain Genetic Diseases by Transplantation*. London, Cogent, 1989, p. 132.

76. Evrard P: Personal communication, 1993.

77. Amir N, Zlotogora J, Bach G: Mucopolipidosis type IV. Clinical spectrum and natural history. *Pediatrics* 79: 953–959, 1987.

78. Johnson WG: Disorders of glycoprotein degradation, in Rosenberg RN, Prusiner SB, Di Mauro S, Barchi RL, Kunkel LM (eds): *The Molecular and Genetic Basis of Neurological Disease*. Boston, Butterworth-Heinemann, 1993, pp. 421–435.

79. Levade T, Graber D, Flurin V, et al.: Human β-mannosidase deficiency associated with peripheral neuropathy. *Ann Neurol* 35: 116–119, 1994.

80. Durand P, Borrone C, Della Cella G: Fucosidosis. *J Pediatr* 75: 665–674, 1971.

81. Van Hoof F, Hers HG: Mucopolysaccharidosis by absence of alpha-fucosidase. *Lancet* 1: 1198, 1968.

82. Willems PJ, Gatti R, Darby JK, et al.: Fucosidosis revisited: a review of 77 patients. *Am J Med Genet* 38: 111–131, 1991.

83. Willems PJ, Garcia CA, De Smedt MC, et al.: Intrafamilial variability in fucosidosis. *Clin Genet* 34: 7–14, 1988.

84. Taylor RM, Farrow BR, Stewart GJ: Amelioration of clinical disease following bone marrow transplantation in fucosidase-deficient dogs. *Am J Med Genet* 42: 628–632, 1992.

85. Occhiodoro T, Hopwood JJ, Morris CP, et al.: Correction of alpha-L-fucosidase deficiency in fucosidosis fibroblasts by retroviral vector-mediated gene transfer. *Hum Gene Ther* 3: 365–369, 1992.

86. Hietala M, Gron K, Syvanen AC, et al.: Prospects of carrier screening of aspartylglucosaminuria in Finland. *Eur J Hum Genet* 1: 296–300, 1993.

87. Voznyi YV, Keulemans JLM, Kleijer WJ, et al.: Applications of a new fluorimetric enzyme assay for the diagnosis of aspartylglucosaminuria. *J Inherit Metab Dis* 16: 929–934, 1993.

88. Jaeken J, Stibler H, Hagberg B: The carbohydrate deficient glycoprotein syndrome: a new inherited multisystemic disease with severe nervous system involvement. *Acta Pediatr Scand Suppl* 375, 1991.

89. Kristiansson B, Anderson M, Tonnby B, et al.: Disialo transferrine developmental deficiency syndrome. *Arch Dis Child* 64: 71–76, 1989.

90. Jaeken J, Van Eijk HG, Van der Heul C, et al.: Sialic acid deficient serum and cerebrospinal fluid transferrine in a newly recognized genetic disease. *Clin Chim Acta* 144: 245–247, 1989.

91. Krasnewich D, Brantly M, Skovby F, et al.: Cases of carbohydrate-deficient glycoprotein syndrome due to abnormal synthesis of dolicho-linked oligosaccharides. *Am J Hum Genet* 55 (suppl): A174, 1994.

92. Hagberg BA, Blennow G, Kristiansson B, et al.: Carbohydrate-deficient glycoprotein syndromes: peculiar group of new disorders. *Pediatr Neurol* 9(4): 255–262, 1993.

93. Stibler H, Skovby F: Failure to diagnose carbohydrate-deficient glycoprotein syndrome prenatally. *Pediatr Neurol* 11: 71–74, 1994.

Chapter 5

CHILDHOOD AND ADOLESCENT HEREDITARY METABOLIC DISORDERS

GENERAL FEATURES

COMMON CLINICAL SYNDROMES

PROGRESSIVE SPASTIC PARAPLEGIAS

PREDOMINANTLY PROGRESSIVE CEREBELLAR ATAXIAS

HMDs PRESENTING WITH ACTION MYOCLONUS, SEIZURES, AND ATAXIA

HEREDITARY, PREDOMINANTLY EXTRAPYRAMIDAL DISORDERS OF LATE CHILDHOOD AND ADOLESCENCE

FAMILIAL POLYNEUROPATHIES IN JUVENILE METABOLIC DISEASE

PROGRESSIVE VISUAL LOSS AS AN INITIAL MANIFESTATION IN JUVENILE HEREDITARY METABOLIC DISORDERS

FAMILIAL METABOLIC ENCEPHALOPATHIES WITH CLINICAL EVIDENCE OF DIFFUSE CNS DISORDER
    Disorders with a Mendelian Mode of Inheritance
    Diseases with a Maternal Mode of Inheritance: Defects
      in Mitochondrial DNA

PROGRESSIVE METABOLIC AND DEGENERATIVE DISEASES WITH SPECIAL NEUROLOGIC AND SOMATIC (ESSENTIALLY CUTANEOUS) FEATURES

PROGRESSIVE GENETIC ENCEPHALOPATHIES LEADING TO STROKE

METABOLIC DISORDERS WITH INTERMITTENT NEUROLOGIC SIGNS

FAMILIAL ENCEPHALOPATHIES IN WHICH PERSONALITY CHANGES, BEHAVIORIAL DISTURBANCES, AND DEMENTIA MAY BE A PRESENTING SIGN

ISOLATED DELAY IN MENTAL AND MOTOR DEVELOPMENT

GENERAL FEATURES

In this age period, which extends from the third or fourth year through adolescence (usually taken as 13 to 18 years), the patient has presumably been normal until the appearance of neurologic symptomatology. More explicitly, there has usually been no obvious impairment of motor skills; language has been acquired at the usual times; and perception, imagination, and intellectual development have apparently been flawless. As a consequence, the patient has been able to acquire a sizable store of memories and knowledge of the world. This allows a large repertoire of nervous functions to become accessible to the neurologist for the assessment of a disease process. Also, this makes possible the more accurate timing of some derangements of the central or peripheral nervous system.

The time course, i.e., temporal profile, of a genetic biochemical disorder of this age period tends to span months and years, far longer than that of an earlier age period. Furthermore, the lesions tend to be more restricted to certain systems of neurons, such as the corticospinal tracts, motor nerve cells of the spinal cord, optic nerves or retina, cerebellum, basal ganglia, or peripheral nerves. Symptoms referable to any one of these structures may stand in relative isolation before a more typical syndrome gradually emerges. Seizures alone may be the initial manifestation. In some diseases, a general impairment of mental function, scholastic failure or an alteration of behavior may indicate the onset of the disorder.

Early neurologic development may have been slow in some children, and for several years the essential criteria of hereditary metabolic disease, namely, progressivity of a disorder of nervous function, may be called into question. Sometimes there are difficulties in determining whether the patient had been altogether normal in the past, especially if the family is unreliable and unobservant. Slight awkwardness or intellectual slowness may have been ignored or attributed to a birth injury, increasing demands of the classroom, learning disability or a developmental language disorder.

Faced with such diagnostic difficulties, the clinician is helped by the discovery of subtle clinical markers—ocular signs, skeletal changes, abnormal facial features—and by radiologic, hematologic, neurophysiologic, or biochemical findings.

A troublesome feature of several of the neurometabolic disorders of this age period is the diversity of expression of any given disease entity. It does not always segregate according to a single phenotypic pattern. The clinical expressions may be as varied as action myoclonus, a Friedreich phenotype, a polyneuropathy, visual failure, or mental deterioration. The reasons for such differences are still poorly understood. The type of mutation, the degree of residual enzymatic activity, the existence of tissue-specific enzymes, and the percentage of mutant to normal genes in different tissues possibly account for some of the diversity of pathologic and clinical expression.

The mode of inheritance of the diseases is diverse. In addition to autosomal recessive, X-linked, and maternal modes of transmission, autosomal dominant disorders are more frequently encountered. Each requires a different plan of family counseling and preventive measures.

In some of the genetic diseases presented below, the biochemical abnormality has not been determined. In current parlance they are called *degenerative diseases*. We have included these here because they pursue a generally progressive course like the known neurometabolic diseases and they have a tendency to

select certain systems of neurons. For most of them, the mutant gene has now been characterized, but its protein product has not been discovered or its action is not fully understood. A definitive diagnosis in these cases relies on DNA studies of affected patients and families.

Any one of the HMDs described here may begin in childhood, preadolescence, or adolescence without there being important symptomatic differences. This variability in the age of onset of a disease may even be found within a single family. It is for this reason that we have brought them together within this one chapter.

COMMON CLINICAL SYNDROMES

Here will be described the neurometabolic diseases that cause manifest derangements of particular parts of the nervous system. Despite the aforementioned diversity of phenotypic expression, most of the diseases have a favored anatomical localization and most nervous structures are susceptible to the effects of some disease processes and not to others. Other organs may be variously affected.

As was stated earlier, this is the basis of our syndromic approach in later epochs of life. Each syndrome serves, therefore, as a standard guideline for the neuropediatrician. Already it was remarked that, although one syndrome for a given disease predominates, there is usually some degree of overlap with other syndromes. The authors have found it useful to group the diseases of this age period into the following syndromes:

A progressive spastic paraplegia (possibly associated with electrophysiologic evidence of a peripheral neuropathy).

Cerebellar ataxia, when associated with other signs of nervous system dysfunction (particularly myoclonus, dystonia, or proprioceptive sensory defects).

Action myoclonus (polymyoclonus).

An extrapyramidal syndrome.

A progressive peripheral neuropathy or motor neuron disease.

A multisystem cerebrospinal syndrome.

Cognitive impairment and behavioral change.

Facial and skeletal dysmorphism with mental and neurologic signs.

Episodic confusion and coma; episodic ataxia.

Successive stroke-like episodes.

Progressive hearing loss.

Progressive visual failure and ophthalmologic abnormalities.

For the convenience of the reader, clinical findings and laboratory tests are presented in Tables 5-1 to 5-5, which appear on pages 180 to 184.

PROGRESSIVE SPASTIC PARAPLEGIAS

In many metabolic disorders of childhood or adolescence, a progressive spastic paraplegia related to bilateral lesions of the pyramidal tracts is one of several signs which may herald the onset of a neurometabolic disease. In *adrenomyeloneuropathy*, a metabolic disorder with demyelination, and in *Strümpell-Lorrain disease*, a neurodegenerative disorder with selective involvement of the pyramidal tracts, a slowly progressive spastic paraplegia is the initial and major neurologic manifestation.

Many other juvenile HMDs may present at first as a spastic paraplegia, including the following:

- X-linked spastic paraplegia with PLP deficiency
- Metachromatic leukodystrophy
- Krabbe leukodystrophy
- The cerebral form of X-linked adrenoleukodystrophy
- Sjögren-Larsson syndrome
- Arginase deficiency
- Hallervorden-Spatz disease

In some of these conditions the bilateral pyramidal syndrome is associated with a peripheral neuropathy.

Sometimes the etiologic diagnosis of an isolated slowly progressive paraplegia is very difficult. A fixed diplegia of pre- or perinatal origin, a spinal tumor, a rare type of familial spastic paraplegia or, in tropical countries, an infection of HTLV-1 virus will come under consideration.

Laboratory investigations useful for the differential diagnosis of a progressive paraplegia or any paraplegia of obscure origin are indicated in Table 5-1.

All the listed disorders are described in other sections of this chapter, except for Strümpell-Lorrain familial spastic paraplegia, other forms of familial spastic paraplegia, and the Sjögren-Larsson syndrome, which will be presented here. Arginase deficiency, a rare dis-

order, will also be included. The semiology and differential diagnosis of all spastic, genetic, and nongenetic paraplegias are described in Chap. 6.

Familial Spastic Paraplegia, Strümpell-Lorrain Type Strümpell-Lorrain familial spastic paraplegia (FSP) is characterized by a slowly progressive paraplegia which remains an isolated clinical manifestation, at least, for many years. Its anatomical basis is a degeneration of the pyramidal tracts and variable involvement of the posterior columns of the spinal cord. It represents a type of systemic neuronal degeneration akin to spinocerebellar degeneration. Its pathogenesis is unknown. It is transmitted generally as a dominant trait, but in some families the mode of inheritance is autosomal recessive. The disease is not uncommon with 104 cases reported in one series in 1977[1] and 32 and 70 patients respectively in two recent reports.[2,3]

Onset of the disease may be at any time from the age of 5 years to the seventh decade. Recessive forms tend to occur earlier. There is a spastic paraplegia with exaggerated tendon reflexes and bilateral Babinski signs. Involvement of the upper limbs usually occurs later in the disease and remains less severe, but the patients are often clumsy. After several years, there may be mild impairment of deep sensation, especially vibration, and slight cerebellar signs. Sphincter disturbances, i.e., urinary urgency and frequency, may occur late in the disease. In some cases we have observed evidence of lower motor affection of the legs; other patients have muscle pain in the lower extremities. Pigmentary degeneration of the retina is not uncommon. Intelligence is normal. Nerve conduction velocities and CSF protein are normal. The initial complaint may be of walking difficulty and frequent falls; there is a tendency to walk on tiptoes. Frequently, however, the clinical symptomatology is quite mild, and the diagnosis is made by the fortuitous discovery of a bipyramidal syndrome in a child with minor complaints, or in a parent or sibling of an affected child. Of the 41 patients reported by Behan and Maia, only seven had sought medical advice.[4]

The course of the usual, dominant, form of the disease is very slow, and many patients retain the ability to walk until late adulthood. Abrupt and transient periods of deterioration may occur. We have observed this in five such patients. Recessive forms of the disease usually have a more severe course. There is no other biological abnormality.

Genetics Inheritance of true Strümpell-Lorrain type of FSP is generally autosomal dominant (Fig. 5-1).

(text continued on page 185)

Table 5-1

Main juvenile hereditary and degenerative disorders presenting with a progressive spastic paraplegia (bipyramidal syndromes)[a]

Important data for diagnosis		Main diseases with other clinical characteristics	
Clinical	Laboratory		
Clinical and electrophysiological evidence of a peripheral neuropathy Ophthalmologic examination Other neurologic signs, mental and motor Family history Rate of progression	MRI NCV, SSEP, ERG CSF protein Plasma VLCFA Sulfatides in urine Sural nerve biopsy Enzymologic and DNA studies	Adrenomyeloneuropathy[b] (X-linked)	Very slow progression; evidence of peripheral neuropathy ($\pm$); cerebral demyelination ($\pm$); VLCFA $\uparrow$ in plasma; female carriers may be symptomatic
		Strümpell-Lorrain familial spastic paraplegia (AR, AD)	Isolated spastic paraplegia; urinary tract dysfunction $\pm$; slow progression; usually no mental retardation; PDR
		Complicated forms of familial spastic paraplegia (FSP)	FSP with additional signs; including X-linked FSP with PLP deficiency and Sjögren-Larsson disease
		Metachromatic leukodystrophy (AR)	Cognitive and behavioral changes; clinical and neurophysiologic evidence of neuropathy; CSF protein $\uparrow$; periventricular cerebral demyelination; sulfatiduria; typical inclusions in Schwann cells
		Juvenile Krabbe leukodystrophy (AR)	Optic atrophy or central blindness ($\pm$); evidence of neuropathy ($\pm$); ataxia; periventricular cerebral demyelination; typical inclusions in Schwann cells ($\pm$)
		Other lysosomal diseases (AR)	Paraplegia rapidly associated with various neurologic, ocular, dysmorphic, and hematologic abnormalities

Abbreviations and symbols: NCV = nerve conduction velocities; PDR = pigmentary degeneration of retina; VLCFA = very long chain fatty acids; FSP = familial spastic paraplegia; PLP = proteolipid protein; AR = autosomal recessive; AD = autosomal dominant; SSEP = somatosensory evoked potentials; ERG = electroretinogram; $\uparrow$ = elevated; ($\pm$) = inconstant.

[a] Two other rare disorders are Sjögren-Larsson syndrome and arginase deficiency.

[b] The cerebral form of X-linked adrenoleukodystrophy may also start with a paraplegia.

Table 5-2

Main juvenile HMDs presenting with progressive cerebellar ataxia (see also Table 6-3 and Chap. 4)

Important data for diagnosis		Main diseases with other clinical characteristics[a]	
Clinical	*Laboratory*		
Presence or not of areflexia, proprioceptive sensory deficit, myoclonus, seizures, extrapyramidal motor abnormalities	Evaluation of cardiac function NCV, EMG CSF protein and lactate	Friedreich ataxia (AR)	Cerebellar and proprioceptive ataxia; tendon areflexia; pyramidal signs; distal amyotrophy ($\pm$); cardiomyopathy; sensory NCV $\downarrow$
Eyes: oculomotricity, conjunctiva, eyegrounds Cardiomyopathy Visceral abnormalities Family history	Serum cholesterol, lipoproteins, vitamin E Acanthocytes MRI Enzyme assays and DNA studies	Disorders with the Friedreich phenotype (maternal or AR mode of transmission)	MERRF (defects of mtDNA): myoclonus, seizures; lactate $\uparrow$ in CSF; RRF. Abetalipoproteinemia: celiac syndrome; pigmentary degeneration of retina; acanthocytosis AVED: primary vit.E deficiency Late-onset G_{M2} gangliosidosis: lower motor neuron disorder
		Other early-onset spinocerebellar degenerations (AD or AR)	Pyramidal signs; DTR not depressed; no proprioceptive deficit; no cardiopathy
		Late-onset sphingolipidoses (AR)	Including G_{M1}, Krabbe leukodystrophy, type C Niemann-Pick disorder, metachromatic leukodystrophy

Abbreviations and symbols: NCV = nerve conduction velocities; EMG = electromyogram; AVED = ataxia with vitamin E deficiency; AR = autosomal recessive; mtDNA = mitochondrial DNA; AD = autosomal dominant; $\uparrow$ = elevated; $\downarrow$ = decreased; ($\pm$) = inconstant.

[a] All disorders with polymyoclonus may also have cerebellar ataxia.

Table 5-3

Main juvenile HMDs presenting with progressive polymyoclonus and seizures (± ataxia) (see also Table 5-6)

Important data for diagnosis		Main diseases with other clinical characteristics	
Clinical	*Laboratory*		
Age of onset	EEG	MERRF (maternal inheritance)	Juvenile onset; mixed cerebellar and proprioceptive ataxia; mental retardation; short stature; deafness; lactate ↑ in CSF (and blood); muscle weakness; muscle RRF
Rate of progression	ERG		
Vision, oculomotricity	Auditory evoked		
Eyegrounds	potentials		
Hearing	MRI		
Presence of cerebellar ataxia	Lactic acid in CSF		
and/or proprioceptive sensory	Hematology	Lafora disease (AR)	Juvenile onset; visual hallucinations (±); rapid mental and motor deterioration; OA; skin biopsy reveals inclusions in sweat glands
deficit	Thin-layer		
Seizures	chromatography for		
	oligosaccharides in		
	urine		
	Skin biopsy, muscle	Unverricht hereditary myoclonus	Usually no mental deterioration; slow course; seizures may be rare
	biopsy	epilepsy (AR)	
	Enzymatic and		
	DNA studies	Sialidosis type I (AR)	Cherry red spot; no visceral abnormality; sialyloligosaccharides in urine; vacuolated lymphocytes
		Neuronal ceroid lipofuscinosis type 2[a] (AR)	Onset at 2 to 4 years; rapid deterioration; pigmentary degeneration of retina; skin biopsy: inclusions in cells
		Late-onset sphingolipidoses (AR)	Various neurologic, ophthalmological, and visual abnormalities

Abbreviations and symbols: ERG = electroretinogram; MERRF = myoclonus epilepsy and ragged red fibers; RRF = ragged red fibers; OA = optic atrophy; AR = autosomal recessive; ↑ = elevated.

[a] Polymyoclonus occurs but is less prominent in the other neuronal ceroid lipofuscinoses.

Table 5-4

Main juvenile HMDs presenting as extrapyramidal diseases (rigidity, athetosis, chorea, dystonia)[a]

Important data for diagnosis		
Clinical	Laboratory	Main diseases with other clinical characteristics
Age of onset Search for associated neurologic, mental or visceral abnormality Dysarthria or not Mental deficit or not Oculomotor abnormalities Examination of cornea, retina Progression of disease Examination of parents In some cases, therapeutic test with dopa	Slit-lamp examination of cornea and lens Hematology: search for acanthocytes MRI ERG Cupruria and ceruloplasmin levels GC/MS for organic acids in urine Evaluation of immunoglobulins Skin biopsy DNA and enzymatic studies	**Wilson disease (AR)** — Neurologic onset after age 8 years; psychic disturbances; dysarthria; mental regression; faciobuccopharyngeal and generalized rigidity; intention tremor; corneal ring; liver disease; abnormal copper metabolism **Huntington disease (AD)** — Psychiatric disturbances, dementia; rigidity, dysarthria; rarely chorea; seizures; atrophy of caudate (CT scan); one parent (father) possibly with "parkinsonism" or "psychoses" **Hallervorden-Spatz disease (AR)** — Dystonia or other extrapyramidal signs; pigmentary degeneration of retina (±); MRI reveals typical changes in globus pallidus **Dystonia muscularis deformans (primary idiopathic torsion dystonia) (AD)** — Clinical diagnosis; unilateral onset (leg); mentation and speech normal; myoclonic jerks (±) **Other primary familial dystonias (AR, AD)** — Clinical diagnosis; family history; persistent or intermittent; response to dopa in one variety **Glutaric aciduria I (AR)** — Early-onset dystonia or choreoathetosis; episodic comas; basal ganglia lesions on MRI; typical organic aciduria with GC/MS **Sulfite oxidase deficiency (AR)** — Early-onset; dislocation of lens; typical metabolites in urine **Familial striatal necrosis** — MRI; possibly with Leber disease **Chorea-acanthocytosis (AR)** — Acanthocytosis **Nonprogressive familial chorea (AD)** — Clinical diagnosis; family tree **Nonprogressive familial athetosis (AD)** — Clinical diagnosis; family tree **Some cases of ataxia-telangiectasia (AR)** — Choreoathetosis; cerebellar signs; typical ocular signs; typical immunologic abnormalities

Table 5-4 (contd.)
Main juvenile HMDs presenting as extrapyramidal diseases (rigidity, athetosis, chorea, dystonia)[a,b]

Important data for diagnosis		
Clinical	Laboratory	Main diseases with other clinical characteristics
	Juvenile lipofuscinosis (AR)	Retinal degeneration; seizures; vacuoles in lymphocytes; inclusions in skin cells

Abbreviations and symbols: ERG = electroretinogram; GC/MS = gas chromatography/mass spectrometry; AR = autosomal recessive; AD = autosomal dominant; (±) = inconstant.

[a,b]In several of these diseases (including Huntington disease) the mutant gene has been cloned.

Table 5-5
Juvenile HMDs presenting as having mental retardation and motor delay, behavioral abnormalities, or intellectual regression[a]

Search for these clinical clues	Perform these laboratory investigations
Mild facial dysmorphic features	Slit-lamp examination of cornea and lens; examination of retina
Progressive dysarthria;	X-rays of skull, spine, hips, and hands
Slight, recent motor impairment	Ultrasound of heart, kidney, liver, and spleen
Visual failure	MRI of brain
Disorder of oculomotricity	Search for vacuolated lymphocytes (and storage cells in bone marrow)
Corneal opacities	
Retinal or macular degeneration; optic atrophy	Evaluation of protein, lactate, and glucose in CSF (also GABA and other amino acids)
Hearing loss	
Hepatomegaly-splenomegaly; cardiac or renal dysfunction	Evaluation of NCV and EMG if areflexia; brain stem auditory potentials
Kyphoscoliosis	
Skin changes	Screening for mucopolysaccharides (MPS) in urine
	Thin-layer chromatography for oligosaccharides, MPS in urine
	GC/MS for organic acids in urine and VLCFA in plasma
	If necessary, ultrastructural examination of conjunctiva or skin biopsy, and fibroblast culture for definitive biochemical studies
	Enzymatic and DNA studies

Abbreviations: VLCFA = very long chain fatty acids; NCV = nerve conduction velocities; EMG = electromyogram.

[a]Disorders with this symptomatology are cited later in this chapter and in Chapter 4.

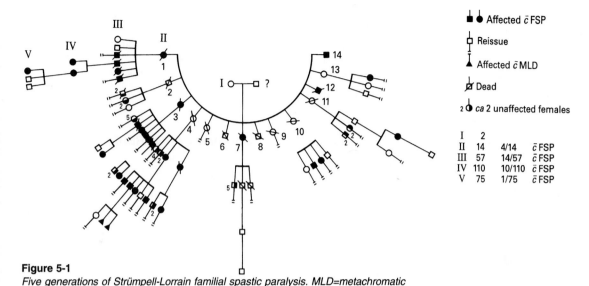

I	2		
II	14	4/14	c̄ FSP
III	57	14/57	c̄ FSP
IV	110	10/110	c̄ FSP
V	75	1/75	c̄ FSP

Figure 5-1
Five generations of Strümpell-Lorrain familial spastic paralysis. MLD=metachromatic leukodystrophy.

It has been linked to chromosome 2p,[5,6] 14q, and 15q.[7] The autosomal recessive form is associated with a chromosome 8 locus.

An *X-linked form* often combined with cerebellar ataxia has been mapped to Xq22 in the region of *the gene locus for proteolipid protein*. Point mutations in this gene have been identified.[8,9] The same gene is defective in some cases of Pelizaeus-Merzbacher disease (PMD) suggesting that X-linked spastic paraplegia and PMD are related allelic disorders.

Diagnosis   Differential diagnosis of FSP may be difficult with a spastic diplegia of pre- or perinatal origin; other metabolic disorders with paraplegia; a tumor of the spinal cord; and some rare cryptogenetic familial disorders with spastic paraplegia (see below).

In one of our patients who had *hyperornithinemia with gyrate atrophy of the retina*, the initial diagnosis was Strümpell-Lorrain disease because of failure in urinary screening of amino acids, and a complete ophthalmologic examination had not been done. It should also be kept in mind that a chronic paraplegia may result from an infection with HTLV-1 which may affect several members in a family.[14]

Other Types of Familial Spastic Paraplegias; Complicated Forms of FSP   In addition to the pure,

isolated form of familial spastic paraplegia, i.e., the true Strümpell-Lorrain disease, a number of familial conditions have been reported in which a very slowly spastic paresis is the main but not the only sign. The list of them is long and their exact classification sometimes uncertain. They are called *complicated forms of FSP*. The associated findings include some degree of ataxia, retinal degeneration, optic atrophy, amyotrophy, sensory neuropathy, ichthyosis, and mental retardation. An autosomal recessive form of hereditary sensory neuropathy has also been associated with spastic paraplegia. There is an axonopathy affecting both myelinated and unmyelinated axons, often leading to a mutilating lower limb acropathy.[10]

In another autosomal recessive condition, the *Kjellin syndrome*, there is mild to moderate mental retardation from birth. Progressive spastic paraplegia develops around age 20 and is associated with neurogenic atrophy, dysarthria and central retinal degeneration.

The Sjögren-Larsson Disease   The Sjögren-Larsson form of spastic paraplegia[11–13] is another complicated form. Here there is a congenital ichthyosis resembling alligator skin. Other features are distal amyotrophy, macular degeneration, and mental retardation. Many patients have glistening white dots in the retina, speech disturbances, seizures, kyphosis, and short stature. A severe leukodystrophy is evident on MR scans. This has been confirmed in neuropathological studies which demonstrate loss of myelinated axons in the central cerebral white matter, corticospinal tracts, and vestibulospinal tracts. Loss of neurons in the cortex and basal ganglia have also been described.

Long-chain fatty alcohols accumulate in plasma due to a deficiency of fatty alcohol:NAD$^+$ oxidoreductase activity. The activity of this enzyme can be assayed in leukocytes and cultured skin fibroblasts.[11] Its level in heterozygotes is intermediate between that found in homozygotes and normal control subjects. Prenatal diagnosis can be achieved by enzymatic studies on chorionic villi or fetal skin biopsies. This autosomal recessive disorder is most prevalent in northern Sweden. The gene believed to be responsible for it has been mapped to chromosome 17 (17p11.2).[13]

Progressive spastic paraparesis also occurs in some of the *spinocerebellar degenerations.*

Arginase Deficiency Arginase deficiency is a rare disorder of urea cycle synthesis. Its symptomatology is very different from the disorders resulting from deficiencies of the other enzymes of the urea cycle which have a neonatal onset (Chap. 2) or advance intermittently (Chap. 3). Only one case of arginase deficiency with a neonatal onset has been reported.

The major symptoms in arginase deficiency consist of a progressive spastic paraplegia, intellectual deterioration, hyperactivity, and growth failure. Choreoathetosis had been added in one child. Vomiting, delayed development, irritability and seizures[15] have apparently been observed in the first year of life in most children. Episodes of hyperammonemia leading to coma may occur.

Laboratory Findings There is mild hyperammonemia, marked hyperargininemia (as high as 1500 μM), high urinary levels of diaminoacids (arginine, lysine, cystine, and ornithine) and orotic aciduria. Urinary excretion of citrulline and glutamine are also increased. The CSF contains very high levels of arginine.

Genetics The gene for arginase has been mapped to band q23 of chromosome 6. A variety of nonsense mutations, microdeletions, and missense mutations for this autosomal recessive disease that reduce arginase activity have been reported.[16]

Treatment Restriction of dietary protein and artificial diets devoid of arginine have been recommended. The mechanism of brain lesions and the exact role of hyperargininemia have not been elucidated.

PREDOMINANTLY PROGRESSIVE CEREBELLAR ATAXIAS

General Remarks

In childhood or adolescence there is a unique category of diseases in which involvement of the nervous system is more or less limited to groups of neurons and selected tracts in the cerebellum and spinal cord. The clinical effect is mainly a progressive incoordination of movements. The prototype of these familial spinocerebellar diseases is *Friedreich ataxia*, in which motor incoordination is of both cerebellar and sensory type. Its cause is genetic but little is known of its pathogenesis. Other types of autosomal recessive spinocerebellar ataxias have also been described in childhood and adolescence. The Friedreich phenotype, i.e., a sensory and cerebellar (tabetocerebellar) ataxia with similar spinocerebellar lesions, is also found in a limited number of known metabolic disorders, such as abetalipoproteinemia, hypobetalipoproteinemia, and AVED, also to be described here. Juvenile G_{M2} gangliosidosis and myoclonic epilepsy and ragged red fibers (MERRF), which may also display clinical and pathological features resembling those of Friedreich ataxia, are presented in another section of this chapter.

In addition to the spinocerebellar degenerations, progressive ataxia may also be an important feature of a number of late childhood or adolescent metabolic encephalopathies in which there is a more diffuse involvement of the nervous system (Tables 5-2 and 6-3). Characteristically, *the ataxia seldom exists for a long time in relatively pure form.* Such signs as spastic weakness, extrapyramidal disorders, abnormalities of oculomotor function, seizures, myoclonus, and dementia soon follow.

Also, some of the infants and young children in whom a seemingly more diffuse disorder of the nervous system had occurred survive into adolescene with cerebellar ataxia as a prominent feature.

Other types of spinocerebellar or cerebellar degeneration of childhood are apparently not related to a metabolic disorder. They include the autosomal dominant spinocerebellar ataxias (SCA I to V) and the auto-somal dominant cerebellar ataxias (ADCA I and II).

There is also a group of pure cerebellar ataxias of genetic origin with a tendency to appear in early life, to progress little or not at all, and to be accompanied by mental retardation and speech defects. They are usually inherited as an autosomal recessive trait. Their anatomical basis is a severe cerebellar atrophy with predominant loss of granule cells. These congenital nonprogressive cerebellar atrophies (or hypoplasia) are described in Chap. 6.

The distinction between cerebellar ataxia and some peripheral nerve diseases in which proprioceptive defects account for the incoordination may be somewhat difficult. Cerebellar incoordination and action myoclonus may also be difficult to distinguish, and they may be conjoined.

Friedreich Ataxia   Friedreich ataxia (FA) is an autosomal recessive inherited spinocerebellar disease, starting before the age of 20, consisting of a sensory and cerebellar ataxia with areflexia, Babinski signs, pes cavus, scoliosis, and cardiomyopathy. Diagnosis is based on clinical findings. There are no definite biochemical abnormalities, although recent evidence suggests a disorder of pyruvate metabolism. The gene mutation for the disorder has been mapped to chromosome 9 (9q13).

Clinical Features   Described in 1861 by Friedreich of Heidelberg,[17] who took pains to separate it from syphilitic locomotor ataxia, i.e., tabes dorsalis, it was from the beginning recognized as a hereditary disease. The onset usually occurs before the age of 20 years, and in half of the patients reported from the Salpetrière by Mollaret, it occurred before the age of 10 years and sometimes as early as 2 years.[18] These figures have since been confirmed. Harding[19] finds a mean age of onset at 10.5 ± 7.4 years. Once begun, the disease advances steadily to the point where walking becomes impossible, usually within 5 to 10 years. Median survival time from onset in one series was reported as 34.7 years with a 30-year survival rate of 75 percent for females and 48 percent for males. Death is ordinarily from cardiac involvement.[20]

Ataxia of gait is nearly always the first symptom, but it may be misidentified by the patient as weakness and fatigue. Clumsiness of the hands follows within a few months or years but incoordination of the upper limbs usually remains moderate. Dysarthria is always present and in some instances an early symptom.

Incoordination of the oropharyngeal and respiratory muscles accounts for slow, sometimes staccato and explosive speech. Pes cavus and kyphoscoliosis develop in most patients.

When the disorder is fully developed, careful analysis of the ataxia discloses both a sensory and a cerebellar component (i.e., it is cerebellotabetic, to use the term of Charcot). In any given case, either may predominate but it usually tends to be the cerebellar component. The ataxia is static in the sense that it is evinced most clearly when the patient is sitting or standing; it presents as tottering and swaying of the body and a rhythmic nodding of the head. In walking, the patient reels, tries to correct imbalance by a wide stance, throws the legs forward abruptly and haphazardly, and may lurch to either side or actually fall. The arms are held out at the sides to help with balance. When a sensory defect has become an important factor, there is an obvious dependence on vision and the Romberg sign is present. Also, instability of posture of outstretched fingers and hands (pseudoathetosis), appearing when the eyes are closed, betrays the defect in proprioception. Finger-nose and heel-knee tests evoke asynergia and dysmetria as well as intention tremor; and rapid alternating movements are irregularly slowed (dysdiadochokinesia).

The tendon reflexes are absent in all four limbs. But since this is the result of a gradual process, their retention is not an entirely valid reason for excluding the diagnosis early in the course of the disease. Recently, three families with FA have been reported, in which some affected members had preserved tendon reflexes.[21] The plantar reflexes are extensor. Position and vibratory senses are typically reduced, especially in the legs, although this may not be evident in the earliest stages. Tactile loss may occur but there is retention of pain, temperature, and pressure sensation. Some patients complain of paresthesias and cramps. Distal weakness and atrophy of the lower limbs are observed at some stage in more than half of the patients.[19] A coarse horizontal nystagmus is noted in one-third of the cases. A defect of voluntary gaze with delay and slowness of saccades is frequently found as well as overshoot dysmetria. Myoclonus and a variety of dyskinesias may be noted in some patients. Cheyne-Stokes respiration has been reported. Optic atrophy (with a normal ERG) has been recorded in approximately 20 percent of the cases. Color vision may be impaired. Deafness is rare. Blindness, retinal changes, and deafness occur much less frequently than in other, essentially dominant, forms of spinocerebellar degenerations. The mental faculties are spared.

A cardiopathy (hypertrophic obstructive cardiomyopathy) is demonstrable in the great majority of cases of Friedreich ataxia and can be said to constitute a major hazard in this disease. Its expression is variable and nonspecific. A systolic murmur, usually the result of subaortic stenosis, tachyarrhythmias with atrial fibrillation, angina pectoris, cardiomegaly, a variety of ECG changes (T-wave changes and abnormalities of the ST segment), and changes in the vectocardiogram are found. Abnormalities of the ECG may exist in the absence of clinical signs of cardiac disorder. The cardiomyopathy evolves toward heart failure or severe dysrhythmias and may give rise to pulmonary or cerebral embolism. These cardiac complications terminate life. In a few cases, signs of heart disease occurred so early that the patient's initial medical contact was with a cardiologist or internist.

An abnormal glucose tolerance test or insulin-dependent diabetes mellitus (in 10 to 25 percent of cases) is another noteworthy feature of FA. Diabetes is either type I or type II.[22] During the preclinical phase of diabetes, a transient excessive secretion of insulin has been recorded. Some patients have died in diabetic coma.

Diagnostic Paraclinical Tests   There is no specific laboratory marker. Electrophysiologic studies have disclosed a slight decrease in sensory nerve conduction velocities. Sensory evoked potentials are of diminished voltage or delayed in practically all patients. The possibility of a disturbance of pyruvate metabolism has been postulated. An abnormal elevation in blood pyruvate in response to an oral glucose load has been observed in some cases. The possibility of a deficiency in the activity of the enzymes, pyruvate dehydrogenase, lipoamide dehydrogenase, or mitochondrial malic enzyme, has been raised. Plasma levels of vitamin E are normal. There is no acanthocytosis. On MRI there may be a mild atrophy of the cerebellum and a thinness of the spinal cord.

Genetics   FA is the most common type of autosomal recessive ataxia. Linkage analyses have localized the gene for the disease to the region q13 of chromosome 9. The gene frequency has been estimated at approximately 1/110 persons in England,[19] and the incidence of the disease at 1/10,000 in Sweden. Although there is clinical heterogeneity in FA, no evidence of genetic heterogeneity has been found. In Acadian families with FA

in which the course of the disease has been much slower, genetic analysis has shown that the mutation is at the same locus. The availability of DNA markers linked to the mutant gene offers the possibility of prenatal diagnosis of the disease. Currently there is no means of identifying heterozygotes.

Pathologic Findings   In the nervous system there is a loss of large sensory ganglion cells in the dorsal root ganglia, of medullated fibers in the posterior columns, and of large myelinated fibers in peripheral sensory nerves, as well as a loss of cells of the Clarke column, a degeneration of the spinocerebellar tracts, and a degeneration of the anterior and lateral corticospinal tracts and Betz cells in the precentral gyrus. Loss of neurons and medullated fibers has also been found in the nucleus and fasciculus solitarius, in the dorsal motor nucleus and root of the vagus, and in glossopharyngeal, vestibular, and hypoglossal nuclei. Loss of anterior horn cells is slight and variable from case to case. Purkinje cells are moderately diminished in number, particularly in the anterior lobes and superior vermis. There is also neuron loss in the dentate nuclei. Rarely are the central tegmental tracts and medial longitudinal fasciculi depleted of fibers.

In the enlarged heart, in addition to various changes and fibrosis in the myocardium, narrowing of the coronary arteries and degeneration of the cardiac nerves and ganglia have been observed, as well as focal lesions of the sinus node.

Physiopathology and Clinicopathologic Correlations   The basic process seems to be a selective degeneration of neurons, essentially in the posterior root ganglia and the spinal cord, as well as Betz cells in the motor cortex and other neurons in the brain stem and cerebellum. The neuronopathy begins within the distal part of the axons, a "dying-back neuropathy," affecting also the long ascending and descending tracts of the spinal cord. The pathogenesis is unknown. The tabetic aspects of the ataxic state correlate with the degeneration of dorsal root ganglia; the cerebellar aspects correlate with degeneration of the spinocerebellar tracts and cerebellar lesions; the pyramidal signs are a manifestation of the degenerated pyramidal tracts; and the reflexes are abolished because of the interruption of the spinal reflex arcs, a consequence of the loss of proprioceptive fibers. The kyphoscoliosis and pes cavus have not been adequately explained.

Diagnosis   Diagnosis of FA is based essentially on the following clinical criteria: age of onset between 3 and 20 years, a tabetocerebellar ataxia, generalized absence of tendon reflexes and Babinski signs, a cardiomyopathy, and an autosomal recessive mode of transmission. The full clinical constellation may take some time to evolve, requiring at various stages differentiation from other early-onset spinocerebellar degenerations (see below). In some patients with FA there is a marked and early distal amyotrophy of the lower limbs, similar to that seen in the hereditary sensorimotor polyneuropathies of the Charcot-Marie-Tooth type, where a tremor may also be present. A historical illustration of these difficulties is to be found in the discussions of the Roussy-Levy syndrome. As described by these authors, this syndrome is characterized by a tabetic type of ataxia in conjunction with proprioceptive sensory loss, areflexia, moderate weakness and distal atrophy of the limbs, pes cavus, and tremor. There is no cerebellar ataxia, dysarthria, pyramidal tract signs, nystagmus, or cardiopathy—the familiar characteristics of FA. The discovery after many years of a hypertrophic neuropathy with onion-bulb formation in one of the original patients of Roussy and Levy[23] resolved the problem: the Roussy-Levy syndrome is in fact a familial polyneuropathy, possibly in combination with a familial tremor.

The presence of myoclonus in rare cases of typical Friedreich ataxia may raise the problem of the definition and limits of Ramsay Hunt syndrome (see below).

Finally, a tabetocerebellar ataxia (the Friedreich phenotype) may be found in a number of metabolic disorders (such as MERRF, abetalipoproteinemia, or late-onset sphingolipidoses). Vitamin E deficiency is the cause of the phenotype resembling Friedreich ataxia in abetalipoproteinemia and in ataxia with vitamin E deficiency (AVED).

Treatment   Only symptomatic treatment is available.

Early-Onset Autosomal Recessive Spinocerebellar Ataxias other than Friedreich Ataxia   Not all autosomal recessively inherited spinocerebellar ataxias starting in childhood or adolescence correspond to the clinical picture of Friedreich ataxia (FA). The distinction in individual cases may be difficult to make on purely clinical grounds, especially early in the disease. The recent availability of a DNA marker linked to the gene of FA on chromosome 9, and linkage studies in non-Friedreich early-onset spinocerebellar degenerations should help in solving this problem.

Early-Onset Cerebellar Ataxia with Retained Tendon Reflexes   In 1981 Harding[24] attracted attention to a type of early-onset spinocerebellar ataxia (EOCA) that differed from Friedreich ataxia. This condition, inherited as an autosomal recessive trait, has a mean age of onset of approximately 10 years of age with a range of 18 months to 20 years. Cerebellar ataxia predominating in the lower limbs and dysarthria are the first and most prominent signs. Tendon reflexes are preserved or frequently exaggerated (with the possible exception of the ankle jerks). There are bilateral Babinski signs. The proprioceptive component of ataxia is mostly lacking (except late in the disease in some cases) and the joint position and vibratory senses are usually retained. There may be moderate distal muscular wasting. Optic atrophy is absent, deafness is rare, scoliosis is infrequent, and there is no evidence of cardiac involvement or diabetes. Intelligence is preserved. Brain stem auditory evoked responses are abnormal in nearly all patients. Sensory action potentials may be reduced but are not absent. Based on electrophysiologic and histologic studies, these patients have been divided into two groups, those with and those without neuropathy.[25] Brain scans are normal or show moderate cerebellar atrophy. The main differences between this disorder and FA are the absence of a cardiomyopathy and diabetes, the preservation of tendon reflexes (although they may exist in a few instances of genetically linked cases of Friedreich ataxia with a typical cardiomyopathy),[25a] the usual absence of a tabetic type of ataxia, lack of kyphoscoliosis, and a slower course. Patients become incapable of walking about 10 years later than in FA. There has been no linkage analysis, and we are unaware of any pathological studies. As the results of neurophysiological studies and the morphological findings of sural neural biopsy in these patients are not uniform, it is likely that EOCA is genetically heterogeneous. In further support of this concept, one of us has observed two siblings with EOCA and a pigmentary retinal degeneration. The determination of the mutant gene will certainly provide an essential diagnostic tool and insight in the nosology of this variety of spinocerebellar degeneration.

Previous reports of non-Friedreich early-onset spinocerebellar degenerations are scarce and their significance uncertain. They differ from the cases described above by the frequency of blindness and mental retardation or dementia. They have been published under the name of Marie hereditary cerebellar ataxia or Familial spastic ataxia. They are briefly discussed below.

Marie Hereditary Cerebellar Ataxia: Cases of Fraser, Nonne, and Sanger Brown; Familial Spastic Ataxia of Childhood

The patients reported by Fraser and Nonne (which were included in Marie hereditary cerebellar ataxia[26]), the family reported by Sanger Brown[26], as well as the patients reported as familial spastic ataxia,[27] were all characterized by cerebellar ataxia, dysarthria, pyramidal signs, and lack of sensory ataxia. There was no evidence of a cardiomyopathy and there was no scoliosis. Choreiform and grimacing movements were observed in some. The disease frequently started in childhood and had a slow progressive course. Optic atrophy, retinal degeneration and mental retardation occurred frequently. Autosomal recessive inheritance was probable in some families, others had an autosomal dominant mode of transmission; the mode of inheritance was uncertain in others. The presence in many patients of optic atrophy, retinal degeneration, mental retardation and dementia seems to differentiate these cases from those reported by Harding. The relationship between familial spastic ataxia and the Strümpell-Lorrain type of familial spastic paraplegia is not always clear.

The postmortem findings provide the basis for a subdivision of the cases into three groups[26]: (1) olivopontocerebellar atrophy (Menzel type); (2) cortical cerebello-olivary atrophy (Holmes type); (3) dentatorubral atrophy (Hunt type). Neuron loss in each of the designated systems and glial replacement are usually the only pathologic changes.

Autosomal Dominant Progressive Cerebellar Ataxia with Retinal Degeneration and Ophthalmoplegia (Types I and II)

An autosomal dominant form of progressive cerebellar ataxia (ADCA) with pyramidal tract signs and defects in vision and oculomotricity has also been reported in adults and occasionally in children.[27a,27b] There is a gradually progressive visual failure associated with pigmentary retinopathy (ADCA type II) as well as supranuclear ophthalmoplegia and marked slowing of saccadic eye movements. Patients who inherit this disorder from their father are more likely to develop the severe infantile form. Thus, there is both anticipation and genetic imprinting, two of the phenomena common to diseases of unstable trinucleotide repeat expansion. It is therefore likely that this will prove to be the underlying genetic mechanism for autosomal dominant cerebellar ataxia with pigmentary macular dystrophy.

Autosomal Dominant Spinocerebellar Ataxia

Autosomal dominant spinocerebellar ataxia (SCA) types 1, 2, 3, 4, and 5 are essentially adult diseases. Pyramidal, extrapyramidal, ocular, and peripheral nerve abnormalities are associated with cerebellar signs. As a result of linkage analysis, the chromosomal location of most SCA (and ADCA) is known. Type 3 SCA has apparently the same clinical profile and expanded CAG repeats as in Machado-Joseph syndrome.[27c] It is also evident that the association, ataxia, pyramidal signs, and mental deterioration may occur in a number of hereditary metabolic disorders listed in Table 6-3.

Abetalipoproteinemia (Bassen-Kornzweig Disease)

Abetalipoproteinemia is a rare autosomal recessive disorder characterized by an absence of very low density lipoproteins (VLDLs) and low density lipoproteins (LDLs) (β-lipoproteins). A celiac syndrome in infancy is followed by a neurologic disorder bearing resemblance to Friedreich ataxia. Retinitis pigmentosa and acanthocytosis are included in this syndrome. Levels of plasma cholesterol and triglycerides are low. Neurological and retinal manifestations are most probably the consequence of a deficiency in vitamin E. The primary abnormality seems to be a defect in the ability of the liver and intestines to assemble or secrete apo B-containing lipoproteins. This has been shown to be due to a lack of activity of a microsomal triglyceride transfer protein (MTP). Mutations in the MTP gene result in defective loading of apo-B with lipids.

Clinical Features Since the first description by Bassen and Kornzweig in 1950,[28] fewer than 100 cases of this condition had been reported up to 1989. The first clinical manifestations are those related to fat malabsorption: steatorrhea, bulky stools, abdominal distention, and vomiting, which are present in early infancy and tend to subside after a few years. Weight gain is slow and growth is delayed. In some children, the first neurologic sign has been depressed tendon reflexes; this has been observed as early as the second year of life. Usually between the ages of 5 and 10 years, but sometimes later, unsteadiness of gait, incoordination, and dysarthria become manifest. Areflexia, proprioceptive sensory disturbances, cerebellar signs, and possibly Babinski signs constitute the usual syndrome. Distal weakness and amyotrophy and evidence of a peripheral neuropathy with distal hypoesthesia are detected in most cases. Supranuclear vertical ophthalmoplegia can occur. Paralysis of the oculomotor muscles with ptosis, facial weakness, and amyotrophy of the tongue have been reported. A myopathy with presence of ceroid pigments in muscle fibers has also been observed. Pes cavus and kyphoscoliosis are present in most cases. The CSF is normal. The locomotor difficulties and deformation of the spine progress slowly so that most patients are unable to stand unaided by the time they have reached late adolescence or adulthood. Intelligence is usually normal but mental retardation has been described in some.

Abnormal pigmentation of the retina, macular or peripheral, appears at various stages of the disease, but visual failure is usually not evident before adolescence. By then, night blindness, constriction of the visual fields, and pigmentary degeneration of the retinas are evident. Lenticular opacities have been reported. The ERG may be extinct despite normal funduscopic appearance.

Acanthocytosis is a constant and apparently early finding. It is best seen in preparations of fresh blood suspended in Dacie's solution or, if necessary, under the scanning microscope. The red blood cells are spiky or thorny and a few have a characteristic long tentacle. Low sedimentation rates and lack of rouleaux formation are other important hematologic changes. Cardiac enlargement, arrhythmia, and ECG abnormalities are commonly found making the disease even more similar to Friedreich ataxia.

The duration of life is variable: some patients die in childhood, while others may live until the third or fourth decade. Cardiac failure or arrhythmia may have been the cause of death in some patients.

Diagnostic Laboratory Tests The crucial biochemical abnormalities for the diagnosis of abetalipoproteinemia include low plasma cholesterol and triglycerides, lack of VLDLs and LDLs in the plasma, absence of chylomicrons and low serum levels of fat soluble vitamins A, E, and K. Biopsy specimens of the jejunal mucosa show normal villi and numerous fat droplets (that are not in the Golgi apparatus) in mucosal cells.[29]

Electrophysiological studies may show a reduction of conduction velocities in the sural nerve and evidence of muscle denervation atrophy. Somatosensory evoked potentials are practically always reduced.

Pathologic Findings The lesions in various organs have to be judged from very few autopsies. In one case they consisted of loss of myelinated fibers in the posterior columns and spinocerebellar tracts, loss of neurons

in the cerebellar hemispheres (both Purkinje cells and granule cells), and loss of anterior horn cells in the spinal cord. In another case there was loss of myelinated fibers in the posterior columns and in the spinocerebellar and corticospinal tracts. Large quantities of lipofuscin were found in cortical neurons. The cerebellum was normal. The number of large myelinated fibers was reduced in the sural nerve.

In biopsies of jejunal mucosa, the villi retain their normal morphology, but the mucosa is filled with lipid droplets containing mostly triglycerides. In one patient there was fiber loss, fibrosis, and an excess of lipochrome in the myocardium, similar to that seen in tocopherol deficiency.

Pathogenesis and Physiopathology There are defects of one or more proteins involved in the processing of B apolipoproteins through the secretory pathway for VLDLs and chylomicrons. The primary defect does not apparently lie within the apo B gene itself, but is related to posttranslational events involving lipidation of apo B.

As a consequence of the deficiency of B apolipoprotein, chylomicrons are not formed and lipids are not transported from the intestinal cells to the lymphatic system. Fat malabsorption results in a deficiency of vitamin E, which is the cause of the neurological, ophthalmological, muscular, and cardiac abnormalities of the disease. The decrease in vitamin E absorption could result in the peroxidation of unsaturated myelin phospholipids.

Differential Diagnosis The resemblance to Friedreich disease may be striking, including the cardiopathy. Some cases hitherto reported as Friedreich disease with pigmentary degeneration of the retina may have been examples of abetalipoproteinemia.

Other neurological syndromes with acanthocytosis include hypoabetalipoproteinemia and choreaacanthocytosis. Choreoamyotrophy and acanthocytosis,[30] and other rare conditions are listed in Table 7-7. There are other causes of chronic vitamin E deficiency that may lead to a neurological disorder mimicking Friedreich ataxia, namely, familial isolated vitamin E deficiency (AVED), hypobetalipoproteinemia, and prolonged cholestasis from congenital biliary artesia.[31]

Treatment A supplement of high doses of vitamin E in the diet (1000 to 2000 mg/day in infants, 5000 to 10,000 mg/day in older children and adults) has a remarkable effect on the development or progression of the neurological and ocular symptoms. A supplementation in vitamin A (2500 IU daily or every other day) and vitamin K is also recommended. Care must be taken to avoid vitamin A toxicity (by measurement of plasma levels of vitamin A). The gastrointestinal symptoms respond to restriction of triglycerides containing long-chain fatty acids. However, because of possible side effects, this treatment should only be used temporarily or in case of severe malabsorption.

Hypobetalipoproteinemia Hypobetalipoproteinemia is a very rare disorder distinct from abetalipoproteinemia. It is caused by mutations in the apolipoprotein B (apo B) gene in most cases.[32] Defects often affect the rate of synthesis or the rate of removal of apo B. In the homozygous state there are usually neurological, ocular, muscular, digestive, and hematologic manifestations, which are indistinguishable from those of abetalipoproteinemia. There are generally no detectable apo B-containing lipoproteins and chylomicrons are deficient. Unlike abetalipoproteinemia, levels of cholesterol and triglycerides are low in heterozygotes. Acanthocytosis, a retinopathy, areflexia, and ataxia occur in some heterozygotes.

Familial Isolated Vitamin E Deficiency with the Neurological Phenotype of Friedreich Ataxia: Ataxia with Vitamin E Deficiency (AVED) Since first described by Burck et al. in 1981,[33] at least 20 patients have been reported with this autosomal recessive condition. It is distinct from Friedreich's disease and from abetalipoproteinemia. Many were brought to light by Ben Hamida et al. from Tunisia.[34] They emphasize the need to measure plasma concentrations of vitamin E in patients with progressive ataxia.

Onset of the disease is in the first or second decade, and its neurologic features are usually indistinguishable from those of Friedreich ataxia: progressive cerebellar ataxia,[38] proprioceptive sensory loss, tendon areflexia, Babinski signs, dysarthria, scoliosis and pes cavus. Neurophysiologic tests reveal a sensory axonal neuropathy.[35] There may be a cardiopathy.

There is no evidence of fat absorption and lipoproteins are normal. Serum levels of a tocopherol are very low. The locus has been mapped to chromosome 8q[36,37] (whereas the locus for Friedreich ataxia is on 9q13.1). The AVED gene codes for an α-tocopherol transfer protein which selects and incorporates α-tocopherol in the VLDLs. It has been suggested that there may be a defective hepatic tocopherol-binding protein underlying this disease.[37]

Supplementation with vitamin E (5 to 10 mg/kg/day) raises plasma concentrations, but clinical results are still uncertain and have to be further investigated.

L-2-Hydroxyglutaric Acidemia An L-2-hydroxyglutaric acidemia (2 OH glu) has been described in more than 20 patients and is probably an autosomal recessive inherited disorder. Onset has been between the ages of 6 and 10 years (30 years in one patient). The disease is characterized by progressive cerebellar ataxia, dysarthria, and moderate to severe mental deterioration. Epileptic seizures occur and there have been mild dystonic or pyramidal signs in some patients as well as stunting of growth and macrocephaly.

MRI characteristically shows cerebellar atrophy, lesions in the subcortical white matter, and abnormal signals in the dentate nuclei and putamens.

Diagnosis rests on the demonstration of high levels of 2 OH glu in the urine and the CSF. The concentrations of lysine in plasma and CSF are also increased. The disease has a protracted course extending well into adolescence or adulthood. A defect in L-2-hydroxyglutaric acid dehydrogenase found in human liver may be the cause.[39]

HMDs PRESENTING WITH ACTION MYOCLONUS, SEIZURES, AND ATAXIA

The Progressive Myoclonic Epilepsies

Polymyoclonus (action myoclonus) is defined here as multiple arrhythmic, asymmetric, asynchronous, involuntary twitches and jerks of various parts of the body caused by the rapid contraction of a single muscle or group of muscles. It is characteristically induced or exaggerated by voluntary movements and proprioceptive stimuli. Unlike chorea, the twitch lasts but a fraction of a second. Polymyoclonia represents a cardinal neurologic sign in several hereditary disorders, some of them of metabolic origin. It is generally associated with seizures of varying types and intensity, with cerebellar ataxia, and sometimes with dementia. In late childhood or adolescence the main diseases with polymyoclonus are the following: (1) progressive familial myoclonus epilepsy of Unverricht-Lundborg, also called Baltic myoclonus, (2) Lafora disease, (3) myoclonus epilepsy with ragged red fibers (MERRF), and (4) late-onset metabolic or "degenerative" diseases, mostly of lysosomal type (e.g., juvenile type I sialidosis).

Table 5-6
Polymyoclonus (action myoclonus) in the hereditary metabolic encephalopathies; seizures and/or cerebellar ataxia are often conjoined

Disease		Notable neurologic signs besides ataxia and seizures
MERRF	+ + +	Proprioceptive sensory deficit; muscle weakness
Unverricht-Lundborg familial myoclonus epilepsy	+ + +	Frequently normal intelligence
Lafora disease	+ + +	Dementia; rapid deterioration; visual hallucinations
Ramsay Hunt syndrome		See text
Sialidosis type I	+ + +	CRS
Sialidosis type II	+ +	CRS (dysmorphia)
Lipofuscinoses, essentially NCL II	+ +	Pigmentary degeneration of retina
Chronic, later-onset G_{M2} gangliosidosis	+ +	Lower motor neuron involvement
Gaucher III disease	+ +	Supranuclear ophthalmoplegia
Dentatorubropallidoluysian atrophy	+ +	Extrapyramdial signs
Primary idiopathic dystonias	+ +	Dystonia
Alpers syndrome	+ +	Rapid brain atrophy; liver disease
Juvenile Farber disease	+	
Juvenile neuroaxonal dystrophy	+	
Schindler disease	+	
Huntington chorea	+	Extrapyramidal syndrome
Ataxia-telangiectasia	+	Disorder of conjugate gaze
Friedreich disease	+	
Benign essential familial myoclonus	+ +	

Abbreviations and symbols: CRS = Macular cherry red spot; + + + = polymyoclonus a constant sign; + + = frequent (between 25 and 50 percent); + = rare or occurring in a rare disease.

In these four main groups of disorders (Table 5-3) the clinical picture is very similar: myoclonus, the denominating sign, is usually associated with epilepsy and/or with cerebellar ataxia. Cerebellar ataxia may be difficult to distinguish from polymyoclonus. The metabolic and neurodegenerative disorders of all ages with myoclonus are listed in Table 5-6. The pathologic anat-omy of polymyoclonus in all these conditions remains uncertain. A relation to lesions in the dentate nuclei and cerebellar cortex seems probable, but in most of the diseases other subcortical structures are also involved. Mention will also be made in this chapter of a benign form of essential familial myoclonus. The differential diagnosis of polymyoclonus will be discussed in Chap. 6.

Unverricht-Lundborg Progressive Familial Myoclonic Epilepsy; Baltic Myoclonus; Degenerative Type of Progressive Familial Myoclonic Epilepsy (Ramsay Hunt Syndrome) In this type of progressive familial myoclonic epilepsy (PME) the neuropathologic lesions consist of a nonspecific type of degeneration of various groups of neurons in the cerebellum, brain stem, and subcortical structures of the brain. No evidence of a metabolic disturbance has as yet been obtained. The disorder is inherited as an autosomal recessive trait. The gene has been localized on the distal part of chromosome 21 (band q22.3).[40] Genetic heterogeneity of the disease cannot be excluded.

At the turn of the century, Unverricht[41] and his student Lundborg[42] were the first to draw attention to a familial form of a progressive encephalopathy of which the main signs were disabling myoclonus and generalized seizures. They presented no pathologic data. Their names are frequently attached to the disorder, even though they did not determine its nature. A large group was subsequently reported from Finland, and the term Baltic myoclonus was later applied. Finally, it was suggested that the syndrome earlier described by Ramsay Hunt might represent the same disease,[43] although there is no pathological evidence to support this opinion.

Clinical Features The Unverricht-Lundborg syndrome occurs worldwide but is particularly frequent in Finland and Estonia, where its incidence is estimated at 1/20,000.[44,45] More than 100 cases have been reported from these countries. A significant number of patients have also been found in the western Mediterranean countries (43 cases in the series of Roger).[46] The onset is in childhood or adolescence (from 6 to 16 years) and begins with generalized seizures, often of the myoclonic type. Absences and drop attacks may be observed. Seizures are more frequent in the morning, on awakening, when massive myoclonic jerks may be most disturbing. Within a few months it becomes apparent that what may have earlier been regarded as a case of idopathic epilepsy is far more serious, for many of the actions of the patient now are marred by irregular arrhythmic myoclonic jerks. This polymyoclonic activity is made worse by voluntary movements, maintenance of posture, and proprioceptive stimuli such as passive mobilization of the limb or even elicitation of tendon reflexes. They are also enhanced by excitement. Intensification and spread of myoclonus can lead to a generalized myoclonic seizure with loss of consciousness. The myoclonus eventually involves the entire musculature, even the

movements required for speech, giving a kind of jerky dysarthria and unpredictable dysphagia.

A more or less marked cerebellar ataxia may appear but is sometimes difficult to distinguish from intention myoclonus. Pyramidal signs may occur later in the disease. Depressed tendon reflexes, wasting of distal musculature, and signs of chronic denervation on the EMG may be seen. Scoliosis is noted in some cases, and there may be evidence of autonomic involvement. There are no ocular abnormalities. Intelligence is relatively well preserved, though in time most patients will exhibit mild mental deterioration. The EEG reveals various degrees of slowing of the background activity with superimposed paroxysmal bursts. Some patients have a background activity that remains normal for several years.[46] Spikes may appear at the vortex during REM sleep. Giant somesthetic evoked potentials are usual.

There are no diagnostic biochemical tests, but membrane-bound vacuoles have been detected in the sweat glands of some patients.[47] The recent finding of DNA markers linked to the defective gene on the distal part of chromosome 21 (21q22.3) both in patients from Finland and the Mediterranean areas[48] will certainly be of considerable help in the identification of this disorder.

The course of the disease is marked by more or less rapid progression, and the severity of the polymyoclonus increases. The frequency of epileptic seizures is usually relatively low and they are fairly well controlled by treatment. On the contrary the action myoclonus progresses relentlessly and after a few years becomes incapacitating. Death occurs in the third or fourth decade.

Pathology Neuropathological studies have shown nonspecific neuronal degeneration in various parts of the central nervous system.[45,49–53] The topography of nerve cell loss is variable from case to case, but lesions predominate in the cerebellar cortex, the dentate nuclei and the thalami; they may also be seen in other structures, such as the basal ganglia, the brain stem, and the anterior horn cells of the spinal cord. In one case,[51] nerve cell loss was said to be restricted to the inferior olives; in another case it mainly involved the olives, substantia nigra, and corpus luysi.[52]

Treatment There is as yet no effective treatment for the polymyoclonus. Periodically one encounters isolated reports of dramatic, but usually transient, improvements with certain drugs (for instance, 5-OH Tryptophan, Piracetam, or Baclofen), whereas improvement is unobtainable in other patients. Phenytoin may aggravate the condition and should not be used.

Lafora Disease: Familial Progressive Myoclonic Epilepsy with Lafora Bodies   Lafora progressive myoclonic epilepsy is an autosomal recessive disease of adolescence with a rapidly progressive course. It is characterized by the presence of specific cytoplasmic inclusions, Lafora bodies,[54] composed of polyglucosans, in the neurons of the central nervous system. Seizures, polymyoclonus, and dementia are the cardinal signs. The biochemical defect is unknown, but the mutant gene has been mapped to chromosome 6. The average course of the disease is 5 years (Fig. 5-2). Detection of Lafora bodies in tissue specimens of skin, liver, and muscle may be of great help in the diagnosis for they are accessible by biopsy.

Clinical Features   Approximately 60 anatomically verified cases had been reported up to 1980. Our clinical experience has been with 3 cases. The disease is inherited as an autosomal recessive trait and is distributed worldwide. A recent report from South India mentions 21 cases in 16 families.[55]

The mean age of onset is 14 years (9 to 20 years) but a few have begun in mid-adulthood. A previously normal individual is most commonly assailed by tonic-clonic or myoclonic seizures, by polymyoclonus or presents as an isolated unexplained mental retardation. Seizures may precede the other signs of the disease by several months or even years, as was observed in one of our patients. The intention myoclonus has the same characteristics as that in Unverricht-Lundborg disease. It rapidly becomes incapacitating. Mental deterioration is a constant feature and usually but not constantly an early sign. Personality changes and bizarre behavior may occur. Occipital seizures with visual signs and visual hallucinatory phenomena have been recorded in 30 to 50 percent of cases.[56] Cerebellar ataxia, distinguishable from intention myoclonus, is a definite finding. Optic atrophy is not rare, and deafness has been an early finding in some cases. Rigidity and exaggerated tendon reflexes may develop later in the disease. The EEG shows polyspike slow-wave complexes and a progressive slowing of background rhythms. However, background activity may remain normal for several years. Photosensitivity is usual. There may be giant somesthetic sensory evoked potentials.

MRI reveals moderate cerebellar atrophy. The detection of Lafora bodies in the epithelium of sweat glands in biopsy specimens of skin (preferentially axil-

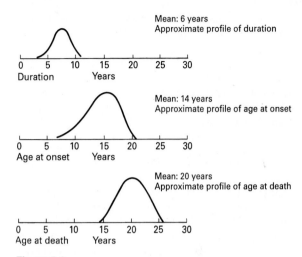

Mean: 6 years
Approximate profile of duration

Mean: 14 years
Approximate profile of age at onset

Mean: 20 years
Approximate profile of age at death

Figure 5-2
Lafora disease: duration, age at onset, age at death.

lary skin) and in the liver, or muscle tissue stands as the only definitive diagnostic test. However, the demonstration of typical inclusions in these tissues is not always possible,[57] so it cannot be fully relied upon. In other words, a negative biopsy does not exclude the diagnosis. In exceptional circumstances a cortical biopsy is justified. There is no effective treatment (see Unverricht-Lundborg disease). The clinical course generally spans 2 to 10 years; 20 years is the mean age of death.

Genetics   The disease is most probably inherited as an autosomal recessive trait. The mutant gene has been mapped to 6q23-25.

Pathology   There is generally moderate atrophy of the cerebellum with loss of Purkinje cells and, to a lesser extent, granule cells. The hallmark of the disease is the intracytoplasmic inclusion body described by Lafora in 1911. They are round basophilic, PAS-positive inclusions measuring 3 to 30 nm in diameter in the cytoplasm of neurons throughout the CNS. They are particularly numerous in the cerebellar cortex, dentate nuclei, thalami, substantia nigra, globus pallidus, and to a lesser degree, in the cerebral cortex. Under the electron microscope they have no surrounding membrane and consist of a central electron-dense granular core and closely packed filaments, which are composed of polyglucosans (glucose polymers). Similar inclusions are found in the skin, skeletal muscle, heart, and liver, seemingly without derangement of their function.

Clinicopathologic Correlation   The myoclonus is usually ascribed to the lesions in the cerebellar cortex and dentate nucleus, but the widespread distribution of the pathologic changes does not allow rigorous clinico-pathologic correlations.

Adult Polyglucosan Disease   In this clinicopatho-logical entity of adulthood, polyglucosans are stored in neuronal and astrocytic processes in the central nervous system and in axons of the peripheral nerves. The rela-tionship of this disorder to Lafora disease is unknown. It may be a variant of Lafora body disease because the cellular chemistry of the inclusions seems to be identical. However, the two conditions do differ clinically.[58,59] The principal neurologic findings have been a progressive weakness and spasticity of the legs, urinary inconti-nence, and a peripheral neuropathy identified by the EMG and measurements of nerve conduction velocity. Sensory deficits develop after some time. Cognitive impairment is present in half the patients. MRI discloses diffuse brain atrophy and a leukodystrophy in some cases. Diagnosis is based on the finding of polyglucosan bodies in axons in peripheral nerve biopsies. A defi-ciency of the glycogen branching enzyme 1,4-glucan 6-glucosyltransferase has been found in leukocytes, nerves, and muscle of Ashkenazic patients, but not in non-Jewish patients, suggesting the possibility of a heteroge-neous disorder.[59,60]

Two boy siblings, aged 14 and 19, with total branching enzyme deficiency have been reported. They had severe deposits of polyglucosan bodies in striated and smooth muscle fibers, histiocytes, fibroblasts, peri-neural cells, axons, and astrocytes.[61] In addition, a fatal infantile form of polyglucosan storage has been described in a hypotonic respirator-dependent newborn, with concomitant deficiencies of branching enzyme and phosphorylase.[62]

Myoclonus Epilepsy and Ragged Red Fibers   The maternally inherited syndrome myoclonus epilepsy and ragged red fibers (MERRF) is described later on.

Lysosomal Disorders with Polymyoclonus, Seizures, and Ataxia   In a number of late childhood lysosomal disorders, polymyoclonus or a syndrome of polymyoclonus, seizures, ataxia, and dementia stand as cardinal features (this has been found in sialidosis type I, late infantile G_{M2} gangliosidosis, and juvenile (type III) Gaucher disease). In these conditions, which are described in other parts of this chapter, there are ocular signs and/or visceral abnormalities.

There exist other familial conditions in late child-hood in which action myoclonus may occur; they are listed in Table 5-6.

The Nosologic Status of the Ramsay Hunt Syndrome (Dyssynergia Cerebellaris Myoclonica)   Too often the term Ramsay Hunt syndrome has been loosely applied to any case of action polymyoclonus with epi-lepsy and cerebellar ataxia, irrespective of its cause. Some writers imply that it is only an example of Unverricht-Lundborg disease. For others, the term is, more appropriately, reserved for diseases in which ataxia and myoclonus are prominent, seizures rare, and demen-tia absent (progressive myoclonic ataxia).[64] In view of this ambiguity, it is important to examine carefully the original description.

In 1921 Ramsay Hunt published his well-known paper on dyssynergia cerebellaris myoclonica with pri-mary atrophy of the dentate system. He described two brothers with signs of Friedreich ataxia who shared an illness that became manifest at age 10 and 19 and was followed, after a period of 5 to 10 years, by epilepsy and intention myoclonus.[65] Autopsy of one brother showed loss of neurons, and gliosis of the dentate nuclei, as well as degeneration of the superior cerebellar peduncles, and loss of myelinated fibers in the dorsal columns of the spinal cord and the spinocerebellar tracts. There were no intracellular inclusions. In the same study Ramsay Hunt gave a purely clinical account of four unrelated patients with myoclonic epilepsy followed later by signs of cerebellar ataxia. As this last sequence of events is common to different types of PME, the term *Ramsay Hunt syndrome* should be restricted to the syndrome exhibited by the first two cases, in which there was clin-ical evidence of spinal cord involvement, like in Friedreich ataxia, and degeneration of the superior cer-ebellar peduncles.

The majority of cases of progressive myoclonus epilepsy can be allocated to specific disease entities such as Unverricht-Lundborg disease, Lafora disease, MERRF (some cases of which appear to conform to the anatomical and clinical description of Ramsay Hunt) and late infantile lysosomal disorders, so that the discussions concerning the specificity of Ramsay Hunt syndrome may seem obsolete.

Other Disorders with Action Myoclonus

Sialidosis type I (Cherry Red Spot-Myoclonus Syndrome)   Sialidosis type I is an autosomal recessive disorder due to an isolated deficiency of α-neuraminidase (coded on chromosome 10).

The disease starts in late childhood or adolescence and is characterized by progressive visual loss, polymyoclonus, and seizures.[66,67] Most of the reported cases come from Italy; we have seen two in Boston. There is a macular cherry red spot in the optic fundi, and some patients have punctuate opacities of the lens. Corneal clouding does not occur. Polymyoclonus is the most striking feature of the disease. Multiple, irregular, asynchronous, myoclonic jerks are precipitated by action and intentional movements, sensory stimuli, or emotional upset. They interfere gravely with all types of motor activity and may eventually become so incapacitating that patients can no longer walk, speak, or feed themselves. Generalized tonic-clonic seizures are added to the clinical picture. Cerebellar ataxia has been reported. Intelligence generally starts out as normal or only slightly impaired, but later deterioration is unmistakable. Blindness and optic atrophy occur in the later stages of the disease. Dysmorphic features, bone or joint abnormalities, or hepatomegaly are entirely absent.

CT scans and MRI permit visualization of cerebral and cerebellar atrophy. Foamy histiocytes in bone marrow smears and a few vacuolated lymphocytes in peripheral blood are usually found. Under the electron microscope, clear vacuoles, some of which are filled with fibrillary material, can be observed in cells from skin, liver (Kupffer cells), and bone marrow. There is an increase of sialic acid containing oligosaccharides in urine. A convenient method of screening for these compounds is thin-layer chromatography.

The disease is caused by a deficiency in α-neuraminidase. Enzyme assays can be made on cultured skin fibroblasts, leukocytes, amniocytes, and chorionic villi. Prenatal diagnosis and detection of carriers are possible.

Attempts to suppress the polymyoclonus by medication have been disappointing. Some benefit has accrued from benzodiazepines, 5-hydroxytryptophan,[68] and carbidopa therapy.

Sialidosis type II has been described in Chap. 3.

Hereditary Dentatorubral-Pallidoluysian Atrophy

Hereditary dentatorubral-pallidoluysian atrophy (DRPLA), a dominantly inherited disease, is known to be a rare cause of progressive myoclonus epilepsy of the degenerative type. The original report came from Japan.

Takahashi et al.[69] described three patients in three generations. The onset was in late childhood. One patient had polymyoclonus, epilepsy, pyramidal signs, and mental deterioration. The second had ataxia, intention myoclonus, dementia, and no seizures. The third had a cerebellar ataxia, choreiform movements, and dementia but neither seizures nor myoclonus. Neuropathological lesions in two cases consisted of nerve cell loss and gliosis in the dentate nucleus, red nucleus, pallidum, and corpus luysi. Degeneration of the striatum, cerebellar cortex, and of the lateral corticospinal tracts were also present.

Additional cases of this autosomal dominant disorder have been described not only from Japan where its prevalence is estimated to be 0.4 to 0.7 per million persons, but also from Europe.[70,71] Age of onset is variable, even within the same family, and there is genetic anticipation. The disease has been linked to chromosome 12pter-p12 and is due to an expanded CAG trinucleotide repeat in the open reading frame of a gene whose product is being termed atrophin-1.[72] The normal range of repeats is 8 to 35, which expands to 49 to 75 in DRPLA patients. Generally, the larger the repeat size, the earlier the onset and more severe the symptoms.[74] Most cases are inherited from the father, but when maternal transmission occurs, symptoms start earlier (mean of 14 years) and are more severe, although the degree of expansion is smaller compared to the case with paternal transmission.

Haw River syndrome, a dominantly inherited disorder affecting five successive generations of a rural African-American family had many similarities to DRPLA. It is characterized by ataxia, chorea, seizures, and dementia. Mental retardation and psychiatric disorders also occur. The neuropathological findings include marked neuronal loss in the dentate nucleus, microcalcification of the basal ganglia, demyelination of the centrum semiovale, and marked neuroaxonal dystrophy of the posterior columns. It is due to the same expanded trinucleotide repeat as DRPLA.[73]

Benign Essential Familial Myoclonus   Essential familial myoclonus is a benign syndrome of unknown cause(s) and of obscure physiopathologic mechanism. At present it can be defined mainly in terms of a few negative criteria. The disease is not significantly progressive, and there is no mental deterioration, epilepsy, or other major neurological sign. This fact alone rules out any relationship to progressive myoclonus epilepsies of known etiology. A dominant pattern of inheritance is usual. Since the initial description of Friedreich "paramyoclonus multiplex," the few reports of this rare syndrome that have appeared in the literature convey the impression that it is not a homogeneous entity.

Age at onset is in the first decade (exceptionally in early infancy); the movement abnormality involves the muscles of the trunk, neck, limbs, and possibly the face, which are intermittently activated by shock-like contractions involving a few fascicles or all of a group of muscles. Some are not sufficiently intense to excite movement, whereas others cause jerking of the entire limb, neck, trunk, face, tongue, pharynx, and larynx, altering the voice in the latter instance. Myoclonus is often present at rest, although it tends to be diminished by relaxation and enhanced by rapid voluntary movement. There is no significant progression of the disease. In some patients there are periods when the involuntary movements seem to be in abeyance. The degree of motor handicap is variable but may be severe in some patients. No significant biochemical abnormalities have been found, and the EEG and brain scans are normal. Focal cerebral blood flow reduction contralateral to the myoclonus symptoms have been demonstrated in one father and son.[75] More than one physiological mechanism may underlie the disorder. Hallett et al.[76] report a family in which isolated benign myoclonus was inherited as an autosomal dominant trait. The EMG showed the myoclonus to be characterized by long complex bursts (50 to 100 ms) often synchronous in different muscles, occurring during ballistic movements (ballistic movement-overflow myoclonus). They may constitute a subtype of essential familial myoclonus. Along with others, we have observed cases of essential myoclonus in association with essential tremor, or with essential tremor in other members of the family.[77] The combination of myoclonus in conjunction with idiopathic dystonia is well documented; its conjunction with ataxia (familial myoclonus and ataxia) has also been recorded.[78] Treatment of essential myoclonus is difficult. Clonazepam, piracetam, primidone, and sodium valproate as well as anticholinergic drugs may be employed in severe forms, sometimes with good results.

Essential Palatal Myoclonus Palatal myoclonus is a rare movement disorder characterized by rhythmic myoclonic jerks of the soft palate. Most cases are related to acquired lesions of the brain stem (tumoral, vascular, infectious). Exceptionally it occurs in a hereditary disorder (such as cholestanolosis) involving the tegmental tracts, inferior olives, or olivodentate system. Other cases are classified as idiopathic and in very rare instances start in childhood. Palatal myoclonus charac-

teristically produces a rhythmic ear click. The movements generally persist during sleep. Childhood forms of palatal myoclonus usually disappear after some time, and are benign, apart from the inconveniences of the auditory click.[79,80]

Conclusions

From the above account it is apparent that the symptomatic triad—seizures, progressive intention myoclonus, and ataxia—should call attention mainly to four metabolic or neurodegenerative disorders: Unverricht-Lundborg disease, Lafora disease, MERRF, and certain juvenile forms of lysosomal disorders (including sialidosis type I) (see Table 5-6). Widely different, these diseases are caused respectively by a nonspecific neuronal degeneration, a nonlysosomal storage disease, a defective mitochondrial DNA, and a lysosomal storage disorder. Each has a unique histopathology but probably shares a common topology, most particularly a lesional predominance in the cerebellar cortex and dentate nucleus, and possibly the red nucleus, inferior olives, and spinal cord. They differ also in their mode of inheritance. MERRF has a maternal pattern of inheritance; the other disorders are autosomal recessive. The chronology of appearance and the relative importance of seizures, myoclonus, ataxia, and dementia is variable. Although a PME may start with polymyoclonus or mental deterioration (Lafora disease), most cases become first manifest as generalized seizures of the tonic-clonic, myoclonic, or myoclonic-astatic type, sometimes the only sign for many months. So, a PME may initially be mistaken for a form of idiopathic epilepsy.

The symptomatology of the different categories of PME may be very similar to start with but some symptoms help to distinguish them. (1) A short stature, deafness, impaired deep sensation and evidence of sensory ataxia, muscular weakness, high levels of lactate in the CSF, and evidence of a maternal pattern of inheritance indisputably point to MERRF. (2) The presence of visual hallucinations and occipital seizures, and a rapid course are observed in Lafora disease. (3) A slow progression and the absence of dementia favor a diagnosis of Unverricht-Lundborg disease. (4) A macular cherry-red spot points to sialidosis type I. (5) Extrapyramidal signs are a feature of DRPLA.

Confirmatory tests of one of the PMEs should include measurement of lactic acid in the CSF; a muscle biopsy to detect ragged red fibers (and possibly Lafora bodies); a skin or liver biopsy to search for Lafora bodies (or other inclusions); a CT scan (basal ganglia calcifications may be present in MERRF); a search for sialic acid containing oligosaccharides in the urine; and according to context, specific enzymatic tests and the study of mtDNA. Benign familial myoclonus is usually easy to recognize because of its typical symptomatology and family history. This condition may pose significant therapeutic problems.

HEREDITARY, PREDOMINANTLY EXTRAPYRAMIDAL DISORDERS OF LATE CHILDHOOD AND ADOLESCENCE

Introduction

The neurologic manifestations of this group include a combination of rigidity, involuntary movements, tremor, muscle spasms, or abnormalities of posture. They are, to use the term introduced by Kinnier Wilson, "extrapyramidal." The commonest combinations are a combination of rigidity-tremor-akinesia — the parkinsonian syndrome; the sudden, rapid, erratic, purposeless movements of chorea; the forceful writhing movements and postures of athetosis; the sustained twisting spasms and abnormal postures of torsion dystonia; the various types of tremor (these movement disorders are also described in Chap. 6).

In the hereditary extrapyramidal disorders, lesions (and/or evidence of an abnormal metabolism) affect predominantly specific groups of neurons in the basal ganglia and upper brain stem, but they tend to become diffuse as the disease advances. Only a minority are related to a known metabolic defect. Some of them are believed to be due to disorders of neurotransmitters. The mechanism of the cellular pathology is still obscure, although the possible action of excitotoxic amino acids has been postulated, especially in Huntington disease. For still other diseases, their morphological as well as the biochemical basis remains unknown. Studies of neurotransmitters with modern techniques may offer promise of solving these problems. The prospect of early diagnosis and prevention have been greatly enhanced by recent and ongoing studies of molecular genetics.

Although the clinical picture of many of the extrapyramidal disorders is apt to vary widely from case to case, in most of them, one sign or syndrome stands out clearly.

Progressive Familial Diseases with a Parkinsonian Syndrome or Some Variant Thereof

Paralysis agitans (Parkinson disease), a degenerative disorder of middle or late adulthood, is the clinical prototype. It is characterized by rigidity, tremor, slowness of movement, and postural imbalance without significant paralysis. Its cause is a loss of cells in the substantia nigra and depletion of dopamine in the substantia nigra and striatum. Paralysis agitans virtually never occurs in childhood and adolescence. However, fragments of its symptomatology are reproduced by certain familial diseases in these early age periods. For diagnostic purposes it is useful (1) to set apart this grouping of familial diseases with elements of the parkinsonian syndrome; and (2) to distinguish them from another group of familial extrapyramidal disorders which are featured by dystonic spasms or choreoathetotic (or athetotic), or more rarely, purely choreic involuntary movements. More specifically, a child who presents with progressive generalized rigidity and tremor should always be suspected of having one of two diseases: familial hepatocerebral degeneration (Wilson disease) or juvenile Huntington disease. Juvenile Parkinson disease, another genetic disorder, is a very rare and probably a heterogeneous entity. Other conditions in which a parkinsonian syndrome may develop are listed in Tables 5-4, 5-7, and 6-5.

Familial Hepatolenticular Degeneration (Wilson Disease; Westphal-Strümpell Pseudosclerosis) Wilson disease (WD) is an autosomal recessive disorder that causes heavy deposition of copper in the liver, the corneas, the kidneys, and the nervous system. The gene for WD is located on chromosome 13 at q14.3 and codes for a copper-transporting protein. The exact mechanism of tissue damage remains unknown, but the primary deficiency of copper transport is thought to be in the liver, whereas the brain, kidneys, and other organs are secondarily affected. Clinically (Fig. 5-3) the disease may present as an isolated hepatic disorder, particularly in childhood, and after 8 to 12 years of age, by neurological signs with evident liver cirrhosis. Either of two major and relatively dissociated symptoms may be the first cerebral manifestations: (1) a generalized rigidity predominating in the facio-oropharyngeal musculature or (2) a gross postural or intention tremor. Behavioral and cognitive changes are often present and may precede other neurologic signs. The Kayser-Fleischer ring results from copper deposition on the limbus of the cornea. It

Table 5-7
Main characteristics of major juvenile genetic extrapyramidal disorders

	Extrapyramidal signs	Other possible neurologic signs	Ocular abnormalities	Mental deterioration; psychiatric signs	Non-neurologic signs	Family history; genetics	Neuroimaging	Biochemistry	Molecular biology	Presymptomatic, prenatal diagnosis	Specific treatment
Wilson disease	Facio-oropharyngeal rigidity* Parkinsonism Intention tremor		Kayser-Fleischer ring*	Present	Liver cirrhosis*	AR	Striatal lesions	Low serum ceruloplasmin Hypercupruria Increased copper content of liver*	Gene cloned on chromosome 13	Possible	Effective copper chelators
Huntington disease	Parkinsonian rigidity Chorea	Myoclonic seizures	Disorder of voluntary gaze	Present	None	AD; one parent (father, in juvenile form) always affected, sometimes subtly*	Atrophy of caudate	None	Gene cloned on chromosome 4	Possible	None
Hallervorden-Spatz disease	Dystonia Choreoathetosis	Pyramidal signs	Retinitis pigmentosa	Present	None	AR	Low signal in globus pallidus in MRI*	None	None	Not possible	None
Idiopathic progressive torsion dystonia (dystonia musculorum deformans)	Dystonia, first local then generalized* One variety is dopa responsive (DR)	Parkinsonian rigidity Myoclonus	None	Absent	None	AD, some AR	No abnormality	None	Gene on chromosome 9 Gene for DR variety on chromosome 14		Effective for DR variety
Chorea-acanthocytosis	Chorea Dysarthria	Dystonia, rigidity, tics Axonal neuropathy	None	Present	Acanthocytosis*	?	Changes in striatum	Lipoproteins normal	None	Not possible	None
Benign familial chorea	Chorea, nonprogressive*	Tremor	None	Absent*	None	AD, AR X-linked	No abnormality	None	None	Not possible	None

Abbreviations and symbols: AD = autosomal dominant; AR = autosomal recessive; DR = dopamine responsive; an asterisk (*) indicates pathognomonic or necessary for the diagnosis.

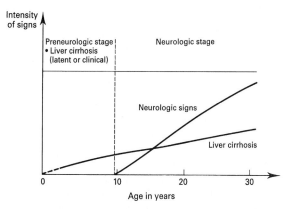

A disease with latent or clinical hepatic cirrhosis, subsequently a complex extrapyramidal syndrome consisting of a constant faciobuccopharyngeal dyskinesia, various combinations of rigidity, intention tremor, involuntary movements and spasms of the limbs and accompanied by a typical pericorneal pigmentation and progressive dementia.
 • Copper accumulates in liver, then in brain and other tissues, causing damage
 • Liver disease precedes neurologic dysfunction

Figure 5-3
Wilson disease: clinical profile and key signs.

stands as a constant and specific hallmark of the disease by the time neurological signs appear, and it may also be seen to a lesser degree even in the purely hepatic form. The finding of low ceruloplasmin and total copper levels in the serum and an excess of copper in the urine are diagnostic. Of even greater validity are a high copper content in biopsied liver tissue and a failure of ceruloplasmin to incorporate radiolabeled copper. The availability of the WD gene cDNA offers the possibility of molecular diagnosis to detect patients at the preclinical stage and prenatally. The use of copper chelators has considerably improved the prognosis of what was earlier a fatal disorder.

Clinical Features Copper deposits in liver and brain may accumulate for a decade or more before causing functional impairment. Either hepatic or neurologic signs may inaugurate the disease.

Liver disease, in the face of minor neurological signs or more often in their absence, is the presenting feature in approximately 30 percent of cases.[83] There is either a chronic cirrhosis with hepatosplenomegaly (sometimes mainly splenomegaly) and occasionally portal hypertension and hypersplenism, or less often, recurrent episodes of jaundice and vomiting that may resolve spontaneously. A Kayser-Fleischer ring (Fig. 5-4) is found in approximately 70 percent of cases in purely

hepatic forms. Evidence of renal tubular dysfunction may be added in some cases. The more florid manifestations of cirrhosis tend to occur in young patients. A fulminating, frequently lethal, liver disorder may be the only expression of the disease in children aged between 4 and 8 years. In numerous cases, however, the hepatic cirrhosis remains more or less asymptomatic and is discovered only after the onset of neurologic signs.

Neurologic Signs Neurologic signs do not become apparent before 8 to 10 years of age and more often appear in adolescence and early adulthood. One of our patients (which number more than 50) experienced onset at the age of 7; three of our patients experienced onset between the ages of 34 and 50.

In the more rapidly developing "Wilsonian" form of the disease (the type of case occurring in late childhood or early adolescence), a faciolinguopharyngeal rigidity causing facial masking, open mouth, grimacing, dysarthria, and dysphagia are the principal manifestations. In the patients whose disease is of slower evolution (Westphal-Strümpell pseudosclerotic form), a tremor that may initially be confined to one arm is often the first sign; it is present when the limb is used voluntarily or is held in a particular posture. And the characteristic slowness of movement and rigidity of the faciobuccopharyngeal musculature is not long in appearing.

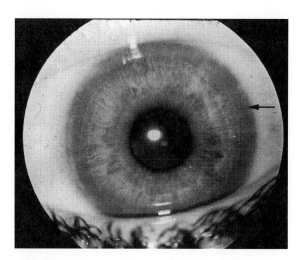

Figure 5-4
Kayser-Fleischer corneal ring (arrow) in Wilson disease.

As the disease advances, the face becomes masked and set in a characteristic grin. Mastication and swallowing become difficult. Speech is increasingly impaired and finally lost. The muscular rigidity becomes generalized with a parkinsonian type of gait; and voluntary movements evoke a gross and irregular tremor (more so in the so-called Westphal-Strümpell variety) that reaches its maximal degree when the limbs are outstretched (wing-beating, "rubral" tremor). Attempts at volitional control as well as emotional excitement may aggravate rigidity and tremor. Bizarre dyskinesias, resulting in unnatural postures of the limbs, tonic spasms of the pterygoid muscles with opening of the jaw or other stereotyped involuntary movements, are not infrequent. Some patients also experience tonic spasms initiated by voluntary movements (tonic innervation).

Other possible extrapyramidal signs that may occur early in some cases include chorea, which may start abruptly, and flagrant choreoathetotic or dystonic symptoms. Rare cases have begun with a cerebellar ataxia or a diffuse intention myoclonus. Seizures may occur and are either of generalized or partial type. There are usually no pyramidal signs.

Psychiatric abnormalities and aberrations of behavior are sometimes the earliest manifestations of the neurologic disorder and may for a time be difficult to interpret, resulting in an incorrect assumption of a primary psychological disorder, early schizophrenia, or other psychopathy. This error sometimes delays therapy. In one series,[84] these early behavioral abnormalities were present in 60 percent of the cases. Loss of emotional control, subtle impairment of intellectual function, and difficulty in conforming to the customs of the family and society are usual. Scholastic failure usually attracts notice in untreated patients, and regrettably, even in some of the successfully treated ones. The intellectual capacities in general fall below the normal level.

In our own personal experience, a slight personality and cognitive change, dysarthria, an open-mouth facies and tremor of an arm have been the most frequent initial signs of the disease.

The *Kayser-Fleischer* corneal ring is invariably associated with the neurologic syndrome. It is the most specific sign of WD. It consists of a greenish brown deposit of copper in the Descemet membrane just within the limbus of the cornea (Fig. 5-4). When fully developed, it is seen with the naked eye, but a slit-lamp examination is required in the early stages of the disease. It is present in 60 percent of children at the stage of acute or subacute liver disease. It may be present in asymptomatic affected individuals.

Other Signs Renal tubular dysfunction leading to hyperaminoaciduria, glucocuria, hyperuricuria, impaired transport of phosphate and calcium (Fanconi syndrome), and occasionally hypophosphatemic rickets are demonstrable. Renal stones may occur. Osteomalacia, osteoporosis, spontaneous fractures, and arthropathy, unexplained epistaxis, acute hemolytic anemia, often associated with liver failure, may somewhat complicate the disease even at an early date. Pigmentation of the lower extremities and azure lunulae of the fingernails have also been reported.

Without treatment the disease progresses slowly towards complete incapacitation and death after 1 to 3 years.

Diagnostic Laboratory Tests Typically there is a greatly reduced level of serum ceruloplasmin (< 20 mg/100 mL in 95 percent of cases, normally 25 to 50 mg/100 mL), a decrease in total serum copper (3 to 10 μM, normally 11 to 24 μM), and an elevation of the proportion of nonceruloplasmin copper (Fig. 5-5). Urinary excretion of copper is increased (100 to 1000 μg/24 h, normally 40 μg/24 h) and is greatly augmented by the administration of penicillamine. The content of liver copper is markedly increased (> 250 μg/g dry weight; normally 20 to 50 μg/g). Liver biopsy with assay of copper content by absorption spectrometry appears to be the most reliable diagnostic laboratory test. The demonstration of a much reduced incorporation of radiolabeled copper (^{64}Cu) into ceruloplasmin serves as a confirmatory test, especially when ceruloplasmin levels are normal, as they may be in a few cases of WD. This is

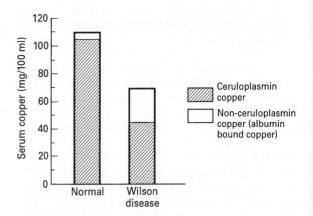

Figure 5-5
Serum copper in Wilson disease.

especially appropriate in the young patient with only liver disease. Also, ceruloplasmin levels may fall during acute liver failure from causes other than WD. Other tests which reveal dysfunction of the liver, kidney, and the other organs are relevant. Thrombocytopenia and neutropenia are frequent.

MRI demonstrates abnormal signals (hypointense on T1-weighted and hyperintense in T2-weighted images) in the caudate nuclei, lenticular nuclei, thalami, and dentate nuclei. Cortical and cerebellar atrophy may be present in long-standing cases. With positron emission tomography (PET scan) the regional cerebral metabolic rate of glucose consumption is reduced, particularly in the striatum, cerebellum, and to a lesser extent, the thalamus and cortex.[85]

Genetics   WD is an autosomal recessive disease. Its incidence is not certain. Estimates place the figure at 1 in 30,000 to 1 in 50,000 live births, with a gene frequency of 1/90. The gene for the disease, located on chromosome 13q14.3, codes for a copper-binding p-type ATPase that is highly homologous to the Menkes disease gene product. Two of the more than 25 mutations described represent 38 percent of the mutations in patients of European origin.[86] Studies of genotype versus phenotype aid in the prediction of disease severity. But the remaining variability suggests that extra factors   affect phenotypic response, that is, factors beyond the type of mutation. Thomas et al.[86] postulate that these might include dietary copper intake, metallothioneine inducibility, and capacity for dealing with copper stress. Heterozygotes are symptom-free but 20 percent of them have lowered levels of ceruloplasmin, whereas their hepatic copper concentration is normal.

Diagnosis and Counseling   WD should be considered in two circumstances. (1) In all children who develop progressive extrapyramidal signs after the age of 7 to 8 years, *not before*. The early predominance of rigidity and akinesia in the faciolinguopharyngeal musculature, the concomitance of liver disease (detected sometimes only by liver function tests) and, above all, the constant presence of a Kayser-Fleischer corneal ring are identifying clinical features. The latter will help differentiate WD from the acquired hepatocerebral degenerations with choreoathetosis, cerebellar ataxia, episodic coma, and dementia. One should also be alert to WD in young patients exhibiting behavioral and psychic abnormalities, especially when they are associated with minor neurologic abnormalities such as dysarthria or limb rigidity. (2) In all patients in childhood, adoles-

cence, or adulthood with isolated chronic or acute liver disease. Experience shows that the diagnosis of Wilson hepatopathy is too frequently overlooked at a time when treatment could prevent the neurologic disorder.

Whatever the mode of presentation, the first laboratory investigations should include measurement of serum ceruloplasmin and total copper, as well as urinary copper excretion (before and after penicillamine). If these tests are negative (as occurs only rarely), but suspicion of the disease is high, one should turn to liver biopsy for the demonstration of pathologic changes and elevated copper content. When available, the demonstration of a marked decrease of radiolabeled copper into ceruloplasmin will firmly establish the diagnosis.

A diagnosis of WD in one sibling should always lead to the full investigation of other siblings in the family. Siblings of a patient with WD have a 1 in 4 risk of developing the disease. To distinguish between a normal and an affected individual, all children in the family should be examined for liver and nervous dysfunction, the corneal ring, and by measurement of serum ceruloplasmin, and urinary copper. If necessary, one should examine the copper content of a liver biopsy. Direct mutation analysis is now available and should help discriminate between presymptomatic and unaffected siblings of affected patients. Prenatal diagnosis by DNA analysis is also available where the mutation(s) is known, or by DNA polymorphism when the mutations have not yet been identified.[87] The sensitivity of molecular tests for potential heterozygotes will depend upon the number of different mutations for which screening is performed, since most mutations occur with only a 1 or 2 percent frequency rate.[86]

Pathologic Findings   In Wilson's original cases, gross cavitation of the lenticular nuclei was observed, but the more usual pathologic change is a shrinkage of these structures due to neuronal degeneration in association with hyperplasia of protoplasmic astrocytes and spongiosis of the tissue. These findings are concentrated in the lenticular nuclei but are found to a lesser degree in the dentate nuclei, the substantia nigra, the cerebellar cortex, and the thalamic and mesencephalic nuclei. Neuron loss alone with gliosis corresponds more closely to the Strümpell-Westphal pseudosclerosis form of the disease. Copper is located in the subcellular soluble fraction, bound to cuproproteins. The liver lesion is one of healed and recurrent, subacute, yellow atrophy resembling postnecrotic cirrhosis. Some of the regenerated lobules are large and a biopsy of one of them may not reveal the cirrhosis. Copper, attached to metallothioneine, is first diffusely spread in the cytoplasm of cells, then later is localized mainly in lysosomes. The pigment in the cornea is a copper salt deposited in the lamina propria of the Descemet membrane.

Pathophysiology and Clinicopathologic Correlations The defect in the transport of copper, allowing it to accumulate in the liver and later in other tissues, results in two fundamental disturbances of copper metabolism: (1) a reduction in the biliary excretion of copper and (2) a decrease in the incorporation of copper into ceruloplasmin (which occurs in the liver). The sequence of events appears to be as follows. The first metabolic effect is the accumulation of copper in the liver. In some children this may lead to serious liver failure, but usually it proceeds for long periods without notable impairment of hepatic function. Eventually concentrations of nonceruloplasmin copper increase and this metal begins to be deposited in the brain and other organs by "overflow."[83] The cerebral lesions apparently always occur after the development of liver cirrhosis and must be linked in some peculiar manner to hepatic dysfunction.

No one has satisfactorily explained the improvement that follows treatment. It could be due to depletion of copper in the brain or in the liver, to improved liver function, or possibly to other unknown factors. The reversibility of part of the neurologic deficit suggests that there is a stage in which the function of neurons is deranged by the metabolic abnormality before neuronal death and tissue necrosis.

The tremor and rigidity correlate with lesions of the substantia nigra and ataxia to lesions of the dentate nuclei (dentatorubrothalamic tracts), but the microscopic changes are actually quite diffuse and do not allow precise clinical correlation.

Treatment Treatment of WD was transformed in 1956 when Walshe introduced a copper-chelating agent, penicillamine.[88] D-penicillamine, now available without the more toxic mixture of the D and L forms, remains the standard treatment. The dose is 1000 mg/day, divided into two doses, but may be increased to 2000 or even 3000 mg/day. For small children, 500 mg/day is adequate. The dose varies with the amounts of urinary copper; amounts of 500 to 1000 mg/day are usually satisfactory. Undesirable side effects occur in 10 percent of patients. These include cutaneous changes, nausea and vomiting, thrombocytopenia and leucope-

nia, hemolysis, arthropathy, and pyridoxine deficiency. The most serious of these are lupus erythematosis or an immune complex nephropathy (nephrosis). A brief course of corticosteroids given at the onset of penicillamine therapy may prevent or alleviate the hypersensibility.

Other effective drugs can be substituted when the results with penicillamine are poor or other reactions, such as aplastic anemia, cannot be controlled. Walshe favors triethylene tetramine (trientine), which is effective and has no known serious side effects. The dose is 400 to 900 mg/day in three divided doses before meals. Zinc salts, preferably zinc acetate (50 to 150 mg/day) or zinc sulphate (660 to 1320 mg/day), which block the intestinal absorption of copper, are used during the maintenance phase and are most valuable in presymptomatic individuals. Tetrathiomolybdate and dimercaprol have occasionally been employed. Tetrathiomolybdate binds free copper when given intravenously. Both penicillamine and trientine have been given safely during pregnancy.

The choice between the major chelators (essentially penicillamine and trientine) is based on personal experience (and availability of trientine). One should monitor the urinary elimination of copper induced by these drugs and the clinical response to treatment. Monitoring of the treatment with zinc is more difficult and necessitates the study of ^{64}Cu uptake. Treatment with zinc sulfate resulted in dramatic improvement in neurological status and resolution in lesions on the T2 MRI study of one patient who had deteriorated significantly while receiving D-penicillamine.[89]

Improvement usually occurs only after 3 to 6 months and a transitory aggravation of several symptoms for weeks after treatment is started is not infrequent. When acute episodes of worsening with very high levels of nonceruloplasmin copper occur, peritoneal dialysis or plasmapheresis may be useful adjuncts.[83]

The results of treatment are on the whole satisfactory. Although the best results can be predicted in presymptomatic patients or those in the early stages of the disease, unexpectedly good responses have been obtained with some severely affected individuals. In a series of 137 patients with WD treated with penicillamine or occasionally with other chelators, 40 percent had become symptom-free; 25 percent were left with some minor neurological deficit; 18 percent had their disorder arrested but remained disabled; and 17 percent died despite an apparently adequate chelating therapy.[88] Liver damage lessens with treatment. MRI abnormal-

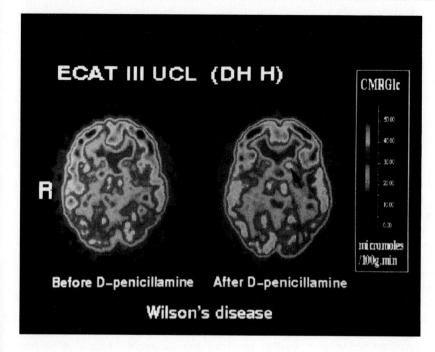

Figure 5-6
Wilson disease. Compare PET scans before and after treatment with D-penicillamine for one year. Reappearance of image of glucose metabolism, using fluorodeoxyglucose (FDG), in caudate nucleus after treatment (arrow) (ref. 95).

ities improve in nearly all patients, but pretreatment brain atrophy does not change.[90] A number of our patients have lived healthy, active lives for 30 to 40 years. Successive PET scans in one patient showed the reappearance of glucose metabolism in the caudate nucleus after treatment (Fig. 5-6). Cessation of therapy is often followed by recrudescence of liver abnormality, which again responds to treatment. For residual neurologic symptoms, a trial of levodopa may be helpful.

Liver transplantation has been used in acute irreversible liver failure and in patients with advanced liver disease. The Kayser-Fleischer ring disappeared in some patients,[91] confirming the primary role of liver dysfunction and supporting the *liver overflow* theory of WD.

Huntington Disease (Huntington Chorea): Childhood and Juvenile Forms Huntington disease (HD) is a degenerative disorder with a dominant pattern of inheritance and unknown biochemical pathogenesis. It usually occurs in middle adult life and presents as a syndrome of chorea, motor apraxia, personality changes, and dementia. Children are affected in some families, but their clinical picture differs in that rigidity, dementia, and seizures are more frequent (Fig. 5-7).

Nerve cell loss in the striatum and, to a moderate degree, the cerebral cortex constitutes the pathologic hallmark of this disease. The site of the genetic defect

has been shown to be on the short arm of chromosome 4, but the pathogenesis of this fatal condition remains uncertain. The availability of DNA markers linked to the Huntington gene, and recently the identification of the gene, allows presymptomatic and prenatal detection, but since there is no effective treatment, this predictive procedure raises important ethical problems.

Clinical Features of Childhood Form The prevalence of the disease in populations of Western European descent is between 3 and 7 in 100,000. The age of onset in childhood has been as early as 3 years but in most

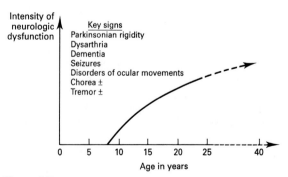

Figure 5-7
Childhood Huntington disease: profile and key signs.

instances has occurred between 5 and 12 years. The proportion of HD starting before age 20 was estimated to be between 6 and 12 percent.[92,93]

Either motor or psychiatric disturbances may first attract attention. Slowness and maladroitness of movements, an abnormal gait, and dysarthria are early signs. Later a more or less typical parkinsonian picture slowly emerges. The gait is slow, stiff, and short-stepped, with the trunk tending to flex. All movements are slow and the patient seems disinclined to move. The face is masked and blinking is reduced; infrequently there may be prolonged blepharospasm. There is dysphagia. The voice is soft (hypophonic) and words are spoken quickly and unevenly; chewing and swallowing become difficult. A tremor (4 to 5 per second) may appear when the limbs assume certain postures, but it is at once abolished by movement, as it is in typical cases of parkinsonism. A fine rapid tremor (7 to 10 per second) may also occur.

Not all cases of childhood HD assume this rigid form. In some, as in the adult, chorea is the initial and predominant manifestation, and (as in Wilson disease) may occasionally be mistaken for Sydenham chorea. Interestingly, rigid children with HD may develop transient chorea when given levodopa, an observation which may prove of some value in differential diagnosis. Seizures are frequent in children in contrast to the adult form and may occur early. They may be of the myoclonic or myoclonic-astatic type. Myoclonic seizures may be quite severe. Action myoclonus (polymyoclonus) may be observed in some patients. Intention tremor and cerebellar signs have been reported. A disturbance of voluntary gaze occurs early but has not been explicitly documented in the childhood form. The main ocular abnormalities consist of prolonged latency and slowness of saccades on commanded movements, and difficulty in gaze-holding. An obligatory blink or head turn may be used to start the lateral eye movement.[94] Visual acuity and optic fundi are always normal, as is hearing. There is no evidence of involvement of the pyramidal system. The CSF is normal.

Whatever the extrapyramidal symptomatology, progressive dementia is a constant feature. Unexplained scholastic failure plus changes in behavior and personality may precede evident motor dysfunction. Irritability and excessive emotionality are other striking features, as are bizarre ideas, negativism, and even catatonic postures. For a time these may be mistaken for a "functional" psychosis. Depression is more common in adults.

In well-developed cases, CT scans and MRI show a characteristic atrophy of the caudate nucleus and putamen. The head of the caudate nucleus is markedly flattened. The anterior horns of the lateral ventricles are moderately enlarged; there is usually evidence of slight atrophy of the frontal lobes and possibly of the cerebellum. The highly characteristic atrophy of the caudate nucleus may be absent early in the disease. Positron emission tomography (PET) using fluorodeoxyglucose demonstrates hypometabolism of glucose in the caudate nucleus even before atrophy of this structure is evident in CT or MR scans, as was recently the case in one of our young patients.[95] One should verify the absence of acanthocytes in the peripheral blood, especially in the choreic form of the disease, since chorea in association with this red blood cell abnormality is a different disease (chorea-acanthocytosis). Duration of the disease is approximately 10 years.

Genetics Huntington disease is inherited as an autosomal dominant trait with complete penetrance. Its exact prevalence has not been precisely determined. Some estimates establish the prevalence rate in populations of Western European descent to 3 to 7 in 100,000 or to 4 in 100,000;[93] but in some areas there are much higher or much lower rates. The mutation rate is extremely low and the overwhelming majority of cases can be confirmed by family history. The infantile disease is much more frequently transmitted by affected fathers than by mothers, an example of genetic imprinting.[96,97]

The genetic marker for HD (a restriction fragment length polymorphism) was mapped to the short arm of chromosome 4 by Gusella, Martin, and associates in 1983.[98] This was of considerable importance for the diagnosis and prediction of HD and constituted the first example of "reverse genetics," an approach in which the mutant gene is identified without knowing the resultant biochemical defect, reversing the traditional approach.

Recently, the gene has been cloned.[99,100] Its exact chromosomal location is 4q16.3 and it codes for a protein, huntingtin, whose function is not yet known. The defect that causes HD is in the open reading frame of the gene with expansion of a segment of CAG repeats from fewer than 32 to 40 or more copies. There is a statistical association between onset at an earlier age and increased numbers of repeats. Also, the expansion is unstable, so that repeat length varies between affected parents and their affected children. Patients with juvenile HD have 50 to 80 or more copies.[101] The discovery of the Huntington gene now makes it possible to identify with much more certainty a person who has the disease.

It also raises hope that a means may be found to diminish expression of the deleterious gene.

Diagnosis and Prediction   Diagnosis of HD is based on clinical analysis, family history, radioimaging, and recombinant DNA techniques. HD should be considered a possibility in all children or adolescents of both sexes who, after a normal period of development, present with the following abnormalities: clumsiness of hands, and gait disturbances with slowness of voluntary movement, rigidity; chorea or choreoathetosis; progressive dysarthria; scholastic failure, mental deterioration, behavioral or psychic abnormalities; and dementia.

The demonstration of atrophy of the caudate nucleus on radioimaging (and if necessary hypometabolism of this nucleus with the PET scan) provide valuable confirmation without which one should hesitate in making the diagnosis, particularly if the disease is well advanced. Huntington disease can practically always be confirmed by family history. However, at the time of a child's disease, the father (or much more rarely, the mother) may be too young to show changes in cognition and behavior, or evidence of motor dysfunction. The disorder in the parent is sometimes misdiagnosed as Parkinson disease, Alzheimer disease, depression, or schizophrenia. Unfortunately, most of the adult members of a family with the disease will not have learned of it until after their marriage and period of childbearing. DNA analysis will offer the possibility of detecting individuals or even fetuses destined to have the disease. In the absence of any treatment, presymptomatic testing may have a negative impact on individuals and families. Counseling, psychological assessment and support, and post-test follow-up are therefore considered essential whenever genetic testing for HD is being offered. Guidelines for the molecular genetics tests in Huntington disease have been put forward.[102,103]

Pathology   The key neuropathologic characteristic of HD consist of severe neuronal degeneration and astrogliosis in the caudate nucleus and, to a lesser degree, the putamen. The volume of these structures is progressively reduced. The nucleus accumbens (at the ventral aspect of the corpus striatum) is usually relatively spared. At the onset of the disease there may be no discernible neuropathological abnormalities.[104] With traditional neuropathological methods, neuronal loss begins and predominates in the small striatal neurons; the large ones are initially spared. Golgi impregnations, immunohistochemical methods, and the measurement of neurotransmitters have confirmed that the degenerative process is not uniformly expressed in all striatal neurons and that it may be patchy. The medium-sized spiny projecting neurons containing substance P, enkephalins, and GABA are preferentially destroyed. These neurons represent 85 percent of the striatal neurons and receive glutaminergic and dopaminergic afferents. In contrast, interneurons containing somatostatin, neuropeptides, and NADPH diaphorase, and aspiny acetylcholesterase containing interneurons, are spared. This selectivity is under investigation as it may be important. Cell degeneration is not confined to the striatum. Lesser degrees of neuronal loss are found in other structures, particularly in the frontotemporal cortex (the midcortical layers), resulting in mild cortical atrophy and enlargement of the lateral ventricles. Various degrees of nerve cell loss have also been reported in the thalamus, brain stem, spinal cord, and cerebellar cortex. Marked cerebellar atrophy has been remarked upon in some childen.[105] The pallidum is reduced in size from loss of putaminopallidal fibers, but the neuronal population is only slightly reduced. The substantia nigra, in which moderate cell loss has been reported in the pars reticulata, was normal in childhood cases.[105] Measurement of neurotransmitters and neuropeptides in postmortem brain tissue is potentially important for the understanding of the disease and its treatment. Initial results have shown that GABA, acetylcholine, substance P, and cholecystokinin are decreased; somatostatin and neuropeptide Y are increased; dopamine and glutamate are normal. *In vivo* studies with SPECT have shown decreased binding of striatal dopamine D2 receptors.

Clinicopathologic Correlation and Pathogenesis   The clinical manifestations reflect the depletion of neuron populations. Dementia, and probably seizures and myoclonus, reflect nerve cell loss in the cerebral cortex, and possibly the caudate nucleus. The chorea appears to relate to the lesions in the caudate and putamen. Cerebellar ataxia in children correlates with the cell loss in the cerebellar cortex. The rigidity remains unexplained. The substantia nigra is apparently normal in the childhood cases and dopamine levels are normal. Brion and Comoy[105a] correctly point out that the ascription of rigidity to shrinkage of the pallidum, as has been proposed, is surely incorrect because (1) the rigidity is relieved, not caused, by stereotaxic lesions and (2) in pallidoluysian degeneration, athetotic and ballistic movements have occurred instead of rigidity.

The exact pathogenesis of brain lesions in HD is unknown. It has been postulated that nerve cell death could be related to the action of endogenous excitotoxic substances acting on NMDA glutamate receptors. The use of antibodies against huntingtin has demonstrated that this protein is present in HD, especially in nerve cells. The increased amount of polyglutamine that it contains may be excitotoxic, causing apoptosis (death) of nerve cells. This has led to the proposal that substances which inhibit the release of excitotoxic neurotransmitters (such as baclofen) might be beneficial.

Treatment Baclofen (a glutamate antagonist) and diltiazem (a calcium channel blocker that might offset the effect of glutamate on calcium fluxes) have been said to attenuate the symptomatology. Phenothiazines, butyrophenones, and clonazepam block the action of dopamine and have been of some help in suppressing the choreic symptoms (levodopa, on the contrary, induces choreic movements). Cysteamine, also undergoing therapeutic trials, blocks the release of somatostatin, which facilitates the release of dopamine.

Juvenile Parkinson Disease; Juvenile Paralysis Agitans (Ramsay Hunt Disease) A typical parkinsonian syndrome has occasionally appeared in a child or adolescent in whom there was no evidence of WD, HD, or any other known extrapyramidal disorder. Tremor at rest, rigidity, bradykinesia, masked face, flexed postures of the body, and monotonous voice characterize a syndrome whose main features are indistinguishable from those of adult paralysis agitans. Intellectual capacities are generally preserved. Most cases have been sporadic. Familial incidence has been reported only once (two brothers were affected at the ages of 10 and 19 years). The disease progresses slowly into middle or late adulthood. One of the authors (RDA) observed a child who had typical parkinsonism for 10 years and later developed a pyramidal syndrome and dementia.

The idea that juvenile parkinsonism may constitute a specific degenerative disease stems from the anatomic findings of Ramsay Hunt[106] in a 40-year-old patient affected since the age of 15 years. Ramsay Hunt found a marked loss of neurons in the pallidum with replacement gliosis and disappearance of the large cells in the putamen and caudate nucleus. The substantia nigra was said to be normal. Disregarding the striatal lesion, Ramsay Hunt concluded that the disease was a primary atrophy of the pallidal efferent system. In another autopsied case,[107] the anatomic findings were similar except for a slight neuron loss in the substantia nigra and corpus luysi. This second patient had a somewhat atypical clinical

history with marked tremor but no rigidity. Onset was at the age of 7 years. Another of Ramsay Hunt's original cases had an onset at age 10 years and died at age 65 years. The postmortem examination conducted by Davison[108] showed pallor of the globus pallidus and striatal lesions that were said to be "typical of Parkinson's disease." We believe these findings are unreliable.

We are uncertain about the identification of juvenile paralysis agitans as a specific disease entity characterized by a primary degeneration of the large cells in the striatum and the pallidum. Only by further clinical examples and by more refined pathologic and biochemical studies can such an entity be established. Note that pallidal lesions differing only slightly from those described here have been found with a completely different clinical picture (see below).

The possible relationship of juvenile parkinsonism and dopa-responsive dystonia deserves comment. Parkinsonian features occur in some patients with this disease and a parkinsonian syndrome, with a good reaction to levodopa, has been observed in members of families with dopa-responsive dystonia. In one patient, autopsy showed the presence of Lewy bodies and focal nerve cell loss in the substantia nigra.[109]

The etiology of juvenile paralysis agitans has not been determined. Some cases are surely examples of the sequelae of encephalitis, head trauma, or the use of drugs (MPTP). In other instances, the parkinsonian syndrome may be the first phase of a more diffuse disorder of the brain, possibly a metabolic encephalopathy. In a subset of patients with Parkinson disease, familial aggregation occurs in a manner suggesting autosomal dominant inheritance with reduced penetrance.[110] The age of onset in the proband generation is earlier by an average of 17 years than in the parental generation, suggesting genetic anticipation.[111] An unstable trinucleotide repeat is therefore one of the possible etiologies for juvenile Parkinson disease, but this hypothesis awaits molecular DNA proof.

A mitochondrial complex I deficiency has also been implicated in the etiology of Parkinson disease.[112] Reduced activity of complex I has been demonstrated in platelets, muscle, and brain of patients. However, studies using rat brains show that chronic administration of levodopa will itself cause significant reduction in complex I activity. It is therefore likely that the observed reduction in complex I activity in Parkinson disease is due to the fact that, when they were tested for complex I activity, most patients were receiving levodopa.[113]

Familial Diseases with Dystonia (Also Athetosis or Choreoathetosis)

In a number of extrapyramidal disorders, the cardinal clinical manifestation consists of slow, sustained, irregular muscle spasms and abnormal postures interspersed with more rapid involuntary movements. They have been described as *dystonia* (torsion dystonia), athetosis, or choreoathetosis. The differences between these conditions may be subtle. In most of the genetic disorders presenting in this way no biochemical abnormality has been found. Some disorders are associated with a more or less systematically distributed neuronal degeneration predominantly in the basal ganglia, whereas in others there are no detectable changes.

In the medical literature, *dystonia* unfortunately has been used in different ways. It may designate a persistent hypertonic state of any kind that results in a fixed abnormality of posture. Thus, Denny-Brown refers to the hemiplegic posture with flexed arm and extended leg as hemiplegic dystonia and the flexed posture of parkinsonism as flexion dystonia. However, in the following pages we are using the term in its original sense, as described below.

Progressive Hereditary Dystonias The term *dystonia* has been applied to two groups of disorders. The first comprises progressive genetic disorders of unknown origin in which this type of movement abnormality is practically the only manifestation, *the primary idiopathic genetic dystonias.* In the second group dystonia is a symptom of several hereditary neurodegenerative and neurometabolic disorders or some acquired or accidental condition, *the secondary dystonias.* We will consider here successively the semiology of dystonia, and then the primary idiopathic dystonias, the secondary dystonias, and the paroxysmal dystonias.

General Clinical Features of Dystonia In this curious neurologic state, a group of muscles begins inexplicably to be involved in involuntary and sustained spasms that cause abnormal, often distorted, postures (torsion dystonia). It may be confined to, or start in, a particular segment of the body, usually the neck, proximal parts of a limb, or the trunk. Eventually it pervades other parts of the musculature. Dystonic spasms may come on intermittently, being initiated by the adoption of a posture or the performance of a voluntary movement. Each spasm persists for a variable period of time. When evoked by a willed movement, it is at first limited to the engaged part of the body (intention spasm) and it

interferes with the voluntary use of that part; with continued effort, it may spread to other muscles not required in the movement. Brusque jerks of muscles frequently interrupt or are superimposed on the dystonic movement.

In the neck, the head is involuntarily turned, tipped, or retracted by a smooth or jerky spasm that the patient attempts to counteract by contraction of antagonistic muscles. Maintenance of posture is important in its evocation, as is shown in many cases by the disappearance of the torticollis or retrocollis on lying down. In the lumbar region, extensor spasms may arch the back and thrust the pelvis forward, at first only when the patient is upright, but later even during recumbency. One or both shoulders may be elevated (hunched); hips may flex when walking. Only very limited groups of muscles may be affected at first or throughout the illness. Blepharospasms, facial contortions, torticollis and retrocollis, tongue protrusion, Breugel facial distortion syndrome, writer's cramp, and spasmodic dysphonia represent some of these restricted or segmental forms. Emotional excitement tends to enhance dystonic spasms. The patient usually invents some postural or sensory tricks to counteract or alleviate the spasms. They are reduced during periods of quiet and solitude, and they disappear during sleep.

In progressive generalized diseases, the dystonic state ultimately spreads to all muscles until the trunk, neck, and the limb girdle muscles are continuously in spasm; and finally it results in fixed deformities (pseudocontractures) that leave the body contorted. Some patients exhibit athetotic movements in distal parts of the limbs and face, suggesting that any distinction between athetosis and dystonia is only relative. Willed movements remain powerful as long as the dystonia does not interfere. The tendon reflexes are not enhanced and the plantar reflexes are flexor. Resistance to passive movements is variable, tending to be plastic in type; equally characteristic, however, is for all muscular tone suddenly to vanish, leaving the limb slack. The movement disorder becomes more difficult to analyze when other motor abnormalities (tremor, myoclonus) are conjoined, as they are in a few diseases.

Primary Idiopathic Hereditary Dystonias We will consider under this heading the following disorders: dystonia musculorum deformans (idiopathic torsion dystonia), idiopathic focal dystonias, dopa-responsive dystonia, and other rare types of hereditary dystonias.

Idiopathic   Torsion   Dystonia;   Dystonia Musculorum Deformans Idiopathic torsion dystonia (ITD) is an autosomal dominant disease in which generalized dystonic spasms and postures constitute the only neurologic abnormality. No biochemical abnormality is known and the pathology of the disease is indeterminate. The gene of ITD has been located on the long arm of chromosome 9.

Clinical Features The symptoms in most instances appear in childhood or adolescence rarely before the age of 6 years. Initially, one limb (foot or hand), rarely the neck, is involved. It is observed that the episodic spasms are induced by movement of that part, leading to a spasm and distorted posture. Voluntary movements are blocked by the spasm. In our experience with more than a hundred such cases, one lower limb was most often initially affected. At first intermittent, when walking or running, spasms of the foot and leg soon become more frequent and finally persist throughout the waking day. Gradually they spread to the thigh muscles, causing the leg to extend or to flex at the hip. Sometimes the knee flexes, so that the foot is removed from the floor, leaving the patient standing helplessly on one leg. Other parts of the body are later involved: the other leg, the trunk (lordosis and scoliosis), arms, neck (torticollis), and face (blepharospasm). Apart from the focal laryngeal forms of dystonia, dysarthria is generally not an early sign in idiopathic torsion dystonia. In exceptional cases, the disease may begin with spasms of the phonatory muscles (laryngeal stridor), imparting a rough, strained quality to the voice or cause staccato-like interruptions. Later, there may then be a marked dysarthria and dysphagia. In another of our cases, the first sign in a student was blepharospasm. Unlike the diseases that cause athetosis, grimacing is seldom observed. Brief myoclonus-like muscular contractions and tremor are frequently associated.[114] Essential tremor has been reported in family members of patients with dystonia.[115]

Other neurologic signs are conspicuously absent. The tendon reflexes are unaltered, although they may be difficult to elicit because of spasms, and the plantar reflexes are flexor. Sphincteric control is fully preserved. There is no evidence of cerebellar dysfunction. Vision, hearing, and somatic sensation are intact. Intelligence is rarely affected, although late in the course of the disease some degree of intellectual decline may take place. Examinations of the CSF and the EEG are uninformative.

No specific abnormalities have been identified by neuroimaging. A reduced glucose metabolism has been demonstrated by PET scans in the basal ganglia, in the frontal projection field of the mediodorsal thalamic nuclei, and in the frontal cortex.[116] In the early stage of the disease, reduction of sleep and an alteration of sleep pattern has been found.

Progression of disease is very variable even within a family; it may be rapid in the first few months or years and later become stabilized or, rarely, may even improve during late adolescence or adulthood. One of our patients, the brother of a girl with typical dystonia, had a dystonia of one leg which disappeared during early adult life. Age of onset is an important factor in determining prognosis: an early onset is generally associated with a poorer outcome.

If treatment fails, retrocollis and lordosis, or curvature of the trunk, eventually force the patient to remain in a chair or in bed and even lying on the back may be impossible. Recumbency does not relieve the spasms; only deep sleep does this. Any effort of will to move one part may aggravate the spasms in all the muscles; strong emotion also may have the same effect. Permanent deformity of the trunk and horrid contortions are the end stage of the disease, until death from pulmonary infection and inanition terminates the illness.

Diagnostic Laboratory Tests   There is no known diagnostic test. Measurements of neurotransmitters have detected no significant or consistent change. Low homovanillic acid (HVA) in the CSF has been reported. Neuroimaging is not contributory. Molecular genetic linkage studies will provide important diagnostic clues.

Genetics   ITD is an autosomal dominant disorder with 30 to 40 percent penetrance; 15 percent of the cases probably represent new mutations. The disease is particularly frequent (5 to 10 times more common) in Ashkenazic Jews, especially those from Lithuania and Byelorussia.[117] A gene marker for the disease has been linked to the q34 region on chromosome 9, both in Jewish and non-Jewish patients. The prevalence of dystonia has been estimated at 3 to 4 in 100,000, and at 6 to 8 in 100,000 for eastern European Jews living in Israel. The mild segmental forms may be allelic variants. A common mutation is probable in the Ashkenazic Jewish population, since an extended haplotype of polymorphic markers around the dystonia gene on chromosome 9q34 is found in greater than 90 percent of all early-onset affected individuals.[117]

Pathologic Findings   The pathologic alterations have been peculiarly elusive. Neuron loss and gliosis in the striatum and thalamus are described in several reports, but experienced neuropathologists agree that they are difficult to interpret and some deny their existence, claiming such alterations to be artifactual.[118] We, too, have noted the difficulty of demonstrating the lesion but have tended to blame the failure on the inadequacy of the nonquantitative, random-section techniques customarily used in neuropathology. The use of specific nerve cell markers has not been attempted, as far as we know. Prolonged phenothiazine-induced extrapyramidal disturbances in animals and tardive dyskinesia in humans currently have no identified cellular basis, which suggests the possibility of a purely biochemical or subcellular lesion.

Clinicopathologic Correlations and Pathogenesis Lack of a consistently demonstrable lesion leaves all relevant questions unanswered. One assumes the central process to occupy the lenticular nucleus and its diencephalic connections. The involvement of basal ganglia is supported by the studies of glucose metabolism in these structures with the PET scan. Although a morphologic marker for ITD is lacking, there is evidence supporting a neurochemical abnormality in the norepinephrine system, specifically in the ventral diencephalon where the concentration of norepinephrine[119] or its metabolite 3-methoxy-4-hydroxyphenylglycol (MHPG) are reduced.[120]

Differential Diagnosis   Although the clinical picture of a progressive isolated dystonia as described above is fairly characteristic, the diagnosis is frequently missed. ITD must be differentiated from acquired dystonias, such as those resulting from birth injury, head trauma, encephalitis, or drugs (see Chap. 6) and from a number of genetic encephalopathies with an extrapyramidal symptomatology (see below and Tables 5-4 and 6-5). A typical progressive torsion dystonia occurs in familial striatal necrosis (see below).

Treatment   Anticholinergic drugs such as trihexiphenidyl have been shown to be effective in some cases. Starting with 1 mg/day, the dose must be increased progressively. Some patients require more than 60 mg/day. Benzodiazepines may be of some benefit. Drugs which block dopamine receptors (pimozide) have been used with unpredictable results, as has tetrabenazine, a presynaptic dopamine-depleting substance. Some patients have benefited from carbamazepine. Because the dopa-

mine-responsive type of dystonia may be indistinguishable from generalized idiopathic torsion dystonia, it is recommended that all children with idiopathic dystonia should have a therapeutic trial with levodopa/carbidopa.

Idiopathic Focal Dystonias   Idiopathic focal dystonias are essentially encountered in the adult. They are more frequent than infantile generalized torsion dystonias. Their prevalence is 29/100,000. They appear to be related to an autosomal dominant gene or genes.[121] Clumsiness and tremor may be observed in other members of the family. Idiopathic focal dystonias take several forms: cervical dystonia (spasmodic torticollis), cranial dystonia (a combination of blepharospasm and oromandibular dystonia), isolated oromandibular dystonia, isolated blepharospasm, distal dystonia of one limb (for instance writer's cramp), spasmodic dysphonia. Treatment of focal dystonia has been markedly improved by the injection of botulinum toxin into the involved muscles. Local injection of the toxin blocks the release of acetylcholine at the motor nerve terminal, causing chemodenervation which lasts for several months.

Dopa-Responsive Dystonia   Approximately 200 cases of dopa-responsive dystonia (DRD) have been reported, 65 from Japan, 55 from North America, and 66 from Europe and other countries. This type of autosomal dominant childhood dystonia is linked to the q22.1-22.2 locus on chromosome 14, the locus for the GTP cyclohydrolase I.[122] An autosomal recessive mode of inheritance has been suggested for some families. The disease is more common in females. Clinically it may not differ significantly from idiopathic torsion dystonia, although the onset is frequently earlier (from infancy to early adolescence).

Dystonic spasms are first manifest in one or both lower extremities, leading to a gait abnormality which may be misinterpreted as cerebral palsy or some degenerative disorder. Later the extrapyramidal signs spread to the trunk, arms, and neck. Tremor and other parkinsonian features may be added to the neurologic picture in some patients, usually when they reach adulthood.[123] A parkinsonian syndrome has been observed in previously unaffected members of families with DRD. About two-thirds of cases have diurnal fluctuations (Segawa disease) as a characteristic feature[124]; dystonic postures and rigidity tend to appear in late afternoon, being much less pronounced in the morning and after sleep. Neuroimaging is uninformative. The hallmark of the disease is its rapid and remarkable response to small doses of levodopa. When combined with carbidopa, some patients have been maintained symptom-free on as little as 25 mg twice a day. This treatment must be maintained indefinitely.

Reduced synthesis of dopamine in DRD is suggested by low levels of homovanillic acid and biopterin in these children. This hypothesis has been borne out by the recent finding of a deficiency in GTP cyclohydrolase I activity in this disease.[122] This is the rate-limiting enzyme for the synthesis of biopterin, a cofactor for tyrosine hydroxylase which, in turn, is the rate-limiting enzyme for dopamine synthesis. It catalyzes the first step in tetrahydrobiopterin biosynthesis, the conversion of GTP to D-erythro-7,8-dehydroneopterin triphosphate. Residual activity of this enzyme in affected patients is only 2 to 20 percent of normal, rather than the expected 50 percent of normal for heterozygous carriers of an autosomal allele. It therefore appears that the mutant allele causes a dominant negative effect on the normal allele. Unaffected gene carriers have higher levels of residual activity and higher levels of neopterin in the spinal fluid than affected heterozygotes.

Four different mutations have thus far been described. Molecular DNA studies should be able to detect individuals who are at risk. However, since penetrance is not 100 percent, assays of enzyme activity will also be needed in order to predict who is likely to express the disease.

Dystonia-Parkinsonian Syndrome   The parkinsonian syndrome which is occasionally associated with idiopathic dystonia may be so marked as to justify the term *dystonia-parkinsonian syndrome*. Levodopa may or may not be helpful. One of these patients with a progressive extrapyramidal syndrome, consisting of parkinsonian rigidity and dystonia since the age of 6 years, died at 38 years of age. His symptoms had been partially responsive to dopa; autopsy showed presence of Lewy bodies in the substantia nigra, together with a reduced melanin content and only a slight focal loss of neurons in this area.[109] (See also juvenile Parkinson disease.)

A rapid-onset autosomal dominant form of dystonia-parkinsonism has been described in one large family with at least 12 affected members. Symptoms, consisting of both dystonia and parkinsonism, began abruptly and progressed over a few days or weeks. The age of onset was between 14 and 30 years and, in one person, at age 45. Brain CT and MR scans were normal. Levels of HVA in the CSF, measured in two patients, were decreased to 17 percent and 37 percent of normal; levels of MHPG and 5-hydroxyindoleacetic acid

(5-HIAA) were normal in both. There were no autopsy studies. Treatment with antiparkinson medications produced mild or no improvement. Linkage analysis excluded the ITD region at chromosome 9q34.[126]

Other Primary Hereditary Dystonias

1. In alcohol-responsive dystonia or myoclonic dystonia, a rare autosomal dominant disorder starting usually in the first or second decade of life, dystonia and myoclonic jerks are more or less confined to the upper limbs and are remarkably, if transitorily, alleviated by the drinking of alcohol. Benzodiapezines may also have beneficial effects.

2. An adult-onset X-linked recessive form of dystonia associated with parkinsonism has been reported on Panay, one of the Philippine Islands, and has been linked to the q13.1 region of the X chromosome.[125]

The Secondary Hereditary Dystonias   Dystonia (as well as athetosis and choreoathetosis) occasionally occurs in Wilson disease, Huntington disease, choreoacanthocytosis, and other conditions listed in Tables 5-4, 5-7, and 6-5. Dystonia also stands as one of the most striking features of Hallervorden-Spatz disease.

Hallervorden-Spatz Disease   Hallervorden-Spatz disease (HSD) is an autosomal recessive hereditary disorder of unknown etiology. It is characterized by a complicated clinical symptomatology comprising progressive extrapyramidal signs and usually dementia. The neuropathologic changes consist of partial destruction and pigmentary deposits of iron in the pallidonigral region and diffuse axonal swellings (spheroids). As no pathogenic biochemical mechanism has yet been detected, diagnosis rests on the demonstration of the characteristic clinical and pathologic findings. During life, MRI is particularly helpful in revealing typical abnormalities in the globus pallidus. Some cases reported as Hallervorden-Spatz disease had atypical features and their classification remains uncertain.

Clinical Features   In a review of the literature in 1974, Dooling and Richardson[127] found 54 cases corresponding to the clinicopathologic prototype. We have personally observed several patients. Aided by MRI, it is now increasingly often that clinicians can diagnose HSD during life with a high probability of being correct. The first sign may develop at any age between 2 and 15 years but may be delayed until adult life. The disease had become apparent in more than 50 percent of the cases by the age of 10 years and in 80 percent by the age of 15 (Fig. 5-8a).

A progressive disorder of locomotion and involuntary movement of extrapyramidal type are usually the initial manifestations. Dystonic postures, choreoathetotic movements, and rigidity are the main findings. Each of these elements may be the original or predominant sign. Onset with dystonia is usual in childhood, and parkinsonian rigidity is more often the main feature in older patients. Dysarthria appears early in the disease. Tremor may occur but is less prominent and its anatomical basis is not easily determined. The majority of patients eventually show signs of corticospinal involvement and in a few patients a progressive spastic paraplegia is the initial manifestation, as we have observed in two adolescents. Seizures are rare and the EEG is generally normal. Progressive intellectual deterioration becomes evident in nearly all cases, and some children will have been mentally retarded since early childhood. A few patients have normal intelligence. Pigmentary degeneration of the retina has been reported in approximately one-third of the patients and optic atrophy in a few others.

MRI studies reveal a remarkable picture on T2-weighted images: pronounced bilateral hypointensity of the globus pallidus (due to iron accumulation), and in typical cases, a central high-signal area (necrosis), the *tiger eye sign* (Fig. 5-8b).[128]

The disease has a relentlessly progressive course and most of the patients die in the second or third decade of life (see Fig. 5-8a).

Variants It has been emphasized that some patients reported as having Hallervorden-Spatz disease had clinically typical features without the usual distribution of lesions in the brain at autopsy (particularly in the substantia nigra). Other patients, although showing the typical topography of lesions, have shown an atypical clinical syndrome. A few had neurologic signs consisting only of progressive mental retardation. Until the basic defect of this disease is known, these cases should be included only provisionally. Neuroaxonal dystrophy has been considered by some to be a late infantile variant of Hallervorden-Spatz disease. We believe these two conditions should be kept separated (see Chap. 4).

Diagnostic Laboratory Tests No specific biochemical test is available. Routine laboratory investigations are normal, including CSF. Acanthocytosis has been reported in a few cases,[127] possibly indicative of a

separate genetic entity (see HARP syndrome). Serum and urine levels of iron are normal. MRI gives the only important diagnostic lead.

Pathologic Findings and Chemical Pathogenesis These consist of (1) symmetric partial destruction of the inner segment of the globus pallidus and of the pars reticularis of the substantia nigra; (2) accumulation in these areas of pigments resulting in brownish discoloration on macroscopic inspection and giving a positive reaction for iron in stained sections; and (3) argyrophilic spheroid bodies due to axonal swellings, which are found not only in the pallidonigral regions but elsewhere in the gray matter, including the cerebral cortex. Significant elevation of iron has been found in tissue from the basal ganglia.

Although an inborn error of metabolism has been postulated in Hallervorden-Spatz disease, the basic mechanism of the disease is unknown. There is nothing to incriminate a metabolic abnormality of iron, or of vitamin E deficiency (which in animals leads to axonal swellings). Recently it has been shown that diffuse axo-

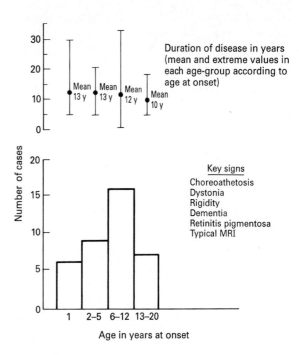

Figure 5-8a

Hallervorden-Spatz disease: age of onset and duration. Key signs.

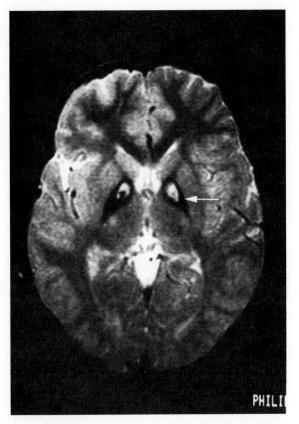

Figure 5-8b
Hallervorden-Spatz disease in an 8-year-old child. MRI T2. Low-signal and central high-signal areas in pallidum (arrow), bilaterally. (Courtesy Dr. C. Gillain.)

nal swellings may also occur in Schindler disease, a metabolic disorder.

A delayed iron disappearance over the basal ganglia after injection of radiolabeled iron (^{59}Fe) has been reported and also an increase of ^{59}Fe uptake by cultured fibroblasts from patients with a normal body iron metabolism. The significance of these findings is uncertain. Studies of the metabolism of biogenic amines have not been informative. A reduced activity of cysteine dioxygenase and low levels of GABA in the pallidum and substantia nigra are of interest.

Involvement of the pallidonigral parts of the brain can be considered as the basis of the extrapyramidal signs. As in neuroaxonal dystrophy, it can be assumed that the abnormalities of terminal axons (spheroids) in the cortex, basal ganglia, and brain stem create a functional disorder which must block synaptic transmission.

This could explain the progressive dementia and other signs. The iron deposits may be secondary to destruction of structures known to be rich in iron.

Differential Diagnosis The diagnosis of Hallervorden-Spatz disease should be considered in a child or adolescent with a progressive extrapyramidal disorder, mental deterioration, retinitis pigmentosa, and characteristic changes on MRI. Other diseases to be considered are all juvenile or adolescent extrapyramidal diseases, especially idiopathic torsion dystonia and juvenile Huntington disease.

Treatment No effective treatment is available. Dopaminergic and anticholinergic drugs have been recommended in cases with a parkinsonian syndrome but the results of such treatment are unimpressive. Benzatropine may occasionally alleviate symptoms. Baclofen may relieve muscle spasm and decrease dystonic posturing, and anticholinergics can control drooling.

The Paroxysmal Dystonias or Choreoathetosis

Transient attacks of dystonic or choreoathetotic involuntary movements occur in several conditions; the patients are normal between attacks. Some are inherited as autosomal dominant traits; others are sporadic. A number of them can be treated effectively. Sometimes it may be difficult to distinguish paroxysmal dystonias from epileptic phenomena. Paroxysmal dystonia (or choreoathetosis) assumes four forms: (1) paroxysmal kinesigenic choreoathetosis (the most frequent), (2) paroxysmal nonkinesigenic choreoathetosis, (3) the rare paroxysmal choreoathetosis induced by prolonged exercise, and (4) hypnogenic paroxysmal choreoathetosis.

Paroxysmal Kinesigenic Choreoathetosis or Dystonia Paroxysmal kinesigenic choreoathetosis or dystonia (PKD) usually starts in childhood and is inherited as an autosomal dominant trait. Males are more often affected than females. Attacks of involuntary movement affecting the limbs conform to the classic descriptions of dystonia, choreoathetosis, chorea, or even ballismus. They are brief, lasting a few seconds to five minutes or more. They are initiated by movement (hence kinesigenic), or upon being startled, especially after a period of rest. They may be unilateral or bilateral. Speech may be impossible, but consciousness always remains normal. Sometimes the attacks are preceded by a brief sensory aura confined to the affected limb. The attack is followed by a brief refractory period. The episodes may occur up to 100 times a day. Between attacks the child is normal. The EEG and brain MRI are not altered. Treatment with anticonvulsant drugs may prevent the attacks. The paroxysmal episodes tend to subside with age.

Paroxysmal Nonkinesigenic Choreoathetosis or Dystonia   Paroxysmal nonkinesigenic choreoathetosis or dystonia (PNKD) is rarer than PKD. Onset is usually in childhood but can begin as late as adult years. Some cases are clearly inherited as an autosomal dominant trait but others have been sporadic. Unilateral or bilateral involuntary movements of the dystonic or choreoathetotic type are not triggered by movement, and the attacks last longer, usually a few minutes to several hours. They, too, may be preceded by a sensory aura. Speech may be arrested, but consciousness is preserved. The paroxysmal episodes are much less frequent than in PKD, and can be separated by intervals of a few days or even months. In one family, relatives of affected patients suffered from painful cramps. Treatment of paroxysmal nonkinesigenic dystonia is generally disappointing. The disorder does not respond to anticonvulsants but may benefit from acetazolamide, a benzodiazepine, or L-tryptophan.

Paroxysmal Choreoathetosis Induced by Exercise   Only very few such families have been reported. The attacks usually develop in the legs, after exercise.

Hypnogenic Paroxysmal Choreoathetosis   In this very rare familial, autosomal dominant disease, attacks of dystonia, choreoathetotis, or ballismic movements occur every night during stages 2 to 4 of non-REM sleep. The EEG is normal. Attacks are usually brief but may last up to one hour. Carbamazepine is generally effective but may not work when the attacks are prolonged. Some individuals also have typical kinesigenic attacks during daytime.

Diagnosis of the Paroxysmal Dystonias   Seizures constitute the main diagnostic problem, particularly those arising from lesions in the frontal region, and especially in the supplementary motor area. Supplementary motor seizures can give rise to tonic posturing of one or more limbs. All sporadic nocturnal attacks of dystonia should be considered of epileptic origin until proven otherwise.

Hereditary Choreas other than Huntington Disease

Apart from the chorea seen in juvenile Huntington disease, choreic movements, combined with other neurological abnormalities, occur in Wilson disease, Hallervorden-Spatz disease, ataxia-telangiectasia, and Lesch-Nyhan disease (Table 6-5). Chorea also stands as the central manifestation of *chorea-acanthocytosis*.

In another group of diseases, chorea is the solitary finding over the lifetime of the patient. The best known example is *benign hereditary chorea*. We have already described paroxysmal kinesigenic choreoathetosis. Chorea from acquired diseases are mentioned in Chap. 6.

Chorea-Acanthocytosis (Neuroacanthocytosis; Levine-Critchley Syndrome)   This is a hereditary disorder with a still uncertain mode of transmission, characterized by the association of chorea and other neurological signs with acanthocytosis of red blood cells. Lipoproteins are normal. Approximately 30 cases have been reported since 1967. We have had occasion to study two of them pathologically.

Clinical Features   Onset is between 8 and 60 years, with a mean age of 32 years. The disorder is slowly progressive and shows many variations in its clinical expression. Chorea is almost always present. Orofaciolingual and pharyngeal dyskinesias give rise to marked dysarthria and dysphagia. The neurological picture is sometimes more complex. Dystonic spasms, akinesia, and parkinsonian rigidity also occur. Uncontrollable vocalizations, ticlike manifestations, and biting of lips and tongue have been observed. Depressed tendon reflexes and distal muscle wasting have been seen in some patients, and electrophysiologic and histologic evidence of an axonal neuropathy were found. Approximately one-third of the patients have seizures. Mental deterioration is a constant feature and psychiatric disturbances and personality changes are frequent.

Neuroimaging studies sometimes show nonspecific signal abnormalities in the caudate and lenticular nucleus. Atrophy and hypometabolism of the caudate nucleus were also reported. In one 40-year-old patient, cerebral blood flow tomography demonstrated severe hypoperfusion in both frontal lobes.[129]

Diagnostic Laboratory Tests   The hallmark of the disease is the presence of red blood cell acanthocytes.

This anomaly of red blood cells is mild in some cases and may be overlooked. Scanning microscopy and other techniques then become useful.[130] Some asymptomatic relatives of patients with neuroacanthocytosis have an isolated acanthocytosis. Serum lipoproteins are normal (contrary to what is seen in abetalipoproteinemia, another neurological disease with acanthocytosis). High levels of creatine phosphokinase in the blood are frequently observed, but the muscles show no histologic abnormality. It has been suggested that an abnormal composition of membrane-bound fatty acids is responsible for acanthocytosis in this disorder.[130]

Genetics The mode of transmission of this hereditary disorder remains uncertain.

Pathology Autopsy in one patient has shown neuronal loss and gliosis in the caudate, putamen, globus pallidus, and the pars reticularis of the substantia nigra. We observed similar findings in our two patients. The cerebral cortex and the spinal cord were spared. In two other patients with clinical parkinsonism, neuronal cell density was reduced in the substantia nigra, most severely in the ventrolateral region. In another patient without parkinsonism, the nigral cell number was at the lower limit of the control range.[132] PET scans using ^{18}F-labeled dopa have provided evidence of a selective loss of dopaminergic projections to the putamen and of D^2 receptor binding sites.

Diagnosis The differential diagnosis involves all other progressive extrapyramidal disorders, particularly Huntington disease. The search for acanthocytes should be undertaken in any patient with this neurologic syndrome. Other disorders with acanthocytosis (including McLeod syndrome[131]) are listed in Table 7-7.

Treatment There is no specific treatment.

Benign Nonprogressive Familial Chorea This disorder is characterized by an isolated nonprogressive chorea starting in infancy or childhood. There are reports on 24 families.[133–137] We have studied 2 families clinically. The inheritance has been autosomal dominant in 20 families, autosomal recessive in 3, and possibly X-linked in 1. Onset is usually in late infancy or early childhood (from 1 to 4 years) or in adolescence. There are typical, rather rapid (jerky), random, purposeless, choreic movements involving the limbs, trunk, neck, and facial musculature. If severe, they may cause difficulty in walking and affect speech.

There may be a postural tremor as well as axial dystonia. The dyskinesia is persistent except during sleep and shows no tendency to worsen as time passes, except occasionally during adolescence. In one of our families, the abnormality of movement was observed in a 5-year-old girl, her 36-year-old father, and 67-year-old grandfather. There are no other neurologic signs, and mental deterioration is conspicuously absent. Although intelligence is generally normal, it was marginally reduced in a few cases. The severity of the disease is variable from case to case, as are the possibilities of adjusting one's life to the disorders. It may occasionally lead to serious motor handicap.[138] Wheeler[138] states that some improvement may be obtained with the use of haloperidol, chlorpromazine, and/or prednisone.

Essential Tremor Essential tremor is relatively common and usually dominantly inherited. It may start in childhood, usually in early adolescence, occasionally as early as 5 years.[81] Tremor is the only sign. Typically the involuntary oscillations (with a frequency of 8 to 10 Hz) predominate in the distal part of the upper extremities; they are absent at rest and increase during voluntary movements and maintenance of posture. The head, neck, lower extremities, and voice are more rarely affected. Shuddering attacks may occur early in the disease.[82] An increased frequency of migraine has been noted. The disorder is slowly progressive. Diagnosis is easy in the presence of a typical family history. Sometimes it needs to be differentiated from cerebellar tremor, and with myoclonus with which it is occasionally conjoined. Essential tremor has also been observed in families with idiopathic dystonia. Most cases of essential tremor do not require treatment. Propanolol, metaprolol, nadolol, primidone, and alcohol have been beneficial. The progressive encephalopathies giving rise to tremor are listed in Table 6-5.

Other Rare Extrapyramidal Disorders

Familial Striatal Necrosis; Familial Dystonias with Putaminal Hypodensities There are cases of childhood familial, slowly progressive dystonia or choreoathetosis with bilateral necrosis of the striatum on neuroimaging or at autopsy, which are apparently unrelated to Leigh syndrome, PDHC deficiency, an organoacidopathy, or some other metabolic disorder. These patients fall into two categories.

In most families with striatal necrosis several children are affected in a sibship, with normal parents, suggesting an autosomal recessive mode of inheritance. There are no other neurological or ocular signs. Mental deterioration is usual but not invariable.[139–143] We have observed three families with this disease. Intelligence was normal in two siblings. In another of our cases, dystonia occurred at the age of 12 years and was for many years unilateral, with radiological evidence of bilateral putaminal necrosis. The dystonia then became generalized. There was no mental deterioration. Recent observations lead us to believe that many cases of familial striatal necrosis are related to mitochondrial disorders.

Striatal necrosis and Leber optic neuropathy has been reported in four families in which a slowly progressive dystonia, starting in childhood with striatal lucencies on CT scans, was associated in some of its affected members with visual failure in early adulthood.[144–146a] Some patients had only amaurosis. The visual failure had a subacute onset, as in Leber optic neuropathy (LHON) and was due to an optic atrophy. Intelligence was conspicuously normal in all cases. Stunting of growth of affected children and nondescript "myopathic signs" were reported in one family.[144] The genetic pattern in these families strongly suggested maternal inheritance. In fact, it has been shown that the variant of LHON with dystonia was associated with point mutation G1 4459A.

Isolated striatal necrosis on MRI and dystonia also occur in some metabolic disorders, particularly glutaric aciduria type I and a few others (Table 5-8). In Leigh disease and other hereditary disorders, necrosis of the striatum is part of a more complex pathologic picture. Acute or subacute striatal necrosis also occurs after an infection or some systemic diseases (Chap. 6).

Table 5-8

Necrosis of the putamen and pallidum in the hereditary metabolic encephalopathies[a]

Leigh disease	Propionic acidemia
PDH E$_1$ deficiency	Methylmalonic acidemia
Leber optic neuropathy	3-Methylglutaconic acidemia[b]
Familial striatal necrosis	Wilson disease
Glutaric aciduria I	

[a]Disorders in which "hypodensities" (lucencies) of the putamen and globus pallidus have been observed on CT scans or MRI as an isolated or dominant morphological abnormality (from the literature and personal observations). This table is not exhaustive.

[b]Case of Dr. G. Ferriere; PDH = pyruvate dehydrogenase.

Familial Bilateral Striopallidodentate Calcinosis (Familial Fahr Disease)   A small number of slowly progressive familial encephalopathies are characterized by isolated bilateral and symmetrical calcifications in the striatum, pallidum, dentate nucleus (and more rarely, the thalamus, cerebral cortex, and cerebellar white matter). The associated neurologic signs are athetosis, dystonia, cerebellar ataxia, seizures and mental retardation in variable combinations. No evidence of hypoparathyroidism, pseudohypoparathyroidism, or kidney disease has been obtained.

The calcifications are seen on CT scans. They can remain clinically silent for years. Neurologic signs usually appear in adolescence or more often in adulthood. In one of our patients, a child with slowly progressive athetosis, the extent of calcification progressed slowly with time. It is likely that this syndrome (frequently called Fahr disease with dubious historic justification) does not represent a homogeneous condition. Nonetheless, a certain number of cases of familial bilateral striopallidodentate calcinosis most likely do represent a distinct entity, with an autosomal dominant mode of inheritance, as was recently pointed out by Manyam et al.[147] In autosomal dominant cases a twofold increase in homocarnosine (a peptide specific to the central nervous system) was found in the CSF, but this abnormality was not detected in sporadic cases in which there were decreased levels of histidine. That the 6-[18]fluoro-L-dopa uptake in the striatum was normal in some cases, despite diffuse calcifications, suggests that the nigrostriatal dopamine pathway was unaltered. Autopsy of patients with striopallidodentate calcinosis has shown that calcifications are mainly located around vessel walls and that neuronal loss is usually mild. The pathogenesis of the calcium deposits and the cause of the neurologic disorder remain unknown.

Numerous disorders occurring during childhood and adolescence are liable to give rise to basal ganglia calcifications. Some are acquired and may be due to infections such as HIV infection, ischemia, or radiotherapy. Others are related to hereditary disorders, such as Cockayne syndrome, mitochondrial encephalopathies, the Aircardi-Goutieres syndrome; or they may be a feature of primary hypoparathyroidism (an X-linked disease characterized by tetany, seizures, cataracts and low calcium and high phosphorus levels in the serum). Pseudohypoparathyroidism is another cause. A rare autosomal recessive disorder, carbonic anhydrase II deficiency, gives rise to extensive brain calcifications in addition to renal acidosis, dense bones, mental retardation, and dysmorphic facial features (marble bone-marble brain disease).[148] A mild degree of perivascular calcifications in the lenticular nucleus may be found at autopsy or by CT scans of individuals devoid of neurological signs.[149] (For brain calcifications see also Chap. 6 and Chap. 8.)

Progressive Athetosis with Skeletal Dysplasia and Keratan Sulfaturia Seven cases have been reported (four belonging to one sibship) of a condition combining progressive athetosis, abnormalities of the vertebral and femoral heads, corneal opacities, and urinary excretion of keratan sulfate.[150] Both sexes were affected. Kyphosis and limitation of mobility of the coxofemoral joints were usually the first signs, followed soon (at the age of 5 to 7 years) by the appearance of athetosis. The involuntary movements increased progressively, eventually affecting the facial musculature and resulting in a severe dysarthria. There were no pyramidal signs. Intelligence has been relatively normal in most cases. Bony abnormalities consisted of anterior beaking of the vertebrae at the thoracolumbar junction and an irregular flattening of the femoral heads. Corneal opacities were observed under the slit-lamp. β-Galactosidase was absent in a liver biopsy specimen in one case. The disease was slowly progressive and was considered as an example of a new form of mucopolysaccharidosis.

Febrile Episodes with Loss of Consciousness in a Family with Athetosis and Mental Retardation Considering the deleterious effect of hyperthermia on individuals with any type of cerebral damage, it is not certain that the fever is an essential part of the syndrome. Nevertheless, the family reported by Harvey et al.[151] included a father and five children who had a progressive athetosis and mental deterioration that worsened intermittently after each episode of fever and coma.

Syndrome of Choreoathetosis, Dystonia, and Pallidal Atrophy A few cases have been reported,[152,153] occurring either sporadically or in siblings (two brothers in one family), of a disease beginning between the ages of 5 and 15 years and characterized by athetosis, torsion spasms, and brusque choreic movements. The disorder started on one side of the body and later became generalized. Grimacing, dysarthria, and dysphagia were prominent. Intellectual faculties were preserved. Progression of the disease was steady, with death occurring after 5 to 10 years. In five autopsied cases the lesions were restricted to the globus pallidus with nerve cell loss and gliosis and disappearance of efferent

nerve fibers. This pure pallidal atrophy has been rather arbitrarily separated from the pallidal atrophy with more diffuse involvement of the basal ganglia described previously as juvenile paralysis agitans. No metabolic basis has been established.

Hypoprebetalipoproteinemia, Acanthocytosis, Retinitis Pigmentosa, and Pallidal Degeneration (HARP Syndrome) An 11-year-old girl presented with dystonia, orofacial dyskinesia, retinitis pigmentosa, and progressive dementia. There was a hypoprebetalipoproteinemia, low serum cholesterol, acanthocytosis, and abnormal signals in the pallidum comparable to those seen in Hallervorden-Spatz disease.[154]

Primary Degeneration of Corpus Luysi In this condition, reported by Malamud and Demmy,[155] two children aged 5 and 6 years developed bilateral choreoathetosis with some elements of severe chorea or ballismus. Mental deterioration and increased emotionality became manifest as the disease advanced. Postmortem examination revealed a selective degeneration of each corpus luysi. Also a Wernicke-like spongy degeneration was seen in the periaqueductal region and mamillary bodies. It seems possible that this disease is a form of subacute necrotizing encephalomyelopathy (Leigh syndrome). Another family with hereditary ballismus attributed to degeneration of the corpus luysi has been reported. Postmortem examination was not performed.[156]

Familial Nonprogressive Athetosis Cases of familial nonprogressive choreoathetosis are extremely rare. In one Swiss family examined by one of the authors (RDA), the disease had severely disabled one small girl (age 3 years) and had reduced the motor activities of her brother (age 8 years) to the point that he could only roll on the floor to get around, and had to turn the pages of a book with his nose. He had to be fed by his parents, and communicated by spelling words indicated with a nod to the appropriate letters of the alphabet. Their two cousins were affected to a lesser degree: one was an 18-year-old girl whose legs were affected but was still able to travel alone by train, to talk, and to study accounting; the other was a 30-year-old man who worked in a factory and was the best marksman in the village. Every postural adjustment and voluntary effort in these individuals evoked a slow mobile spasm that spread to much of the musculature of the body. There was a more or less continuous rigidity of the limbs. The facial and bulbar muscles usually tended to be involved and made it difficult to speak, chew, and swallow. No ataxia, tremor, myoclonus, dystonic deformity of trunk, or pyramidal signs were present. Mentation was little affected, if at all.

The pathology of such conditions is unknown and it is unwarranted to conclude that familial athetosis corresponds to the disease called *état dysmyelinique* (status dysmyelinisatus) described by Vogt and Vogt, which is discussed below.

Status Dysmyelinisatus of Vogt Vogt and Vogt[157] reported these pathologic findings in two related children. One was born after a 7-months gestation and never sat up or walked; he displayed athetosis and had frequent seizures. Intelligence was said to be normal at the time of death at age 10 years. The second child was born after an 8-months gestation and showed spasticity in the first year of life in conjunction with athetosis, dysarthria, dysphagia, and seizures. Death occurred at 8 years. In neither case was there progressivity of the disease under consideration. The first child had a small brain; in both children there was marked atrophy of the pallidum and corpus luysi, and loss of medullated striopallidal and pallidoluysian fibers. Because of the paucity of the neuronal loss, the Vogts decided to call this condition status dysmyelinisatus, but their description lacks precision. Many neuropathologists are of the opinion that the pathologic picture does not represent a progressive degenerative disease but instead the sequelae of acute damage consequent to anoxia or kernicterus.

Summarizing Remarks on Progressive Genetic Extrapyramidal Disorders From this account of the progressive genetic extrapyramidal diseases of childhood and adolescence, it is clear that Wilson disease is the most frequent and easily recognized as it has specific corneal and biochemical abnormalities. Diagnosis of Huntington disease is based on a positive family history, which is constantly present, and on modern techniques of neuroimaging and molecular genetics. The diagnosis of the primary progressive dystonias rests essentially on clinical findings, response to treatment (levodopa), and on the availability of DNA markers linked to the gene. Hallervorden-Spatz disease is also a consistent clinicopathologic entity. As the major clinical signs—choreoathetosis, dystonia, pyramidal signs, retinitis pigmentosa, dementia—are not specific, diagnosis is based on typical MRI findings. Dystonia and other extrapyramidal manifestations may also be a feature of a number of metabolic encephalopathies, such as Leigh disease, juvenile lipofuscinosis, and other lysosomal diseases. The differential characteristic of the most

important genetic extrapyramidal disorders are summarized in Tables 5-4, 5-7, and 6-5.

Only Wilson disease and a form of dopa-responsive torsion dystonia can be successfully treated. One must be prepared to diagnose them early in their course. Presymptomatic and prenatal detection are possible in Wilson disease and in Huntington disease. But in the absence of treatment, difficult psychological and ethical problems may be raised when this procedure is applied to the latter disease.

Of the the many rare extrapyramidal disorders, it will be impossible to list them all. Some constitute distinct entities and have recognizable features. This is true of dystonias with striatal necrosis and of choreaacanthocytosis. The presence of an apparently isolated dystonic syndrome indicates a therapeutic trial with levodopa; brain scans should be repeated as striatal lesions may be found only in the advanced stages of the disease, and acanthocytosis should be systematically searched for in all progressive diseases with chorea or other extrapyramidal signs.

It is obvious also that a number of other families with progressive extrapyramidal disorders have been described whose illnesses do not fit into the above categories, although they bear clinical resemblance to certain of them. Frequently only one family has been reported. One major difficulty in classifying these diseases is that at present they are identified solely on clinical and pathologic grounds, and specificity of pathologic findings may be lacking. To increase the complexity of the problem, clinicoanatomic correlations are so inexact that they do not serve in diagnosis. For example, the so-called pallidal atrophies are alleged to occur in connection with several different clinical pictures; grouping of cases purely according to the described phenotype is frequently inadequate because of the careless usage of such terms as tremor, chorea, athetosis, and dystonia. One must assume that the classification of these conditions will remain difficult and their nosology uncertain until the biochemical pathogenesis is better known and specific biochemical and pharmacological tests and DNA markers become available.

FAMILIAL POLYNEUROPATHIES IN JUVENILE METABOLIC DISEASE

Involvement of the peripheral nervous system occurs in a number of metabolic diseases *in infancy and early childhood*, and in most of them (such as Krabbe leukodystrophy and metachromatic leukodystrophy), it is associated with clinical manifestations of a disorder of the central nervous system. Even if not predominant, the affection of the nerves assumes diagnostic importance. Often the clinical evidence of a peripheral neuropathy is slight and needs electrophysiological (by measurement of nerve conduction velocities) and in some cases histologic (biopsy) confirmation. (See Chaps. 3 and 4.)

In a few of the *juvenile and adult metabolic disorders*, a polyneuropathy is a prominent feature and may exist for some time before obvious signs of involvement of other parts of the nervous system or visceral organs become apparent. This is true of Refsum disease, familial amyloid polyneuropathy, Tangier disease, Fabry disease, some cases of giant axonal neuropathy, juvenile metachromatic leukodystrophy, adult polyglucosan disease, and more rarely, mitochondrial disorders and peroxisomal disorders. All are conditions in which evidence of other neurologic and visceral disturbances invariably appear in the course of the disease.

In Charcot-Marie-Tooth disease and Déjerine-Sottas disease, a distal sensorimotor neuropathy is the only manifestation. This group of disorders, by far the most frequent type of hereditary sensorimotor polyneuropathy, was presented as a differential diagnosis of the metabolic neuropathies in the first edition of this book. It is now known that they may have a metabolic origin, since it has been discovered recently that most cases of the Charcot-Marie-Tooth syndrome and also Déjerine-Sottas disease are related to a genetic defect of myelin proteins. They will therefore be discussed here.

Metabolic disorders in which there is evidence of either a polyneuropathy or lower motor neuron disease are listed in Table 6-9.

The hereditary sensory neuropathies, including Riley-Day syndrome, will be considered in Chap. 6.

Refsum Disease (Phytanic Acid Storage Disease; Heredopathia Atactica Polyneuritiformis)

Refsum disease[158] is an autosomal recessive disorder associated with a defect in the α oxidation of phytanic acid; this results in the accumulation of this substance in the nervous system and other tissues. The cardinal manifestations of the disease are retinitis pigmentosa and a progressive, often remitting, polyneuropathy with high CSF protein; a neurosensory deafness; and more rarely, a cerebellar ataxia. Intelligence remains normal. Ichthyosis, cardiac involvement, and bone changes are found in some cases. Dietary restriction of phytanate has beneficial effects.

Clinical Features   Onset of the disease is usually in the second or third decade of life. Approximately one-third of the cases become apparent before the age of 10 years, some as early as 4 or 5 years; onset as late as the fifth decade has also been reported. The disease usually evolves slowly and progressively. Visual failure frequently precedes the gait disturbance due to the polyneuropathy. Night blindness (nyctalopia) due to the pigmentary degeneration of the retina often constitutes the first, frequently neglected, symptom. Only the peripheral parts of the visual fields are at first affected and there is still a fairly good diurnal visual acuity. Photophobia may occur. Extinction of the ERG may precede typical ophthalmologic signs of pigmentary degeneration of the retina. Cataracts may later contribute to the visual impairment. Miosis and poor pupillary response to light are noted in some cases.

The peripheral neuropathy develops insidiously and may pursue an unremitting course. With the passage of time weakness, atrophy of the limb musculature, and distal sensory disturbances, particularly of proprioception, appear. Tendon reflexes are abolished. Peripheral nerves may be palpably enlarged. Nerve conduction velocities are low. The CSF protein concentration is elevated. In more than half the patients there are dramatic subacute exacerbations of the polyneuropathy (with no cells in the CSF), which may last for a few weeks. The symptoms thereafter gradually recede, only to recur a few months or years later, mimicking an idiopathic chronic relapsing polyneuritis of inflammatory origin.

Cerebellar ataxia may be superimposed on the sensory ataxia and weakness, being manifested by slurred speech, intention tremor, and dyssynergia. Nystagmus may be present but is usually of a type that accompanies amaurosis. The incoordination and unsteadiness observed in a number of patients with Refsum disease are probably more related to the sensorimotor neuropathy than to cerebellar dysfunction.

Hypoacusis or deafness is detected in approximately two-thirds of the cases and may be an early sign. Results of discrimination tests suggest that the hearing loss is of sensorineural (cochlear) type. Anosmia is a frequent abnormality. The intelligence level is usually normal and does not change.

Rough, scaly thickening of the skin over the extremities is seen in a number of patients. Involvement of the heart is evidenced by ECG abnormalities such as impaired atrioventricular conduction and bundle branch block. Progressive heart failure has been reported, and some of the few reported cases of sudden death in this disease may have been of cardiac origin. Some patients have had a shortening of the metacarpal or metatarsal bones or an epiphyseal dysplasia.

Phytanic acid concentrations are constantly elevated in the serum and urine, and this constitutes a specific abnormality that is pathognomonic of Refsum disease.

The course of the disease extends over many years, frequently several decades, with periods of dramatic remission and exacerbation of the neuropathy. Exacerbation of the neuropathy sometimes appears to be evoked by an infectious illness. Death has usually been due to respiratory paralysis or cardiac failure.

Diagnostic Laboratory Tests   Plasma levels of phytanic acid (measured by gas-liquid chromatography) are considerably elevated (5 mg/dL to over 100 mg/dL; normal never over 0.5 mg/dL), and there is a marked reduction of the ability of a patient's cultured fibroblasts to oxidize phytanic acid.

Genetics   Refsum disease is inherited as an autosomal recessive trait. There is no ethnic prevalence. Heterozygotes show a 50 percent reduction in phytanic acid oxidation by cultured fibroblasts. They have no clinical manifestations.

Pathologic Findings   Peripheral nerve lesions consist of an overall increase in the diameter of the nerves, a loss of myelinated fibers, and onion-bulb formations of Schwann cells, like those in Charcot-Marie-Tooth and in Déjerine-Sottas diseases. Lipid inclusions and intramitochondrial crystalline deposits, none of which are specific, have been reported in Schwann cell cytoplasm. The CNS lesions are neither constant nor specific. In some cases there has been a degeneration of Purkinje cells, and of neurons in the dentate nuclei, inferior olives, and vestibular, cochlear, and red nuclei. The pigmentary and sensory epithelium of the retina are partly destroyed. Lipid inclusions are noted in hepatocytes. Phytanic acid has been found in excess in the brain, peripheral nerves, kidneys, and other organs.

Pathogenesis   Refsum disease is almost certainly due to a single gene defect involving an enzyme responsible for the α oxidation of phytanic acid,[160] a substance entirely derived from exogenous sources. The mechanism by which phytanic acid accumulation creates lesions in the nervous system and other organs remains unresolved. One possibility is that the incorporation of phytanic acid into membrane structures alters their properties and impairs their function. Phytanic acid

also accumulates in the serum of patients with peroxisomal disorders such as Zellweger disease, neonatal adrenoleukodystrophy, and infantile Refsum disease (completely different from Refsum disease). The total lack of peroxisomes in these disorders strongly suggests that they play a role in phytanic acid catabolism. While mitochondria are able to metabolize phytanic acid, the rate of oxidation in peroxisomes is 20 times greater.[161] In the Zellweger syndrome, a global defect of peroxisomal function results in multiple biochemical abnormalities, including defects in the metabolism of pristanic acid (a derivative of phytanic acid) and other fatty acids. In this syndrome, there is a secondary defect of phytanic acid α oxidation. Instead, in classic Refsum disease there is most probably a selective defect of the enzyme(s) responsible for α oxidation of phytanic acid.

Differential Diagnosis   A definitive diagnosis of Refsum disease requires the demonstration of markedly elevated levels of phytanic acid in plasma and a reduction in the ability to oxidize phytanic acid in a patient's cultured fibroblasts.

The following conditions must be differentiated: all types of hereditary pigmentary degenerations of the retina; the hereditary sensorimotor polyneuropathies of Charcot-Marie-Tooth type, metabolic diseases with polyneuropathies, and chronic idiopathic relapsing polyneuritis.

Treatment   All phytanic acid comes from dietary sources, and dietary restriction reduces the plasma and tissue levels. Treatment of Refsum disease requires drastic reduction of phytanic acid intake.[160] On a low phytanate diet, plasma levels may be slow to fall (because of large stores of phytanic acid in adipose tissues). Plasmapheresis or plasma exchange has been advised in some cases, especially when starting the dietary treatment and possibly during subacute relapses. Dietary restriction has had remarkable but partial results on the polyneuropathy and possibly on the ECG.

It is important to screen the siblings of an affected individual to find the presymptomatic or paucisymptomatic stage of the disease and to initiate early treatment. Prenatal diagnosis is possible.

Familial Amyloid Neuropathies   Familial amyloid neuropathies (FAP), first described by Andrade in 1952, constitute a group of autosomal dominant disorders characterized by the extracellular accumulation of abnormal forms of prealbumin (transthyretin) in peripheral nerves and other organs such as the heart, eyes, and kidneys. Several mutations leading to substitutions of single amino acids in the transthyretin molecule coded on chromosome 18 have been detected. The most frequent substitution is methionine for valine at position 30 of the transthyretin molecule (Met 30).

The familial amyloid neuropathies (FAN) occur almost exclusively in adults with onset between 20 and 35 years, sometimes later. But the diagnosis cannot be excluded when an adolescent or a child develops a polyneuropathy.

The disease is endemic in northern Portugal (where 517 kindreds have been discovered), and clusters of cases have been found in many parts of the world in individuals of Portuguese ancestry. But the same type of disease has been encountered in non-Portuguese families in various countries, particularly in Sweden and Japan and in the United States.

The hallmark of the disease is a progressive sensory and autonomic polyneuropathy.

Clinical Features   The first and major manifestation of the "Portuguese type" of FAN consists of a predominantly sensory neuropathy with pain and parathesias, starting generally in the distal portion of the lower limbs and spreading progressively and symmetrically to the hands and arms (FAP I). In some cases, onset is in the upper limbs. An isolated carpal tunnel syndrome occurs in one type (FAP II). Loss of pain, temperature, and touch sensation is more prominent than loss of vibratory and position sense (some cases have been misdiagnosed as syringomyelia). Neurogenic plantar ulcers and trophic arthropathies occur late in the disease.

Sensory disturbances precede weakness and amyotrophy by 2 to 3 years. The tendon reflexes are abolished.

An autonomic impairment is always present to some degree and may be the first to attract attention. Its manifestations include gastrointestinal symptoms (diarrhea alternating with constipation, vomiting, and gastric distension), a hypotonic bladder, sphincter dysfunction, orthostatic hypotension, and impotence. Pupils frequently fail to react to light and may be irregular. The CSF protein is generally elevated. Mental function is normal.

There are also manifestations of systemic amyloidosis. Cardiovascular disturbances are common. There may be a cardiomyopathy with conduction disturbances, such as atrioventricular and left bundle block (which can require pacemaker implantation), and heart failure. Amyloid vitreous opacities are characteristic and may

lead to a loss of vision that can be relieved by vitrectomy. There may be albuminuria, and later in the disease, a nephrotic syndrome and renal failure, especially in cases of apolipoprotein A-1 deposition (FAP III) and with defects in the fibrinogen α chain. A corneal lattice dystrophy together with a progressive cranial and peripheral neuropathy are characteristic of the Finnish type of FAN (FAP IV).

Malnutrition and a marked weight loss are usual. Death occurs after 10 to 15 years, sometimes longer, from renal and cardiac failure and cachexia.

Clinical Diagnosis   The main signs raising suspicion of HAN are the following:

1.   A patient of Portuguese origin.

2.   A sensory polyneuropathy with analgesia and thermoanesthesia and less prominent motor paralysis.

3.   Other medical findings such as gastrointestinal symptoms, bladder dysfunction, orthostatic hypotension, an abolished pupillary photomotor reflex (attributable to an autonomic neuropathy) signs of renal failure, and clinical and ECG evidence of myocardial disease.

4.   The presence of ocular findings such as amyloid opacities in the vitreous humor and a corneal lattice dystrophy.

Genetics   At least four different genes have been implicated in the etiology of the hereditary amyloid neuropathies.

1.   Transthyretin, coded on chromosome 18

2.   Apolipoprotein A-1 (apo A-1), located on chromosome 3

3.   Gelsolin, which maps to chromosome 9

4.   The α chain of fibrinogen A on chromosome 4

Although more than 40 different mutations have been found in the transthyretin gene, the only mutations thus far described in the gelsolin gene have been confined to codon 187; similarly, for the Apo A-1 and fibrinogen α genes only two mutations are so far known. Amyloid fibril deposition occurs in the heterozygous state so that these mutations act as dominant alleles.

Laboratory Tests   On biopsies of the sural nerve the presence of deposits within the nerve structure which are stained with antitransthyretin antibodies proves the diagnosis of FAN.

For further characterization of the disease and detection of gene carriers for preclinical and prenatal diagnosis two methods can be employed. (1) Isolation and characterization of the abnormal transthyretin in the plasma. The Met 30 prealbumin test can be done on small amounts of plasma. (2) Direct DNA analysis using the Southern blot technique to detect abnormal transthyretin genes. Also DNA tests have been devised for several of the transthyretin variant genes including Met 30, offering excellent possibilities of presymptomatic and prenatal diagnosis. If these are normal, DNA analyses for mutations in the Apo A-1, gelsolin and fibrinogen α chain genes should be carried out.

Pathology   The peripheral nerves, which are usually not enlarged, contain extracellular deposits of amyloid in the endoneurium, walls of blood vessels and in the basal lamina of Schwann cells. Infiltrates also occur in the epineurium and perineurium.

Analysis of fiber sizes[162] reveals that the nonmedullated and small medullated fibers are disproportionately depleted, whereas the large ones tend to be preserved. This is the converse of most types of neuropathy and explains the unusual sensory pattern of analgesia and dysautonomia.

The spinal and autonomic ganglia are also involved. Heavy amyloid deposits may be found in the meninges, but the brain tissue is spared.

Usually moderate deposits of amyloid are seen in various tissues: kidneys, heart, gastrointestinal tract, endocrine glands, skin, etc.

Variants   As noted, in addition to the Met 30 mutation—the most commonly reported gene defect—a number of other mutations (substitutions of a single amino acid) in the transthyretin gene have been identified.[162] Some have tended to be associated with a clinical picture differing from the common Portuguese type with respect to age of onset, rate of progression, and relative distribution of organ involvement. A particularly early-onset aggressive form of the disease has been observed in a family with the transthyretin Pro[55] variant.[163] Mutations in the transthyretin gene may also give rise to amyloid cardiomyopathies without a neuropathy.

Treatment   Treatment of FANs remains purely symptomatic. Detection of carriers, prenatal diagnosis, and genetic counseling are essential.

Tangier Disease (Familial High-Density Lipoprotein Deficiency)   Tangier disease is a rare autosomal recessive hereditary disorder characterized by a severe deficiency of high-density lipoproteins (HDLs) in the plasma and storage of cholesterol esters in many tissues. Clinically, the most important deposits of cholesterol esters are found in the faucial tonsils, spleen, liver, bone marrow, and corneas. A peculiar polyneuropathy has been present in most cases. The unique appearance of the enlarged yellow-orange tonsils and the low plasma cholesterol with normal or elevated triglycerides are characteristic.

The primary defect underlying the disease is unknown, but is believed to involve defective translocation of lipids from Golgi structures. This disruption in the movement though intracellular organelles results in accumulation within macrophages of triglycerides, phospholipids, and cholesterol esters, and a failure of these cells to assemble HDLs with intracellular lipids.

Clinical Features   Tangier disease was first described in 1960. Approximately 40 cases had been reported in 1989 from several different countries. Most but not all of them had a neuropathy which was first manifest in childhood or adolescence. The form of the polyneuropathy has been most unusual. In some patients, the most striking sign is analgesia. Pain and temperature sensation are abolished, especially in the arms and head. This is associated with a slight degree of weakness of the face and muscles of the upper extremities. The tendon reflexes are diminished or absent. Loss of pain and temperature sensation may be found over most of the body. This symptomatology is suggestive of syringomyelia. Other patients have developed asymmetric, fluctuating parasthesias and tactile loss. A single limb may be affected. Cranial nerves may be involved. The clinical picture may be that of a relapsing multiple mononeuropathy. A slowly progressing symmetrical polyneuropathy occurs in other cases. Changes in the EMG and nerve conduction velocities are inconstant and variable. CSF proteins may be slightly elevated. Biopsies of the sural nerve reveal vacuoles in Schwann cells, mostly in the unmyelinated fibers.

Deposits of orange-colored cholesterol esters on the tonsils or oropharyngeal mucosa are a unique manifestation of Tangier disease. Most patients have had splenomegaly with thrombocytopenia and foam cells in bone marrow smears and skin biopsies. Hepatomegaly, lymphadenopathy, and corneal opacities on slit-lamp examination are more rarely observed. Intestinal function is normal and there is no acanthocytosis. By proctoscopy one may see orange spots in the intestinal mucosa.

The course of Tangier disease seems to be relatively benign. The greatest threat to life is atherosclerosis. Several of our patients have had coronary thromboses at an early age, so life expectancy cannot be considered normal.

Diagnostic Laboratory Tests Lipoprotein electrophoresis shows a virtual absence of HDLs. Plasma apolipoprotein A-1 is extremely low. Fasting chylomicronemia is often observed. Total plasma cholesterol is low, and the level of triglycerides normal or elevated.

Heterozygotes in families with known homozygotes have low HDL concentrations.

Pathological Findings Very few postmortem studies of the peripheral nervous system have been reported. Loss of myelinated fibers has been observed. In the syringomyelia-like form, degeneration of small myelinated and unmyelinated fibers prevails and spinal ganglion cells contain numerous membrane-bound lipid inclusions.[164] Lipid storage has not been found in the central nervous system.

Foam cells are present in supravital preparations of the bone marrow and the reticuloendothelial system of various other organs; they are seen to contain doubly refractile, sudanophilic, PAS-negative droplets. They give a positive reaction with the Schultz stain for cholesterol. The lipid deposits are generally extralysosomal.

Clinicopathologic Correlations The nature of the primary defect in Tangier disease and the pathogenesis of the polyneuropathy are unknown.

The mechanism by which cholesterol esters accumulate in the tissue is certainly related to the normal role of HDLs in reverse cholesterol transport, and therein lies a point of great interest in this rare disease.

Treatment No specific treatment is known.

Fabry Disease (α-Galactosidase Deficiency) Fabry disease is an X-linked inherited disorder caused by a deficiency of the lysosomal hydrolase α-galactosidase A. The enzymatic defect leads to the accumulation of glycosphingolipids with α-galactosyl moieties—predominantly globotriaosylceramide (trihexosylceramide: Gal-Gal-Glc-Cer), to a lesser extent galabiosylceramide (digalactosyl ceramide: Gal-Gal-Cer), and blood group B substances—in body fluids and tissues, especially in blood vessels, central and peripheral autonomic nervous system, and corneas. The accumulation of glycosphingolipids in kidneys and cerebral vessels leads in adulthood to renal failure and strokes; these are the main causes of death.

Neurologic involvement results in recurrent attacks of burning pains of the extremities, frequently associated with physical activity and fever. These begin in childhood and continue throughout life. Typical telangiectatic skin lesions, called angiokeratomas, and corneal opacities are the most easily recognizable stigmata of this disease. Heterozygous females may have an attenuated form.

The gene encoding α-galactosidase has been localized to the long arm of the X chromosome at Xq22.1. More than 50 different mutations have been described, most confined to a single pedigree.[165]

Clinical Features Over 400 cases have been reported. Hemizygous males display the full-blown pathologic picture. The disease becomes evident at any time in late childhood or adolescence. Either neurologic or cutaneous manifestations may be the first to attract attention. The principal neurologic sign is recurrent episodes of burning or lancinating pain in the extremities, mostly in the fingers and toes, accompanied by paresthesias. Pain and discomfort may be extreme. In some patients they are induced by changes in body temperature due either to physical activity, infection, or other causes. During episodes of pain, which may last several days or weeks, fever and elevation of erythrocyte sedimentation rate are frequently found. Edema of the hands and feet may occur. Crises of abdominal pain and episodes of diarrhea are not uncommon. After the attack is over, the neurologic examination may be virtually normal.

Hypohydrosis is reported. The small cutaneous telangiectasias of angiokeratoma appear as punctate, dark red, flat or slightly raised lesions symmetrically distributed especially between the umbilicus and the knee. Telangiectases are also seen in the oral mucosa. Although not present in every case, they occur with high density in skin surfaces exposed to frequent stretching or stress.

There are also corneal opacities, which have been observed as early as the age of 6 months. They are located in the deep layers of the epithelium and appear initially as a diffuse haze (seen only with the slit-lamp) and later as fine, straight, or curved lines radiating from the periphery toward the center of the cornea in a very characteristic pattern. A peculiar type of cataract in the form of feathery white lines radiating from the posterior capsule of the lens has been reported. There may also be tortuosities of conjunctival and retinal vessels (Fig. 5-9).[166] Cutaneous and ocular signs may be concomitant with the neurologic manifestations, but are also observed before the attacks of pain, especially when systematically searched for in the kindred of a patient affected with Fabry disease.

Signs of incipient renal dysfunction appear in late childhood, but severe renal insufficiency and hypertension usually do not develop before adulthood. Thrombotic cerebrovascular lesions are most likely to appear during early or middle adulthood. They cause focal cerebral signs, such as aphasia and hemiplegia, and also seizures.

Joint and bone lesions are not exceptional. Arthritis of the distal interphalangeal joints and necrosis of the femoral heads have been reported. Chronic pulmonary insufficiency is another possible complication of the disease. Intestinal diverticuli may develop, a potentially serious complication.

Foam cells can be found in bone marrow preparations and lipid-laden cells are seen in the urine sediment.

Death occurs most often as a result of uremia or cerebrovascular disease, usually between the ages of 40 and 50 years.

Atypical Variants and Mild Forms   Mild forms of Fabry disease, with sufficient residual activity of α-galactosidase A to prevent or markedly delay and reduce the major manifestations of the disease, have been reported in adults.[167] These individuals were either asymptomatic or presented with proteinuria, heart disease, or isolated acroparesthesias. In several patients the clinical manifestations and evidence of substrate accumulations were restricted to the heart (cardiomyopathy).

Diagnostic Laboratory Tests   Confirmation of the clinical diagnosis in hemizygotes requires (1) demonstration of a deficient α-galactosidase A activity in plasma, leukocytes, tears, or cultured skin fibroblasts; there is generally no detectable activity of this enzyme in affected males; in some atypical cases (see under "Variants") some residual activity of α-galactosidase may be detected; and (2) demonstration of increased levels of globotriaosylceramide in plasma and urinary sediment. In atypical cases skin, conjuctiva, or kidney biopsies may serve to detect the typical intralysosomal inclusions.

The biochemical tests should be performed in all siblings and in the parents and relatives of an affected boy in order to find preclinical hemizygotes and hetero-

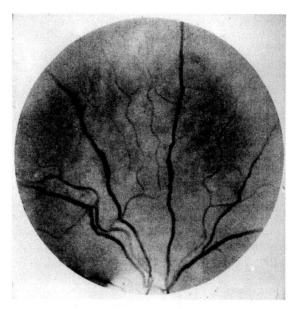

Figure 5-9
Fabry disease: focal dilatations of retinal vessels.

zygote female carriers. These data, as well as the result of genetic molecular studies in the affected child and his relatives, are essential for prenatal diagnosis.

Heterozygous females, because of random X-chromosome inactivation, may have levels of α-galactosidase A ranging from zero to normal. There may also be an increase of globotriaosylceramide in the urine. Skin or conjuctival biopsies may also help in their detection. However, more accurate diagnosis of heterozygotes can be accomplished by the demonstration of a molecular lesion in the α-galactosidase gene or by restriction fragment length polymorphism (RFLP) analysis.

Prenatal diagnosis can be accomplished in male fetuses by the demonstration of a deficient activity of α-galactosidase A, or by molecular analysis of chorionic villi or amniocytes.

Genetics   Fabry disease is an X-linked disorder. Heterozygote females are asymptomatic or develop minor symptoms of the disease. The most frequent and often the only manifestation in them is the characteristic corneal opacity. Intermittent pain, angiokeratoma, proteinuria, and cardiac involvement are much rarer. Exceptionally, the expression of the disease has been comparable to that of the hemizygous male.

The gene coding for α-galactosidase A is located at Xq22.1. Several types of molecular lesions have been identified, including partial deletions, duplications, splice-junction defects, insertions, and point mutations.

Pathologic Findings Glycosphingolipids are distributed in the endothelial, perithelial, and smooth muscle cells of all vessels in the body, including vessels in the central nervous system. This predilection is unique among the glycosphingolipidoses. They also accumulate in the glomerular and tubular cells of the kidney, the epithelial cells of the cornea, and the muscle fibers and endocardium of the heart.

In the nervous system, storage is seen mainly in neurons of the central and peripheral autonomic system. Lipid granules have been observed, in particular, in the neurons of the intermediolateral columns of the spinal cord, the nucleus gracilis, the nucleus cuneatus, the dorsal vagal and salivary nuclei, the nucleus ambiguus, the substantia nigra, the hypothalamus, the dorsal root ganglia, the myenteric plexus, and perineural cells. Loss of small myelinated and nonmyelinated fibers has also been reported.

When the lipid-laden cells from various sites—skin, conjunctiva, and kidney—are examined with the electron microscope, all the deposits exhibit a lamellated concentric pattern. Within dermal nerves, axons of the smaller unmyelinated fibers are more susceptible to lipid infiltrations; there is no accumulation in Schwann cells.[168]

The glycosphingolipids with terminal α-galactosyl moieties that accumulate in the tissues consist of globotriaosylceramide and galabiosylceramide. Blood group B substances, which have terminal α-galactosyl moieties, are also stored. Note that patients with blood group B or AB tend to be more severely affected by the disease.

Clinicopathologic Correlations The involvement of the autonomic neurons in the central and peripheral nervous system, and possibly also peripheral nerve ischemia, may be responsible for the sensory disturbances, hypohydrosis, and abdominal pains, and it could account for alterations of vasomotor control. The relation between hypothalamic lesions and febrile episodes remains a matter for speculation.

The widespread involvement of the vasculature—endothelial cell proliferation leading to small vessel obstruction and microaneurysms—causes ischemia and infarctions in the brain, heart, and other organs. Kidney involvement results in systemic hypertension. Lipid deposits on the mitral valve, in the myocardium, in the conduction system of the heart, and in coronary arteries are the basis of the cardiac abnormalities and brain embolism.

Differential Diagnosis Rheumatic fever, appendicitis, renal colic, and porphyria must be ruled out during febrile attacks of pain. Other causes of angiokeratoma in the HMDs are listed in Table 7-6.

Treatment The incapacitating episodes of pain and acroparesthesia have been significantly alleviated by the use of diphenylhydantoin and carbamazepine. Avoidance of sunshine and hot weather are recommended. Administration of an antipyretic and drinking large quantities of water are also helpful. Since platelet aggregation is enhanced in Fabry disease and may be partly responsible for the increased incidence of stroke as well as cardiac and renal vascular thrombosis, antiplatelet agents such as ticlopidine and aspirin may be used prophylactically.

Renal transplantation has proved to be valuable in correcting renal failure. It also provides an in situ source of the normal enzyme and has led to clinical and biological improvement in some, but not all, patients.

Replacement therapy using a human enzyme has proved biochemically effective in preliminary trials, but only when large amounts of the recombinant enzyme are available will it be possible to evaluate long-term clinical effects of this treatment. Liver transplantation may also become a useful therapeutic measure; its effects have not yet been fully evaluated.

Prevention of the disease and adequate genetic counseling is based on the possibility of detecting heterozygotes, prenatal screening, and the knowledge of the mode of transmission of the disease. All the sons of an affected male will be normal, but all daughters will be obligate carriers of the gene. Statistically half the sons of a heterozygous female will have the disease and half the daughters will be carriers.

Acute Intermittent Porphyria Acute intermittent porphyria (AIP) is an autosomal dominant disorder resulting from a deficiency in the activity of porphobilinogen (PBG) deaminase. This is one of the enzymes involved in the biosynthetic pathway of heme (ferroprotoporphyrin IX). The disease declares itself by acute intermittent attacks of abdominal pain, psychic disturbances, and polyneuropathy, attacks which may be provoked by the administration of barbiturates and certain other drugs. Waldenström,[169] who in 1957 wrote one of the most authoritative accounts of acute intermittent porphyria, stated that clinical symptoms do not occur before puberty and in only 15 percent of his series of 321 cases did the disease begin before 20 years of age. Nevertheless, AIP has been seen in childhood[170,171] and may be more frequent at that age than generally believed. Thirty-seven pediatric cases were reported up to 1974.[170]

The majority of individuals with PBG deaminase deficiency remain clinically normal.

Clinical Features   Abdominal pain is generally the first sign of the disease. It may be localized or generalized and is frequently accompanied by nausea, vomiting, and constipation. Abdominal distension and diarrhea may occur. Pain in the chest and back have also been noted. In severe cases the symptoms may raise questions of an acute surgical abdomen and lead to unnecessary laparotomy; coupled with the use of barbiturates for induction of anesthesia, this may provoke a disastrous exacerbation of the attack.

Other possible symptoms include urinary retention or incontinence, tachycardia, hypertension, and occasionally fever. A few patients continue to have chronic, fluctuating abdominal pain. Restlessness, crying, insomnia or confusional psychosis, hallucinations, and violent behavior may precede or accompany the polyneuropathy. Seizures are not rare.

A predominantly motor polyneuropathy is a common feature of AIP. It is localized first in the arms or legs but may extend to other parts of the body. Involvement may be symmetric or asymmetric and either the proximal or distal parts of the limbs are more affected. Distal weakness of the fingers and wrist extensors (pseudoradial paralysis) may be the presenting symptom. Sensory changes are often combined with the motor deficit. There may be parathesias, dysesthesias, or anesthesia to touch and pain. Pain in the limbs is a frequent symptom. Tendon reflexes are rapidly lost, but muscle bulk is preserved unless the paralysis persists for months.

Progression of the polyneuropathy is variable. Mild cases are restricted to the limbs, but the trunk may be involved, with the danger of acute respiratory failure, and there may be paralysis of cranial nerves, particularly the VIIth and the Xth nerves, causing a potentially dangerous dysphagia. Oculomotor disturbances are rare. Transitory amaurosis or visual field defects of cerebral origin have been recorded. Tachycardia, hypertension, vomiting, and bladder dysfunction may result from involvement of the autonomic nerves. The CSF proteins are rarely elevated.

Complete recovery of the polyneuropathy is usual after a few weeks. In severe cases, recovery may require several months or years and residual signs may occasionally persist. Evidence of denervation atrophy in EMGs and low nerve conduction velocities are usual. The acute attacks are apt to recur, after more or less asymptomatic intervening periods. A few patients develop a chronic fluctuating syndrome. Among patients with chronic or recurrent mental symptoms that lead to admission to psychiatric institutions, there have been a few with AIP.[172]

Asymptomatic   PBG   Deaminase   Deficiency. Precipitating Factors   Approximately 90 percent of individuals with a deficiency in PBG deaminase activity remain asymptomatic during their lifetime. This has been established by extensive screening of the families of patients. Such asymptomatic heterozygotes may display no biochemical abnormality, or may have an increased production and excretion of heme pathway metabolites (PBG) and δ-aminolevulinic acid (ALA) but without clinical expression (latent AIP).

Individuals with latent, or clinically expressed AIP, may be precipitated into an acute attack by a number of drugs, endocrine factors, inadequate nutrition, and infections. Among the potentially harmful medications, barbiturates are the best known. Most of the other antiepileptic drugs, sulfonamides, ergotamine, chloroquine, are also apt to trigger an attack. A complete list of potentially dangerous drugs can be found in the chapter on porphyrias in *The Metabolic and Molecular Bases of Inherited Disease.*[173] In many instances, however, no precipitating factors of an acute attack of AIP can be identified.

Diagnostic Laboratory Tests   Patients with AIP (and some individuals with latent AIP) excrete increased amounts of δ-aminolevulinic acid (ALA) and porphobilinogen (PBG) in the urine during and between attacks. These compounds should be measured by quantitative methods. The classical port-wine coloration of urine is due to the presence of porphyrins and a high content of porphobilin, an autooxidized product of PBG. An excessive urinary concentration of PBG and ALA is not always present in AIP, and may also be seen in coproporphyria and variegate porphyria. Measurement of urinary and stool porphyrins will differentiate these conditions from AIP.

The definitive diagnosis rests on the demonstrations of reduced PBG deaminase activity in erythrocytes and also in cultured fibroblasts and lymphocytes. The enzyme activity is approximately 50 percent of normal (consistent with the heterozygous state). The interpretation of the results of enzymatic assays may be complicated by the wide variations of normal values.

Other laboratory findings include hypercholesterolemia and increased amount of β-lipoproteins, inappropriate secretion of antidiuretic hormone, and renal involvement.

All family members of a patient with AIP should be investigated, using assays of erythrocyte PBG deaminase and determination of urinary ALA and PBG levels. When such analyses are made, most individuals with a deficiency in PBG deaminase will be found to have no clinical symptoms and either normal or elevated levels of ALA and PBG.

Prenatal diagnosis can be achieved by enzymatic assays of amniocytes.

Genetics   AIP is an autosomal dominant disease. The incidence of the defective gene has been estimated at between 5 and 10 in 100,000. The highest incidence of the disease appears to be in Scandinavia and the United Kingdom. In Sweden (where clinical forms occur in only 10 percent of those with the carrier state), it was estimated that it was 1.5 in 100,000, on the basis of PBG and ALA determinations. There are no large-scale collections of epidemiologic data based on the measurement of erythrocyte PBG deaminase.

The gene locus of PBG deaminase has been assigned to chromosome 11 (11q24.1-q24.2). CRIM-negative mutations are found in 85 percent of affected individuals (CRIM is cross-reacting immunologic material).

Differential Diagnosis   AIP should be considered in the presence of an attack of an acute surgical abdominal disorder, an acute polyneuropathy of the Guillain-Barré type, and a confusional psychosis. Tyrosinemia and polyarteritis nodosa are the only other diseases in which there is abdominal pain and mononeuritis multiplex or polyneuritis.

In patients with chronic or fluctuating psychiatric manifestations, the diagnosis has frequently been missed, and the incidence of AIP in psychiatric populations is higher than in the normal population.[174] AIP must be differentiated from other varieties of familial porphyrinuria with a similar neurological symptomatology (see below).

Pathologic Findings   The nerves at autopsy may show no change if death occurred in the acute phase. In the patients who lived for a longer time with polyneuropathy, there is a segmental demyelination and also Wallerian degeneration. Cerebral lesions, some of ischemic type, are inconsistent.

The pathogenesis of the disease and especially of its neurologic manifestations remains obscure.

Treatment   All patients with AIP should be provided with warning bracelets. They should maintain a balanced diet and should avoid illicit drugs. Infections and other intercurrent disorders should be treated promptly. An incipient attack may be aborted by oral or intravenous administration of glucose. During the attack, intravenous administration of carbohydrate may improve the symptomatology. Hyponatremia may occur and should be reversed.

Intravenous administration of hematin, which is effective in reducing levels of ALA and PBG, is generally recommended, although it can induce phlebitis and thrombophlebitis. (Haemarginate and other heme products are available.) Chlorpromazine and narcotic analgesics can be used safely to combat severe abdominal pain, as are phenothiazines for vomiting, and propanolol for severe hypertension. Seizures should be treated with gabapentin and other anticonvulsants which are not metabolized by the liver.

Other Genetic Porphyrias with a Neurologic Symptomatology   Three familial porphyrias that are genetically distinct from AIP also have a prominent neurologic symptomatology.

Hereditary coproporphyria (HCP) is an autosomal dominant disorder caused by a heterozygous deficiency of coproporphyrinogen oxidase (COPRO). Its neurovisceral symptomatology is indistinguishable from that of AIP. Cutaneous photosensitivity is a prominent feature and there may be involvement of the liver. The biological hallmark of the disease is an excessive excretion of coproporphyrin in urine and feces. High levels of ALA and PBG are found in the urine between attacks. The activity of COPRO is found to be reduced by 50 percent. The gene for COPRO is coded on chromosome 9. Mutations have been described in two cases.[175,176]

Variegate porphyria (VP) is caused by a heterozygous deficiency in protoporphyrinogen oxidase (PROTO) and is inherited as an autosomal dominant trait. The disease is frequent in South Africa but occurs worldwide. The neurological and visceral symptomatology of VP is similar to that of AIP and HCP. Cutaneous manifestations are typical. During attacks, patients excrete abnormal quantities of coproporphyrin, ALA, and PBG in the urine. PROTO deficiency can be measured in fibroblasts or lymphocytes, but this assay is usually not available. Differentiation between VP and HCP may be achieved by fecal porphyrin analysis. Linkage between VP and α_1-antitrypsin suggests that the gene for PROTO is on chromosome 14.

δ-Aminolevulinic acid (ALA) dehydratase deficiency porphyria is a rare autosomal recessive disorder that has been reported in six patients, four of them with a severe neuropathy. Onset in one child was at the age of 2 years. The gene for ALA dehydratase has been assigned to 9q34.[177]

Hereditary Tyrosinemia I   Hereditary tyrosinemia type I is an autosomal recessive disorder due to a deficiency of fumarylacetoacetate hydrolase (FAH). More than 100 cases have been reported. Mitchell et al.[177a] have studied 48 cases diagnosed by neonatal screening at birth. The disease begins in infancy and leads to chronic liver failure, renal tubular dysfunction, and occasionally hypertrophic cardiomyopathy. In some patients acute liver failure necessitates liver transplant. There are frequent episodes of acute polyneuropathy associated with abdominal pain, and sometimes psychic symptoms. Respiratory assistance may be required. The clinical picture closely resembles that of acute intermittent porphyria. Indeed, the genetic defect results in the accumulation of succinylacetone, which inhibits ALA dehydratase and causes ALA levels to increase, as in acute intermittent porphyria. Urinary tests for succinylacetone and tissue assays for fumarylacetoacetate hydrolase establish the diagnosis. Electrodiagnostic studies and nerve biopsies have apparently shown the polyneuropathy to be of axonal type. Death usually occurs during the first decade of life. Mutations in the FAH gene, which maps to 15q23-q25, have been described. RFLP analysis can be used for carrier detection and prenatal diagnosis in families with an affected child.

Charcot-Marie-Tooth Disease; Déjerine-Sottas Disease (The Hereditary Motor and Sensory Neuropathies)

Charcot-Marie-Tooth (CMT) disease is a slowly progressive hereditary polyneuropathy of childhood and adolescence causing distal symmetrical weakness and atrophy of the lower limbs, and to a lesser extent, of the hands and forearms. Its course is relatively benign and life expectancy is normal. The central nervous system and other organs are not involved. With an esti-

mated frequency of 1/2500, CMT is the most common of the inherited polyneuropathies. Differences in peripheral nerve lesions and in their neurophysiological correlates have led to the distinction of two main entities within the CMT phenotype.

CMT I, or hereditary motor and sensory neuropathy I (HMSN I), is characterized by demyelination, Schwann cell onion-bulb formation, and nerve trunk hypertrophy, suggesting a defect of myelin formation by Schwann cells. Motor and sensory nerve conduction velocities are markedly reduced.

CMT II (or HMSN II) is a neuroaxonal neuropathy without primary demyelination or enlargement of peripheral nerves. Nerve conduction velocities are in the normal range but sensory action potentials are decreased.

CMT I and CMT II are clinically indistinguishable in practice. Both are autosomal dominant diseases, but exceptionally are transmitted as autosomal recessive or X-linked traits.

A third variety of inherited polyneuropathy, Déjerine-Sottas disease, or HMSN type III, differs from the usual Charcot-Marie-Tooth phenotype by an early onset, often in infancy, and a much more severe course. An autosomal recessive type of inheritance has been postulated, but recent findings show that transmission may follow an autosomal dominant pattern. Lesions of the peripheral nerves are of the same type as in CMT I, although more severe. Nerve conduction velocities are very low.

Recent advances in molecular biology, while justifying this classification and confirming the heterogeneity of CMT disease, have brought considerable clarification in the exact delineation and etiopathogenesis of this group of disorders.

Charcot-Marie-Tooth Disease (CMT I and CMT II)

CMT Disease Type I (Demyelinating Type)   It is by far the most frequent variety of the Charcot-Marie-Tooth syndrome. We have personally examined approximately 200 patients.

Clinical Features   The disease starts insidiously and may remain unnoticed for some time. It is usually recognized between the ages of 6 and 18 years. The onset may also be as late as the third or fourth decades, or before the age of 5 years. Children and adolescents come to medical attention because of increasing difficulties in walking and maintaining balance, or because of deformities of the feet. Foot deformities may lead first to an orthopedic consultation.

On examination, a constant finding is a bilateral weakness of dorsiflexion and eversion of the feet, which result in foot drop and steppage gait. The extensors of the toes are weak, except for relative sparing of the long extensor of the first toe, and there is a more or less important retraction of the Achilles tendon. These findings reflect the selective involvement of the pretibial and peroneal muscles. Internal rotation of the foot, and muscular strength of the thigh are normal. Unlike the paraparesis of spinal or cerebral origin, genu recurvatum (related to weakness of the anterior thigh muscles) does not occur in our experience. This might be of diagnostic help. Ankle reflexes are abolished early, but knee jerks may remain normal or slightly reduced for some time. Distal sensory loss is usually mild and may be impossible to ascertain in young patients. Although proprioceptive sensation is somewhat impaired in adolescents and adults, sensory ataxia is minimal or absent. Muscle cramps and pain in the legs after exercise are relatively common complaints.

Deformities of the feet develop, particularly pes cavus and hammer toes, which may or may not be present at the time of the first examination. Although the feet tend to be cold, there are no important trophic changes such as plantar ulcers. There is no disturbance of the urinary sphincters.

Amyotrophy of the hands and distal part of the forearms usually develop later and may remain quite mild, with little or no functional inconvenience. A mild tremor of the upper limbs may appear in some patients. In adolescents and adults, enlargement of nerve trunks is perceptible, particularly in the ulnar and peroneal regions. Cranial nerves are not involved, but miosis and poor pupillary reactions to light are observed in rare cases. Scoliosis may occur in the more severely affected patients. Intelligence is normal.

Motor and sensory nerve conduction velocities are markedly reduced. (Motor nerve conduction velocities are usually below 30 m/s.) CSF protein concentration is usually elevated.

Analysis of a biopsy specimen of the sural nerve (generally not required for diagnosis), by optical and electron microscopy, teasing of nerve fibers, and histometry, reveal what is essentially a marked loss of large myelinated fibers, myelin breakdown, some degree of remyelination, and onion bulbs. These are formed by concentric lamellae of Schwann cell cytoplasm entrapping collagen around an affected myelinated fiber, and leading to an overall increase in the endoneurial surface.

In most instances the disease progresses very slowly and the condition remains benign, with only mild to moderate functional handicap and a normal life expectancy. A minority of patients with scoliosis and marked involvement of the hands become severely incapacitated in late adolescence and adulthood. One of us has seen two brothers (aged 9 and 17), with very early-onset CMT I. They were homozygous for a mutation in the P_0 peripheral myelin protein gene. They were delayed in walking and had thin extremities. The older boy was wheelchair-bound with severe muscle wasting hypotonia, areflexia, dysmetria, and absent vibration sense below the shoulders. Both parents, who were distantly related, had minimal signs of CMT.

The frequency of the "formes frustes" of CMT I disease cannot be overemphasized. They are usually detected upon examination of the parents and other relatives of a patient. Affected individuals often do not complain of any trouble and lead normal lives. The disease is manifested by slightly arched feet, absent ankle reflexes, and reduced nerve conduction velocities. Such findings in one parent corroborate the diagnosis of dominant CMT disease.

Genetics and Pathophysiology   CMT I is inherited as an autosomal dominant trait in approximately 85 percent of patients. Autosomal recessive, X-linked dominant, and X-linked recessive mode of inheritance have been documented, but only in a few families.

To establish the mode of inheritance and to detect gene carriers, a thorough clinical and electrophysiological examination of both parents and as many members of the family as possible is indispensable, keeping in mind that many affected individuals will display only minor clinical signs. The genetic diagnosis is further elucidated by DNA studies of a number of family members. In counseling families of a patient with CMT, it should always be remembered that this is essentially a benign disorder.

(1) Two autosomal dominant loci have been identified. Most patients with dominant CMT I (referred to as CMT IA) have a 1.5 Mb DNA duplication of chromosome 17 in the region of p11.2, which contains the gene encoding peripheral myelin protein 22 (PMP22). Some patients have no duplication but instead have point mutations of the PMP22 gene. In a small number of families (CMT IB), the defective gene maps to chromosome 1 in the region 1q22-23.1, and deletions or point mutations have been identified in the peripheral myelin protein, P_0. The P_0 protein, which is expressed strictly in the myelin-forming Schwann cells, is an adhesion glycoprotein involved in the compaction of the mul-

tilamellar myelin sheet. It accounts for more than half the peripheral myelin protein content.

These findings indicate that CMT I is related to two different genetically determined defects of peripheral myelin proteins, confirming the hypothesis based on pathological findings that CMT I is a disorder of myelin-forming Schwann cells. (It is noteworthy that the PMP22 gene is also mutated in the trembler mouse, which has served as a model for the study of CMT.)

(2) An autosomal recessive form[178] and an X-linked dominant form of the disease[179] have been reported in a few families with a phenotype indistinguishable from that of the usual autosomal dominant variety of CMT I. In the X-linked dominant families, there is no male-to-male transmission, and males are more affected than females. Female carriers may display mild clinical and electrophysiological abnormalities.

(3) CMT X, the very rare X-linked recessive form of CMT I,[180] has its onset in early infancy. It also produces mental retardation and deafness. Female carriers are normal. The disease appears to be related to a defect of the gene for connexin 32 mapped on chromosome Xq31.1. Several different mutations in this gene have been identified.[181,182] Connexins are gap junction proteins.

CMT Disease Type II CMT II is found in about one-third of all cases of CMT disease. It is indistinguishable from CMT I on clinical grounds. The onset is usually insidious, and the disease becomes manifest in the second or third decade of life or later, but many patients have been noted to be clumsy since childhood. Sensory deficits may be marked with proprioceptive ataxia and tremor in some cases. Although areflexia is the usual finding, knee jerks may remain normal for some years. Scoliosis and involvement of the hands are rare. There is no hypertrophy of nerve trunks. "Formes frustes" are frequent. On the whole, the disease is mildly or moderately incapacitating and life expectancy is normal. The only major differences between this disease and CMT I are in the electrophysiologic and pathologic findings. Nerve conduction velocities are normal or minimally slowed, whereas sensory evoked potentials are decreased or absent. This distinguishes CMT II from the distal form of spinal muscular atrophy. The EMG shows evidence of denervation atrophy. Analysis of a sural nerve biopsy reveals a marked loss of large myelinated fibers without significant alterations of myelin sheaths of the remaining fibers. Degenerating axons are rare and dispersed through the nerves; onion bulbs

are not present. CSF protein may be elevated but less regularly than in CMT I.

Genetics CMT II is essentially an autosomal dominant disease, but autosomal recessive forms have been reported.[183] It is important to examine the affected parent who may exhibit only minimal clinical signs. Sensory evoked potentials should be studied in parents and siblings in order to establish the mode of inheritance. Sporadic cases are not rare. In the near future, genetic counseling will be greatly facilitated by molecular biological techniques. In counseled families it must again be kept in mind that CMT is a benign disease.

Recent DNA linkage studies[184] have established that CMT II is genetically distinct from CMT I. Charcot-Marie-Tooth disease type II can be secondary to a defect in at least two different genes on the short arm of chromosome 1. Approximately 50 percent of CMT II families map to 1p36.[185] In other families the locus has been mapped to 3q13-22.

Variant of CMT II Ouvrier in Australia has described an autosomal recessive variety of CMT II with early onset and a rapid course leading to serious motor handicap.[186]

Differential Diagnosis of Charcot-Marie-Tooth Disease (CMT I and CMT II) The diagnosis of Charcot-Marie-Tooth disease is based on clinical examination of the patient and the patient's family and on electrophysiological studies. Electrophysiological studies should involve measurements of motor and sensory nerve conduction velocities and sensory evoked potentials. The EMG, always a painful test, should be reserved for cases of CMT II if the diagnosis is uncertain. A sural nerve biopsy is practically never necessary for diagnostic purposes in typical dominant CMT I. Occasionally it can be useful in CMT II.

Since many patients are first seen for pes cavus, they may be considered as having a purely orthopedic problem. When tremor and/or a proprioceptive deficit with some degree of ataxia are present, the possibility of Friedreich ataxia or another form of spinocerebellar degeneration may be raised. The association of tremor and a peripheral neuropathy is discussed under Roussy-Levy syndrome. Differentiation between distal spinal muscular atrophy and CMT may be difficult because both diseases have a very similar clinical picture. Sensory evoked potentials are decreased or absent in CMT, whereas they are normal in spinal muscular atrophy. Differentiation from a chronic inflammatory polyneuropathy has been a problem in some sporadic cases.

When a sporadic distal polyneuropathy with decreased nerve conduction velocities and a high protein content of the CSF begins in the second or third year of life, a metabolic disorder such as a metachromatic leukodystrophy and Krabbe disease must be considered.

Treatment Patients with weak ankles and foot drop benefit from braces, tendon transplants, and ankylosing procedures.

Déjerine-Sottas Disease The term Déjerine-Sottas (DS) disease, or hereditary motor and sensory neuropathy type III (HMSN III), should be reserved for cases that differ from the usual Charcot-Marie-Tooth phenotype because of an earlier onset and a much more severe disability. Here, as in CMT I, there is a demyelinating hypertrophic neuropathy with onion-bulb formation, suggesting a defect in myelin-forming Schwann cells.

The disease starts in infancy, causing much delay in motor development. Walking is usually not achieved before the ages of 3 or 4 years, or even later in our experience. Muscle weakness of the limbs is predominantly distal; thigh muscles may be involved; genu recurvatum may be found. The upper limbs are affected as well, and the use of the hands becomes difficult. Proprioceptive sensory loss may be manifest, contributing to the difficulty of locomotion. Tendon reflexes are always absent. The facial muscles are often affected. A sluggish response of the pupils to light may be noted. The enlarged nerves may be felt and seen as salient cords beneath the skin by late childhood and adolescence. Intelligence is normal. Nerve conduction velocities are always very low (motor nerve conduction velocities may be below 20 m/s in the lower limbs). Protein levels are high in the CSF. Scoliosis frequently occurs after some years. A sural nerve biopsy shows marked hypomyelination, myelin breakdown, and onion bulbs. There is an important reduction of large myelinated fibers. On the whole, lesions are of the same kind as in CMT I but they are more severe. Children with DS disease usually make slow motor progress during childhood but they remain seriously incapacitated.

Genetics Transmission of DS disease is usually said to conform to an autosomal recessive pattern. However, DS disease has been found associated with point mutations in the peripheral myelin protein 22 (PMP22) gene,[187,188] as well as in the myelin P_0

gene[189]; in both instances patients were heterozygous. These findings suggest that the inheritance pattern of DS is actually autosomal dominant and that de novo mutations in more than one myelin protein gene can give rise to the DS phenotype.

Rare patients homozygous for the CMT IA gene duplication have been found to exhibit the Déjerine-Sottas phenotype.

Differential Diagnosis Krabbe leukodystrophy and in late infancy metachromatic should be excluded by appropriate biochemical and enzymatic studies.

Congenital Hypomyelinating Polyneuropathy Is Possibly an Extreme Variant of DS Disease Several cases of this polyneuropathy have been reported. We have observed six children with this condition.[190,191] They had severe hypotonia and limb weakness in early infancy. The muscular deficit predominated on distal muscles. There was no involvement of the respiratory muscles or facial muscles, features which distinguish it from Werdnig-Hoffman disease and congenital myopathies. In most cases the tendon reflexes were absent, nerve conduction velocities very slow, and protein levels elevated in the CSF. Peripheral nerve biopsies showed a considerable reduction in the number of myelin sheaths, and there were onion bulbs, composed of concentric layers of basement membrane. The prognosis has been variable, though most children have made slow but significant progress. The cases probably represent extreme forms of HMSN III.

In particularly severe forms of congenital hypomyelination (or amyelination) neuropathy, arthrogryposis is present at birth.[192] Central nervous system defects may be associated. These newborns require ventilatory support and generally do not survive more than a few weeks. In an autopsied case the immunocytochemistry demonstrated a pronounced decrease in immunostaining of the P_2, P_0, and myelin basic protein (MBP) proteins in the peripheral nerve root, moderate deficiency of myelin associated glycoprotein (MAG), and no selective dropout of any one of the myelin proteins tested. The authors concluded that the hypomyelination was the result of a developmental arrest at the promyelin stage.

Addendum There is a certain terminological confusion concerning Déjerine-Sottas disease. Déjerine and Sottas described a disease starting in early childhood or infancy, which they found to be related to a hypertrophic neuropathy, whereas Charcot and Marie described a similar disease in adults and adolescents, which they mistakenly thought to represent a myelopathy. The two conditions were therefore initially believed to be fundamentally different. Later, all cases with a hypertrophic neuropathy were labeled Déjerine-Sottas disease. It is now known that a hypertrophic demyelinating neuropathy is a feature of the majority of patients with the Charcot-Marie-Tooth phenotype, as well as those with the infantile, and more severe, form of polyneuropathy to which the term Déjerine-Sottas disease should be restricted. Hypertrophy may also be found in Refsum disease and in chronic and recurrent polyneuritis.

Giant Axonal Neuropathy Giant axonal neuropathy is a generalized disorder of cellular intermediate filaments affecting essentially the peripheral and central nervous system. It is probably transmitted as an autosomal recessive trait. Since it was first described by Asbury et al. in 1972, approximately 30 patients have been reported. The onset of the disease is generally between the ages of 2 and 7 years with progressive difficulty in walking due to a peripheral neuropathy. There is a weakness and later atrophy of the distal parts of the lower limbs, spreading gradually to the upper limbs. The tendon reflexes are depressed. Sensation, particularly vibratory and proprioceptive sensation, is impaired distally. Peripheral nerves are not enlarged. Facial weakness and mild ptosis have been reported. Motor nerve conduction velocities are normal or mildly decreased, and sensory action potentials are absent. The presence of bilateral Babinski sign provides evidence of pyramidal tract involvement. A cerebellar ataxia, dysarthria, and horizontal and vertical nystagmus appear after some time, or may be the initial manifestation of the disease. Marked dysphagia may become a major problem. Seizures have been reported in some cases, as well as optic atrophy. Patients are usually moderately retarded mentally and a progressive mental decline has been observed in some of them. Scoliosis is generally present after the age of 10 years. Small stature is usual. A remarkable but not quite constant feature is the presence of tightly curled hair in patients of all ethnic backgrounds. CT scans show hypodense defects in the cerebral and cerebellar white matter and a generalized atrophy.[193]

Diagnosis Diagnosis rests on the detection of the characteristic accumulation of neurofilaments in axons and other cells. A skin biopsy alone may be sufficient because of the ubiquitous accumulation of microfilaments in nerve trunks and nonnervous structures. In

sural nerve biopsies examined with the light microscope, there are numerous fusiform swellings of axons, which may measure up to 350 nm in diameter. Myelin sheaths surrounding the axonal spheroids are thin and may be absent. There is a moderate reduction in the number of myelinated and unmyelinated fibers. Under the electron microscope the axonal spheroids are seen to contain tightly packed neurofilaments and a few neurotubules and other organelles. The average neurofilament diameter was found to be 12.4 nm compared with 10.1 nm in controls.[194] Cross-bridging of side arms is rare.

Focal increases in intermediate filaments are also observed in Schwann cells, endothelial cells, endoneural and perineural cells, and cultured skin fibroblasts.

Pathology of the Central Nervous System Large axonal swellings and marked astrocytosis with Rosenthal fiber formation are seen throughout the central nervous system, particularly in the white matter of the cerebral hemispheres, pyramidal tracts, corpus callosum, cerebellar white matter, middle cerebellar peduncles, and posterior columns of the spinal cord. The number of Purkinje cells and granule cells in the cerebellum is much decreased, and there is severe loss of neurons and gliosis in the inferior olives, the nucleus gracilis, and the nucleus cuneatus.

Differential Diagnosis Differential diagnosis may be very difficult. The disease may be confused with Friedreich ataxia and the other childhood spinocerebellar degenerations, and early on, with other forms of progressive polyneuropathy. The diagnosis may be suspected clinically on the basis of the special appearance of the hair. It is established by a nerve biopsy. However, multifocal increases in the density of neurofilaments in peripheral axons can be observed in the neuropathies due to intoxication with acrylamide or with industrial solvents (glue sniffers).

Pathogenesis The fundamental defect of this disorder of cellular intermediate filaments is not known.

Treatment Clinical improvement was reported in a patient treated with penicillamine. This observation, together with experimental studies, raises the possibility of a disorder of thiol metabolism.

Summarizing Remarks Concerning the Juvenile Metabolic Polyneuropathies

Lesions of the peripheral nervous system occur in a significant number of known juvenile HMDs, where they may contribute to the clinical symptomatology and assume diagnostic importance (see Table 6-9). In only a few of them is the polyneuropathy a major presenting sign and the central point of the diagnostic discussion.

To this category belong Refsum disease, juvenile metachromatic leukodystrophy, familial amyloid neuropathy, porphyric neuropathy, and Tangier disease. The final three are only rarely encountered in children. They are relatively easily recognized because of the type of peripheral nerve involvement and accompanying neurologic and visceral signs. In familial amyloid disease, a sensory and autonomic polyneuropathy with motor signs in the background is usually associated with a cardiomyopathy. Most patients are of Portuguese descent. Acute intermittent porphyria is characterized by an acute relapsing or more chronic, essentially motor neuropathy, accompanied by episodes of abdominal pain and psychiatric manifestations. In the rare Tangier disease, peripheral nerve involvement may take the form of a multiple mononeuropathy, a progressive polyneuropathy, or a syringomyelia-like syndrome; the orange coloration of the tonsils and low blood cholesterol are characteristic. Refsum disease patients exhibit a slowly evolving (at times, relapsing) sensorimotor, distal areflexic syndrome resembling Charcot-Marie-Tooth syndrome. Deafness, retinitis pigmentosa, and ECG changes, which may have preceded the neuropathy, are important clues. In metachromatic leukodystrophy, demyelination on MRI and increased sulfatiduria are characteristic.

Fabry disease is unique with respect to the severe pain, worsened by hyperthermia, and virtually no objective sensory-motor involvement. This striking symptomatology is the consequence of lesions in the peripheral and central autonomic nervous system. Giant axonal neuropathy is a generalized disorder of intermediate filaments frequently starting as a polyneuropathy. Table 6-9 lists the other known metabolic disorders which may occasionally present for some time as an isolated sensorimotor neuropathy.

The most common form of Charcot-Marie-Tooth disease I (CMT I) and Déjerine-Sottas disease (HMSN III) have finally been proved to be metabolic disorders. They are related to genetically determined defects of peripheral myelin proteins, which are strictly expressed in Schwann cells. They can be considered the peripheral equivalent of Pelizaeus-Merzbacher disease, which is due to a defect of a central nervous system myelin protein, proteolipid protein. The cause of the neuroaxonal form of the disease (CMT II) has not yet been determined. The clinical manifestations of Charcot-Marie-Tooth disease are not always obvious. They may be minimal in some patients. The differential diagnosis includes such conditions as spinocerebellar degeneration, distal spinal muscular atrophy, a chronic inflammatory neuropathy, or an orthopedic deformity.

PROGRESSIVE VISUAL LOSS AS AN INITIAL MANIFESTATION IN JUVENILE HEREDITARY METABOLIC DISORDERS

Progressive visual loss in childhood or adolescence may result from three types of disorders.

1. A tumor infiltrating or compressing the optic nerves or chiasm.

2. A purely ophthalmologic disorder (primary retinal degeneration, cataracts, glaucoma, myopia).

3. A progressive neurometabolic disease.

In HMDs blindness may result either from retinal or macular degeneration, from optic atrophy (demyelination of optic nerves), or from lesions of the geniculocalcarine (i.e., central) optic pathways. Cataracts and corneal opacities may be added factors. A recently acquired squint (if not paralytic) and a pendular nystagmus should always suggest amblyopia. HMDs in which progressive visual failure is frequently an early manifestation are the following:

- Juvenile lipofuscinosis (pigmentary degeneration of the retina)
- Sialidosis I (macular degeneration: cherry red spot)
- Adrenoleukodystrophy (central blindness or optic atrophy)
- Krabbe disease (optic atrophy or central blindness)
- MELAS (focal necrosis of visual cortices)
- Leber optic neuropathy (subacute retinal lesions)

Several of these disorders are described in this chapter. Other HMDs which may give rise to blindness, and problems in differential diagnosis are mentioned in Chap. 6 and listed in Table 6-11.

FAMILIAL METABOLIC ENCEPHALOPATHIES WITH CLINICAL EVIDENCE OF DIFFUSE CNS DISORDER

A number of hereditary metabolic encephalopathies at this age period resemble those of infancy and early childhood insofar as they exert their effects on the nervous system more diffusely, sometimes in multiple foci. The symptoms and signs are therefore more varied, even within a single disease entity. A bipyramidal syndrome, cerebellar incoordination, dystonia, choreoathetosis, dementia, seizures, myoclonus, motor neuron disease, visual failure, and oculomotor abnormalities occur in many combinations and in variable chronologies. Of all the clinical findings, the ophthalmologic findings may assume particular importance when they occur early or dominate the clinical picture.

(1) The following genetic *metabolic diseases with a Mendelian mode of inheritance* may evolve clinically in this fashion: (1) lysosomal storage diseases with primarily neuronal involvement including later-onset G_{M2} gangliosidosis and G_{M1} gangliosidosis, Niemann-Pick type C disease, Gaucher type III disease, juvenile Farber disease, Spielmeyer-Vogt disease, sialidosis type II, and galactosialidosis; (2) leukodystrophies such as juvenile metachromatic leukodystrophy, juvenile Krabbe leukodystrophy, and X-linked adrenoleukodystrophy; (3) most cases of Leigh syndrome; (4) nuclear encoded defects in mtDNA (defects of intergenomic signaling); (5) cholestanolosis; (6) juvenile neuroaxonal dystrophy; (7) neuronal intranuclear inclusion disease. We will here describe these diseases briefly and then try to extract from the clinical data certain guidelines that may be useful for their differentiation.

(2) *Maternally inherited defects of mtDNA*, which are also multisystem disorders that display a wide range of neurological manifestations, will be presented separately.

Disorders with a Mendelian Mode of Inheritance

Late-Onset G_{M2} Gangliosidosis (Childhood, Adolescent, and Adult Forms)   The G_{M2} gangliosidoses are a group of autosomal recessive disorders characterized by the intralysosomal accumulation of G_{M2} ganglioside in nerve cells, as a result of a deficiency of hexosaminidase A, or exceptionally, of the G_{M2} protein activator. The great majority of G_{M2} gangliosidoses occur in early infancy and have been described in Chap. 3. Most late-onset G_{M2} gangliosidoses are related

to a deficiency in hexosaminidase A. A significant number belong to the so-called B1 variant. The B1 variant results in an altered substrate specificity of hexosaminidase A: the mutated enzyme retains the ability to degrade most conventional artificial substrates (a peculiarity that may lead to diagnostic errors), but not sulfated substrate or the natural substrate, G_{M2} ganglioside. Two point mutations have been found to be the cause of the B1 variant phenotype in at least three hexosaminidase A (HEXA) sites, Arg^{178}, Val^{192}, and Asp^{258}.

Late-onset forms of G_{M2} gangliosidoses can occur at any time during childhood, adolescence, or even adulthood, and their clinical expression is extraordinarily variable even within sibships, in contrast to early infantile G_{M2} gangliosidoses. They can be divided into two broad categories: childhood "subacute" G_{M2} gangliosidosis (also called juvenile G_{M2} gangliosidosis) and a more chronic G_{M2} gangliosidosis (the so-called adult-onset form).

Clinical Features   Approximately 20 patients with *childhood subacute G_{M2} gangliosidosis* have been reported; there is no ethnic prevalence. Onset is generally between the ages of 3 and 6, and deterioration is severe and rapid. Neurological signs are those of a diffuse encephalopathy. Among the first and most important manifestations are progressive loss of speech, dysarthria, walking difficulties due to a spastic paraparesis with pyramidal signs, and cerebellar ataxia; more generally there is a combination of these signs. Dystonia and choreoathetosis have also been reported.[195,196] An abnormal startle response is seen occasionally. Tonico-clonic or myoclonic seizures and myoclonus are prominent features in some children. Irritability and aggressivity, and periods either of adynamia, apathy, and disinterest or bizarre behavior may occasionally be observed as early signs. Mental deterioration is always present but may not be discernible at first. Loss of vision and retinal changes are inconstant or, when present, are likely to have developed late. Optic atrophy, macular degeneration, macular cherry red spots[197] and pigmentary degeneration of the retina have all been described. Signs of denervation atrophy in the EMG have been recorded.[196] Nerve conduction velocities and the CSF are normal. Neuroimaging does not aid in diagnosis.

After a period of approximately 3 to 10 years the patient is usually bedridden and demented.

A few patients with an onset at 2 or 3 years of age and a rapid downhill course have cherry red spots and a startle response as in Tay-Sachs disease. They may represent compound heterozygotes with a B1 and a Tay-Sachs allele (see below).

The first manifestation of *chronic G_{M2} gangliosidosis* occurs at any time between early childhood and adulthood. In one-third of the cases, onset is before the age of 10 and as early as 3 years. (When the term adult form is employed as a synonym for chronic form, this is manifestly a misnomer.) A number of cases have not been recognized until middle or even late adulthood, even though minor neurological abnormalities may have existed for many years before. Two affected siblings in the same family may have different clinical presentations with variation in the age of onset and severity of symptoms. The majority of patients are of Ashkenazic Jewish origin.

Clinical expression of the chronic form is extremely variable, but signs of lower motor neuron and spinocerebellar dysfunction are prominent. Progressive dystonia and psychiatric manifestations are also common. The onset is insidious and the progression is slow. More than 40 cases have been tabulated in recent reviews.[196,198,199] At the Shriver Laboratory we have seen more than 20 cases. Initial development is generally normal, although some children are said always to have been clumsy and to have had some difficulty at school. Slowly progressive speech difficulties with a dysarthric and stuttering voice of nasal quality or difficulties in walking and coordination of limb movements may inaugurate the disease. Cerebellar ataxia and pyramidal signs may be prominent. Some patients have been reported to have the clinical picture of an atypical spinocerebellar degeneration[200] or atypical Friedreich disease.[201] Dystonia[195] and supranuclear ophthalmoplegia with oculomotor apraxia[196,202] have also been reported. Vision is not impaired and optic fundi are normal. A remarkable feature, found in all patients, is the involvement of lower motor neurons, leading to a proximal and later distal weakness and amyotrophy of the limbs (Fig. 5-10), fasciculations, and signs of denervation atrophy in the EMG. There is no sensory loss and sensory nerve conduction velocities are normal. Some patients mimic spinal muscular atrophy or amyotrophic lateral sclerosis.[196,199] Evidence of neurogenic atrophy usually coexists with other neurologic signs, resulting in a complex "multisystem" neurological disease.

Psychiatric disturbances are present in approximately half the patients. Bizarre, irrational behavior, episodes of depression, and bouts of psychosis with hallucinations can occur at various stages of the disease, occasionally as one of the first manifestations.

Intellectual deterioration is frequent but not constant and may not be an early sign.

Cerebellar atrophy can be seen with MRI. The CSF is normal and EEG abnormalities variable and nonspecific. Sensory nerve conduction velocities are normal.

The course of the disease is protracted and may extend over several decades, sometimes until middle adulthood. Fertility is preserved in both men and women, and some have children.

Diagnostic Laboratory Tests   In view of its extraordinary diversity, diagnosis of late-onset G_{M2} gangliosidosis rests uniquely on enzymatic screening. Skin or rectal biopsies may be helpful in detecting typical intralysosomal inclusions, but may fail to reveal any abnormality. Most patients have the ordinary type of hexosaminidase A deficiency, with low but measurable enzyme activity in cultured fibroblasts.

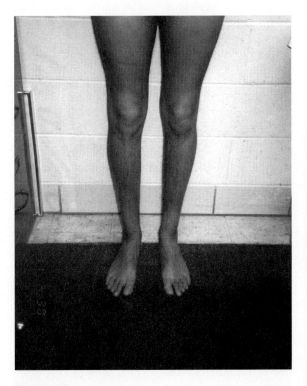

Figure 5-10

Late-onset G_{M2} gangliosidosis in an adolescent presenting with signs of motor neuron disorder. Note amyotrophy of legs. Areflexia, denervation atrophy, and normal nerve conduction velocities were present.

A number of patients, especially those with the childhood form, have the enzymatic changes typical of the *B1 variant*. It is possible that some of the most severely affected cases of childhood G_{M2} gangliosidosis with cherry red spots and a rapid course are compound heterozygotes with one B1 allele and a second allele commonly associated with the classic early infantile Tay-Sachs disease. One of the authors has examined the brains of two patients, 10 and 14 years of age, with this variety of G_{M2} gangliosidosis. Lipid deposits were found in nerve cells of all cortical and subcortical gray structures. They were predominantly located in the axon hillock, extending into and dilating the proximal segment of the axon (meganeurite), whereas the modestly dilated perikaryon was essentially filled with lipofuscin. In two brothers who died in their late forties and in a 52-year-old woman with late-onset G_{M2} gangliosidosis, followed by one of us, autopsy studies showed storage of all neurons, with predominant involvement of layer 3 of the cerebral cortex, the limbic system, and cerebellar Purkinje cells. The degree of cell loss was not as extreme as in classic late infantile forms of G_{M2} gangliosidosis. It seems probable that some cases thought in the past to belong to the Bielschowsky-Janksy type of lipofuscinosis were in fact examples of the B1 variant of G_{M2} gangliosidosis.

A virtual absence of hexosaminidase B and a profound but not total absence of hexosaminidase A, representing the childhood (juvenile) form of *Sandhoff disease*, have been observed in a few children with a clinical picture similar to that of childhood G_{M2} gangliosidosis due to hexosaminidase A deficiency.[203]

Adult-Onset Cases of G_{M2} Gangliosidosis   Here the symptomatology is that of the chronic form of the disease described above. Onset is usually insidious and progression slow. Some patients may have only mild neurological symptoms and may live to an advanced age. Navon has reported a woman whose clumsiness was noted at the age of 35, but progression was so slow that, even by age 76, she had only moderate difficulty in coordinating hand movements and in full movements of the eyes.[204] She had no gait ataxia, weakness or atrophy; her speech and mentation were normal. We have observed a patient with similar features.

Adult G_{M2} gangliosidosis is also inherited as an autosomal recessive trait and is caused by marked deficiency of hexosaminidase A. Most patients have been of Ashkenazic Jewish ancestry. Nearly all have a point mutation in exon 7 of their HEXA α-chain alleles, causing a substitution of serine for glycine at position 269 of the peptide. Their other α-chain allele usually contains one of the mutations of classical Tay-Sachs disease. However, three individuals with onset of their disease in mid-adulthood were found to be homozygous for the exon 7 mutation. Their symptomatology was even milder and the progression of their disease slower than in the usual case of adult onset G_{M2} gangliosidosis.[204]

Late-Onset Chronic Form of G_{M1} Gangliosidosis
G_{M1} gangliosidosis is an autosomal recessive disorder caused by a deficiency in lysosomal β-galactosidase. For practical purposes it can be divided into an early infantile form, the most common (Chap. 3), a late infantile form starting during the second year of life (Chap. 4), and a more chronic form starting at various ages from childhood to adolescence and adulthood. The term *adult form of G_{M1} gangliosidosis* is improperly employed as a synonym for *chronic form*. We will describe here only the *chronic late-onset form of G_{M1} gangliosidosis*.

Clinical Features   Onset is usually in late childhood or adolescence but may occur as early as 4 years of age or as late as the third or fourth decade. This phenotype has been observed in different ethnic groups but appears to be especially frequent in the Japanese.

The slowly progressive neurological signs that are most frequently observed are dysarthria and extrapyramidal signs, especially dystonia. Seizures are uncommon. Cerebellar ataxia or myoclonus are generally not seen. Retinal changes, macular cherry red spots, and corneal opacities are absent. There is no dysmorphism or organomegaly. Intellectual impairment when present is slight or moderate. Mild bone changes such as flattening of the vertebral bodies may be observed. Occasionally they may cause a spinal compression. The course of the disease usually extends over several decades.

It is obvious that the clinical diagnosis is difficult, if not impossible. Assays of β-galactosidase should therefore be systematically included in the screening procedures of all progressive motor disorders of uncertain origin during this age period (especially when extrapyramidal signs are present).

Laboratory Tests   The urine contains excessive amounts of a keratan sulfate-like substance, and galactose-containing products derived from glycoproteins.

The diagnosis is based on the demonstration of a deficiency of acid β-galactosidase in leukocytes and cultured fibroblasts. (Note that a deficiency of β-galactosidase is also found in Morquio B disease and galacto-sialidosis.) A small number of specific mutations in the β-galactosidase gene have been shown for each phenotype, the late infantile, juvenile, and adult forms of G_{M1} gangliosidosis and for Morquio B disease.

Pathological and Biochemical Changes They are qualitatively similar to those of the earlier forms of the disease.

Juvenile Niemann-Pick Type C Disease Niemann-Pick type C (NPC) disease is an autosomal recessive disorder that is distinct from NPA and NPB, described in Chap. 4. NPA and NPB are caused by a primary deficiency of sphingomyelinase, whereas NPC is due to an abnormality in the intracellular processing of exogenous cholesterol, which may result in a secondary partial reduction of sphingomyelinase activity. The primary biochemical deficit of NPC remains to be elucidated.

In about one-third of the NPC cases[205,206] onset occurs in the second year of life (late infancy) with the uncharacteristic neurological picture of a diffuse rapidly progressive encephalopathy, manifest by loss of motor and mental functions and a bipyramidal syndrome. The liver and spleen are generally enlarged, and foam cells are found in the bone marrow. Epilepsy is rare. Vision is usually normal, and there is no evidence of a peripheral neuropathy or elevated protein levels in the CSF. Most children with this variant die between the ages of 3 and 5 years (see Chap. 4). The other two-thirds of the NPC cases begin during childhood or adolescence (juvenile form). Not to be omitted is a neonatal form with a severe cholestatic *liver disease* without neurological involvement and pursuing a rapidly fatal course. Prenatal liver failure (fetal ascites) has been documented.

Clinical Features of Childhood or Adolescent (Juvenile) NP Type C Disease In approximately 70 percent of cases,[205] the clinical symptoms appear between the third and eighth year, less often between the tenth and fifteenth year, and in a few cases not until adulthood. Previous psychomotor development is normal or slightly delayed. Cerebellar ataxia, incoordination, intention tremor, and dysarthria are among the major signs. Dystonia and choreoathetosis are prominent in some patients, but the neurological hallmark of the syndrome is a supranuclear paralysis of vertical eye movements. There may be a complaint of an inability to see low-placed objects, which results in the head being tilted downwards. There are occasional episodes during

which the eyes become fixed in an upward position (oculogyric crises). More precisely, there is an impairment of upward and even more of downward eye movements on command and on the fixating and following of objects, but with persistence of these movements on passive vertical motions of the head. Vertical optokinetic nystagmus is abolished. Horizontal eye movements are generally normal or impaired only at a later stage. Vertical supranuclear palsy is a nearly constant finding after the age of 7 years. Other neurological signs include tonico-clonic or complex partial seizures in about one-third of the patients, and cataplexic attacks (falling when emotionally excited). Spasticity and frank pyramidal signs are usually not in the foreground but can be detected in the later stages of the disease. Mental deterioration is usual but may occur relatively late; behavioral problems may also be observed. We have examined two brothers with dystonia signs and supranuclear ophthalmologia and normal intelligence. Cerebellar atrophy is frequently shown by MRI. Retinal changes, visual failure, and evidence of lower motor neuron disease or polyneuropathy are lacking or exceptional. The CSF is normal.

There is moderate enlargement of the spleen and, to a lesser degree, of the liver in most but not all cases. A prolonged neonatal jaundice or a transient self-limiting episode of early infantile icterus with conjugate hyperbilirubinemia, which regresses between ages 2 and 4 months, has been recorded in about half the patients.

The presence of peculiar storage cells in the bone marrow is of diagnostic importance. Giemsa stain reveals cells containing voluminous vacuoles and a few coarse, dark inclusions; and cells containing numerous minute, strikingly blue granules characteristic of the sea-blue histiocyte (Fig. 5-11).

Neither skeletal abnormalities (on x-ray films) nor facial dysmorphism have been reported.

Death occurs usually in the second or third decade from aspiration pneumonia, but some individuals have lived longer.

Diagnosis and Laboratory Tests A vertical supranuclear gaze paralysis, foam cells and sea-blue histiocytes in the bone marrow, hepatosplenomegaly, and when present, an antecedent history of prolonged neonatal or transient infantile jaundice, virtually establish the clinical diagnosis of NP type C disease. Skin, conjunctival, or rectal biopsy may be of some help in detecting intralysosomal lamellar cytoplasmic bodies. The activity of sphingomyelinase in leukocytes is normal, but a partial deficiency may be found in cultured fibro-

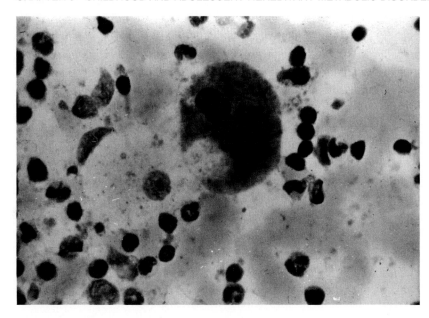

Figure 5-11
Niemann-Pick disease type C: bone marrow smear shows sea-blue histiocyte (dark cell) and foamy histiocyte.

blasts, a secondary consequence of lysosomal cholesterol sequestration. The diagnosis rests on the demonstration of unique abnormalities of intracellular translocation of exogenous cholesterol. This can be done on cultured skin fibroblasts or lymphocytes by demonstrating an impaired cholesterol esterification and the intralysosomal storage of unesterified cholesterol, as demonstrated by intense perinuclear fluorescence in filipin-stained fibroblasts. These methods may permit prenatal diagnosis.

Pathology Neuropathologic data are scant. Neurons in the brain and autonomic ganglia of the myenteric plexuses contain inclusions causing cytoplasmic distension. Under the electron microscope the lipid deposits have been described as intralysosomal pleiomorphic cytoplasmic inclusions, differing from the lamellar inclusion of the other lipidoses. Neurons in the basal ganglia, thalamus, and brain stem are particularly involved. Lipid storage in Purkinje cells and dentate nuclei has also been reported.

The spleen is filled with PAS-positive vacuolated storage cells. Clear membranous vacuoles with scanty granular material are found in Kupffer cells and hepatocytes.

Sea-blue histiocytes in the bone marrow are not specific. They are also found in a number of nonneurological conditions, such as idiopathic thrombocytic purpura, chronic granulocytic leukemia, a form of albin-

ism, type V hyperlipoproteinemia, and lecithin:cholesterol acyltransferase deficiency. Sea-blue histiocytes were also reported before 1973 in a few patients with poorly defined neurological syndromes or retinal degeneration.[207]

Chemical Pathology In contrast with the massive storage of sphingomyelin in spleen and liver seen in NP disease types A and B, in type C there are unesterified cholesterol, phospholipids, and a moderate quantity of sphingomyelin. No significant increase of cholesterol or sphingomyelin is found in the brain. The gray matter exhibits an elevation of G_{M2} and G_{M3} gangliosides between fivefold and tenfold, and a considerable increase of glucosylceramide.

A characteristic abnormality of intracellular translocation of exogenous cholesterol in cultured skin fibroblasts derived from patients with NP type C disease is demonstrable. The primary biochemical defect remains to be elucidated, but knowledge of an anomalous intracellular cholesterol deposition may have important therapeutic implications.

The gene that is defective in this disease has been linked to chromosome 18.[208]

Treatment No specific therapy is currently available. A therapeutic trial in 25 patients placed on a diet restricted in cholesterol and the administration of cholesterol-lowering agents has resulted in reduction in hepatic and plasma cholesterol levels, but its effect on the course of the neurological disorder remains to be assessed.[209] One 9-month-old boy with progressive hepatosplenomegaly and neurodevelopmental delay was treated with cholesterol-lowering agents and reevaluated at 13 and 19 months of age: the neurologic development was considered to be normalized and the lipid resonance defect in the magnetic resonance spectra had disappeared.[210]

Subacute Neuropathic (Juvenile) Gaucher Disease (Type III Gaucher Disease)   In this rare form of Gaucher disease, involvement of the spleen, liver, and bone marrow is similar to that of the chronic nonneuropathic type I form of the disease. Splenomegaly and liver enlargement are usually present at birth or during early infancy, and when there are no neurologic signs it may be impossible to distinguish between the much more frequent type I and the neuropathic type III Gaucher disease. Neurological signs develop between 6 and 15 years of age, sometimes as late as early adulthood. The clinical syndrome is complex but some symptoms and signs stand out: frequent action myoclonus (polymyoclonus) or tonico-clonic seizures, and a supranuclear palsy of horizontal gaze, which is present in the majority of cases and is therefore of great diagnostic importance. A generalized extrapyramidal rigidity, trismus, and facial grimacing may be observed. Progressive mental deterioration is almost invariable. In a British family, where three siblings were affected,[211] the neurological disease began at 8 years. Convulsions, continuous irregular myoclonic jerks, dysarthria, slow mental deterioration, and a striking limitation of lateral gaze and ocular fixation and pursuit were the main signs.

A splenomegaly, Gaucher cells in the bone marrow, and an increased serum acid phosphatase activity are always present. Typical bone lesions, the same as those in type I Gaucher disease appear after several years. The severity and progressivity of the systemic disease is variable.

Some patients may have a supranuclear palsy of horizontal gaze as the sole neurological manifestation at an early age, and the more serious neurologic complications develop many years later. In a 10-month-old child with the visceral signs of Gaucher disease, who was examined by one of us, a paresis of conjugate lateral gaze was already present at that age. Slow mental deterioration and clumsiness appeared by the age of 10 years. In a group of patients with this type of isolated ophthalmologic manifestation in early childhood, the systemic disease may sometimes progress rapidly, with

death in late childhood or adolescence from hepatic and pulmonary complications of the storage process.[212]

An unusual number of cases of type III Gaucher disease have been found in the Norrbottnian region of northern Sweden (22 cases were reported in 1991).[213] In some of them, neurological manifestations appeared after or were seemingly exaggerated by splenectomy, possibly as a result of a rapid increase in the level of glucocerebrosides.

Neuropathology   Brain lesions are similar to those found in the acute early-onset neuropathic form of the disease (type II). They consist essentially of neuron loss with neuronophagia and perivascular Gaucher cells.

Genetics   Type III Gaucher disease is probably genetically distinct from types I and II. It has only once been reported in Jews (whereas type I is particularly frequent in Ashkenazic Jews).

The human glucocerebroside gene has been located on the long arm of chromosome 1 at band q21. More than 40 mutations in this gene have been identified. The most common are in exon 9 and exon 10. One mutation in exon 10, Leu[444]→Pro, is most prevalent in type III patients, appearing in the homozygous state in the Norrbottnian cases. In types I and II it is present only in the heterozygote state.[214,215] A deficiency of a glucocerebroside activator was reported in two patients with type III.[216]

Diagnosis   In view of the frequency of type I Gaucher disease, its coincidence with an unrelated neurological disorder is always a theoretical possibility. Also notable is the fact that vertebral lesions in the type I disease may lead to compression of spinal nerve roots or the spinal cord.

Treatment   In view of the severity and relentless progressivity of neurologic signs, type III Gaucher disease is a candidate for therapeutic trials such as enzyme replacement, organ transplantation, and bone marrow transplantation. Good results with bone marrow transplantation have been reported from Sweden.[213]

The Late-Onset Form of Farber Disease   In three patients belonging to two families, the disease started in the second or third year of life and consisted of severe and rapidly progressive mental deterioration, ataxia, pyramidal signs, seizures, polymyoclonia, and macular cherry red spots. There were subcutaneous nodules and arthropathy but no visceral involvement. The disease was rapidly lethal.[216a] (See also Chap. 3.)

Juvenile Neuronal Ceroid Lipofuscinosis (JNCL; NCL III; Spielmeyer-Vogt Disease; Late-Onset Batten Disease)

Juvenile neuronal ceroid lipofuscinosis (JNCL) is an autosomal recessive disorder with world-wide distribution. The disease begins in the juvenile period and pursues a protracted course (Fig. 5-12). Failure of vision with typical ophthalmoscopic and electroretinographic (ERG) changes appear in the early phase of the disease. Slow intellectual deterioration, seizures, a peculiar disorder of speech, and finally, an extrapyramidal rigidity follow as the disease progresses. The presence of vacuoles in lymphocytes is a useful diagnostic aid (Fig. 5-13). Typical intralysosomal inclusions are found in cutaneous and conjuctival tissue obtained by biopsy. An overview of the NCLs and a description of the infantile forms are to be found in Chap. 4.

Clinical Features   The disease starts between the ages of 5 and 10 years, sometimes as late as 12 to 13 years, but so far not earlier than 4 years. Until then, psychomotor development and language are normal or only slightly retarded. Age at onset and clinical course are more or less the same in a given family. Failure of vision, dementia, dysarthria, and seizures may appear in close succession, and any one of them may be the initial or predominant manifestation.

Decrease in visual acuity, generally the first manifestation of the disease, may begin in either the central or the peripheral parts of the visual fields. It progresses after several years to total blindness. The ophthalmologic findings are somewhat variable, although the basis for visual failure is always a degeneration of the sensory epithelium of the retina (Fig. 5-13). In most cases there is evidence of chorioretinal atrophy with attenuated blood vessels, pigmentary changes, and often optic atrophy (retinitis pigmentosa). Degeneration of the macula is a prominent finding. Loss of the foveal reflex has been mentioned as an early sign. The ERG is extinct. A posterior cortical cataract has been described. The ophthalmoscopic changes are not always present, even in the presence of amblyopia; but ERG changes are constant.

Intellectual decline, sometimes an early event, usually becomes manifest two or more years after onset of the visual signs and proceeds slowly to dementia. Short attention span, memory loss, and alternate periods of restlessness and adynamia are common manifestations. Delusions and hallucinations as well as episodes of psychotic behavior have been observed but are infrequent. When they do occur without preceding or associated visual failure, the disease raises many of the problems discussed below in the section on behavioral disturbances and dementia. Dysarthria is generally observed at this stage but may be present earlier. It takes the form of slurred, mumbled speech and a kind of stuttering. The dysarthria is often a reflection of muscular rigidity. Stereotyped repetitions of words or sentences (palilalia) are frequent.[217]

Seizures, ordinarily grand mal in type, usually appear several years after the visual signs; in some patients they are the first neurologic symptom. They tend to become progressively more frequent, although

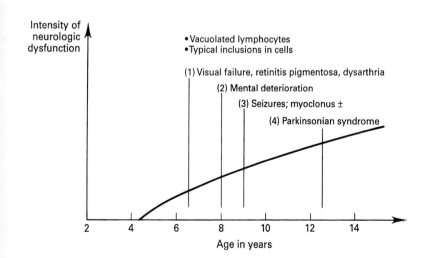

• Vacuolated lymphocytes
• Typical inclusions in cells

(1) Visual failure, retinitis pigmentosa, dysarthria

(2) Mental deterioration

(3) Seizures; myoclonus ±

(4) Parkinsonian syndrome

Intensity of neurologic dysfunction

Age in years

Figure 5-12
Juvenile neuronal ceroid lipofuscinosis: clinical evolution and life profile.

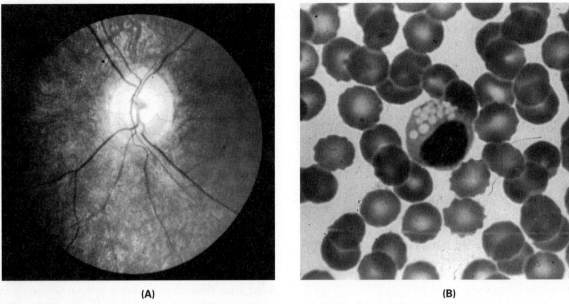

(A)   **(B)**

Figure 5-13
*Juvenile neuronal ceroid lipofuscinosis. **A.** Pigmentary degeneration of retina. **B.** Vacuolated lymphocyte in peripheral blood.*

rarely do they pose a major therapeutic problem. Interictal myoclonic jerking may be present in a few patients but they are not predominant or an early manifestation, as they are in earlier forms of NCL.

After several years, motor dysfunction is added to the clinical picture. It takes mostly the form of a generalized extrapyramidal rigidity with concomitant abnormalities of posture and locomotion, resembling the parkinsonian syndrome. The extrapyramidal signs and associated amblyopia understandably lead to severe disturbance of gait and equilibrium. Sometimes parkinsonian rigidity may be an early sign of the disease. Choreoathetosis is much less frequent. Cerebellar ataxia may be present, but rarely is it an early or prominent manifestation. Pyramidal signs are elicitable more often in the later stages of the disease and occasionally are asymmetric, causing a relative hemiparesis.

At later stages the patient is totally blind, paralyzed, and demented, and death ensues after 10 to 20 years.

Electroencephalic abnormalities are present in nearly all cases and may precede the onset of seizures. The tracings consist of diffuse bursts of slow waves or slow waves and spikes superimposed on a background of disorganized activity. Low frequencies of photic stimulation do not evoke the high-amplitude occipital

spikes seen in Bielschowsky disease. Visual evoked and sensory evoked cortical responses are reduced. Leukocytes in the peripheral blood contain abnormal inclusions of two types, which may or may not be combined in the same cell: translucent vacuoles in 10 to 30 percent of lymphocytes and azurophilic hypergranulations in neutrophils. The presence of vacuolated lymphocytes (Fig. 5-13), although nonspecific, is a constant feature and therefore of great help in diagnosis, especially in the initial phases of the disease. On neuroradiological imaging there is a moderate diffuse brain atrophy and an increased thickness of the calvarium.

Inclusions may be demonstrated by electron microscopy in cutaneous and conjunctival tissue (and autonomic nerve cells of the myenteric plexuses), obtained by biopsy. Intralysosomal deposits have a fingerprint-like lamellar formation, but curvilinear bodies and granular deposits may also be present.

The gene for JNCL is located on chromosome 16 in the p12.1 band.[219]

Pathologic Findings In all parts of the more or less atrophic brain, neurons are seen to be moderately distended by Sudan black-positive, PAS-positive, and autofluorescent granules. Granule cells and Purkinje cells in the cerebellum are severely depleted. Under the electron microscope the neuronal inclusions are membrane-bound and closely resemble lipofuscin. Aggregates of membranous bodies of fingerprint appearance are prominent. Some curvilinear inclusions may also be seen. This material accumulates in the perikaryon, particularly in the part between cell body and axon hillock, and may extend into the proximal axon (meganeurites). Similar inclusions also exist in neurons of the autonomic nervous system (particularly the myenteric plexuses) and in Schwann cells. They have also been found in the cells of the spleen, liver, muscle fibers, sweat glands, skin, and conjuctivas. The main changes in the retina consist of a degeneration of the rods and cones and pigmentary epithelium and an invasion of the retina by pigment-containing histiocytes. Lamellar inclusions have been observed in electron micrographs of lymphocytes.

Diagnosis   A child aged between 7 and 10 years with visual failure, retinitis pigmentosa, mental changes, seizures, and vacuolated lymphocytes stands a large chance of having JNCL. When the disease is initially monosymptomatic, the numerous causes of pigmentary degeneration of the retina (including purely ophthalmologic disorders), dementia with or without seizures, progressive dysarthria, a parkinsonian syndrome, or even primary epilepsy must all be considered. An ultrastructural study of a skin biopsy is certainly warranted under all these clinical circumstances. Definitive diagnosis rests on the demonstration of the typical intralysosomal inclusions and on the result of DNA studies. In the Jansky-Bielschowsky disease (late infantile NCL) there are no vacuoles in lymphocytes but characteristic electrophysiologic findings. Curvilinear lysosomal inclusions are typical. For a consensus on diagnostic criteria of the NCL see Kohlschutter et al.[218]

Treatment   There is no specific treatment. The use of antioxidants has brought temporary relief to some children. A trial in six children by supplementation of the diet with polyunsaturated fatty acids, with a follow-up lasting $2\frac{1}{2}$ to 7 years, suggests possible benefits.[220]

Kufs Adult Type of Neuronal Ceroid Lipofuscinosis
This is a rare disorder starting as late as the third or fourth decade. Indeed, more than half of reported cases cannot in fact be accepted as examples of adult neuronal lipofuscinosis but probably represent various other conditions. Berkovic et al. recognize two different clinical types[218]: type A which presents with epilepsy, myoclonus, ataxia, dementia, and extrapyramidal

signs; and type B with behavioral disturbances, dementia, facial dyskinesia, and various motor abnormalities. Amblyopia or retinal changes do not occur in Kufs disease. This condition is generally inherited as an autosomal recessive trait, but an autosomal dominant inheritance has been reported in two families.

The EEG shows various uncharacteristic changes. There is a marked response to photic stimulation. The ERG is normal. The diagnosis rests on the ultrastructural analysis of biopsied skin (especially sweat glands), muscle, or myenteric plexuses, which reveals intralysosomal accumulations of curvilinear profiles, fingerprintlike deposits, and other lamellar inclusions. Caution in the interpretation of the inclusions is necessary because of the ultrastructural heterogeneity of neuronal lipofuscin which is found in normal cells. Neuropathologic studies have shown intraneuronal inclusions typical of the lipofuscinoses.

Childhood and Juvenile Type II Sialidosis and Galactosialidosis   Type II sialidosis (see also Chap. 4 for clinical description and bibliography) is an autosomal recessive disorder essentially characterized by neurologic, ocular, visceral, skeletal, and facial abnormalities, an excretion of sialylated oligosaccharides and a marked deficiency of the activity of α-neuraminidase (which is encoded on chromosome 10 (10p ter→q23)). A similar clinical picture is caused by a genetically distinct disorder, *galactosialidosis*, in which there is a deficiency of both α-neuraminidase and β-galactosidase due to a deficiency of a protective protein, encoded on chromosome 20 in the q13.1 region. It is probable that some patients reported as having type II sialidosis are in fact cases of galactosialidosis, and the relative frequency of isolated neuraminidase deficiency (sialidosis type II) and galactosialidosis is not known. The chronic "juvenile" form of the disease apparently falls into the category of galactosialidosis. In view of the fact that similar clinical pictures comprising neurologic, ocular, skeletal, dysmorphic, and visceral involvement have been reported as having either type II sialidosis or galactosialidosis, a common clinical description will be given here.

Sialidosis type II and galactosialidosis have been divided into congenital, early infantile, late infantile, and juvenile forms.

The congenital and early infantile forms of type II sialidosis and galactosialidosis have been described in Chap. 3. The late infantile and juvenile (chronic) forms follow this pattern.

(1) In some patients the disease appears in the *first years of life*. Motor development is generally delayed.

Most children walk late with an unsteady gait and are clumsy. Mental retardation rapidly becomes evident. Seizures and myoclonus are often added. Characteristic facial features consist of a mild gargoyle-like appearance, short stature, clinical and radiologic evidence of dysostosis multiplex, and macular cherry red spots. Punctuate lens opacities may also be seen. Hepatosplenomegaly is observed and often there are angiokeratomas. Some children have been troubled by hernias and recurrent respiratory infections during the first months of life. Renal failure with proteinuria is a possible threat. The course of the disease is relatively rapid, and most children do not survive beyond late childhood or early adolescence.

(2) A less dramatic neurological syndrome is found in the *chronic form of galactosialidosis*, usually referred to as the juvenile/adult form of galactosialidosis. Its first manifestations may become apparent as early as the third year of life. This phenotype appears to have a much higher incidence in Japan but has also been reported in other countries. Neurologic abnormalities include myoclonic seizures, action myoclonus, myoclonic epilepsy, ataxia, macular cherry red spots, and corneal clouding. Neurological deterioration may be very slow, and the mental function of half the patients is normal. Angiokeratoma, coarse facial features, and skeletal changes are other characterisic features. Visceromegaly is exceptional. Patients survive well into adulthood.

Laboratory Tests

- Thin-layer chromatography of the urine demonstrates a high concentration of sialylated oligosaccharides (several hundred times greater than normal).

- Under the electron microscope, clear membrane-bound inclusions are found in biopsies of skin fibroblasts, liver (Kupffer cells), and in bone marrow histiocytes.

- In *type II sialidosis* a marked deficiency of the activity of α-neuraminidase is found in cultured fibroblasts, leukocytes, amniocytes, and chorionic villi.

- In *galactosialidosis* there is a combined deficiency of both α-neuraminidase and β-galactosidase. These enzymes can be assayed in leukocytes or fibroblasts, but when using leukocytes, isolated lymphocytes are preferred because the type of α-neuraminidase that is deficient in this disease predominates in lymphocytes. Assays of the protective protein are not entirely reliable.[222]

- Prenatal diagnosis can be accomplished by enzyme analysis of amniotic fluid cells and thin-layer chromatography of deproteinized amniotic fluid for the detection of sialyl oligosaccharides.

- Several mutations in the gene of the protective protein have been reported in the severe juvenile and mild adult forms of galactosialidosis in Japan. Another mutation has been described in four Caucasian patients with the late infantile form.[221]

Late-Onset Metachromatic Leukodystrophy: Juvenile and Adult Forms The reader is referred to the general remarks about the more common forms of late infantile metachromatic leukodystrophy (MLD) in Chap. 4. Late-onset MLD can begin at any age from childhood (3 to 10 years) to adolescence and even adulthood. In general, it can be said that the neurologic signs in later forms tend to be more diversified, involvement of peripheral nerves and increased CSF protein less constant, and behavioral abnormalities and dementia more prominent.

In childhood and in preadolescence (3 to 12 years), the disease may begin, as it does in the late infantile variety, by progressive difficulties in walking with evidence of pyramidal signs and involvement of the peripheral nerves (depressed tendon reflexes and/or low nerve conduction velocities). There may be an early period when only a polyneuropathy is demonstrable. The concentration of protein in the CSF may be elevated. Mental deterioration may be immediately evident or develop sometime after onset of the motor signs. However, in some cases, neurological signs are less typical: onset with a hemiplegia, cerebellar signs, dystonia, and choreoathetosis have all been observed. Abnormalities of nerve conduction and CSF protein may be lacking or are less evident. Behavioral changes and cognitive deficits are common and have been striking in several personally observed patients; seizures can occur but they are rare. The course of the disease is somewhat longer than in the late infantile form.

In adolescents and adults, failure in school or difficulties in vocational or professional work, peculiarities in behavior, or disturbance of cognitive function frequently call attention to the disease, and motor abnormalities such as a bipyramidal syndrome, ataxia, or extrapyramidal signs may not be detected until some time later. MRI reveals alteration of white matter, usually less pronounced than in the earlier form of the disease.

From this description it is clear that MLD in late childhood, adolescence, or in the adult may have a varied presentation. MLD should be considered as a diagnostic possibility in all patients in this age range who exhibit a deterioration of behavior and mental capacities, a progressive disorder of locomotion or coordination, or a progressive polyneuropathy. In all these circumstances, enzymatic assay of arylsulfatase A (ASA) on leukocytes or cultured fibroblasts and the search for excessive sulfatiduria should be systematically performed. Sulfatiduria is constant; as in late infantile MLD, levels of ASA are very low, at the limits of detection by the usual assay methods. (However, studies of substrate turnover in tissue culture suggest that some functional enzyme is retained.) Sometimes the demonstration of typical inclusions in Schwann cells and macrophages in peripheral nerve biopsies proves to be helpful in diagnosis.

Exceptionally, ASA activity is normal in a patient who excretes abnormal amounts of sulfatides in the urine and has the characteristic intralysosomal deposits in Schwann cells. In these patients, six of which have been reported in the literature, there is a complete deficiency of the cerebroside sulfate activator protein (saposin B). This can be demonstrated in leukocytes and cultured fibroblasts.

In screening siblings and parents of individuals affected with MLD, one may find individuals with no evidence of neurological disease (or with a disease not resembling MLD) but with low levels of ASA activity. The activity of their ASA may be only 10 to 15 percent of normal, much lower than the level of activity usually found in heterozygotes. This state of "pseudo-deficiency" has been traced to a gene (*Pd*), which is an allele of the MLD gene, and which occurs in approximately 10 percent of the general population (see also Chap. 4).

It is essential to differentiate the pseudo-deficiency state from presymptomatic MLD or fetal MLD. A first orientation is given by the fact that patients with the *Pd* gene do not excrete excessive amounts of sulfatides. An extensive family screening for ASA activity, special biochemical tests (for instance, sulfatide loading tests in tissue culture) and DNA studies, are required to differentiate the two states.

The course of adolescent or adult MLD is variable. A 5 to 10 year survival is not unusual, but in a few patients, evolution is much more rapid.

As described in Chap. 4, two groups of mutations, I and A, have been shown to induce the lesions of MLD. Individuals with one copy of allele A usually have a late infantile or juvenile onset, and those homozygous for allele A have a late adolescent or adult form.

The results of bone marrow transplantations are discussed in Chap. 9.

Late-Onset Krabbe Disease (Late Infantile and Juvenile Form)   Krabbe leukodystrophy (KL) is an autosomal recessive disorder due to a deficiency of galactosylceramide β-galactosidase. The great majority of patients are affected with the disease before the end of the first year of life, usually between 3 and 6 months. This early infantile form has been described in Chap. 3. In some patients, however, the first signs of the disorder appear in late childhood or adolescence.

Late-onset KL has long been considered quite rare. Between 1906 and 1987, only 23 cases were reported. However, since the increased availability of reliable enzymatic assays in recent years, this late form of the disease is found to be not at all exceptional. Between 1987 and 1990, approximately 40 new cases were reported worldwide.[223] Late-onset forms could possibly represent as many as 10 to 15 percent of all cases of KL. The authors, particularly EK, have diagnosed and treated more than a dozen such patients.

Clinical Features   The symptomatology of 50 cases of late-onset KL was reviewed in 1991 by Lyon and Hagberg.[223] Of those 50, 23 had been reported between 1906 and 1987, and the other 27 were mostly unpublished cases collected in Europe in 1987. The findings in this series duplicated those described in a series of patients by Kolodny et al.[224]

Late-onset KL has a worldwide distribution. It seems particularly frequent in southern Italy and Sicily and is notably very rare in Sweden (1 case compared to 100 cases of the early infantile form reported in 1990).[225]

The disorder starts between the ages of 15 months and 10 years, mostly before the age of 5 years (Fig. 5-14). There is no significant difference in symptomatology between late infantile and juvenile forms (Fig. 5-15). A clearly progressive equinovarus deformity of the feet may be present for several years before other signs of motor disability are appreciated. Progressive difficulties in walking in a previously normal or mildly retarded child were generally the first indication of the disease. A spastic paraparesis with pyramidal signs, a cerebellar ataxia, or a combination of the two dominated the neurological picture. Sometimes a spastic hemiplegia, mainly affecting one lower limb, was the initial sign of the disease, followed after a few weeks or months by a bilateralization of the pyramidal signs. Dystonia has occasionally been reported. Some patients present with obvious clinical signs of a polyneuropathy at the onset of their disease. Involvement of the peripheral nerves (absent deep tendon reflexes and/or low nerve conduction velocities) was found in approximately half the patients with spastic paraparesis or other neurological signs. Evidence of a neuropathy tended to become more obvious with advancing age.

Visual failure usually with optic atrophy was present in most patients at an advanced stage of the disease. In 20 percent of patients in one series[223] it was the initial and only finding for several months. The blindness was usually related to optic atrophy in the earlier-onset cases and to demyelination of the optic radiation in the later-onset variant.[224] Seizures were infrequent. However, in two of our patients the first indications were severe convulsions and they remained a major therapeutic problem. The time of onset and severity of mental deterioration and behavioral abnormalities was variable, even among affected siblings in the same family. In most instances, evidence of dementia appeared progressively some time after the onset of motor signs. Others retained a normal intelligence for many years. The first signs in two children were behavioral changes, irritability, and intellectual impairment.

A high protein content in the CSF was found in half the patients, usually but not constantly associated with low nerve conduction velocities. Predominantly periventricular parieto-occipital areas of demyelination were visible by MRI of the brain (Fig. 5-16). CT scans tended to be normal in the early stages of the disease. In

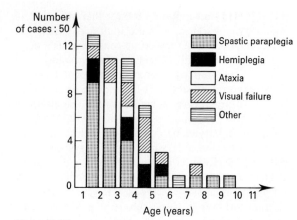

Figure 5-15
Late-onset Krabbe leukodystrophy: inaugural signs. (Courtesy Dev. Neurosci. 13. 1991, ref. 223.)

sural nerve biopsies there was segmental demyelination and typical ultrastructural inclusions in Schwann cells. These were associated with clinical signs of a neuropathy and low nerve conduction velocities. In other patients with normal NCV, no morphological abnormality could be detected. It is notable that the clinical symptomatology of some patients appeared to have been acutely aggravated by an infectious disease.

The course of the disease has been quite variable and unpredictable, possibly because of various exogenous factors. Most patients become tetraplegic and demented after a period of 2 to 5 years, but others can still be alive after one or two decades. It is remarkable that in 35 percent of patients, mostly under 3 years of age, there was a catastrophic decline in neurologic function within 3 months, possibly related to an intercurrent infection. These children had become tetraplegic and demented.

Genetics and Intrafamilial Variations   Late-onset KL is an autosomal recessive disorder. In the series of 50 patients (26 males and 24 females), consanguinity was present in 6 families and two siblings were affected in 12 families. Consanguinity was also present in 2 of the 11 families reported by Kolodny.[224] There was little variation in age of onset within a family and the symptomatology tended to be the same. A few exceptions were noted. In one family, for instance, one child's first sign at the age of 5 years was a gradual loss of vision, whereas the other presented at the age of 2 years with ataxia. There may also be intrafamilial differences with respect to intellectual abilities. In 3 families, one child

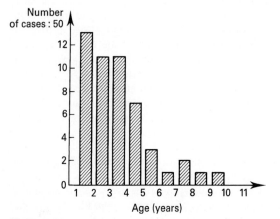

Figure 5-14
Late-onset Krabbe leukodystrophy: age of onset. (Courtesy Dev. Neurosci. 13, 1991, ref. 223.)

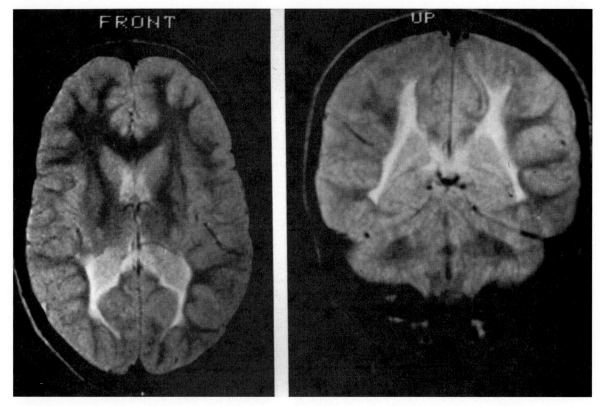

Figure 5-16
Late-onset Krabbe disease in a 6-year-old child. MRI. Symmetrical periventricular demyelination in the parieto-occipital region.

had late-onset KL, whereas another had an early infantile form of the disease.

Pathological Findings and Biochemistry The lesions in the brain are similar to those seen in the classical early infantile disease (cf. Chap. 3). Typical ultrastructural inclusions in Schwann cells in sural nerve biopsies may be lacking.

The deficiency of galactocerebroside β-galactosidase in leukocytes or fibroblasts is markedly reduced and is usually as severe as in the early infantile disease.

Complementation studies suggest that early- and late-onset forms of KL arise from allelic mutations in the same gene. Late-onset KL could represent a state of compound heterozygosity with one allele of early infantile KL, combined with another less deleterious allele. This has been confirmed in molecular studies. One common mutation is a C→T transition at nucleotide base 502, causing an Arg[168]→Cys substitution (which is pre-

sent in both classical and late-onset cases). This common mutation is found in combination with other rare mutations, a feature unique to the late-onset patients.[225a]

Diagnosis The clinical picture of late-onset KL is in no way specific. The diagnosis of the disease should be considered as a possibility in a child or adolescent with one of the following signs: a progressive spastic paraplegia, progressive cerebellar ataxia, progressive visual failure with optic atrophy or cortical blindness, slowly progressive hemiplegia, a peripheral neuropathy, all in the absence of visceral involvement. None exist for long in pure form, which is helpful in differential diagnosis. Low nerve conduction velocities and a high protein content of the CSF, constant findings in the early form of the disease, are lacking in 50 percent of the cases. The diagnosis rests on the discovery of the specific enzymatic deficit.

Adult Forms A few cases of late-onset KL have been reported in the adult. The symptomatology is extremely variable and includes such presentations as a spinocerebellar degeneration[226] or a peripheral neuropathy.[227]

Treatment The results of bone marrow transplantations are discussed in Chap. 9.

X-linked Adrenoleukodystrophy Adrenoleukodystrophy is an X-linked disorder characterized by progressive demyelination of the central nervous system and adrenal insufficiency. The incidence is 1/20,000 male births. Saturated very long chain fatty acids (VLCFAs) accumulate in tissues and body fluids because of an impairment in the peroxisomal oxidation of these fatty acids. The activity of lignoceroyl-CoA synthetase is reduced as the consequence of the deficiency of a peroxisomal membrane protein, ALDP, which is involved in the active transport of enzyme cofactors and/or substrates required for β-oxidation of VLCFAs. ALDP is encoded by an ATP-binding cassette-transporter gene that has been mapped to Xq28, close to the color vision genes. Diagnosis currently rests on the demonstration of an excess of VLCFAs in tissues and body fluids.

The clinical phenotype is variable. Neurological signs are most often the first to appear and are in the foreground. According to Moser,[228] half of the patients have a rapidly progressive encephalopathy starting in childhood, adolescence, or more rarely, in adulthood, characterized by cognitive disturbances, mental deterioration, central loss of vision and hearing, occasionally a progressive hemiplegia, and parieto-occipital areas of demyelination with peripheral contrast enhancement on neuroradiologic imaging. Twenty-five percent of patients, adults more than adolescents, suffer from a slowly progressive paraparesis called adrenomyeloneuropathy. Overt or occult biologic evidence of adrenal insufficiency is present in the great majority but not all cases. It may precede the onset of the neurologic syndrome by many years. In 10 to 15 percent of cases, Addison disease stands as the only manifestation. Some individuals are asymptomatic. Female carriers may develop a spastic paraparesis.

Clinical Features In the great majority of patients, neurological signs are the first to attract attention. There are two neurologic syndromes: the cerebral (infantile, juvenile, or adult form) and adrenomyeloneuropathy.

More than 50 percent of male patients are affected with the common infantile or juvenile *cerebral form of adrenoleukodystrophy* (ALD). The age of onset in most cases is between 3 and 10 years, with a mean age of 8 years. In 5 percent of patients the first signs appear between 11 and 21 years, and in 3 percent they appear during adulthood.

Slow mentation, lack of interest or hyperactivity, dysphasia, dysarthria, and occasionally a psychotic behavior may mark the early stages of the disease. A possible attention deficit disorder or psychosis of indeterminate type was the first diagnosis in a few of our cases. In some older patients, evidence of parietal lobe dysfunction (constructional or dressing apraxia) or evidence of a frontal lobe-type of dementia have also been described.

Hemianopia and progressive impairment of vision are usual and may be among the first signs. The blindness is of central origin, due to the interruption of the geniculostriate radiations. Less often there is involvement of the optic nerve with optic atrophy. Hearing loss, also of central origin, is usually present and frequently an early sign. A progressive hemiplegia may also appear as one of the first manifestations, mimicking multiple sclerosis or a brain tumor. Focal or generalized seizures have been reported in approximately one-third of the patients, rarely as an initial sign.

Evidence of demyelination is demonstrated on MRI in practically all cases (Fig. 5-17). Areas of demyelination are predominantly located in the parieto-occipital regions of both hemispheres and have a caudorostral progression. Lesions are occasionally unilateral, at least initially. Frontal areas are much more rarely affected. Contrast enhancement can be demonstrated at the periphery of the demyelinated zone. Protein concentration is generally elevated in the CSF with normal gamma globulins.

Whatever the initial abnormality, after some months a complex and disabling neurologic picture with dementia, blindness, deafness, and bilateral pyramidal signs develops. After a period of 1 to 2 years, many of the patients have deteriorated to a vegetative state. There is no significant difference between the duration of the disease in children and in adults.

Adrenomyeloneuropathy (AMN) occurs mainly in young adults, less often in adolescents. The neurologic syndrome is one of a very slowly progressive spastic paraparesis without significant involvement of the upper limbs. A bilateral pyramidal syndrome is combined with impaired vibration and position sense, urinary disturbances, and sexual dysfunction—a cluster of

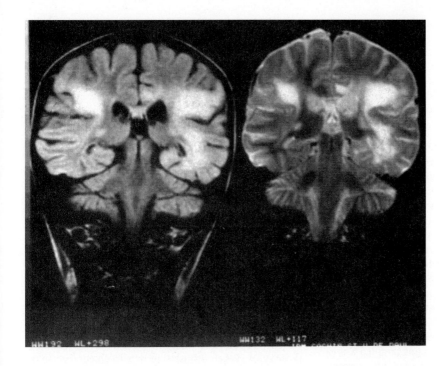

Figure 5-17
*X-linked adrenoleukodystrophy.
MRI shows bilateral asymmetric
lesions of cerebral white matter.
(Courtesy Dr. G. Ponsot.)*

findings indicative of a myelopathy. The only sign of peripheral nerve involvement generally consists of moderate slowing of motor and sensory nerve velocities. Somatosensory evoked potentials and brain stem auditory evoked potentials are also slowed. Hypogonadism is another feature of the disease and may occasionally be observed before the onset of neurologic signs. Vision and mental function are generally intact. However, some evidence of cognitive decline has occasionally been observed, presumably attributable to abnormalities in cerebral white matter. The course of the disease may fluctuate. After 5 to 15 years the patients usually become severely incapacitated and unable to walk. Death occurs in the third or fourth decade. A symptom complex resembling AMD is also observed in female heterozygotes.

Clinical or biological evidence of *adrenal insufficiency* is present in the great majority of cases of ALD and AMN. The manifestations of the endocrine disorder and its chronological relation with the neurologic disorder are variable. Adrenal insufficiency in ALD may take the form of a typical Addison disease, or of an isolated, focal, or diffuse melanodermia. The adrenal dysfunction may also be clinically latent, brought to light solely by endocrinological tests showing an impaired adrenocortical response to adrenocorticotropic hormone (ACTH)

stimulation, and elevated baseline levels of endogenous ACTH.

In the great majority of cases, evidence of adrenal insufficiency is obtained after onset of neurologic signs. There may be an isolated, very mild melanodermia disclosed only when carefully searched for at selective cutaneous and mucosal sites. In a few patients with the typical form of ALD or in adults or adolescents with AMN, a diffuse skin pigmentation has been present since early childhood. Asthma has been associated with this type of adrenal insufficiency. More often the adrenal insufficiency is detected (or confirmed) only by laboratory tests evaluating the response of cortisol to ACTH stimulation.

Rarely, signs of Addison disease antedate the neurologic syndrome, sometimes by several years (as many as 20). In approximately 10 percent of patients, Addison disease constitutes the only manifestation of ALD. Possibly the neurologic disorder may develop later. Finally, it is important to know that all clinical and biological evidence of adrenal insufficiency may be lacking, especially in patients with AMN, and this may complicate the diagnosis.

Symptomatic ALD Heterozygotes Approximately 10 to 15 percent of women who are heterozygous for ALD will manifest typical signs of adrenomyelo-neuropathy. Brain MRI may show white matter abnormalities. Adrenal function is almost always intact. The course of the disease is usually, but not constantly, milder than in hemizygous patients. A small population of women with AMN and typical abnormalities of VLCFAs did not have an affected male relative.

Intrafamilial Variability Different phenotypes may coexist in the same kindred. A boy with a complete picture of cerebral adrenoleukodystrophy may have a brother, cousin, or uncle affected with what seems to be an isolated adrenal insufficiency; the childhood cerebral form and AMN may occur in the same sibship; or a grandfather with a slowly progressive paraplegia may have a grandson with the most devastating form of cerebral disease. Some male individuals with elevated levels of VLCFAs in families with adrenoleukodystrophy may be asymptomatic.

We have observed an interesting family with two affected brothers. One, aged 12, had the classical form with no melanodermia; the other, aged 25, was diffusely melanodermic, without neurologic signs, and led a normal life. The maternal grandfather had a diffuse melanodermia since childhood and died at the age of 50 from a rapidly progressive cerebral disorder.

Mutation analysis of the ALD gene confirms the lack of genotype-phenotype correlations and raises the possibility of a modifier gene to explain phenotypic variability within a single kindred.[229]

Diagnosis The definitive diagnosis of ALD rests at present on the demonstration of abnormally high levels of saturated VLCFAs in plasma, erythrocytes, leukocytes, or cultured fibroblasts, using gas chromatography/mass spectrometry. High plasma levels are already present in the neonate and do not vary significantly with age. Assays of VLCFAs in all female members of a family with an affected boy are essential for the detection of heterozygotes and for genetic counseling. VLCFA assays combined with linkage analysis using the DXS52 probe allow the detection of female carriers in nearly 100 percent of cases. Small deviations from normal may however be difficult to interpret. Strategies to detect mutations in ALD are presently being developed.[230] This should make screening for heterozygotes more certain. *Prenatal diagnosis* is possible using VLCFA assays on amniocytes or cultures of chorionic villus. The DXS52 DNA probe has also been used to identify affected male fetuses.

The clinical diagnosis of ALD is difficult in view of the protean nature of the disease. In the common cerebral form of the disease, a diagnosis of learning disability or psychiatric problem may be made initially, and other causes of amblyopia, deafness, dementia, or progressive hemiplegia may need to be considered. Fortunately, the characteristic abnormalities of the cerebral white matter on MRI direct one to the correct diagnosis in most such cases. The possibility of sporadic Schilder disease must be considered in some instances (see Chap. 6).

Diagnosis is much more difficult in males or females with *adrenomyeloneuropathy*; other metabolic or degenerative disorders, such as the late-onset sphingolipidoses, Strümpell familial paraplegia, and multiple sclerosis, need to be considered. The absence of manifest adrenal insufficiency in one-third of the patients with AMN[228] and the uncertainty of the results of VLCFA analysis in a number of symptomatic female heterozygotes (some of which may have no affected male relatives) adds to the diagnostic difficulty. Molecular biology techniques will solve this problem in the future. Biopsies of skin or peripheral nerve could be of help in those cases. When diffuse skin hyperpigmentation is the only manifestation of the disease, other causes of melanodermia must be considered.

All boys with Addison disease must be systematically screened for ALD. But one should keep in mind that X-linked adrenal insufficiency is seen in glycerol kinase deficiency and has been reported in other families.[231] Families with Addison disease and pure spastic paraplegia have also been reported.[232]

X-linked adrenoleukodystrophy and neonatal adrenoleukodystrophy (see Chap. 2) are entirely unrelated conditions.

Pathology Brain lesions are restricted to the white matter. They predominate in the parieto-occipital regions and tend to progress caudorostrally. In the demyelinated areas are sudanophilic and PAS-positive macrophages, as well as prominent perivascular lymphocytic cuffing, particularly in the peripheral zones of the lesion. Myelin is affected out of proportion to axis cylinders. The appearance is similar to that of sporadic Schilder disease and the cerebral forms of multiple sclerosis. In AMN, lesions are essentially in the spinal cord. Demyelination and inflammatory signs are less marked. There is severe fiber loss, perhaps consistent with a distal axonopathy. Peripheral nerve involvement is minimal. In the adrenal cortex, cells of the inner fasciculate and reticular zone are ballooned and have a striated appearance, due to the accumulation of lipids. At an advanced stage, the adrenal cortex becomes atrophic. Leydig cells are affected in the testicles. Ultrastructural changes are remarkable: lamellar inclusions representing VLCFAs are seen in brain macrophages, Schwann cells, adrenal cells, and Leydig cells. Peroxisomes are normal in the liver and other organs.

Treatment Dietary VLCFA restriction combined with the oral administration of a 4:1 mixture of glyceryl trioleate and glyceryl trierucate lowers plasma VLCFA levels but does not prevent or reverse the neurologic disorder of X-linked adrenoleukodystrophy. Recently, however, bone marrow transplantations have had some effect (see Chap. 9). Steroid replacement therapy for adrenal insufficiency is effective, but the correction of the endocrine disorder does not alter the course of the neurologic disease. Various methods to suppress the inflammatory response in cerebral lesions have been tested, with uncertain results.

Juvenile (Childhood and Adolescence) Leigh Syndrome; Juvenile PDHC Deficiency   The great majority of cases of Leigh syndrome (subacute necrotizing encephalopathy) develop before the age of 2, mostly in the first year of life (see Chaps. 3 and 4). Approximately 17 percent start between the ages of 3 and 15 years, and 2 percent after 15 years.

The clinical picture of the juvenile form is variable and frequently uncharacteristic. It takes the form of a diffuse progressive encephalopathy with mental regression, unilateral or bilateral pyramidal signs, athetoid or dystonic disorders of motility, cerebellar ataxia, and oculomotor abnormalities. The bouts of hyperventilation so typical of infantile Leigh syndrome are less conspicuous here or occur only later in the disease, if at all. The clinical picture may suggest the possibility of a brain stem tumor. An optic atrophy and a peripheral neuropathy may appear. Seizures are rare. CSF proteins are occasionally elevated. The course of the disease is either unremitting or relapsing with transient episodes of sudden worsening of neurological signs, or even a metabolic coma after an infection. Lactate is usually increased in the CSF. There is no evidence of a myopathy, and muscle biopsies are normal.

The diagnosis of late-onset Leigh syndrome, as in the other forms of the disease, depends on the demonstration of the typical symmetrical MRI foci of disease in the basal ganglia and brain stem, and possibly cerebellum and cerebral white matter. Several biochemical abnormalities have been found in the various forms of

Leigh syndrome with a Mendelian mode of inheritance: deficiency of complex IV of the respiratory chain (cytochrome-*c* oxidase deficiency), of the pyruvate dehydrogenase complex (PDHC), much more rarely of complex I, of complex II, and of biotinidase. The maternally inherited Leigh syndrome (MILS) is mentioned below, and in Chap. 3.

The duration of childhood and adolescent Leigh syndrome is variable. Death usually occurs after 3 to 10 years. An acute course, not exceeding a few weeks, has been reported.

Diagnosis The characteristic morphologic picture by radioimaging (or autopsy) is, in principle, required for firm diagnosis of Leigh disease (LD). The differentiation of LD in childhood and adolescence, from sporadic or familial cases of progressive encephalopathies with isolated *bilateral striatal necrosis* may be difficult. Some conditions reported under the heading of bilateral striatal necrosis or striatal lucencies are apparently of a different nature (see Table 5-8 and Chap. 6). Other cases may, however, be related to LD. We have seen young children who initially showed isolated lesions in the putamen on MRI and a few years later developed the full lesional pattern. Lesions may also be atypical. We have observed two brothers aged 10 and 13 years with widespread demyelination of the cerebral white matter, mimicking a leukodystrophy on CT scans, who at autopsy had the typical symmetrical foci of necrosis in the basal ganglia and brain stem. Finally, in one of our patients with PDH deficiency, the clinical picture was indistinguishable from that of LD, and MRI was normal.

Treatment No specific treatment is available. Systemic lactic acidosis in PDH deficiency may be reversed by a ketogenic diet or the use of dichloroacetate. In the very rare patient with a thiamine-responsive form of the disease, thiamine may allay symptoms.

Defects of Intergenomic Signaling   Defects of intergenomic signaling[248] include qualitative and quantitative defects of mtDNA which are the result of mutations in nuclear genes necessary to the integrity of the mitochondrial genome. They are transmitted by Mendelian inheritance.

Dominantly inherited mitochondrial myopathy or encephalomyopathy with multiple deletions of mtDNA. Adults from three generations of one family presented with *progressive external ophthalmoplegia* (PEO), dysphagia, exercise intolerance, cataracts, ragged red fibers in skeletal muscles, and lactic acidosis.[257] There was no retinitis pigmentosa. A child from another family had repeated attacks of incoordination, drowsiness, and coma with ketoacidosis, lactacidemia, and hypoglycemia followed by persistent ataxia, pyramidal signs, oculomotor palsies, and deafness. Ragged red muscle fibers were present. Multiple deletions were found in the asymptomatic mother and maternal aunt. Members of another family exhibited optic atrophy and ptosis. The locus of one such gene has been mapped to chromosome 10q23.3-24.3.[258]

Rare cases of *autosomal recessive PEO* with cardiomyopathy have been related to multiple deletions in mtDNA.

At least 10 cases have been reported of *mtDNA depletion syndrome with variable tissue expression.*[259] It presents either as a fatal congenital condition with muscle weakness, external ophthalmoplegia, nephropathy, liver disease, lactic acidosis and RRF in variable proportions, or as an infantile myopathy. This condition is inherited as an autosomal recessive trait.

Cerebrotendinous Xanthomotosis (Cholestanolosis) Cerebrotendinous xanthomotosis (CTX) is a rare autosomal recessive disorder caused by defective bile acid synthesis, secondary to a lack of the hepatic mitochondrial enzyme sterol 27-hydroxylase. As a result, cholestanol (the 5α-dihydroderivative of cholesterol) accumulates in the nervous system, lens, tendon sheaths, and other tissues. The major clinical manifestations consist of tendon xanthomas, juvenile cataracts, and a progressive neurological disorder in which cerebellar ataxia and progressive mental degeneration are usually combined. Approximately 150 patients have been reported worldwide. The disease starts usually in late childhood or adolescence. The onset of the neurological disorder is insidious. Mental retardation, later dementia, and frequently behavioral abnormalities are observed. Cerebellar ataxia and dysarthria are prominent features. A palatal rhythmic myoclonus may occur as a consequence of tegmental brain stem lesions involving rubro-olivary tracts. Progressive pyramidal signs, leading to a pseudobulbar syndrome, develop with time. Seizures are not rare, and most patients show a diffuse slowing and paroxysmal bursts in the EEG. A mild peripheral neuropathy is a frequent finding.

In the presence of this slowly progressive syndrome of diffuse nervous system involvement, the presence of cataracts and of tendon xanthomas mainly located in the Achilles tendons are of major diagnostic importance. Other features of the disease include osteoporosis with a tendency towards spontaneous fractures,

pes cavus, elongated facies and large paranasal sinuses, and accelerated atherosclerosis. High incidences of spontaneous abortions and early infantile mortality have been reported in some families. MRI brain scans show demyelination especially in the cerebellum and brain stem, atrophy of the cerebellum, brain stem and spinal cord, and other focal abnormalities, all of which are related to the presence of xanthomatous deposits.

A purely spinal form of the disease has been reported.

Laboratory Findings of Diagnostic Importance Laboratory findings of diagnostic importance include the following:

- Low plasma cholesterol concentrations
- Increased levels of cholestanol in plasma and tissues (tendon biopsy)
- Virtual absence of chenodeoxycholic acid in the bile
- High levels of cholestanol and apolipoprotein B in the CSF[233]
- Large amounts of bile alcohol glucuronides in plasma, urine, and bile

If these results are uncertain, tests of bile acid synthesis stimulated with cholestyramine, are worthwhile. This results in an increase in urinary bile alcohol in both affected patients and carriers. The biochemical abnormalities precede the appearance of neurologic signs and should be searched for in screening the family of a clinically affected patient.[234]

The sterol 27-hydroxylase gene has been localized on chromosome 2q33-qter. Several mutations have been detected. Knowledge of a specific mutation within a family may permit the molecular diagnosis of asymptomatic cases.[235]

Pathology The neuropathologic characteristics of CTX were first described by Van Bogaert, Epstein, and Scherer in 1937.[236] Widespread demyelination and presence of xanthomas are found in the cerebellum, brain stem, spinal cord, and to a lesser extent, the cerebral hemispheres. The concentration of cholestanol is high in the brain, as first pointed out by Moser. A severe demyelinating neuropathy has been documented.

Clinicopathological Correlations The neurological dysfunction is clearly related to the lesions of the cerebellum and brain stem.

Treatment Lifelong treatment with oral cheno-deoxycholic acid (chenodiol 750 mg/day) may be highly effective, especially when given early, in the presymptomatic stage.[237] The use of a HMG-CoA reductase inhibitor such as mevinolin, an inhibitor of cholesterol synthesis, may also be effective. Treated patients exhibit significant improvements in clinical symptoms and evoked potentials.[238] Administration of CoQ_{10} has also been advised.

Juvenile Neuroaxonal Dystrophy Dorfman and associates[239] have reported the case histories of two male siblings who at the ages of 10 and 12 years began to have polymyoclonus of increasing severity and generalized seizures. In the years that followed, the myoclonus reached such a degree of severity that it could be activated by the slightest voluntary movement (but not by sound or visual stimulation). Gradually there was added a cerebellar ataxia and a slow decline in intellectual function. Paroxysms of irregular delta activity were found on EEG tracings. Death occurred in one patient at the age of 23 years, and on postmortem examination the typical spheroids of multiple membranous lamellae were found in cerebral cortex, thalamus, and brain stem reticular formation. On pathologic grounds, the case was classified as neuroaxonal dystrophy and resembled other cases of the infantile form of the disease. There appeared to be none of the characteristic features of Hallervorden-Spatz disease, in which axonal spheroids are also present.

A few other cases have been reported as juvenile NAD or juvenile/adult NAD; most patients also had severe polymyoclonus and cerebellar ataxia. One child[240] started walking at the age of 2 years. He fell frequently but developed pretty well until the age of 24 years, when generalized myoclonus, ataxia, and dysarthria appeared. The tendon reflexes were absent and the lower limbs hypotonic, without evidence of pyramidal signs. The patient died at the age of 38 years. Autopsy showed diffuse axonal spheroids, cerebellar atrophy, and normal basal ganglia and substantia nigra. Vuia[241] reported a female patient whose disease started at 12 with an ataxic gait. At 18 she had severe cerebellar signs, polymyoclonus, weakness and wasting of the peroneal muscles, and atrophy of the cerebellum. Later there appeared a generalized extrapyramidal rigidity, choreoathetosis, and a tremor. She died at the age of 25 years. Scattered axonal spheroids mainly in the brain stem and spinal cord, and loss of Purkinje cells were found. The basal ganglia and substantia nigra appeared to be normal. By electron microscopic examination the axonal spheroids were not exactly like those of the infantile NAD. Scheithauer[242] described another case of protracted NAD with myoclonus epilepsy and Schwendemann et al.[243] added the case of a 14-year-old child with progressive dysarthria, clumsiness, and slow intellectual deterioration. Dystonic movements appeared at age 23. There were no pyramidal signs. The optokinetic nystagmus was abnormal. No abnormality was noted by CT scan. Rectal and skin biopsies showed axonal spheroids filled with granular and vesicular material, and a few lamellar structures, which appeared to differ from typical NAD inclusions.

The relationship between juvenile NAD and typical infantile NAD remains to be determined.

Neuronal Intranuclear Inclusion Disease Neuronal intranuclear inclusion disease is a rare progressive neurological disorder of unknown cause, characterized by the presence of intranuclear inclusions in the neurons of the central and autonomic nervous system.[244] Fifteen cases had been reported in 1994.[245]

The disease begins clinically between the ages of 1 and 13 years with signs of diffuse, progressive dysfunction of the nervous system. Progressive cerebellar ataxia and extrapyramidal movement disorder, dystonia, choreoathetosis or rigidity, and dysarthria are prominent, and there are usually bilateral pyramidal tract signs. Evidence of lesions of the peripheral motor neurons with amyotrophy, fasciculations, absent tendon reflexes, and/or signs of denervation atrophy on the EMG constitute one of the notable features of the disease. It is common to find cranial nerve palsies involving the Xth, XIIth, and VIIth nerves (dysphagia, atrophy of the tongue, facial palsy) and ophthalmoparesis. Nystagmus and oculogyric crises are reported. There are variable degrees of intellectual deterioration and frequently severe behavioral disturbances with violent temper tantrums. Death occurs in the second or third decade.

One of us has observed a boy who presented at age 3 years with difficulty in walking, mild incoordination, and loss of speech. A brain MRI at age 6 years disclosed mild cortical atrophy, a small cerebellum, and atrophy of the cerebral peduncles and medullary olives. He became increasingly tremulous. As he deteriorated, he exhibited progressive pseudobulbar palsy, cerebellar ataxia, and a pyramidal tract disorder, sparing cognitive functions but with a labile affect and violent mood swings. Ptosis and a skew deviation were observed, and there was mild dystonic posturing. At age 8, he developed congestive heart failure with mitral regurgitation; he died at age 9 of pneumonia.

The combination of progressive signs of diffuse central nervous system dysfunction (usually with ataxia and extrapyramidal signs) and evidence of anterior horn cell disorder, is characteristic of neuronal intranuclear inclusion disease. A similar picture is seen in G_{M2} gangliosidosis. Diagnosis of neuronal intranuclear inclusion disease is possible by the detection of typical hyalin intranuclear inclusions in the neurons of the myenteric plexus in rectal biopsy specimens.[246] They consist of round eosinophilic bodies measuring 4 to 5 μm, which under the electron microscope are seen to take the form of nonmembrane-bound granular and filamentous material in a lattice-like arrangement. Intranuclear inclusions have been found at autopsy in most neurons of the central nervous system (including anterior horn cells of the spinal cord) and autonomic nervous system. The population of nerve cells is depleted.

The cause of the disease is unknown, but its hereditary nature and an autosomal recessive mode of inheritance seems established: two siblings (including a pair of monozygote twins) were affected in three of the reported families.

There is no treatment.

Diseases with a Maternal Mode of Inheritance: Defects in Mitochondrial DNA

The Juvenile Mitochondrial Encephalomyopathies

Herein are described a group of plurisystemic disorders with a multiform neurologic symptomatology—the juvenile mitochondrial encephalomyopathies. Although some of their manifestations could warrant their inclusion in the section on strokes or on myoclonus epilepsy, the fact that they are all associated with defects in the mitochondrial DNA (mtDNA) and a certain degree of overlap between their different forms, justifies their common description in this section. Juvenile and adulthood mitochondrial encephalomyopathies comprise a wide variety of clinical manifestations and have been divided into a number of syndromes, the most important of which are *Kearns-Sayre syndrome* (KSS), *progressive external ophthalmoplegia* (PEO), *mitochondrial encephalomyopathy with lactic acidosis and strokes* (MELAS), and *myoclonus epilepsy and ragged red fibers* (MERRF).

KSS and one variety of PEO are sporadic conditions caused by large-scale rearrangements (deletions and duplications) of mtDNA, whereas MELAS and MERRF are maternally inherited disorders due to point mutations of the mtDNA.

Other disorders related to point mutations in the mtDNA include Leber hereditary optic neuropathy (LHON), the syndrome of neuropathy, ataxia, and retinitis pigmentosa (NARP), maternally inherited PEO, and maternally inherited Leigh syndrome (MILS).

Although clinical experience and molecular analyses tend to confirm the autonomy of these syndromes, each of them displays a great variety of clinical expressions and there is some degree of overlap between them. The variations of phenotypes are probably explained in part by the fact that the cells of patients contain a variable proportion of normal mtDNA and mutant mitochondrial mtDNA (heteroplasmia). The possibility of manifest disease is determined in part by the proportion of normal to mutated mtDNA. This so-called threshold effect is also influenced by the energy demands of various tissues (high in brain and muscle), by age, and by other factors.[247,248]

Defects of mtDNA related to mutations in nuclear genes with a Mendelian mode of inheritance (multiple deletions of mtDNA and depletion of mtDNA) have been described above. DeVivo[248] has written a recent review on the mitochondrial encephalopathies.

Although there is at present no specific treatment for any one of these fatal disorders, their precise identification is essential for genetic counseling and prevention. The following clinical signs should always draw attention to the possibility of a juvenile mitochondrial encephalopathy in a previously normal child, adolescent or young adult:

1. A progressive multisystem disorder involving, in variable proportion and chronology, the central nervous system, the peripheral nervous system, the eyes, the ears, the muscles, and the heart.

2. A progressive external ophthalmoplegia (especially when retinitis pigmentosa is also present).

3. Polymyoclonus, i.e., multiple erratic, asynchronous, myoclonic jerks enhanced by voluntary movements, usually associated with, but independent from, myoclonic seizures and ataxia.

4. The association of cerebellar ataxia and proprioceptive sensory deficit.

5. Muscular weakness and exercise intolerance associated with a neurologic syndrome.

6. Recurrent, acute, partially regressive neurologic episodes (strokelike episodes) such as hemiparesis, hemianopia, cortical blindness, migraine. They convey the idea of multiple brain infarcts, but actually probably

represent foci of tissue degeneration. These can usually be visualized by neuroradiological imaging.

7. A short stature and progressive hearing loss, which are common to most juvenile mitochondrial encephalomyopathies, and may also be found in the mother in maternally inherited disorders.

Two essential paraclinical findings will confirm the clinical impression of a mitochondrial encephalomyopathy: high levels of lactate in serum and CSF, and the presence of "ragged red fibers" in skeletal muscle biopsy samples. Ragged red muscle fibers (RRF) are characterized by large, essentially subsarcolemmal aggregates of mitochondria, easily revealed under the light microscope with a modification of the Gomori trichrome stain, and with stains for oxidative enzymes. When examined with the electron microscope, the mitochondria appear normal or display only slight abnormalities. RRF are the morphological signature of primary or secondary mtDNA lesions that affect intramitochondrial protein synthesis,[248,249] i.e., large-scale rearrangements of mtDNA or point mutations affecting mtDNA genes and mtDNA defects induced by mutations in nuclear genes. Specialized biochemical and DNA studies of muscle, and possibly also of leukocytes, cultured fibroblasts, and other tissues are needed for the exact definition of the disease and consequently for family guidance.

Kearns-Sayre Syndrome   Kearns-Sayre syndrome (KSS) starts in childhood or adolescence and affects both boys and girls. Most, if not all, cases have been sporadic. There have been very few well-documented examples of familial KSS.

A constant clinical feature, and generally the first sign, is progressive ocular palsies (ptosis and limitations of ocular movements). A pigmentary degeneration of the retina and cerebellar ataxia are the two other cardinal neurological signs. Progressive mental deterioration is usual and there is frequently a progressive sensorineural hearing loss. The illness may be punctuated by episodes of stupor or coma. Seizures are rare. High levels of CSF protein ($> 100 \, mg/dL$) are generally observed. A heart block is the major extraneurologic feature of the disease. Initially there is a left anterior fascicular block and occasionally a right bundle branch block. Complete heart block may result in sudden death, hence the desirability of implanting a pacemaker. Muscle weakness and intolerance to exercise (sometimes with myalgia) is usual. A short stature is practically always present. Hypoparathyroidism, diabetes mellitus, and growth hormone deficiency have all been observed. Elevated values of lactate and pyruvate are found in plasma and CSF, and RRF are practically always present. Neuroradiologic imaging usually shows white matter abnormalities (perhaps a correlate to spongy degeneration) and occasionally calcifications in the basal ganglia. Magnetic resonance spectroscopy will reveal an increase in brain lactate. Spongiosis has been described at autopsy in various structures of the central nervous system.

Molecular Biology and Biochemistry   Molecular rearrangements of mtDNA are found in all patients with KSS. Both duplications and large-scale deletions of mtDNA have been characterized.[250] The size and location of the deletions vary widely and do not correlate with the clinical phenotype. These deletions account for multiple partial defects of respiratory chain enzymes (complexes IV, I, and III).

Variants   The availability of molecular markers now makes it possible to identify incomplete forms and variants of KSS. Heteroplasmic deletions of mtDNA of the same type as those found in KSS have been detected in patients with isolated sporadic *progressive external ophthalmoplegia* with RRF (and occasionally limb muscle weakness and minor neurologic signs) and in children with *combined features of KSS and MELAS* (recurrent stroke-like episodes).[253]

Treatment   Administration of CoQ_{10} and carnitine have been recommended.

Progressive External Ophthalmoplegia   Sporadic cases of progressive external ophthalmoplegia (PEO) and proximal limb weakness with RRF may represent minor forms of KSS when mtDNA deletions are demonstrated.

Sporadic PEO must be distinguished from dominantly inherited PEO with multiple mtDNA deletions (see above), and from *maternally inherited PEO*. Here, ocular palsies are variably associated with ataxia, deafness, pigmentary retinopathy, and heart block. Ragged red fibers are present. The most common cause is a mtDNA A3243G point mutation (typically seen in MELAS).

Pearson Syndrome   This condition affecting bone marrow and pancreatic function may be fatal in infancy. Patients who survive may later develop clinical features of KSS. The genetic lesion is identical to that found in KSS.

Mitochondrial Encephalomyopathy with Lactic Acidosis and Stroke-like Episodes Mitochondrial encephalomyopathy with lactic acidosis and stroke-like episodes (MELAS) begins in childhood, adolescence, or early adulthood after a previously normal development. In 80 percent of cases onset is before the age of 20.

The most distinctive characteristic of the disorder is a series of sudden, partially regressive neurologic attacks, resembling strokes and suggesting cerebral infarcts. Hemiparesis, hemianopia, abrupt onset of cortical blindness, and aphasia are all well documented. Periods of confusion and hallucinations are not infrequent. These episodes may be triggered by a febrile illness. Recurrent migraine-like headaches and episodes of vomiting are common accompaniments. Other neurologic signs include progressive deafness, seizures, mental deterioration, and progressive external ophthalmoplegia (10 percent) (see above). A short stature, muscle weakness, and intolerance to exercise are usual. Severe gastrointestinal derangement has been reported. CT scans and MRI show several areas of parenchymal destruction, essentially in the cortex and white matter of the parieto-occipital lobes and in the basal ganglia (Fig. 5-18). One-third of the patients have basal ganglia calcifications. Lactic acid concentrations are high in blood and CSF. RRF are present in muscle. One-quarter of the patients have a positive family history that is consistent with maternal inheritance. Mothers may also have short stature and deafness.

Molecular Biology and Biochemistry Four point mutations have been shown to be related to MELAS in the majority of patients. Three mutations at nucleotide pairs 3243, 3250, 3271 affect the mtDNA gene for tRNA$^{\text{Leu (UUR)}}$. The other mutation involves the coding region for subunit 4 of complex I. Combined defects of respiratory chain enzymes have been demonstrated, involving complex I, complex IV, and complex III.[251]

Neuropathology The most remarkable abnormalities consist in circumscribed areas of cortical and white matter destruction, essentially in the parieto-occipital lobes. Lesions have been said to resemble ischemic infarcts. Narrowing of brain capillaries with an increased number of mitochondria in endothelial and smooth muscle cells of small arteries and arterioles was reported,[252] suggesting that the stroke-like episodes could be related to a small vessel vasculopathy. However, in one of our cases, the cortical lesions in less affected areas were limited to the superficial layers,

where there was vascular proliferation, and relative preservation of neurons; the arterioles and veins were patent. These peculiarities are similar to those of Leigh disease. There were also fine perivascular calcifications in the striatum and pallidum without neuronal destruction, not at all what one would expect from the massive basal ganglia calcifications on the CT scan.

Myoclonus Epilepsy with Ragged Red Fibers The main, and usually the first, manifestation of myoclonus epilepsy with ragged red fibers (MERRF), starting before the age of 20 years, is the constellation of action myoclonus, seizures, and ataxia. The myoclonus—or "polymyoclonus"—is induced or exaggerated by voluntary movements. Seizures are mostly of the myoclonic type. On neurological examination, impaired deep sensation in the lower limbs can be the basis of a tabeto-cerebellar ataxia, similar to that of Friedreich ataxia. In view of this striking symptomatology, some patients

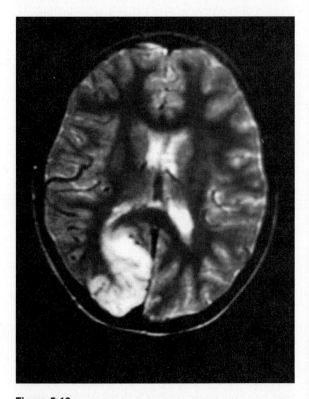

Figure 5-18
MELAS: MRI shows an area of corticosubcortical necrosis in the left occipital region involving the visual cortex.

with MERRF have been described as having Ramsay Hunt syndrome (for a discussion of this condition, see above). Other abnormalities include dementia, neurosensory deafness, optic atrophy, short stature, and muscle weakness. Lactic acidosis and the presence of RRF are essential features of the disorder. Basal ganglia calcifications may be found on CT scans. The EEG is characterized by irregular generalized spike and wave discharges appearing on a background of abnormal activity. The somatosensory evoked potentials have large amplitudes.[254]

Molecular Genetics and Biochemistry MERRF is a familial disease with a pattern of inheritance compatible with a maternal transmission. A point mutation at position 8344 of the mitochondrial gene for tRNA[Lys] has been found in most if not all cases.[254a] There is a combined partial deficiency of complexes I, IV, and III of the respiratory cycle.

Neuropathology Neuronal degeneration of the dentate nuclei and the superior cerebellar peduncles, and degeneration of the posterior columns and spinocerebellar tracts have been reported. These lesions correlate well with the presence of polymyoclonus, cerebellar signs, and posterior column sensory deficits and they are similar to those described by Ramsay Hunt in his classical 1921 report on "dyssynergia cerebellaris myoclonica." Spongy changes have also been reported in the brain and brain stem.

Variants: Overlap between MELAS and MERRF Several patients have been described who have features of both MERRF and MELAS, i.e., the presence in the same patient of myoclonus and ataxia together with recurrent vomiting, recurrent headaches, or transient strokes with cortical softenings on the CT scan. Some patients with either syndrome have also had a pigmentary retinopathy.

The Neuropathy, Ataxia, and Retinitis Pigmentosa (NARP) Syndrome This maternally inherited disease was first described in a family in which four patients in three generations were affected with various combinations of ataxia, sensory neuropathy, pigmentary degeneration of the retina, pyramidal signs, mental deterioration, and proximal limb weakness.[255] Onset is usually in adolescents or young adults. In the most affected patient the disease is already evident at the age of 3 years. Lactic acidosis and RRF in skeletal muscles were not present. This condition has been found to be associated with an mtDNA point mutation at base pair 8993 (T8993G) involving the gene for subunit 6 of mitochondrial ATPase. The same mutation has since been found in other families. There was a great variability of clinical expression. Some patients had the NARP syndrome, others were typical of Leigh syndrome (MILS, see below). A correlation was found between the amount of mutated DNA in skeletal muscles and the severity and symptomatology of the disease.

Maternally Inherited Leigh Syndrome Retinitis pigmentosa is the hallmark of maternally inherited Leigh syndrome (MILS). It is caused by ATP6 NARP 8993 (T to G) mutation. Maternal relatives may have the NARP syndrome. Onset is usually in infancy (see Chap. 3).

Leber Hereditary Optic Neuropathy Leber hereditary optic neuropathy (LHON) is characterized by the sudden onset of visual loss in adolescents or young adults. Younger children, some of them as young as 5 years, have also been affected. Blindness is generally bilateral, but may at first be unilateral, the second eye being affected several weeks or months later. Papillary (optic nerve head) edema and tortuosity of retinal vessels are characteristic. The condition is usually static and vision may improve with time. Neurological signs may be found in some cases, including ataxia, choreoathetosis, pyramidal signs, a peripheral neuropathy, psychiatric disorders, and cardiac dysrhythmias. There are no ragged red fibers in skeletal muscles, and blood and CSF lactate are in the normal range. Leber optic neuropathy is a maternally inherited disease. The fact that 85 percent of patients have been males has not received a satisfactory explanation. At least 15 mtDNA point mutations have been described in this disease; half of them involve a single base change in nucleotide position 11778.[256] As pointed out above, bilateral striatal lucencies on MRI, usually associated with dystonia, may be found in patients with LHON or in members of their family without ocular signs. The LHON variant with dystonia is associated with point mutation G14459A.

Wolfram Syndrome Recently a deletion in mtDNA has been found in this syndrome. It is characterized by the association of diabetes mellitus, optic atrophy, deafness, mental retardation, external ophthalmoplegia, ataxia, extrapyramidal signs and mild lactic acidosis.[256a]

Concluding Remarks about the Encephalopathies with Clinical Evidence of Diffuse CNS Disorders in the Juvenile Period

From this array of diffuse or multifocal diseases of the nervous system the following clusterings appear to be of practical diagnostic value:

G_{M2} *gangliosidosis*: signs of lower motor neuron disease, or a Friedreich-like syndrome, or dystonia, retinal degeneration.

G_{M1} *gangliosidosis*: dystonia.

Gaucher disease type III: supranuclear ophthalmoplegia, seizures, myoclonus, splenomegaly.

Niemann-Pick type C disease: supranuclear ophthalmoplegia, foam cells and sea-blue histiocytes in bone marrow smears, transient episodes of early neonatal jaundice.

Spielmeyer-Vogt disease: onset with visual failure due to pigmentary degeneration of the retina, mental deterioration, psychotic manifestations, extrapyramidal signs, vacuolated lymphocytes.

Type II sialidosis and galactosialidosis: Hurler phenotype, macular cherry red spots, myoclonus, possible renal failure. (Type I sialidosis produces cherry red macula and myoclonus without the Hurler phenotype.)

The leukodystrophies: metachromatic leukodystrophy and Krabbe leukodystrophy produce a progressive paraplegia or hemiplegia, amblyopia due to optic atrophy (or lesions of the central visual pathways), cerebellar ataxia, mental symptoms, a peripheral neuropathy. White matter lesions are detected on MRI.

X-linked adrenoleukodystrophy: mental deterioration or psychiatric manifestations, progressive hemiplegia, central blindness and deafness, evidence of adrenocortical insufficiency. White matter lesions are detected with peripheral enhancement on MRI.

Adrenomyeloneuropathy: slowly progressive paraplegia (and neuropathy), abnormalities of cerebral white matter on MRI.

Leigh disease: brain stem signs (cranial nerve palsies, disturbance of oculomotricity, nystagmus, respiratory dysrhythmias), extrapyramidal signs, optic atrophy, relapsing course, typical MRI, lactic acid elevated in CSF, no RRF.

Cholestanolosis: cataracts, cerebellar ataxia, bipyramidal signs, tendon xanthomas.

Juvenile Farber disease and juvenile neuroaxonal dystrophy: very rare diseases in which polymyoclonus is prominent.

Neuronal intranuclear inclusion disease: signs of lower motor neuron disorder associated with evidence of central nervous system involvement (extrapyramidal and cerebellar signs).

Mitochondrial encephalomyopathies with defects of mtDNA: differential characteristics described in text.

PROGRESSIVE METABOLIC AND DEGENERATIVE DISEASES WITH SPECIAL NEUROLOGIC AND SOMATIC (ESSENTIALLY CUTANEOUS) FEATURES

In this section we include three diseases which do not fit adequately into the previous categories.

- *Lesch-Nyhan disease*: its most distinctive features are painful oral mutilations and an extrapyramidal disorder.
- *Cockayne syndrome*: which produces skin photosensitivity, special facial appearance, dwarfism, and microcephaly.
- *Xeroderma pigmentosum with neurologic complications* (DeSanctis-Cacchione syndrome).

Lesch-Nyhan Disease: HPRT Deficiency Lesch-Nyhan disease is an X-linked inherited disorder of purine metabolism. There is a complete deficiency of hypoxanthine-guanine-phosphoribosyltransferase (HPRT), leading to an overproduction of uric acid and a characteristic neurologic syndrome. Neurologic signs follow a fairly uniform pattern and consist of motor retardation and athetosis, compulsive oral self-mutilation, and mental retardation (Fig. 5-19). The pathogenesis is unknown. Manifestations of hyperuricemia include crystalluria, nephrolithiasis, gout, and obstructive uropathy. Allopurinol prevents renal complications of hyperuricuria but is without effect on the neuropsychiatric disorder. Partial deficiency of HPRT is associated with hyperuricemia and variable degrees of neurologic dysfunction. The gene for HPRT has been mapped to the long arm of chromosome X. A number of different mutations have been linked to the disease.

Clinical Features The incidence of Lesch-Nyhan disease (LND) has been estimated at 1/100,000 to 1/

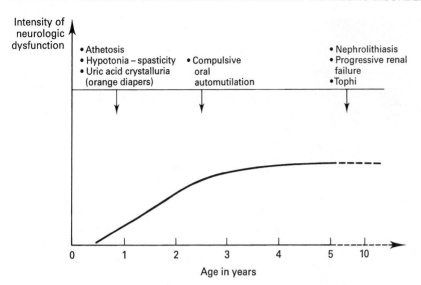

Figure 5-19
Lesch-Nyhan disease: clinical course.

380,000.[260] The infant is normal at birth and during the first months of life, except in a few cases in which there is hypotonia, recurrent vomiting, and difficulty with secretions. A delay in motor development becomes apparent between 3 and 6 months of age.

Between 12 and 18 months of age, involuntary movements appear, usually taking the form of jerky choreiform movements and facial grimacing, and less often, athetosis. Axial hypotonia and bilateral corticospinal tract signs with variable degrees of spasticity and tonic spasms appear most often at the end of the first year.

Between the age of 2 and 4 years, the affected boys begin to bite their lips, tongue, and cheeks. This painful oral automutilation is practically a unique feature of this disease (except for the Riley-Day syndrome); it may result in horrid disfigurements (Fig. 5-20). Later there is irrepressible finger biting of one or both hands. Many self-inflicted wounds result from this, sometimes necessitating extraction of teeth and nearly always immobilization of one or both arms, a measure often welcomed by the child. Other aspects of self-injury include head banging and attempts at mutilation of the eyes and legs. There may also be aggressiveness toward others, wherein the patient tries to strike anyone in the vicinity. Spitting at others and the use of abusive language are other aspects of the compulsive behavior at a later stage.

Although a highly characteristic feature, automutilation is not invariable in Lesch-Nyhan disease. It may be present in one boy and absent in another in the same sibship. It may appear only between 6 and 8 years or much later during adolescence, but usually there is a tendency for it to improve with age and to disappear by the end of the first decade.

Mental retardation is common but of variable degree and is often difficult to evaluate because of behavioral and motor abnormalities. IQs below 50 are not unusual, but some children have nearly normal intelligence. There is no progressive dementia. Speech is usually retarded and remains limited. Some patients seem to benefit significantly from appropriate training and education.

There is a severe dysarthria, dysphagia, and a tendency to vomit. Growth is stunted. Motor performance varies according to the relative prominence of either involuntary movements or spasticity, which tend to emerge in the second and third year of life. Practically every patient remains incapable of standing or walking, and most do not learn to sit alone or they lose this ability if it has been acquired. They must be kept in bed or a wheelchair. Approximately half the patients are subject to seizures.

Secondary microcephaly has been reported. There is no evidence of any sensory disturbance or of peripheral nerve involvement to explain the compulsive self-mutilative tendency. Nerve conduction velocities are normal. Corneas, lenses, and optic fundi are normal. The CSF is unaltered and contains no increase in levels of uric acid. The EEG is usually normal.

Clinical Manifestations of Hyperuricemia Lesch-Nyhan disease results in an overproduction of uric acid,

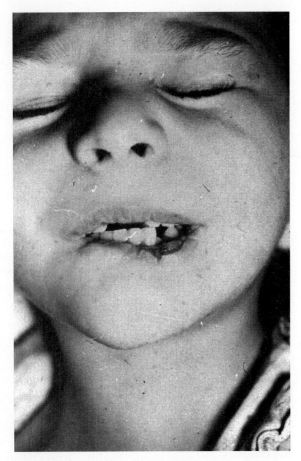

Figure 5-20
Lesch-Nyhan disease: automutilation of lips. (Courtesy Dr. P. Royer.)

reflected by a constant and easily detectable hyperuricuria, and usually by hyperuricemia. The values of urinary uric acid are most usefully expressed in relation to creatininuria: 3 to 4 mg uric acid/mg creatinine instead of less than 1 mg as in normal children. Serum urate concentrations usually range between 7 and 10 mg/dL but tend to show daily variations and can at times fall to normal levels. Patients generally excrete 40–69 mg uric acid per kg of body weight per day, instead of 18 mg as in normal children.

Because of the hyperuricuria, orange crystals of uric acid may color the diapers of infants and young children, but this early mark of the disease may pass unnoticed. Nephrolithiasis develops later in many children and is manifested by abdominal pains and hema-

turia. If untreated, it leads to obstructive uropathy and renal failure. Tophi and arthritis also occur but rarely before the age of 12.

Megaloblastic anemia prior to the occurrence of renal insufficiency is not uncommon. Periods of repeated vomiting have been a problem in some children.

Diagnostic Laboratory Tests These include mainly the determination of the level of uric acid in the urine (expressed in relation to creatinine excretion) and blood, and the assay of HPRT in erythrocytes or cultured fibroblasts.

When a child has a serum level of more than 4 to 5 mg of uric acid/dL and a urine uric acid/creatinine ratio of 3 to 4, this is highly suggestive of LN disease. However, a definitive diagnosis requires an analysis of HPRT activity. Assays are usually done on erythrocyte lysates. Patients with classic LN disease have an enzyme activity close to zero.

A more complicated assay of HPRT activity in intact cultured fibroblasts may be useful in assessing patients with partial HPRT deficiency. Molecular techniques are also employed, especially for carrier detection and prenatal diagnosis.

Partial Deficiency of HPRT In patients with partial deficiency of HPRT, the typical automutilative behavior is absent; sometimes hyperuricemia and its clinical consequences are the only manifestations of the disease. They often present in childhood or adolescence with evidence of nephrolithiasis (hematuria, abdominal pain, ureteral obstruction) or later with gout. In a few patients the hyperuricemia is accompanied by mild neurological manifestations such as choreoathetosis[261] or spasticity and mental retardation. One of us has observed a 12-year-old child with hematuria, auricular tophi, mild but typical choreic movements, and moderate mental retardation. Another group of reported patients have had all the motor features of classical Lesch-Nyhan disease, but with normal intelligence and behavior.[260] Also, a partial deficiency of HPRT has been reported in four members of a family with spasticity, pyramidal signs, mental retardation, and dysmorphic facial features, including proximally placed thumbs and clinodactyly.

When the activity of HPRT is measured in intact cultured fibroblasts (not red cell lysates), an inverse correlation is found between residual activity of the enzyme and severity of clinical symptoms in patients with partial HPRT deficiency. The "intelligent Lesch-Nyhan" patients had activities between 1.4 and 1.6 percent, and the purely hyperuricemic group had activities between 8 and 60 percent.

Genetics   Lesch-Nyhan disease is an X-linked inherited disorder with no geographic or ethnic prevalence. Only boys are affected. Female carriers are asymptomatic. However, some of them may have elevated levels of serum uric acid, and some experience gout after menopause, attributable to heterozygosity of HPRT deficiency.[262] Female heterozygotes for classic LN disease have normal activity of HPRT in erythrocytes. Detection of carriers must be made by enzyme assays on cultured fibroblasts or by enzymatic studies on the hair follicles (hair follicles express only one of the two X chromosomes, and if HPRT is assayed in several hair roots, a clear pattern of mosaicism is found). Molecular methods may also be used.

Prenatal diagnosis can be performed by enzymatic analysis or DNA studies on amniocytes or chorionic villus cells. Because of the wide spectrum of mutations causing HPRT deficiency, one can depend upon molecular methods for carrier detection and prenatal analysis, only if the particular mutation is known in the family.

The gene for HPRT is encoded on chromosome X and has been mapped on the long arm at Xq26-Xq27. The genetic lesions which cause HPRT deficiency are heterogeneous. They consist of point mutations, partial deletions, large deletions, insertions, and duplications. One female with all the features of the disease had a microdeletion in the HPRT gene.[263] Similar cases without DNA studies had apparently been published in 1968.[264]

Neuropathologic Changes and Biochemical Pathology   Approximately 10 patients have been subjected to neuropathologic examination.[265] No specific changes have been found by routine methods. Necrotic brain lesions, said to be related to renal failure, have been reported. (We have not found such lesions in the brains of other uremic patients.)

In biochemical studies of postmortem brain tissue, several indices of dopamine function were reduced by 70 to 90 percent in the basal ganglia. These included homovanillic acid, dopa decarboxylase, and tyrosine hydroxylase. There is a deficit of HPRT in all tissues, including the brain.

Pathophysiology   Pathogenesis of neurological abnormalities is unclear. However, several studies suggest abnormalities in the metabolism of neurotransmitters, particularly in the dopaminergic pathways. Arguments in favor of this hypothesis include evidence of depressed dopamine function in the basal ganglia, where HPRT activity is normally high; participation of guanine nucleotides in the regulation of dopamine-agonist receptor binding, which allows HPRT deficiency to affect dopaminergic functions; and self-mutilation by dopamine agonists produced in experimental animals.

High concentrations of oxypurines and uric acid found in the brain and CSF apparently play no role in the genesis of neurologic signs.

Uric acid overproduction in Lesch-Nyhan disease is the result of an accelerated rate of purine biosynthesis de novo. HPRT, an enzyme of the purine salvage pathway, catalyzes the reaction in which hypoxanthine and guanine are reutilized to form their respective nucleotides, inosinic acid and guanylic acid. This does not happen in HPRT deficiency, hence there is a reduced feedback inhibition, and consequently an acceleration of the de novo pathway of purine synthesis. Possibly more important is a mechanism related to the elevated levels of 5-phosphoribosyl-1-pyrophosphate, the material available for purine biosynthesis in cells that lack HPRT. Consequently, there is an increase of de novo purine synthesis and hyperuricemia. Hyperuricemia is responsible for the renal dysfunction in LN disease.

Diagnosis   The combination of oral automutilation, choreoathetosis, and hyperuricuria in a boy is extremely characteristic. (Oral mutilation also occurs in the Riley-Day syndrome.) Hand biting is nonspecific; it is seen in many types of mental retardation and in children with congenital analgesia.

Typical automutilation behavior may be lacking or may have a late occurrence. Therefore, the possibility of LN disease should be raised in any young boy with choreoathetosis apparently not related to pre- or perinatal injuries.

Complications of hyperuricemia, i.e., nephrolithiasis, obstructive nephropathy, and gout, in a child should also raise suspicion of partial HPRT deficiency. These cases should be differentiated from other genetically determined congenital diseases with hyperuricemia (see below).

Treatment   Treatment with allopurinol is effective for the prevention of renal failure due to hyperuricemia. Reduction of uric acid is paralleled by an increase in urinary levels of hypoxanthine and xanthine, which these patients cannot reutilize, and there is a possible risk of xanthine stone formation. The concentration of these substances in the urine should be monitored during treatment with allopurinol. Alkalinization of the urine may be useful.

There is no specific treatment of the nervous disorder. Allopurinol and related drugs have been without effect even when given in the neonatal period.

The most effective management of automutilation behavior is physical restraint. Some clinicians have advised extraction of teeth, but we find this unnecessary. No drug has proved to be really helpful for long periods. L-5-hydroxytryptophan and fluphenazine have short-term effects in alleviating self-injurious behavior. Bone marrow transplantation and enzyme replacement therapy have failed to influence neurologic symptoms.

Other Purine Enzymopathies with Neurologic Manifestations

In addition to the deficiency of HPRT in Lesch-Nyhan disease, defects of several other enzymes of purine biosynthesis have been found in association with neurologic dysfunction.

1. *Phosphoribosylpyrophosphatase (PP-ribose-P) synthetase deficiency* is a cause of congenital hyperuricemia and has been associated with mental retardation.

2. *PP-ribose-P synthetase overactivity* is another cause of congenital hyperuricemia; it leads to developmental delay and sensorineural deafness in the most severe phenotype. Heterozygous female carriers of this X-linked trait may develop gout and occasionally deafness. Patients with the late juvenile-adult variety may have gout but are neurologically normal.

3. *Adenylosuccinate lyase (ASL) deficiency* was described by Jaeken and Van den Berghe in 1984.[266] Large amounts of succinylaminoimidazolecarboxamide riboside (succinyl Z riboside) and succinyloadenosine accumulate in body fluids and can be detected in the urine by thin-layer chromatography or cation-exchange chromatography. This substrate accumulation is the consequence of a deficiency of ASL. Affected children are profoundly retarded and may display autistic features. A bipyramidal syndrome and epilepsy are also reported. A low protein content of the CSF and hypoplasia of the cerebellar vermis have been observed. A rapid diagnostic test in the urine has been developed.[267] The gene for ASL has been cloned and maps to 22q13.1-q13.2. A point mutation in this gene has been identified in three children of one family with a deficiency of ASL.[268]

4. *Type I glycogen storage disease* frequently causes hyperuricemia and gout. They have also been reported in three glycogen storage diseases with muscle involvement: type III, type V, and type VII glycogenosis.

Cockayne Syndrome

Cockayne syndrome is an autosomal recessive hereditary disorder caused by defective repair of transcriptionally active DNA. There are conjoined microcephaly, dwarfism, retinitis pigmentosa, nerve deafness, special facial features, skin photosensitivity, and delayed psychomotor development. A leukodystrophy in combination with striocerebellar calcifications is characteristic. These abnormalities emerge progressively and the illness pursues a chronic course over a decade or more. There is a characteristic abnormality in DNA and RNA synthesis in cultured skin fibroblasts after exposure to sunlight.

Clinical Features More than 150 cases of this type have been reported. Nance and Berry have reviewed 140 of them.[269] At birth, head size, body weight, and body height are usually normal, although intrauterine growth retardation has been mentioned. Stunting of growth becomes evident in the second or third year and usually continues to severe dwarfism, sometimes with disproportionately long limbs and large extremities. Skeletal maturation is usually normal.

There are characteristic, although somewhat variable, facial features: sunken eyes, loss of subcutaneous fat, large ears, prominent nose, thin, atrophic, and pigmented skin as well as anomalies of the mandible (prognathism or retrognathism). Dental caries are frequent. The combination of changes gives the patient a more or less wizened appearance, remotely resembling progeria. Cutaneous photosensitivity is a major feature that may be detected in early infancy, and it may be quite severe. But there is no actinically induced skin cancer, as seen in xeroderma pigmentosum. There may be anhydrosis and poor lacrimation.

Microcephaly is always marked (head size ranges from 3 to 6 standard deviations below normal) and is proportionately more severe than the stunting of statural growth. It is an early sign. A pigmentary retinopathy with extinction of the ERG is part of the syndrome. It is often associated with cataracts and leads to blindness and pendular nystagmus. Nerve deafness is almost invariable and becomes apparent early in the disease.

Psychomotor development is retarded. Walking and speaking are delayed. Most children do not acquire normal language and communicative skills, and their IQs remain under 30. The progressive mental and motor deterioration proceeds so slowly that it becomes evident only after several years. The ultimate neurologic syndrome, indicating a diffuse involvement of the brain, comprises bilateral pyramidal signs, ataxia, tremor, and occasionally athetosis and seizures. Many patients experience a peripheral neuropathy manifested by abolished tendon reflexes, amyotrophy, and diminished conduction velocities.

CAT scans characteristically reveal calcifications in the basal ganglia and dentate nuclei, and MRI scans show white matter abnormalities. The CSF is normal and the EEG is noncontributory.

Hepatomegaly, renal insufficiency,[269] arterial hypertension, sexual infantilism, and various nonspecific bone changes have been noted in a few cases, but their interpretation is difficult. Unlike other diseases in which there is defective DNA repair, the incidence of cancer in Cockayne syndrome is not increased.

Death may be expected in the second or third decade. The mean age of death in the series of Nance and Berry was $12\frac{1}{4}$ years.[269]

Laboratory Tests   A characteristic of cultured fibroblasts is that DNA replication and RNA synthesis fail to recover from inhibition by UV damage. The repair of total genomic DNA after UV damage is normal, but cells are unable to repair the normally transcribed strands of active genes. Four complementation groups have been delineated using UV sensitivity, suggesting that the disease may be genetically heterogeneous.

The DNA (or RNA) helicase coded by the *ERCC6* gene normally directs its activity toward nucleotide excision repair of actively transcribed genes. Mutations in this gene are associated with Cockayne syndrome complementation group B, which is the most common form of the disease. The gene has been localized to 10q11-q21.[271]

Hyperbetalipoproteinemia, defective blood glucose regulation, and hyperinsulinism have been reported.

Testing the sensitivity of cultured amniocytes to UV light may offer a possibility of prenatal diagnosis.[270]

Pathologic Findings   The few reported neuropathologic studies all describe similar findings, consisting of microcephaly, patchy destruction of white matter in the cerebrum, and perivascular calcification, mainly in the dentate and lenticular nuclei.[274,275] Segmental

demyelination of peripheral nerves with remyelination and formation of onion bulbs has also been found. Membrane-bound granular osmiophilic inclusions have been seen in endoneural and Schwann cells.[272,273]

Variants   Some patients have been described with early infantile sun sensitivity, failure to thrive, microcephaly, cataracts, deep-set eyes, and a rapidly fatal course, with the same RNA synthesis abnormality after UV exposure as in Cockayne syndrome. Neuropathological findings were also consistent with the diagnosis.[276] Two patients with early infantile Cockayne syndrome exhibited DNA repair defects similar to those of the xeroderma pigmentosum complementation group A.[277] An overlapping clinical and biochemical phenotype of Cockayne syndrome and xeroderma pigmentosum has been described.[279] Cockayne disease may also appear in the adult.[278]

Some cases previously reported under descriptive names of leukodystrophy with striocerebellar calcifications, or as Pelizaeus-Merzbacher disease, probably belong to Cockayne syndrome.

Treatment   No treatment is available.

Xeroderma Pigmentosum; DeSanctis-Cacchione Syndrome   Xeroderma pigmentosum (XP) is a rare autosomal recessive cutaneous disorder caused by an inability to repair DNA damaged by ultraviolet radiation. It is characterized by a dermatitis and skin cancer after exposure to sunlight. Neurological manifestations exist in approximately 20 percent of the patients (DeSanctis-Cacchione syndrome). The disease is genetically heterogeneous. Several complementation groups have been described. In the great majority of cases the DNA repair defect is related to a deficient "excision repair" after UV exposure (excision repair deficient form of XP). In about 10 percent of cases the deficit is in the postreplication repair of DNA (excision repair proficient variant of XP). XP with neurological manifestations beginning in childhood or adolescence relates to the "excision repair" deficiency form, i.e., complementation group A in which the XPA gene, coded on chromosome 9q34.1 is defective. The protein product of this gene has a much higher affinity for UV-damaged DNA than for undamaged DNA, suggesting that its role is in "damage recognition." Mutations in this gene in group A patients have been identified. Other complementation groups have also been described. They are generally associated with less severe symptoms.

The genes associated with them and their chromosomal localization are reviewed by Cleaver and Kraemer.[280]

Dermatologic Manifestations   Usually in the first years of life exposure to ultraviolet rays of sunlight gives rise to an abnormal erythema that proceeds to intense redness, edema, and blistering. Repeated reactions of this type cause irregular pigmentation, freckling, keratoses, scarring, and skin cancers (squamous and basal cell carcinomas, melanomas, angiomas, and sarcomas). Exposure of the eyes excites photophobia and conjuctival erythema.

Neurologic Manifestations   They usually appear in late childhood or early adolescence, but evidence of motor and mental retardation may have been detected as early as age 6 months. The syndrome consists of progressive mental deterioration, microcephaly, sensorineural deafness, choreoathetosis, cerebellar ataxia, peripheral axonal polyneuropathy, retarded growth, eventually a spastic quadriplegia. Neuropathological lesions have been shown to be diffuse, including nonspecific neuronal loss in the cerebellar cortex and central nuclei, cerebral cortex, brain stem, spinal cord, and peripheral nerves.[279a]

Cockayne syndrome differs essentially from XP by the existence of a leukodystrophy and striodentate calcifications, the absence of skin tumors, and a different type of DNA repair defect.

PROGRESSIVE GENETIC ENCEPHALOPATHIES LEADING TO STROKE

- Two genetic metabolic diseases that have the property of involving the cerebral vessels and causing ischemic strokes are homocystinuria and Fabry disease. In *homocystinuria* cerebrovascular complications are apt to occur late in childhood or adolescence after earlier evidence of a more generalized brain involvement in the form of mental retardation. In *Fabry disease* the accumulation of glycosphingolipids in cerebral blood vessels and heart do not usually result in brain infarction until early adulthood after a long history of painful dysesthesias, and other signs of peripheral nerve and autonomic involvement. Rare metabolic disorders involving cerebral blood vessels are listed in Table 6-6.

- *Mitochondrial encephalomyopathies* with lactic acidosis and strokelike episodes (MELAS) also exhibit foci of brain damage. It is not yet known if they result from small vessel disease or from nonischemic tissue necrosis.

- Vascular lesions during infancy are a feature of *Menkes disease*.

- In any metabolic disease involving the *heart*, embolisms to the brain may occur.

The most common clinical manifestation of strokes in the metabolic encephalopathies consists of a hemiplegia of acute onset. Acute hemiplegias of other origins are much more frequent. They are described in Chap. 6 (Table 6-6).

Fabry disease and MELAS are described above. Only homocystinuria will be considered here.

Homocystinuria   Different genetic abnormalities may lead to the excessive excretion of urinary homocystine. Most patients with homocystinuria have a deficiency of cystathionine β-synthase. Other causes, related to a deficiency of 5-methyltetrahydrofolate homocysteine methylation, include 5,10-methylenetetrahydrofolate reductase deficiency, defects of cobalamine and folate metabolism, and nutritional deficiencies of vitamin B_{12} and folate (Chaps. 2 and 3).

Homocystinuria due to Cystathionine β-Synthase Deficiency   Cystathionine β-synthase deficiency (CSD) is an autosomal recessive inherited disorder. Its main clinical features are mental retardation and psychiatric disturbances, ectopia lentis, osteoporosis, and life-threatening arterial and venous thromboses. The main biological abnormalities consists of homocystinuria and elevated plasma concentrations of homocystine and methionine. The genetic disorder underlying CSD is probably heterogeneous. Approximately half of the patients are responsive to pyridoxine administration.

Clinical Features   The eyes, brain, vascular system, and the skeleton are the targets of CSD. An international survey of more than 600 cases was published in 1985.[281] While the initial complaint may be the ophthalmologic complication, or more rarely arterial or venous occlusions, mental retardation is usually present from early life. Affected children are slow in sitting, standing, walking, and speaking, and by mid-childhood many of them are obviously mentally retarded. For patients recorded in the 1982–1983 international survey, IQ scores ranged from 10 to 138 with the median being 64. There is usually no evidence of mental regression. Some patients came to medical attention because of psychiatric difficulties, consisting of disorders of behavior, personality peculiarities, episodic depression, and obsessive-compulsive neurosis. One of our patients had an anorexia of obscure origin.

About 20 percent of patients have seizures, and there is a high incidence of EEG abnormalities in patients without seizures. Dystonia has been observed in a few patients. Ectopia lentis, giving the iris a tremulous appearance (iridodonesis) is a hallmark of the disease (Fig. 5-22). The lenses tend to dislocate downwards in contrast to the upward displacement in Marfan syndrome. Dislocation of the lens has very rarely been noted before the age of 2 to 3 years. Half the patients have the defect by the age of 10 years, and the great majority of adults are affected. Myopia is usual and can precede lenticular dislocation. Glaucoma, retinal detachment, and cataracts have also been observed. These ophthalmologic abnormalities are the source of serious visual disturbances and may be difficult to manage.

Children and adolescents tend to be tall and slender, and their appearance may simulate Marfan syndrome—increased length of long bones (dolichostenomelia), decreased upper/lower segment ratio, arachnodactyly (less frequently), pectus excavatus or pectus carinatum. Genu valgum, flat feet, and a shuffling gait are other abnormalities. A highly arched palate

and crowded teeth are frequently observed. Progressive scoliosis is another noteworthy feature. A susceptibility to fracture has been noted. Skeletal x-rays characteristically reveal osteoporosis, especially of the vertebrae and long bones. Other radiological abnormalities include biconcave vertebrae, metaphyseal spicules, and abnormal size and shape of the epiphyses. Patients may have light-colored hair, a malar flush, and livedo reticularis over the limbs. Premature graying of the hair has been reported.

Some neurologic events are clearly the consequence of cerebrovascular (i.e., thromboembolic) accidents. Acute hemiplegias due to arterial or venous thromboses develop in childhood or adolescence. Bilateral carotid thromboses (Fig. 5-21) and occlusion of the central retinal arteries have been reported. Some patients have died from carotid occlusion in the second decade of life. Arterial and venous thromboses have also occurred at multiple sites outside the nervous system. These may be serious and life-threatening. Such vascular complications include thrombophlebitis with pulmonary embolism, thrombosis of the coronary and renal arteries (and hypertension), of the inferior vena cava, and of the arteries serving the limbs (leading to gangrene).

Vascular occlusion can occur at any age. At the end of the second decade the risk of a thromboembolic event has been be estimated at 25 percent.[281] The risk of postoperative thromboembolism is not apparently increased.

Figure 5-21
*Homocystinuria: carotid angiography. **A.** Thrombosis of intracranial carotid artery. **B.** Irregular aspect of carotid artery in neck (arrow) possibly due to degenerative changes. (Courtesy Dr. P. Evrard.)*

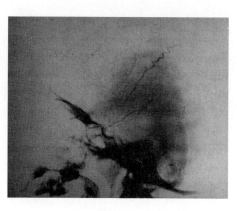

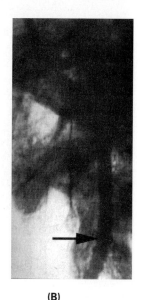

(A)   **(B)**

Among the less frequent abnormalities are hepatomegaly and abnormal glucose tolerance.

Life expectancy in nontreated homocystinuria is reduced. In 1971 McKusick et al.[282] stated that 50 percent of the patients died in their early twenties. But the overall outlook in the 1982–1983 international survey seemed more favorable: mortality by the age of 20 years was 20 percent among pyridoxine nonresponsive patients and 5 percent among responsive patients. Death usually occurred from thromboembolic accidents.

On the whole, untreated pyridoxine-responsive patients are more mildly affected than nonresponsive patients.

Diagnosis Many young children with CSD first present with simple mental retardation or behavioral abnormalities in the absence of lenticular dislocation. A few patients may attract attention through malar flush, a Marfan-life morphology, but in most cases there are no orienting clues. Then the diagnosis is liable to be missed if the cyanide-nitroprusside test for the detection of homocystine in the urine is not systematically performed in all children with mental retardation of uncertain cause. It is known that this test may give both false positive and false negative results, so other biochemical methods are required for definitive diagnosis. The presence of ectopia lentis

is highly suggestive of the disease, but there are other genetic causes of this ocular abnormality, including Marfan syndrome and a few metabolic conditions (see Table 6-11). Homocystinuria is certainly one of the main causes of cerebrovascular accidents without renal disease in childhood and adolescence, but other acquired or genetically determined causes of acute vascular hemiplegia are much more frequent (see Chap. 6, Table 6.6).

Laboratory Tests In CSD the most constant biochemical abnormality is homocystinuria, which is found in all patients beyond early infancy. Hypermethioninemia is also an important finding. The presence of homocystine in the urine is readily detected by the cyanide-nitroprusside test. As this reaction is also positive for cystinuria and other disulfatidurias, homocystine must be further identified by using more specific tests such as various techniques of chromatography. Homocystinuria may be present in other disorders, as stated above, and may be induced by bacterial contamination of urine in cystathionuria. Therefore, to further establish the diagnosis of CSD, amino acids should also be measured in the serum of suspected patients. This procedure will reveal high levels of homocystine and of methionine, as well as markedly reduced concentrations of cystine. Methionine is not elevated in the serum of

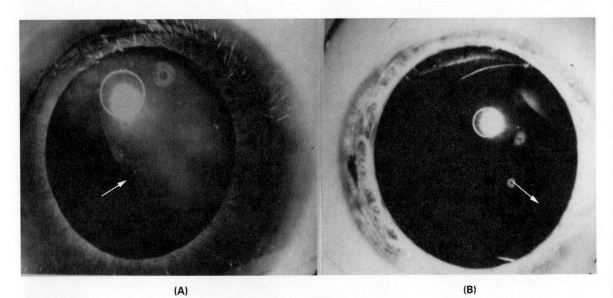

(A)   (B)

Figure 5-22
*Dislocation of lens (slit-lamp). **A.** Marfan disease (upward dislocation) (arrow). **B.** Homocystinuria (downward dislocation) (arrow). (Courtesy Dr. Shirley Wray.)*

patients with homocystinuria related to defects in homocystine methylation. False negative results may also be obtained in testing for homocystinuria when the patient has ingested even very small doses of vitamin B_6.[283]

The diagnosis is confirmed by assays of cystathionine β-synthase in cultured fibroblasts, lymphoblasts, or liver biopsy specimens. Patients have either no detectable activity of the enzyme or a small residual amount. The presence of residual activity of cystathionine β-synthase is essentially found in pyridoxine-responsive patients and may be a necessary but not sufficient requisite for predicting responsiveness to pyridoxine therapy.

Genetics Cystathionine β-synthase deficiency is inherited as an autosomal recessive trait. As determined by newborn screening for hypermethioninemia, its incidence is 1 in 344,000. However, the pyridoxine-responsive form that comprises approximately half the total is usually missed in newborn screening, because hypermethioninemia is generally not yet present at birth. The incidence of the disease is therefore probably 1 in 150,000.[283a] The genetic deficit seems to be heterogeneous. The gene for cystathionine β-synthase maps to chromosome 21q22.3. A variety of mutations have been found, most patients being compound heterozygotes for two different alleles. There is a lack of genotype-phenotype correlation, and surprisingly, some patients with no detectable CS protein have very mild pyridoxine-responsive homocystinuria.[284]

Obligate heterozygotes have 20 to 45 percent of mean control levels of cystathionine β-synthase. It has been suggested that the heterozygotic state may be associated with an increased risk of premature occlusive arterial disease.[285,286]

Prenatal diagnosis can be achieved by enzymatic assays of amniocytes or chorionic villus cells.

Individuals with CSD may be detected by routine screening of newborns for hypermethioninemia, but as noted above, most of them have been of the pyridoxine-nonresponsive type, although, in the total population of patients with homocystinuria, pyridoxine-responsive and pyridoxine-unresponsive patients are equally represented.

Pathologic Findings The most obvious brain lesions are those of vascular occlusion and infarct necrosis. Numerous arteries of the body exhibit degenerative changes of the muscular and elastic fibers as well as intimal thickening. Some of these changes appear to be related to fresh or organized thrombi. Fatty degeneration of the liver has been reported. The zonular fibers of the lens and the ciliary muscles also show degenerative changes. The basis of the mental retardation is not revealed by current histiopathologic methods.

There is virtual absence of cystathionine in the brain (normally it is high). An absence of the specific enzyme has also been demonstrated in the brain as well as in the liver.

Clinicopathologic Correlation The mechanism of vascular occlusion is not known. Enhanced platelet adhesiveness and lesions of the vascular endothelium due to homocystine accumulation have both been postulated. Homocystine interferes with normal cross-linking of collagen. It can potentiate the oxidation of low-density lipoprotein cholesterol.

Treatment In patients detected in childhood or adolescence, the oral administration of large doses of pyridoxine in the form of pyridoxine hydrochloride is effective in reducing or eliminating the biochemical abnormalities in CSD in approximately 50 percent of them. Levels of methionine in plasma and of homocystine in urine are considerably reduced or normalized. Daily maintenance doses of 150 to 500 mg are usually required. A patient should not be considered unresponsive to pyridoxine until a dose approaching 500 to 1000 mg/day has been given for several weeks.[283] Folic acid levels must be normal to obtain a response to pyridoxine. Pyridoxine toxicity (sensory neuropathy, ataxia) does not usually occur with doses under 2000 mg/day.

Pyridoxine therapy has been proven statistically effective in preventing the initial thromboembolic events, and possibly also in preventing lens dislocation. Favorable effects on mentation and behavior have also been reported. It has been suggested that pyridoxine therapy is more effective when combined with a methionine-restricted diet.

Patients detected in childhood or adolescence who are not responsive to pyridoxine should be given a low-methionine, high-cystine diet in order to reduce methionine and homocystine levels in the body. Acceptance of and adherence to such a diet are often resisted. The value of strict methionine restriction on the prevention of thromboembolic complications and on neuropsychiatric signs is still debatable.[283]

Another therapeutic approach has been the use of betaine to lower levels of plasma homocystine and to raise methionine levels. Preliminary reports of this treatment appear to be encouraging.

The great majority of patients detected through routine neonatal screening and treated by low-methionine formulas supplemented in L-cystine, have not developed mental retardation, and seizures have been prevented. Prevention of lens dislocation also appears to be possible. This group of patients is still too young to allow a full evaluation of the dietary treatment on the prevention of thrombosis and embolism. Few pyridoxine-responsive patients have been detected in the newborn period. Some of them received additional vitamin B_6 therapy.

Symptomatic treatment is important, especially for the prevention of ophthalmologic abnormalities.

METABOLIC DISORDERS WITH INTERMITTENT NEUROLOGIC SIGNS

- Disorders of mitochondrial fatty acid β-oxidation and the carnitine cycle, and other mitochondrial disorders, inherited disorders of amino acid and organic acid metabolism, and disorders of carbohydrate metabolism are apt to produce acute neurological attacks, some with ataxia, respiratory abnormalities, stupor and coma, and vomiting. These episodes, which may be life-threatening and have a propensity to recur, are usually recognized in infancy or childhood and will have responded to adequate therapy. Their first recognition in late childhood and adolescence is rare. They are described in Chaps. 3 and 4.

- Leigh syndrome often shows a relapsing course.

- Reversible bouts of ataxia and psychological derangement are seen in Hartnup disease, described next.

Hartnup Disease Hartnup disease (HD) is an autosomal recessive hereditary disorder characterized by a defect in renal tubular reabsorption and intestinal transport of a group of monoamine-monocarboxylic amino acids (neutral amino acids). It leads to a specific aminoaciduria and to the retention of the same specific amino acids, including tryptophan in the intestine. Most affected individuals also excrete excessive amounts of indolic compounds, which originate in the gut from bacterial degradation of unabsorbed tryptophan. Reduced intestinal absorption and urinary loss of tryptophan lead to a reduced availability of this amino acid for the synthesis of niacin. It is believed that the main clinical abnormalities are a consequence of niacin deficiency. However, most individuals with the typical biochemical disorder—detected by neonatal screening or familial screening of an affected child—have been clinically normal. Therefore, although HD appears to be monogenic, additional environmental influences and possible polygenic factors are probably necessary for the overt expressions of the disease.

The clinical manifestations are intermittent and variable, and they show a tendency toward spontaneous improvement with age. They include a pellagra-like skin rash and *reversible* episodes of neurologic dysfunction, the most frequent of which are bouts of cerebellar ataxia and psychologic derangement. Mental retardation is variable and inconstant. Dementia does not occur.

The detection of the typical urinary amino acid pattern is necessary for confirmation of the diagnosis.

Cutaneous and neuropsychiatric aspects of the disease are responsive to nicotinamide therapy.

Clinical Findings The skin changes are usually the first to become apparent. They occur in the late infantile or juvenile period and occasionally in early infancy. A red, scaly rash appears over the face, neck, hands, external surface of the arms, knees, anteroexternal surface of the legs, and dorsal surface of the feet (Fig. 5-23). It resembles the dermatitis of endemic pellagra. The skin is photosensitive and the typical rash appears after exposure to the rays of sunlight. Following the acute erythematous phase, the skin becomes dry and desquamates, leaving depigmentated areas. The episodic neurologic and pyschiatric derangements become manifest for the first time at a variable stage of the disease, either early, in the first or second year, or as late as the tenth year after dermatologic changes have become apparent. Their frequency and pattern of recurrence vary from case to case.

Neuropsychiatric disorders may be precipitated by inadequate or irregular diet and also by such factors as exposure to sunlight, fever, or diarrhea. But identifiable precipitating factors are frequently lacking. Neurologic signs may or may not be concomitant with an exacerbation of the cutaneous lesions. The most frequent neurological sign is a typical cerebellar ataxia, which develops acutely and lasts for a period of a few days or weeks. Although unsteady gait, asynergia, intention tremor, and dysarthria may be severe, they are always fully reversible. Attacks of vertigo and nystagmus are also recorded, sometimes associated with cerebellar signs. Diplopia and ptosis have been observed. Unexplained "slumping" or fainting attacks are an occasional feature. Severe headache and pain in the limbs, back, or chest are commonly experienced during exacer-

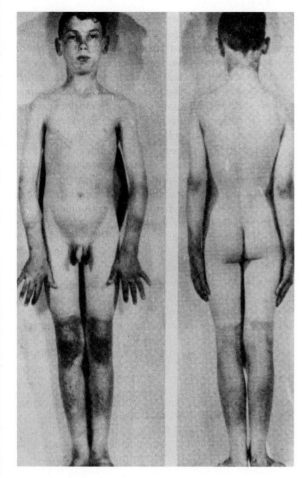

Figure 5-23

Hartnup disease: pellagra-like skin rash in young boy. (Reprinted from Baron et al., Lancet 2: 421, 1956.)

bations of the disease. Diarrhea may occur. There are no sensory disturbances or significant modifications of the reflexes. The optic fundi are normal. The EEG is noncontributory and the CSF protein level is usually normal.

The episodic psychiatric disorders range from emotional lability—inexplicable anxiety, fear, and violent temper—to acute psychoses with confusion, hallucinations, depersonalization, or depression with suicidal tendency. Indeed, these psychiatric disturbances may be the cause for referral to the hospital and may appear in the absence of neurologic signs. The mental status is variable. Some patients are mentally retarded to a slight degree, whereas others have normal intelligence. In gen-

eral, it may be said that progressive mental deterioration is not a feature of Hartnup disease.

The *basic biological abnormality* is a specific aminoaciduria due to a diminished renal tubular and intestinal absorption of a group of monoamino-monocarboxylic amino acids. Its detection is necessary for diagnosis. The free amino acids that are excreted in abnormal amounts (i.e., 5 to 20 times normal) in the urine include alanine, serine, threonine, valine, leucine, isoleucine, phenylalanine, tyrosine, tryptophan, histidine, and citrulline as well as glutamine and asparagine, all of which are neutral monoaminodicarboxylic amides. Proline is not increased (the absence of proline is notable). The amino acid excretion pattern is remarkably constant and is unchanged by nicotinamide. All other tests of renal function are normal. Plasma amino acids are not increased. Most patients, but not all, have an increased excretion of indolic compounds, particularly indican (indoxyl sulfate) and indoleacetic acid.

Although some patients on a normal diet have no excessive excretion of indican in the urine, indicanuria rises dramatically in all patients after an oral dose of tryptophan. Urinary indoxyl derivatives are the final excretion products formed in the liver from indole absorbed in the colon. In Hartnup disease they arise from the action of intestinal microorganisms on colonic tryptophan which has not been absorbed from the jejunum because of the specific transport defect.

Routine newborn screening for Hartnup disease as well as screening of siblings of affected individuals has led to two important findings. (1) The biochemical phenotype of HD is not rare. Based on recent screening data its incidence has been estimated at 1/30,000, demonstrating that HD is one of the most frequent aminoacidopathies. (2) The great majority of children with the biochemical phenotype of HD remain clinically normal.

In one series of 15 children with the biological markers of HD, detected through routine newborn urine screening, all had normal intelligence and none had abnormal neurologic signs. A photosensitive rash developed in one child.[287] In another series of 21 children, 2 developed the typical clinical syndrome, 5 developed nonphotosensitive skin lesions, and 1 had seizures. School performances were normal in all of them. None had received continuous nicotinamide therapy.[288]

To explain why some individuals develop the disease and others do not, it is postulated that environmental factors (poor diet, diarrhea) and possibly polygenic factors (low plasma amino acid levels) interacting with a primary monogenic transport defect are determinative for the expression of the characteristic cutaneous and neuropsychiatric disorders. Clinical signs are believed more likely to appear if the aggregate value of plasma amino acids is below normal.[289]

Variants   There may be patients with isolated renal tubular or intestinal defects.

Diagnostic Laboratory Tests   They consist essentially of chromatography of the urine for the detection of the specific aminoaciduria, the presence of which is necessary for diagnosis, and a search for indoluria after oral loading with L-tryptophan.

Genetics   HD is an autosomal recessive inherited disorder with a widespread geographical distribution. Heterozygotes are normal and have shown no evidence of a renal defect. The specific carrier for neutral amino acid transport, which is probably located in the brush border membrane of renal and intestinal epithelium, has not been identified. The mutant gene responsible for the disorder is not known.

Diagnosis   Intermittent relapsing ataxias and acute reversible neuropsychiatric disturbances may also occur in porphyria, some of the hyperammonemias, and organoacidopathies, and in the mitochondrial disorders. The photosensitive skin lesions are similar to those of pellagra.

There have been reports of rare disorders with a pellegra-like skin rash, ataxia, and other neurologic manifestations, probably related to defects in tryptophan catabolism.[290,291] In none of these conditions is there any evidence of a disorder of renal and intestinal transport.

Treatment   Nicotinamide therapy has given remarkable improvement in the dermatitis and generally in the neuropsychiatric signs as well. Evaluation of the results of long-term treatment has been difficult because of the tendency towards spontaneous improvement.

A high-protein diet is beneficial in patients with low levels of plasma amino acids and it may prevent clinical manifestations of the disease. All clinical symptoms tend to become milder with increasing age. Systematic treatment of asymptomatic individuals with nicotinamide is probably not warranted. HD apparently does not adversely affect pregnancy and seems to do no harm to the fetus.

FAMILIAL ENCEPHALOPATHIES IN WHICH PERSONALITY CHANGES, BEHAVIORAL DISTURBANCES, AND DEMENTIA MAY BE A PRESENTING SIGN

Personality and character changes, behavioral disturbances, and mental regression may precede, by several months or years, all the other abnormalities of the nervous system. This happens in a large number of diseases and particularly in those listed below. The clinical problem may be difficult to resolve for some time, requiring differentiation of such states from developmental delay, learning disorders, social maladjustment problems, autism, and genetic psychoses. It is important for the neuropsychiatrist (1) to be alert to the possibility that certain of these intellectual peculiarities and personality disorders may herald the beginning of any one of the following metabolic diseases (and possibly a few others); and (2) to be prepared to search for subtle organic neurologic signs and utilize appropriate laboratory tests (see Tables 5-5 and 5-9). The principal diseases that may begin with personality changes or dementia are as follows:

X-linked adrenoleukodystrophy

Huntington chorea

Wilson disease

Juvenile neuronal ceroid lipofuscinosis

Juvenile metachromatic leukodystrophy

Juvenile (and adult) G_{M2} gangliosidosis

Juvenile Leigh disease

Hallervorden-Spatz disease

Lafora disease

Sanfilippo disease (MPS III)

Aspartylglucosaminuria

Hartnup disease

Acute intermittent porphyria

Homocystinuria

Other disorders of amino acid and organic acid metabolism

Cholestanolosis

Lesch-Nyhan disease

Each of these disorders has been presented in earlier sections of the book.

Accurate descriptions of personality and behavioral alterations in the published accounts of these diseases are couched in rather vague terms, and it is sometimes difficult to obtain a clear idea of the nature of the changes just by reading about them. They have not been studied adequately by neuropsychologists. In our experience, irritability, agitation, violent behavior, impulsive and irrational acts, or on the contrary, a tendency to be withdrawn, abnormally quiet and indifferent, are the most frequent behavioral patterns. A neurologic basis for these personality and behavior changes should be most carefully sought, when there is an ongoing impairment of cognitive functions. In a child with a previously normal intellectual level, one becomes suspicious when he shows increasing degrees of distractibility and inattentiveness, failing memory, a reduced vocabulary, errors in syntax, poor spatiotemporal orientation, and visuomotor impairment. Unfortunately, some of these signs may be initially mistaken for simple attention disorders, developmental dysphasia, or other types of learning disabilities. In children who have always shown a subnormal mental development, the significance of these abnormalities is at first particularly difficult, and they may be thought to be the consequence of the mental deficit.

In some of these patients the inaugural manifestation of a hereditary metabolic or neurodegenerative disease is a frank psychiatric outbreak: a "psychotic" syndrome, depression, or even a delusional-hallucinatory syndrome. The authors have been confronted with the difficult problem of detecting an HMD when examining patients in psychiatric wards or institutions for the mentally retarded. Many individuals with X-linked adrenoleukodystrophy, Huntington disease,

Wilson disease, later-onset G_{M2} gangliosidosis, metachromatic leukodystrophy, acute intermittent porphyria, homocystinuria, and Hartnup disease have first been hospitalized in psychiatric wards. Visual hallucinations are not rare in Lafora disease. Serious personality changes and acute psychotic or schizophrenia-like episodes can occur intermittently in Hartnup disease, acute intermittent porphyria, combined deficiency of methylmalonyl-CoA mutase and methyltetrahydrofolate:homocysteine methyltransferase, methylenetetrahydrofolate reductase deficiency, and disorders of cobalamin and folate metabolism.

Dementia is a rather broad and inclusive term that embraces all conditions in which there is a decline in intellectual functions from a previously normal or higher level. There is loss of retentive memory, an inability to solve problems, loss of verbal and arithmetical skills, and poor judgment. When frequent seizures are present, there is always the possibility that the seizures themselves, subclinical epileptic discharges, or drugs for their control are responsible for an apparent mental regression. Here again, precise descriptions are generally lacking, and it is presently impossible to correlate the nature of any cognitive profile of a patient with the disease that affects them.

In the presence of progressive behavioral or cognitive changes, the most important clue to the entire group of metabolic diseases of this age period comes from the discovery of the insidious development of subtle neurologic signs, including speech disorders, essentially dysarthria, changes in the quality of voice

Table 5-9

Recommended paraclinical investigations in patients with a fixed encephalopathy of uncertain origin or with behavioral or cognitive abnormalities[a,b]

MRI of brain
X-rays of spine, hips, and hands
Ultrasound scanning of kidney, heart, liver, and spleen
Search for vacuoles and inclusions in blood and, if necessary, bone marrow cells
Measurement of protein, lactic acid, sugar, amino acids, including GABA and homocarnosine, in CSF
Ophthalmologic examination, including slit-lamp study of cornea and lens, and if visual failure, ERG
NCV and EMG if absent DTR
Auditory evoked potentials if suspicion of deafness
Serum cholesterol and lipoproteins
Evaluation of amino acids, organic acids, mucopolysaccharides, and oligosaccharides in urine
Evaluation of VLCFA in plasma
Test for adenylosuccinate lyase in urine
If necessary, skin biopsy in search for inclusions in fibroblasts and sweat glands

---

[a]See also Chap. 4.

[b]Modulated according to context.

and melody of speech, and also stuttering, because they may constitute early indications of a brain disorder. Also, visual failure, disorders of conjugate eye movements, exaggerated tendon reflexes or areflexia and Babinski signs, tremor, elements of an incipient extrapyramidal disorder, abnormal facial features, and deterioration of the background activity on the EEG are valuable diagnostic leads to an HMD. The main clinical and laboratory investigations useful for the diagnosis of metabolic disorders in patients with behavioral changes and dementia are indicated in Tables 5-5 and 5-9.

ISOLATED DELAY IN MENTAL AND MOTOR DEVELOPMENT

In a number of inherited metabolic encephalopathies of childhood, the disease does not cause detectable regression, at least in its incipient stage; it merely causes mental retardation, delay in motor development, and poor motor performances. It may be difficult to distinguish between such conditions and simple motor retardation or cerebral palsy. This problem has already been discussed in Chap. 4.

Such a situation may occur in individual patients in practically all of the metabolic encephalopathies, so their enumeration here is superfluous. Suspicions of a metabolic disorder may be raised by the presence of characteristic ophthalmologic signs, such as a retinal degeneration, corneal opacities, or a disorder of conjugate eye movements, or subtle extraneurologic abnormalities of facial features, skeleton, skin, liver, spleen, or heart. But clinical examination of some patients offers no clue, so the diagnosis has to depend on a limited number of radiological, biological, electrophysiological, and histologic tests, listed in Table 5-9 and 5-5.

We believe these investigations should be systematically performed in a stepwise manner in any patient with an apparently fixed encephalopathy of uncertain origin and with a normal karyotype. The potential advantage for the diagnosis and prevention of metabolic disorders probably outweighs the financial implications of such a strategy.

If all clinical and paraclinical studies remain negative, the possible genetic nature of a cryptogenetic encephalopathy should always be kept in mind, and the parents should be informed.

REFERENCES

1. Holmes GL, Shaywitz BA: Strümpell's pure familial spastic paraplegia: case study and review of the literature. *J Neurol Neurosurg Psych* 40: 1003–1008, 1977.

2. Hazan J, Lamy C, Melki J, et al.: Autosomal dominant familial spastic paraplegia is genetically heterogeneous and one locus maps to chromosome 14q. *Nature Genet* 5: 163–167, 1993.

3. Durr A, Brice A, Serdaru M, et al.: The phenotype of "pure" autosomal dominant spastic paraplegia. *Neurology* 44: 1274–1277, 1994.

4. Behan WMH, Maia M: Strümpell's familial spastic paraplegia: genetics and neuropathology. *J Neurol Neurosurg Psych* 37: 8–20, 1974.

5. Hentati A, Pericak-Vance M, Lennon F, et al.: Linkage of a locus for autosomal dominant familial spastic paraplegia to chromosome 2p markers. *Hum Mol Genet* 3: 1867–1871, 1994.

6. Gispert S, Santos N, Damen R, et al.: Autosomal dominant familial spastic paraplegia: reduction of the FSPI candidate region on chromosome 14q to 7 cM and locus heterogeneity. *Am J Hum Genet* 56: 183–187, 1995.

7. Fink J, Brocade WC, Jones S, et al.: Autosomal dominant familial spastic paraplegia: tight linkage to chromosome 15q. *Am J Hum Genet* 56: 188–192, 1995.

8. Saugier-Veber P, Munnich A, Bonneau D, et al.: X-linked spastic paraplegia and Pelizaeus-Merzbacher disease are allelic disorders at the proteolipid protein locus. *Nature Genet* 6: 257–261, 1994.

9. Marks H, Kobayashi H, Hoffman E: New mutation of proteolipid protein in complicated form of X-linked spastic paraplegia. *Ann Neurol* 36: 535, 1994 (abstract).

10. Thomas PK, Misra VP, King RHM, et al.: Autosomal recessive hereditary sensory neuropathy with spastic paraplega. *Brain* 117: 651–659, 1994.

11. Rizzo W, Dammann A, Craft D, et al.: Sjögren-Larsson syndrome: inherited defect in the fatty alcohol cycle. *J Pediatr* 115: 228–234, 1989.

12. Di Rocco M, Filocamo M, Tortori-Donati P, et al.: Sjögren-Larsson syndrome: nuclear magnetic resonance imaging of the brain in a 4-year-old boy. *J Inherit Metab Dis* 17: 112–114, 1994.

13. Pigg M, Jagell S, Sillen A, et al.: The Sjögren-Larsson syndrome gene is close to D17S805 as determined by linkage analysis and allelic association. *Am J Hum Genet* 8: 361–364, 1994.

14. Salazar-Grueso EF, Holzer TJ, Gutierrez RA, et al.: Familial spastic paraparesis syndrome associated with HTLV1 infection. *New Engl J Med* 323: 732–737, 1990.

15. Patel JS, Van't Hoff W, Leonard JV: Arginase deficiency presenting with convulsions. *J Inherit Metab Dis* 17: 254, 1994.

16. Vockley J, Tabor D, Kern R, et al.: Identification of mutations (D128G, H141L) in the liver arginase gene of patients with hyperargininemia. *Hum Mut* 4: 150–154, 1994.

17. Friedreich N: Über degenerative Atrophie der spinalen Hinterstrange. *Virchow's Arch Path Anat* 26: 391–419, 1863.

18. Mollaret T: *La maladie de Friedreich*. Paris, Legrand, 1929.

19. Harding AE: Friedreich's ataxia: a clinical and genetic study of 90 families with an analysis of early diagnostic criteria and intrafamilial clustering of clinical features. *Brain* 104: 584–620, 1981.

20. Leone M, Rocca WA, Rosso MG, et al.: Friedreich's disease: survival analysis in an Italian population. *Neurology* 38: 1433–1438, 1988.

21. Filla A, De Michele G, Cavalcanti F: Intrafamilial phenotype variation in Friedreich's disease: possible exception to diagnostic criteria. *J Neurol Sci* 238: 147–150, 1991.

22. Finocchiaro G, Baio G, Micossi P, et al.: Glucose metabolism alterations in Friedreich's ataxia. *Neurology* 38: 1292–1296, 1988.

23. Lapresle J, Salisachs P: Onion bulbs in a nerve biopsy specimen from an original case of Roussy-Levy disease. *Arch Neurol* 29: 346–348, 1973.

24. Harding AE: Early onset cerebellar ataxia with retained tendon reflexes. A clinical and genetic study of a disorder distinct from Friedreich's ataxia. *J Neurol Neurosurg Psych* 44: 503–508, 1981.

25. Santoro L, Perretti A, Filla A, et al.: Is early onset cerebellar ataxia with retained tendon reflexes identifiable by electrophysiologic and histologic profiles? A comparison with Friedreich's ataxia. *J Neurol Sci* 113: 43–49, 1992.

25a. Palau F, Demichele G, Vilchez JJ, et al.: Early-onset ataxia with cardiomyopathy and retained tendon reflexes maps to the Friedreich's ataxia locus on chromosome 9q. *Ann Neurol* 37: 359–362, 1995.

26. Greenfield JG: *The Spino-Cerebellar Degenerations*. Oxford, Blackwell, 1954.

27. Hogan GR, Baum MC: Familial spastic ataxia in childhood. *Neurology* 27: 520–526, 1977.

27a. Benomar A, Le Guern E, Durr A, et al.: Autosomal dominant cerebellar ataxia with retinal degeneration (ADCA type II) is genetically different from ADCA type I. *Ann Neurol* 35: 439–444, 1994.

27b. Enevoldson TP, Sanders MD, Harding AE: Autosomal dominant cerebellar ataxia with pigmentary macular dystrophy. A clinical and genetic study of eight families. *Brain* 117: 445–460, 1994.

27c. Rosenberg RN: Autosomal dominant cerebellar phenotypes. The genotype has settled the issue. *Neurology* 45: 1–5, 1995.

28. Bassen FA, Kornzweig AL: Malformation of erythrocytes in a case of retinitis pigmentosa. *Blood* 5: 381–387, 1950.

29. Kane JP, Havel RJ: Disorders of the biogenesis and secretion of lipoproteins containing the beta-apolipoproteins, in Scriver CR, Baudet AL, Sly WS, Valle D (eds):

The Metabolic and Molecular Bases of Inherited Disease. New York, McGraw-Hill, 1995, pp. 1853–1885.

30. Spencer SE, Walter FO, Moore SA: Choreo-amyotrophy with chronic hemolytic anemia: a variant of chorea-amyotrophy with acanthocytosis. *Neurology* 37: 645–649, 1987.

31. Sokol RJ, Guggenheim MA, Heubi JE, et al.: Frequency and clinical progression of the vitamin E deficiency neurologic disorder in children with prolonged neonatal cholestasis. *Am J Dis Child* 139: 1211–1215, 1985.

32. Malloy MJ, Kane JP: Disorders of lipoproteins, in Rosenberg RN, Prusiner SB, Di Mauro S, Barchi RL, Kunkel LM (eds): *The Molecular and Genetic Basis of Neurologic Disease*. Boston, Butterworth-Heinemann, 1993, pp. 286–287.

33. Burck V, Goebel HH, Kuhlendahl HD, et al.: Neuromyopathy and vitamin E deficiency in man. *Neuropediatrics* 12: 267–278, 1981.

34. Ben Hamida M, Belal S, Sirugo G, et al.: Friedreich's ataxia phenotype not linked to chromosome 9 and associated with selective autosomal recessive vitamin E deficiency in two inbred Tunisian families. *Neurology* 43: 2179–2183, 1993.

35. Sabouraud P: Personal communication, 1994.

36. Ben Hamida C, Doerflinger N, Belal S, et al.: Localization of Friedreich ataxia phenotype with selective vitamin E deficiency to chromosome 8q by homozygote mapping. *Nature Genet* 5: 195–200, 1993.

37. Di Donato S: Can we avoid AVED? *Nature Genet* 9: 106–107, 1995.

38. Kayden HJ: The neurologic syndrome of vitamin E deficiency: a significant cause of ataxia. *Neurology* 43: 2167–2169, 1993.

39. Barth PG, Hoffmann GF, Jackson J, et al.: L-2-hydroxyglutaric acidaemia: clinical and biochemical findings in 12 patients and preliminary report on L-2-hydroxyglutaric acid dehydrogenase. *J Inherit Metab Dis* 16: 753–761, 1993.

40. Lehesjoki AE, Koskiniemi M, Pandolfo M, et al.: Linkage studies in progressive myoclonus epilepsy: Unverricht-Lundborg and Lafora diseases. *Neurology* 42: 1545–1550, 1992.

41. Unverricht H: Über familiäre Myoclonie. *Dtsch Z Nervenheilk* 7: 32–67, 1895.

42. Lundborg H: *Die progressive Myoklonus Epilepsie*. Uppsala, Almquist and Wilsell, 1903.

43. Roger J, Genton P, Bureau M, et al.: Dyssinergia cerebellaris myoclonica (Ramsay Hunt Syndrome). A study of 32 cases. *Neuropediatrics* 18: 117, 1987 (abstract).

44. Norio R, Koskiniemi MZ: Progressive myoclonus epilepsy: genetic and nosologic aspects, with special reference to 107 Finnish patients. *Clin Genet* 15: 382–398, 1979.

45. Koskiniemi M, Donner M, Majuri H, et al.: Progressive myoclonus epilepsy—a clinical and histopathological study. *Acta Neurol Scand* 50: 307–332, 1974.

46. Aicardi J: *Diseases of the Nervous System in Childhood.* New York, Cambridge University Press, 1992, pp. 547–549.

47. Cochius J, Carpenter S, Andermann E, et al.: Sweat gland vacuoles in Unverricht-Lundborg disease: a clue to diagnosis? *Neurology* 44: 2372–2375, 1994.

48. Malafosse A, Lebesjoki AE, Genton P, et al.: Identical genetic locus for Baltic and Mediterranean myoclonus. *Lancet* 339: 1080–1081, 1992.

49. Haltia M, Kristensson K, Sourander P: Neuropathological studies in three Scandinavian cases of progressive myoclonus epilepsy. *Acta Neurol Scand* 45: 63–77, 1968.

50. Harriman DGF, Millar JHD, Stevenson AC: Progressive familial myoclonic epilepsy in three families: its clinical features and pathological basis. *Brain* 78: 325–349, 1955.

51. Ammerman T: Isolierte Schädigung der unteren Oliven bei Myoklonus-Epilepsie. *Arch Psychiatr Nervenkr* 111: 213–232, 1940.

52. Van Bogaert L: Sur l'épilepsie myoclonie progressive d'Unverricht-Lundborg. Etude d'un cas anatomique et de la sémiologie du syndrome amyostatique terminal. *Monatsschr Psychiatr Neurol* 118: 170–191, 1949.

53. Yokoi S, Kobori H, Yoshihara H: Clinical and neuropathological studies of myoclonic epilepsy. A report of two cases. *Acta Neuropathol* 4: 370–379, 1965.

54. Lafora GR: Über das Vorkommen amyloider Körperchen in innern der ganglien zellen. *Virchows Arch Pathol Anat* 205: 295–303, 1911.

55. Archarya JN, Satischandra P, Asha T, et al.: Lafora's disease in South India. A clinical, electrophysiologic and pathologic study. *Epilepsia* 34: 476–487, 1993.

56. Roger J, Pelissier JF, Bureau M, et al.: Le diagnostic précoce de la maladie de Lafora. Importance des manifestations paroxystiques visuelles et intérêt de la biopsie cutanée. *Rev Neurol* 139: 115–124, 1983.

57. Drury I, Blaivas M, Abou-Khalil BW, et al.: Biopsy results in a kindred with Lafora disease. *Arch Neurol* 50: 102–105, 1993.

58. Vos AJM, Joosten EMG, Gabreels-Festen RAWM: Adult polyglucosan-body disease, clinical and nerve biopsy findings in 2 cases. *Ann Neurol* 13: 440–44, 1983.

59. Lossos A, Barash V, Soffer D: Hereditary branching enzyme dysfunction in adult polyglucosan disease, a possible metabolic cause in two patients. *Ann Neurol* 30: 655–662, 1991.

60. Bruno C, Servidei S, Shanske S, et al.: Glycogen branching enzyme deficiency in adult polyglucosan-body disease. *Ann Neurol* 33: 88–93, 1993.

61. Schroder JM, May R, Shin YS, et al.: Juvenile hereditary polyglucosan-body disease with complete branching enzyme deficiency (type IV glycogenosis). *Acta Neuropath* 85: 419–430, 1993.

62. Herrik MK, Twiss JL, Vladutiu GD, et al.: Concomitant branching enzyme and phosphorylase deficiencies. An unusual glycogenosis with extensive neuronal polyglucosan storage. *J Neuropathol Exp Neurol* 53: 239–246, 1994.

64. Marsden CD, Harding AD, Obeso JA, et al.: Progressive myoclonic ataxia (the Ramsay Hunt syndrome). *Arch Neurol* 47: 1121–1125, 1990.

65. Hunt JR: Dyssynergia cerebellaris myoclonica. *Brain* 44: 490–538, 1921.

66. Rapin I, Goldfischer S, Katzman R, et al.: The cherry-red spot-myoclonus syndrome. *Ann Neurol* 3: 234–242, 1978.

67. Lowden JA, O'Brien JS: Sialidosis, a review of human neuraminidase deficiency. *Am J Hum Genet* 31: 1–18, 1979.

68. Gascon G, Wallenberg B, Daif AK, et al.: Successful treatment of cherry-red spot myoclonus syndrome with 5-hydroxytryptophan. *Ann Neurol* 24: 453–455, 1988.

69. Takahashi H, Ohama E, Naito H, et al.: Hereditary dentatorubral-pallidoluysian atrophy: clinical and pathologic variants in a family. *Neurology* 38: 1065–1070, 1988.

70. Warner T, Williams L, Harding A: DRPLA in Europe. *Nature Genet* 6: 225, 1994.

71. Potter NT, Meyer MA, Zimmerman AW, et al.: Molecular and clinical findings in a family with dentato-rubral-pallidoluysian atrophy. *Ann Neurol* 37: 273–277, 1995.

72. Margolis RL, Li SH, Li XJ, et al.: Trinucleotide repeat expansion on DRPLA: molecular characterisation of atrophin 1. *Am J Hum Genet* 55: A230, 1994.

73. Burke JR, Wingfield MS, Lewis KE, et al.: The Haw River syndrome: dentatorubropallidoluysian atrophy (DRPLA) in an African-American family. *Nature Genet* 7: 521–524, 1994.

74. Ikeuchi T, Koide R, Tanaka H, et al.: Dentatorubral-pallidoluysian atrophy: clinical features are closely related to unstable expansions of trinucleotide (CAG) repeat. *Ann. Neurol* 37: 769–775, 1995.

75. Delecluse F, Waldemar G, Vestermark S, et al.: Cerebral blood flow deficits in hereditary essential myoclonus. *Arch Neurol* 49: 179–182, 1992.

76. Hallet M, Marsden CD: Ballistic overflow movement myoclonus. A form of essential myoclonus. *Brain* 100: 299–312, 1977.

77. Korten JJ, Notermans SLH, Frenken CWGM, et al.: Familial essential myoclonus. *Brain* 97: 131–138, 1974.

78. Gilbert GJ, McEntee WJ, Glaser GH: Familial myoclonus and ataxia. Pathophysiological implications. *Neurology* 13: 365–372, 1963.

79. Deutschl G, Mischke G, Schenk E, et al.: Symptomatic and essential rhythmic palatal myoclonus. *Brain* 13: 1645–1672, 1990.

80. Boulloche J, Aicardi J: Syndrome des myoclonies du voile spontanément régressif chez l'enfant. *Arch Fr Pediatr* 41: 645–647, 1984.

81. Paulson GW: Benign essential tremor in childhood. *Clin Pediatr* 15: 67–70, 1987.

82. Vanesse M, Bedard P, Anderman F: Shuddering attacks in children: an early clinical manifestation of essential tremor. *Neurology* 26: 1027–1030, 1976.

83. Danks DM: Disorders of copper transport, in Scriver CR, Beaudet AL, Sly WS, Valle D (eds): *The Metabolic and Molecular Bases of Inherited Disease*. New York, McGraw-Hill, 1995, pp. 2211–2223.

84. Scheinberg H, Sternlieb I, Richman J: Psychiatric manifestations in patients with Wilson disease. *Birth Defects* 4: 85–89, 1968.

85. Kuwert T, Hefter H, Scholz D, et al.: Regional cerebral glucose consumption measured by positron emission tomography in patients with Wilson disease. *Eur J Nucl Med* 19: 96–101, 1992.

86. Thomas GR, Forbes JR, Roberts EA, et al.: The Wilson disease gene: spectrum of mutations and their consequences. *Nature Genet* 9: 210, 1995.

87. Cossu P, et al.: Prenatal diagnosis of Wilson disease by the analysis of DNA polymorphism. *New Engl J Med* 327: 57, 1992.

88. Walshe JM, Yealland M: Chelation treatment of neurologic Wilson disease. *Q J Med* 86: 197–204, 1993.

89. Heckmann JM, Eastman RW, De Villiers JC, et al.: Wilson's disease: neurological and magnetic resonance imaging improvement on zinc treatment. *J Neurol Neurosurg Psych* 57: 1273–1274, 1994.

90. Roh JK, Lee TG, Wie BA, et al.: Initial and follow-up brain MRI findings and correlation with the clinical course in Wilson's disease. *Neurol* 44: 1064–1068, 1994.

91. Song HS, Ku WC, Chen CL: Disappearance of Kayser-Fleischer rings following liver transplantation. *Transplant Proc* 24: 1483–1485, 1992.

92. Martin JB: Huntington's disease in young people. *Eur Neurol* 3: 278–289, 1970.

93. Harper PS: The epidemiology of Huntington's disease. *Hum Genet* 89: 365–376, 1992.

94. Leigh RJ, Zee DS: *The Neurology of Eye Movements*. Philadelphia, FA Davis, 1983, pp. 234–235.

95. De Volder A, Bol A, Michel C, et al.: Brain glucose utilization in childhood Huntington disease studied with positron emission tomography (PET). *Brain Dev* 10: 47–50, 1988.

96. Ridley RM, Farrer LA, Frith CD, et al.: A test of the hypothesis that age at onset in Huntington disease is controlled by an X-linked recessive modifier. *Am J Hum Genet* 50: 536–543, 1992.

97. Farrer LA, Cupples LA, Wiater P, et al.: The normal Huntington disease (HD) allele, or a closely linked gene, influences age at onset of HD. *Am J Hum Genet* 53: 125–130, 1993.

98. Gusella JF, Wexler NS, Conneally PM, et al.: A polymorphic DNA marker genetically linked to Huntington's disease. *Nature* 306: 234–238, 1983.

99. Morell V: Huntington's gene finally found. *Science* 260: 28–30, 1993.

100. A novel gene containing a trinucleotide repeat that is expanded and unstable on Huntington's disease chromosome. The Huntington's Disease Collaborative Research Group. *Cell* 72: 971–983, 1993.

101. Kieburtz K, MacDonald M, Shih C, et al.: Trinucleotide repeat length and progression of illness in Huntington's disease. *J Med Genet* 31: 872–874, 1994.

102. Wiggins S, Whyte P, Huggins M, et al.: The psychological consequences of predictive testing for Huntington's disease. *New Engl J Med* 327: 1401–1405, 1992.

103. Tyler A, Walker R, Went L, et al.: Guidelines for the molecular genetics predictive test in Huntington's disease. *J Med Genet* 31: 555–559, 1994.

104. Vonsattel JP, Myers R, Stevens T, et al.: Neuropathological classification of Huntington's disease. *J Neuropathol Exptl Neurol* 44: 559–577, 1985.

105. Byers R, Gilles F, Fung C: Huntington's disease in children. Neuropathologic study of four cases. *Neurology* 23: 561–569, 1973.

105a. Brion S, Comoy C: Rigidité dans la forme infantile de la maladie de Huntington (étude anatomoclinique d'un cas). *Rev Neurol* 112: 183–199, 1965.

106. Hunt JR: Progressive atrophy of the globus pallidus (primary atrophy of the pallidal system). A system disease of the paralysis agitans type characterized by atrophy of the motor cells of the corpus striatum. A contribution to the functions of the corpus striatum. *Brain* 40: 58–148, 1921.

107. Van Bogaert L: Contribution clinique et anatomique à l'étude de la paralysie agitante juvénile primitive (atrophie progressive du globe pâle de Ramsay Hunt). *Rev Neurol* 37: 315–326, 1930.

108. Davison C: Pallido-pyramidal disease. *J Neuropathol Exptl Neurol* 13: 50–59, 1954.

109. Gibb WR, Narabayashi H, Yokochi M, et al.: New pathologic observations in juvenile onset parkinsonism with dystonia. *Neurology* 41: 820–822, 1991.

110. Lazzarini AM, Myers RH, Zimmerman TR, et al.: A clinical genetic study of Parkinson's disease: evidence for dominant transmission. *Neurology* 44: 499–506, 1994.

111. Payami H, Bernard S, Larsen K, et al.: Genetic anticipation in Parkinson's disease. *Neurology* 45: 135–138, 1995.

112. Di Mauro S: Mitochondrial involvement in Parkinson's disease: the controversy continues. *Neurology* 43: 2170–2172, 1993.

113. Przedborski S, Jackson-Lewis V, Muthane U, et al.: Chronic levodopa administration alters cerebral mitochondrial respiratory chain activity. *Ann Neurol* 34: 715–723, 1993.

114. Stacy M, Jankovic J: Childhood dystonia. *Pediatr Ann* 22: 53–58, 1993.

115. Lou JS, Jankovic J: Essential tremor: clinical correlates in 350 patients. *Neurology* 41: 234–238, 1991.

116. Karbe H, Holthoff VA, Rudolf J, et al.: Positron emission tomography demonstrates frontal cortex and basal

ganglia hypometabolism in dystonia. *Neurology* 42: 1540–1544, 1992.

117. Risch N, De Leon D, Ozelius L, et al.: Genetic analysis of idiopathic torsion dystonia in Ashkenazi Jews and their recent descent from a small founder population. *Nature Genet* 9: 152–159, 1995.

118. Zeman W: Pathology of the torsion dystonias (dystonia musculorum deformans). *Neurology* 20: 79–88, 1970.

119. Hornykiewicz O, Kish S, Becker L, et al.: Brain neurotransmitters in dystonia musculorum deformans. *New Engl J Med* 315: 347–353, 1986.

120. Wolfson L, Sharpless N, Thal L, et al.: Decreased ventricular fluid of norepinephrine metabolite in childhood-onset dystonia. *Neurology* 33: 369–372, 1983.

121. Waddy HM, Fletcher NA, Harding AE, et al.: A genetic study of idiopathic focal dystonias. *Ann Neurol* 29: 320–324, 1991.

122. Ichinose H, Ohye T, Takahashi EI, et al.: Hereditary progressive dystonia with marked diurnal fluctuation caused by mutations in the GTP cyclohydrolase I gene. *Nature Genet* 8: 236–242, 1994.

123. Nygaard TG, Trugman JM, De Yebenes JG, et al.: Dopa-responsive dystonia: the spectrum of clinical manifestations in a large North American family. *Neurology* 40: 66–69, 1990.

124. Segawa M, Hosaka A, Miyagawa F, et al.: Hereditary progressive dystonia with marked diurnal fluctuations. *Adv in Neurol* 14: 215–233, 1975.

125. Muller U, Haberhausen G, Wagner T, et al.: DXS106 and DXS559 flank the X-linked dystonia-parkinsonism syndrome locus (DYT3). *Genomics* 23: 114–117, 1994.

126. Dobyns WB, Ozelius LJ, Kramer PL, et al.: Rapid-onset dystonia-parkinsonism. *Neurology* 43: 2596–2602, 1993.

127. Dooling EC, Schoene WC, Richardson EP: Hallervorden-Spatz syndrome. *Arch Neurol* 30: 70–83, 1974.

128. Østergaard JR, Christensen T, Hansen KN: In vivo diagnosis of Hallervorden-Spatz disease. *Dev Med Child Neurol* 37: 227–233, 1995.

129. Delecluse F, Deleval J, Gerard JM, et al.: Frontal impairment and hypoperfusion in neuroacanthocytosis. *Arch Neurol* 48: 232–234, 1991.

130. Sakai T, Antoku Y, Iwashita H, et al.: Chorea-acanthocytosis: abnormal composition of covalently bound fatty acids of erythrocyte membrane proteins. *Ann Neurol* 29: 664–669, 1991.

131. Ho M, Chelly J, Carter N, et al.: Isolation of the gene for McLeod syndrome that encodes a novel membrane transport protein. *Cell* 77: 869–880, 1994.

132. Rinne JO, Daniel SE, Scaravilli F, et al.: Nigral degeneration in neuroacanthocytosis. *Neurology* 44: 1629–1632, 1994.

133. Chun RW, Daly RF, Mansheim BJ, et al.: Benign familial chorea with onset in childhood. *JAMA* 225: 1603–1607, 1973.

134. Haerer AF, Currier RC, Jackson JF: Hereditary nonprogressive chorea of early onset. *New Engl J Med* 276: 1220–1224, 1968.

135. Nutting PA, Cole BR, Schimke RN: Benign recessively inherited choreo-athetosis. *J Med Genet* 6: 408–410, 1969.

136. Pincus JH, Chutorian A: Familial benign chorea with intention tremor. A clinical entity. *J Pediatr* 70: 724–729, 1967.

137. Klawans HL, Brandabur M: Chorea in childhood. *Pediatr Ann* 22: 41–50, 1993.

138. Wheeler PG, Weaver DD, Dobyns WB: Benign hereditary chorea. *Pediatr Neurol* 9: 337–340, 1993.

139. Carmichael EA, Patterson D: A form of familial cerebral degeneration chiefly affecting the lenticular nucleus. *Brain* 47: 207, 1924.

140. Roessmann U, Schwartz J: Familial striatal degeneration. *Arch Neurol* 29: 314–317, 1973.

141. Miyoshi K, Matsuoka T, Mizushima S: Familial holotopistic striatal necrosis. *Acta Neuropathol* 13: 240–249, 1969.

142. Pebenito R, Ferreti C, Chandry RR, et al.: Idiopathic dystonia associated with lesions of the basal ganglia. *Clin Pediatr* 23: 232–235, 1989.

143. Berkovic SF, Karpati G, Carpenter S, et al.: Progressive dystonia with bilateral putaminal hypodensities. *Arch Neurol* 44: 1184–1187, 1987.

144. Novotry EJ, Singh G, Wallace DC, et al.: Leber's disease and dystonia: a mitochondrial disease. *Neurology* 36: 1053–1060, 1986.

145. Marsden CD, Long AE, Quinn NP, et al.: Familial dystonia and visual failure with striatal CT lucencies. *J Neurol Neurosurg Psych* 49: 500–509, 1986.

146. Leuzzi V, Bertini E, De Negri AM: Bilateral striatal necrosis, dystonia and optic atrophy in two siblings. *J Neurol Neurosurg Psych* 55: 16–19, 1992.

146a Van Coster R: Personal communication, 1994.

147. Manyam BV, Bhatt MH, Moore WD: Bilateral striopallidodentate calcinosis: cerebrospinal fluid, imaging and electrophysiological studies. *Ann Neurol* 91: 379–384, 1992.

148. Sly WS, Whyte MP, Sindaram B, et al.: Carbonic anhydrase II deficiency in 12 families with the autosomal recessive syndrome of osteopetrosis with renal tubular acidosis and cerebral calcification. *New Engl J Med* 313: 139–145, 1985.

149. Kendall B, Cavanagh N: Intracranial calcifications in paediatric computed tomography. *Neuroradiology* 28: 324–330, 1986.

150. Maroteaux P: Un nouveau type de mucopolysacchoridose avec athétose et élimination de keratan sulfate. *Nouv Presse Med* 2: 975–979, 1973.

151. Harvey CC, Haworth JC, Lorber J: A new heredofamilial neurological syndrome. *Arch Dis Child* 30: 338–344, 1955.

152. Van Bogaert L: Aspects cliniques et pathologiques des atrophies pallidales et pallidoluysiennes progressives. *J Neurol Neurosurg Psych* 9: 125–157, 1946.

153. Jellinger K: Progressive pallidumatrophie. *J Neurol Sci* 6: 19–44, 1968.

154. Higgins JJ, Patterson MC, Papadopoulos NM: Hypoprebetalipoproteinemia, acanthocytosis, retinitis pigmentosa, and pallidal degeneration (HARP syndrome). *Neurology* 42: 194–198, 1992.

155. Malamud N, Demmy N: Degenerative disease of the subthalamic bodies. *J Neuropathol Exptl Neurol* 19: 96, 1960.

156. Rakonitz E: Die Eigenerkrangkung des Corpus Luysi. Der erste Heredodegenerative Biballismus fall. *Z Neurol Psychiatr* 144: 255, 1933.

157. Vogt C, Vogt O: Zur Lehre der Erkrankungen des Striaten Systems. *J Psychol Neurol* 25: 631–846, 1920.

158. Refsum S, Salomonsen L, Skatvedt M: Heredopathia atactica polyneuritiformis in children: preliminary communication. *J Pediatr* 35: 335–343, 1949.

160. Steinberg D: Refsum disease, in Rosenberg RN, Prusiner SB, Di Mauro S, Barchi RL, Kunkel LM (eds): *The Molecular and Genetic Basis of Neurological Disease.* Boston, Butterworth-Heinemann, 1993, pp. 389–398.

161. Singh J, Pahan K, Dhannsi GS, et al.: Phytanic acid α-oxidation. *J Biol Chem* 268: 9972–9979, 1993.

162. Mascarenhas Saraiva MJ, Pinho Costa P, De Witt S: Goodman Transthyretin and familial amygloidatic polyneuropathy, in Rosenberg RN, Prusiner SB, Di Mauro S, Barchi RL, Kunkel LM (eds): *The Molecular and Genetic Basis of Neurological Disease.* Boston, Butterworth-Heinemann, 1993, 889–894.

163. Jacobson DR, McFarlin DE, Kane I, et al.: Transthyretin Pro[55], a variant associated with early-onset, aggressive, diffuse amyloidosis with cardiac and neurologic involvement. *Hum Genet* 89: 353–356, 1992.

164. Schmalbruch H, Stender S, Boysen G: Abnormalities in spinal neurons and dorsal root ganglion cells in Tangier disease presenting with a syringomelia-like syndrome. *J Neuropathol Exptl Neurol* 46: 533–543, 1987.

165. Eng CM, Desnick RJ: Molecular basis of Fabry disease: mutations and polymorphisms in the human α-galactosidase A gene. *Hum Mut* 3: 103–111, 1994.

166. Scher NA, Letson RD, Desnick RJ: The ocular manifestations of Fabry's disease. *Arch Ophthalmol* 97: 671–676, 1979.

167. Desnick RJ, Ioannou YA, Eng CH: Fabry disease: alpha-galactosidase deficiency, in: Scriver CR, Beaudet AL, Sly WS, Valle D (eds): *The Metabolic and Molecular Bases of Inherited Disease.* New York, McGraw-Hill, 1995, pp. 2741–2784.

168. Cable WJL, Dvorak AM, Osage JE, et al.: Fabry disease: significance of ultrastructural localization of lipid inclusions in dermal nerves. *Neurology* 32: 347–353, 1982.

169. Waldenström J: Studien über Porphyria. *Acta Med Scand* suppl 82, 1937.

170. Barclay N: Acute intermittent porphyria in childhood. A neglected diagnosis? *Arch Dis Child* 49: 403–407, 1974.

171. Becker DM, Kramer S: The neurological manifestations of porphyria: a review. *Medicine* 56: 411–423, 1977.

172. Karpas A, Sassa S, Galbraith RA: The porphyrias, in Scriver CR, Beaudet AL, Sly WS, Valle D (eds): *The Metabolic Basis of Inherited Disease.* New York, McGraw-Hill, 1989, pp. 1320–1329.

173. Karpas A, Sassa S, Galbraith RA: The porphyrias, in Scriver CR, Beaudet AL, Sly WS, Valle D (eds): *The Metabolic and Molecular Bases of Inherited Disease.* New York, McGraw-Hill, 1995, p. 2124.

174. Tishler PV, Woodward B, O'Connor J, et al.: High prevalence of intermittent acute porphyria in a psychiatric patient population. *Am J Psych* 142: 1430–1436, 1985.

175. Fujita H, Kondo M, Taketani S, et al.: Characterization and expression of cDNA encoding coproporphyrinogen oxidase from a patient with hereditary coproporphyria. *Hum Molec Genet* 3: 1807–1810, 1994.

176. Martasek P, Normann Y, Grandchamp B: Homozygous hereditary coproporphyria caused by an arginine to tryptophan substitution in coproporphyrinogen oxidase and common intragenic polymorphism. *Hum Molec Genet* 3: 477–480, 1994.

177. Mercelis R, Hassoun A, Verstraeten L, et al.: Porphyric neuropathy and hereditary delta-aminolevulinic acid dehydratase deficiency in an adult. *J Neurol Sci* 95: 39–47, 1990.

177a. Mitchell G, Larochelle J, Lambert M, et al.: Neurologic crises in hereditary tyrosinemia. *New Engl J Med* 332: 432–437, 1990.

178. Gabreels-Festen AAWM, Gabreels FJM, Jennekens FGI, et al.: Autosomal recessive form of hereditary motor and sensory neuropathy type I. *Neurology* 42: 1755–1761, 1992.

179. Ionasescu VV, Trofatter J, Haines JL, et al.: Mapping of the gene for X-linked dominant Charcot-Marie-Tooth neuropathy. *Neurology* 42: 903–908, 1992.

180. Ionasescu VV, Trofatter J, Haines JL, et al.: Heterogeneity in X-linked recessive Charcot-Marie-Tooth neuropathy. *Am J Genet* 48: 1075–1083, 1991.

181. Bergoffen J, Scherer SS, Wang S, et al.: Connexin mutations in X-linked Charcot-Marie-Tooth disease. *Science* 262: 2039–2042, 1993.

182. Ionasescu VV, Searby CC, Ionasescu R: X-linked Charcot-Marie-Tooth (CMT) neuropathies (CMTX1, CMTX2, CTMX3) show different clinical phenotypes and molecular genetics. *Am J Hum Genet* 55 suppl A, 224, 1994.

183. Harding AE, Thomas PK: Autosomal recessive forms of hereditary motor and sensory neuropathy. *J Neurol Neurosurg Psych* 43: 669–678, 1980.

184. Loprest LJ, Pericak-Vance MA, Stajich J, et al.: Linkage studies in Charcot-Marie-Tooth disease type 2: Evidence that CMT types 1 and 2 are distinct genetic entities. *Neurology* 42: 597–601, 1992.

185. Denton P, Gere S, Wolpert C, et al.: Mapping of the chromosome 1p36 region surrounding the Charcot Marie-Tooth disease type 2A locus. *Am J Hum Genet* 55 suppl A, 257, 1994.

186. Ouvrier RA, McLeod JG, Morgan GJ, et al.: Hereditary motor and sensory neuropathy of the neuronal type with onset in early childhood. *J Neurol Sci* 51: 181–197, 1981.

187. Roa BB, Dyck PJ, Marks HG, et al.: Déjerine-Sottas syndrome associated with point mutation in the peripheral myelin protein 22 (PMP22) gene. *Nature Genet* 5: 269–273, 1993.

188. Valentijn LJ, Ouvrier RA, Norbert HA, et al.: Déjerine-Sottas neuropathy is associated with a de novo PMP22 mutation. *Hum Mut* 5: 76–80, 1995.

189. Hayasaka K, Himoro M, Sawaishi Y, et al.: De novo mutation of the myelin P_0 gene in Déjerine-Sottas disease (hereditary motor and sensory neuropathy type III). *Nature Genet* 5: 266–268, 1993.

190. Lyon G: Ultrastructural study of a nerve biopsy from a case of early infantile chronic neuropathy. *Acta Neuropathol* 13: 131–142, 1969.

191. Guzzetta F, Ferrière G, Lyon G: Congenital hypomyelination polyneuropathy. Pathological findings compared to polyneuropathies in later life. *Brain* 105: 395–916, 1982.

192. Boylan KB, Ferriero DM, Greco CM, et al.: Congenital hypomyelination neuropathy with arthrogryposis multiplex congenital. *Ann Neurol* 31: 337–340, 1992.

193. Stollhoff K, Albani M, Goebel HH: Giant axonal neuropathy and leukodystrophy. *Pediatr Neurol* 7: 69–71, 1991.

194. Donhagy M, King RHM, Thomas PK, et al.: Abnormalities in the axonal cytoskeleton in giant axonal neuropathy. *J Neurocytol* 17: 197–208, 1988.

195. Meek D, Wolfe LS, Andermann E, et al.: Juvenile progressive dystonia: a new phenotype of G_{M2} gangliosidosis. *Ann Neurol* 15: 348–352, 1984.

196. Specola N, Vanier MT, Goutieres F, et al.: The juvenile and chronic forms of G_{M2} gangliosidosis: clinical and enzymatic heterogeneity. *Neurology* 40: 145–150, 1990.

197. Brett EM, Ellis RB, Haas L, et al.: Late onset G_{M2} gangliosidosis: clinical, pathological and biochemical studies on eight patients. *Arch Dis Child* 48: 775–785, 1973.

198. Navon R, Argov Z, Frisch A: Hexosaminidase A deficiency in adults. *Am J Med Genet* 24: 179–196, 1986.

199. Federico A, Palmeri A, Malandrini G, et al.: The clinical aspects of adult hexosaminidase deficiency. *Dev Neurosci* 13: 280–287, 1991.

200. Rapin I, Suzuki K, Suzuki K, et al.: Adult (chronic) G_{M2} gangliosidosis. Atypical spinocerebellar degeneration in a Jewish sibship. *Arch Neurol* 33: 120–130, 1976.

201. Willner JP, Grabowski GA, Gordon RE, et al.: Chronic gangliosidosis masquerading as atypical Friedreich ataxia: clinical, morphologic and biochemical studies of nine cases. *Neurology* 31: 787–798, 1981.

202. Harding AE, Young EP, Schon F: Adult onset supranuclear ophthalmoplegia, cerebellar ataxia and neurogenic proximal muscle weakness in a brother and sister: another hexosaminidase A deficiency syndrome. *J Neurol Psychiat* 50: 687–690, 1987.

203. Rubin M, Kayati G, Wolfe LS, et al.: Adult onset motor neuropathy in the juvenile type of hexosaminidase A and B deficiency. *J Neurol Sci* 87: 103–119, 1988.

204. Navon R, Kolodny EH, Mitsumoto H, et al.: Ashkenazi-Jewish and Non-Jewish adult G_{M2} gangliosidosis patients share a common genetic defect. *Am J Hum Genet* 46: 817–821, 1990.

205. Vanier MT, Pentchev P, Rodrigue-Lafrasse C, et al.: Niemann-Pick C disease: an update. *J Inherit Metab Dis* 14: 580–595, 1991.

206. Pentchev PG, Vanier MT, Suzuki K, et al.: Niemann-Pick disease type C: a cellular cholesterol lipidosis, in Scriver CR, Beaudet AL, Sly WS, Valle D (eds): *The Metabolic and Molecular Bases of Inherited Disease.* New York, McGraw-Hill, 1995, pp. 2625–2639.

207. Silverstein MN, Elefson RD: The syndrome of the sea-blue histiocyte. *Semin Hematol* 9: 299–302, 1972.

208. Carstea ED, Polymeropoulos MH, Parker CC, et al.: Linkage of Niemann-Pick disease type C to human chromosome 18. *Proc Natl Acad Sci* 90: 2002–2004, 1993.

209. Patterson MC, Di Bisceglie AM, Higgins JJ, et al.: The effect of cholesterol-lowering agents on hepatic and plasma cholesterol in Niemann-Pick disease type C. *Neurology* 43: 61–64, 1993.

210. Sylvain M, Arnold DL, Scriver CR, et al.: Magnetic resonance spectroscopy in Niemann-Pick disease type C: correlation with diagnosis and clinical response to cholestyramine and lovastatin. *Pediatr Neurol* 10: 228–232, 1994.

211. Brett EM: Personal communication, 1980.

212. Yu KT, Merrick HFW, Verderese C, et al.: Horizontal supranuclear gaze palsy: A marker for severe systemic involvement in type III Gaucher's disease. *Neurology* 40: 357, 884P, 1990 (abstract).

213. Svennerholm L, Erikson A, Groth CG, et al.: Norrbottnian type of Gaucher disease. Clinical, biochemical and molecular biology aspects. Successful treatment with bone marrow transplantation. *Dev Neurosci* 13: 345–351, 1991.

214. Dahl N, Lagerstrom M, Erikson A, et al.: Gaucher disease type III (Norrbottnian type) is caused by a single mutation in exon 10 of the glucocerebrosidase gene. *Am J Hum Genet* 47: 275–278, 1990.

215. Horowitz M, Zimran A: Mutations causing Gaucher disease. *Hum Mut* 3: 1–11, 1994.

216. Brady OR, O'Neill RR, Barton NW: Glucosylceramide lipidosis: Gaucher disease, in Rosenberg RN, Prusiner SB, Di Mauro S, Barchi RL, Kunkel LM (eds): *The Molecular and Genetic Basis of Neurological Disease.* Boston, Butterworth-Heinemann, 1993, pp. 467–484.

216a. Eviatar L, Sklower SL, Wisniewski K, et al.: Farber disease (lipogranulomatosis): an unusual presentation in a black child. *Pediatr Neurol* 2: 371–374, 1986.

217. Schain R, Willey J: Evolution of characteristic speech disorder in juvenile cerebral lipidosis. *Trans Am Neurol Assoc* 90: 290–291, 1965.

218. Kohlschutter A, Gardiner RM, Goebel HH: Human forms of neuronal ceroid-lipofuscinosis (Batten disease): consensus on diagnostic criteria, Hamburg 1992. *J Inherit Metab Dis* 16: 241–244, 1993.

219. Lerner TJ, Boustany RMN, McCormack K, et al.: Linkage disequilibrium between the juvenile neuronal ceroid-lipofuscinosis gene and marker loci on chromosome 16p12.1. *Am J Hum Genet* 54: 88–94, 1994.

220. Bennett MJ, Gayton AR, Rittey CDC, et al.: Juvenile neuronal ceroid-lipofuscinosis: developmental progress after supplementation with polyunsaturated fatty acids. *Dev Med Child Neurol* 36: 630–638, 1994.

221. Zhon XY, Willemsen R, Gillemans N, et al.: Common point mutations in four patients with late infantile form of galactosialidosis. *Am J Hum Genet* 53: suppl 966A, 1993.

222. Ozand PT, Gascon GG: Heterogeneity of carboxypeptidase activity in infantile-onset galactosialidosis. *J Child Neurol* 7: S31–S40, 1992.

223. Lyon G, Hagberg B, Evrard P, et al.: Symptomatology of late onset Krabbe's leukodystrophy. The European experience. *Dev Neurosci* 13: 240–244, 1991.

224. Kolodny EH, Raghavan S, Kriwit W: Late-onset Krabbe disease (globoid cell leukodystrophy). Clinical and biochemical features of 15 cases. *Dev Neurosci* 13: 232–239, 1991.

225. Hagberg B: Personal communication, 1993.

225a. Kolodny EH, Gamasosa HA, Battistani S: Molecular genetics of late onset Krabbe disease. *Am J Hum Genet* 57 (suppl): A217, 1995.

226. Thomas PK, Halpern JP, King RHM, et al.: Galactosyl ceramide lipidosis: Novel presentation as a slowly progressive spino-cerebellar degeneration. *Ann Neurol* 16: 618–620, 1984.

227. Hedley-White ET, Boustany RM, Riskind P, et al.: Peripheral neuropathy due to galactosylceramide-beta-galactosidase deficiency (Krabbe disease) in a 73-year-old woman. *Neuropathol Appl Neurobiol* 14: 515–516, 1988.

228. Moser HW: Peroxisomal disorders, in Rosenberg RN, Prusiner SB, Di Mauro S, Barchi RL, Kunkel LM (eds): *The Molecular and Genetic Basis of Neurological Disease.* Boston, Butterworth-Heinemann, 1993, pp. 364–372.

229. McGuinness MC, Griffin DE, Power JM: Semi-quantitive analysis of cytokins in inflammatory demyelinative lesions in X-linked adrenoleukodystrophy and multiple sclerosis. *Am J Hum Genet* 57 (suppl): A339, 1995.

230. Ligtenberg MJ, Kemp S, Sarde CO, et al.: Spectrum of mutations in the gene encoding the adrenoleukodystrophy protein. *Am J Hum Genet* 56: 44–50, 1995.

231. Wakefield MA, Brown RS: X-linked congenital Addison's disease. *Arch Dis Child* 56: 73–74, 1981.

232. Penman RW: Addison's disease in association with spastic paraplegia. *Br Med J* 1: 402, 1960.

233. Salen G, Tint S, Shefer S: Increased cerebrospinal fluid cholestanol and apolipoprotein B concentrations in CTX. Effect of chenodeoxycholic acid. *Abstract IX, International Bile Acid Meeting, Basel,* p. 59, 1986.

234. Wevers RA, Cruysberg JR, Van Heijst AF, et al.: Paediatric cerebrotendinous xanthomatosis. *J Inherit Metab Dis* 15: 374–376, 1992.

235. Meiner V, Meiner Z, Reshef A, et al.: Cerebrotendinous xanthomatosis: molecular diagnosis enables presymptomatic detection of a treatable disease. *Neurology* 44: 288–290, 1994.

236. Van Bogaert L, Scherer HJ, Epstein E: *Une forme cérébrale de la cholestérinose généralisée.* Masson, Paris, 1937.

237. Berginer VM, Salen G, Shefer S: Long-term treatment of cerebrotendinous xanthomatosis with chenodeoxycholic acid. *New Engl J Med* 311: 1649–1652, 1984.

238. Mondelli M, Rossi A, Scarpini C, et al.: Evoked potentials in cerebrotendinous xanthomatosis and effect induced by chenodeoxycholic acid. *Arch Neurol* 49: 469–475, 1992.

239. Dorfman LJ, Pedley TH, Tharp BR, et al.: Juvenile neuroaxonal dystrophy. Clinical electrophysiological and neuropathologic features. *Ann Neurol* 3: 419–428, 1978.

240. Thibault J: Neuroaxonal dystrophy. A case of nonpigmented type and protracted course. *Acta Neuropathol* 21: 232–238, 1972.

241. Vuia O: Neuroaxonal dystrophy, juvenile adult form. *Clin Neurol Neurosurg* 79: 307–315, 1977.

242. Scheithauer BW, Forno LS, Dorfman LJ, et al.: Neuroaxonal dystrophy (Seitelberger's disease) with late onset, protracted course and myoclonic epilepsy. *J Neurol Sci* 36: 247–258, 1978.

243. Schwendeman G, Arendt G, Noth J, et al.: Diagnosis of juvenile adult form of neuro-axonal dystrophy with electron microscopy of rectum and skin biopsy. *J Neurol Neurosurg Psych* 50: 818–821, 1987.

244. Haltia M, Somer H, Palo J, et al.: Neuronal intranuclear inclusions disease in identical twins. *Ann Neurol* 15: 316–321, 1984.

245. Sloane AE, Becker LE, Ang LC, et al.: Neuronal intranuclear hyaline inclusion disease with progressive cerebellar ataxia. *Pediatr Neurol* 10: 61–66, 1994.

246. Goutieres F, Mikol J, Aicardi J: Neuronal intranuclear inclusion disease in a child. Diagnosis by rectal biopsy. *Ann Neurol* 27: 103–106, 1990.

247. Shoffner JM, Lott MT, Wallace DC: MERRF: a model disease for understanding the principles of mitochondrial genetics. *Rev Neurol* 147: 431–435, 1991.

248. De Vivo DC: The expanding spectrum of mitochondrial disease. *Brain Develop* 15: 1–22, 1993.

249. Rowland LP, Blake DM, Hirano S, et al.: Clinical syndromes associated with ragged red fibers. *Rev Neurol* 147: 467–473, 1991.

250. Poulton J, Holt IJ: Mitochondrial DNA. Does more lead to less? *Nature Genet* 8: 313–315, 1994.

251. Hirano M, Pavlakis SG: Mitochondrial myopathy, encephalopathy, lactic acidosis and strokelike episodes (MELAS): current concepts. *J Child Neurol* 9: 4–13, 1994.

252. Kishi M, Yoshinori Y, Kurihara T, et al.: An autopsy case of mitochondrial encephalopathy: biochemical and electron microscopy study of the brain. *J Neurol Sci* 86: 31–40, 1988.

253. Zupanc ML, Moraes CT, Shanske S, et al.: Deletion on mitochondrial DNA in patients with combined features of Kearns-Sayre and MELAS syndromes. *Ann Neurol* 29: 680–683, 1991.

254. So N, Berkovic S, Andermann F: Myoclonus epilepsy and ragged-red fibres (MERRF): electrophysiological studies and comparison with other progressive myoclonus epilepsies. *Brain* 112: 1261–1276, 1989.

254a. Silvestri G, Ciafaloni E, Santorelli FM, et al.: Clinical features associated with the A→G transition at nucleotide 8344 of mtDNA (MERRF mutation). *Neurology* 43: 1200–1206, 1993.

255. Holt JJ, Hardiny AE, Petty RK, et al.: A new mitochondrial disease associated with mitochondrial DNA heteroplasmy. *Am J Hum Genet* 46: 428–433, 1990.

256. Obermaier-Kusser B, Lorenz B, Schubring S, et al.: Features of mtDNA mutation patterns in European pedigrees and sporadic cases with Leber hereditary optic neuropathy. *Am J Hum Genet* 55: 1063–1066, 1994.

256a. Prötig A, Cormier V, Chatelain P, et al.: Deletion of mitochondrial DNA in a case of early-onset diabetes mellitus, optic atrophy and deafness. *J Inherit Metab Dis* 16: 527–530, 1993.

257. Servidei S, Zeviani M, Manfredi G, et al.: Dominantly inherited mitochondrial myopathy with multiple deletions of mitochondrial DNA. Clinical, morphologic and biochemical studies. *Neurology* 41: 1053–1059, 1991.

258. Suomalainen A, Kaukonen J, Amati P, et al.: An autosomal locus predisposing to deletions of mitochondrial DNA. *Nature Genet* 9: 146–149, 1995.

259. Moraes CT, Shanske S, Trischler HJ, et al.: mtDNA depletion with variable tissue expression: a novel genetic abnormality in mitochondrial diseases. *Am J Hum Genet* 48: 492–501, 1991.

260. Sege-Peterson K, Nyhan WL, Page T: Lesch-Nyhan disease and HPRT deficiency, in Rosenberg RN, Prusiner SB, Di Mauro S, Barchi RL, Kunkel LM (eds): *The Molecular and Genetic Basis of Neurological Disease.* Boston, Butterworth-Heinemann, 1993, pp. 241–259.

261. Gottlieb RP, Koppel MM, Nyhan WL, et al.: Hyperuricemia and choreoathetosis in a child without

262. Emmerson BT, Wyngaarden JB: Purine metabolism in heterozygous carriers of hypoxanthine-guanine phosphoribosyltransferase deficiency. *Science* 166: 1533–1535, 1969.

263. Ogasawara N, Stout JT, Goto H, et al.: Molecular analysis of a female Lesch-Nyhan patient. *J Clin Invest* 84: 1024–1027, 1989.

264. Bazelon M, Stevens H, Davis M, et al.: Mental retardation, self-mutilation and hyperuricemia in females. *Trans Am Neurol Assoc* 93: 187–188, 1968.

265. Watts RWE, Spellacy E, Gibbs DA, et al.: Clinical, postmortem, biochemical and therapeutic observations on the Lesch-Nyhan syndrome with special reference to the neurologic manifestations. *Q J Med* 51: 43–78, 1982.

266. Jaeken J, Van Den Berghe G: An infantile autistic syndrome characterized by the presence of succinyl purines in body fluids. *Lancet* 2: 1058–1061, 1984.

267. Maddocks J, Reed T: Urine test for adenylsuccinase deficiency in autistic children. *Lancet* 1: 158–159, 1989.

268. Stone RL, Aimi J, Barshop BA, et al.: A mutation in adenylosuccinate lyase associated with mental retardation and autistic features. *Nature Genet* 1: 59–62, 1992.

269. Nance MA, Berry SA: Cockayne syndrome: review of 140 cases. *Am J Med Genet* 42: 68–84, 1992.

270. Lehman AR, Francis A, Gianelli F: Prenatal diagnosis of Cockayne syndrome. *Lancet* 1: 486–488, 1985.

271. Troelstra C, Hesen W, Bootsma D, et al.: Structure and expression of the excision repair gene *ERCC6* involved in the human disorder Cockayne syndrome group B. *Nucleic Acid Mes* 21: 419–426, 1993.

272. Ohnishi A, Mitsudome A, Murai Y: Primary segmental demyelination in the sural nerve in Cockayne's syndrome. *Muscle and Nerve* 10: 163–167, 1987.

273. Susaki K, Tachi N, Shinada M, et al.: Demyelinating peripheral neuropathy in Cockayne syndrome: a histopathologic and morphometric study. *Brain Develop* 14: 114–117, 1992.

274. Moossy J: The neuropathology of Cockayne's syndrome. *J Neuropathol Exptl Neurol* 26: 654–660, 1967.

275. Lyon G, Robain O, Philippart M, et al.: Leucodystrophie avec calcifications strio-cérébelleuses, microcéphalie et nanisme. *Rev Neurol* 119: 197–210, 1968.

276. Patton MA, Gianelli F, Baraister M, et al.: Early onset Cockayne's syndrome: case reports with neuropathological and fibroblast studies. *J Med Genet* 26: 154–159, 1989.

277. Jaeken J, Klocker H, Schwaiger H, et al.: Clinical and biochemical studies in three patients with severe early infantile Cockayne syndrome. *Hum Gen* 83: 339–346, 1989.

278. Kennedy RM, Rowe W, Kepes J: Cockayne syndrome: an atypical case. *Neurology* 30: 1268–1272, 1980.

279. Greenshaw GA, Hebert A, Duke-Woodside ME, et al.: Xeroderma pigmentosum and Cockayne syndrome:

mental retardation or self-mutilation. A new HPRT variant. *J Inherit Metab Dis* 5: 183–186, 1982.

overlapping clinical and biochemical phenotypes. *Am J Hum Genet* 50: 677–689, 1992.

279a. Roytta M, Anttinen A: Xeroderma pigmentosum with neurological abnormalities. *Acta Neurol Sci* 73: 191–199, 1986.

280. Cleaver JE, Kramer KH: Xeroderma pigmentosum and Cockayne syndrome, in Scriver CR, Beaudet AL, Sly WS, Valle D (eds): *The Metabolic and Molecular Bases of Inherited Disease.* New York, McGraw-Hill, 1995, pp. 4393–4419.

281. Mudd SH, Skovby F, Levy HL, et al.: The natural history of homocystinuria due to cystathionine β-synthase deficiency. *Am J Hum Genet* 37: 1–31, 1985.

282. McKusic VA, Hall JG, Char F: The clinical and genetic characteristics of homocystinuria, in Carson NA, Raine DN (eds): *Inherited Disorders of Sulphur Metabolism.* London, Livingstone, 1971, pp. 179–203.

283. Mudd SH, Levy HC, Skovby F: Disorders of transsulfuration, in Scriver CR, Beaudet AL, Sly WS, Valle D (eds): *The Metabolic and Molecular Bases of Inherited Disease.* New York, McGraw-Hill, 1995, pp. 1279–1327.

283a. Levy HC: Personal communication, 1995.

284. Kraus JP: Molecular basis of phenotype expression in homocystinuria. *J Inherit Metab Dis* 17: 383–390, 1994.

285. Boers GHJ, Smals AGH, Trijbels FJM, et al.: Heterozygosity for homocystinuria in premature peripheral and cerebral occlusive arterial disease. *New Engl J Med* 313: 709–715, 1985.

286. Clarke R, Daly L, Mohinson K: Hyperhomocysteinemia, an independent risk factor for vascular disease. *New Engl J Med* 324: 1149–1155, 1991.

287. Wilcken B, Yu JS, Brown DA: Natural history of Hartnup disease. *Arch Dis Child* 52: 38–40, 1977.

288. Scriver CR, Mahon B, Levy HL, et al.: The Hartnup phenotype: Mendelian transport disorder, multifactorial disease. *Am J Hum Genet* 40: 401, 1987.

289. Levy HL: Hartnup disease, in Scriver CR, Beaudet AL, Sly WS, Valle D (eds): *The Metabolic and Molecular Bases of Inherited Disease.* New York, McGraw-Hill, 1995, p. 3639.

290. Freundlich E, Statter M, Yatziv S: Familial pellagra-like skin rash with neurologic manifestations. *Arch Dis Child* 56: 146–151, 1981.

291. Fenton DA, Wilkinson JD, Tascland PA: Family exhibiting cerebellar-like ataxia, photosensitivity and short stature. A new inborn error of tryptophan metabolism. *J R Soc Med* 76: 736, 1983.

Chapter 6

DISTINCTION BETWEEN HEREDITARY METABOLIC DISEASES AND OTHER DISEASES OF THE CHILD'S NERVOUS SYSTEM

DIFFERENTIAL DIAGNOSIS OF GENETIC NEUROMETABOLIC DISEASES IN THE NEONATAL PERIOD
    Perinatal Hypoxia and Circulatory Insufficiency: Hypoxic-Ischemic Encephalopathy of the Newborn
    Intracranial Hemorrhage
    Kernicterus
    Prenatal Encephalitis; Neonatal Bacterial Meningitis
    Prenatal Developmental Abnormalities of the Brain
    Other Neonatal Conditions

DIFFERENTIATION OF HEREDITARY METABOLIC DISEASES FROM STATIC ENCEPHALOPATHIES AND DEVELOPMENTAL ABNORMALITIES IN INFANCY AND EARLY CHILDHOOD
    Cerebral Palsies and their Differentiation from HMDs
    Prenatal Developmental Brain Defects
    Psychomotor Retardation, Developmental Delay, Mental Retardation
    Behavioral Syndromes: Autism and Rett Syndrome

DIFFERENTIAL DIAGNOSIS OF NEUROLOGIC SYNDROMES ENCOUNTERED IN THE HEREDITARY METABOLIC AND DEGENERATIVE ENCEPHALOPATHIES OF CHILDHOOD AND ADOLESCENCE
    Ataxias
    Basal Ganglia Disorders
    Spastic Paraplegia
    Hemiplegias
    Epilepsy
    Differential Diagnostic of Action Myoclonus (Polymyoclonus)

PRINCIPAL FEATURES AND DIFFERENTIAL DIAGNOSIS OF HEREDITARY METABOLIC AND DEGENERATIVE NEUROPATHIES
    Sensorimotor Neuropathies
    Lower Motor Neuronopathies in HMDs
    Involvement of Cranial Nerves in HMDs

OCULAR ABNORMALITIES
    Visual Failure
    Derangement of Ocular Movements
    Characteristic Morphological Changes of the Eyes

DEAFNESS

One of the most exacting tests of clinical skill in neuropediatrics is the distinction of the comparatively rare hereditary metabolic diseases from the many nonmetabolic diseases and developmental anomalies to which the child's nervous system is subject. The task is not an easy one. There are so many variants of the known hereditary metabolic and degenerative diseases which do not conform precisely to their common prototype that one is often left in a quandary. In clinics devoted to the diagnosis and treatment of developmental disorders and metabolic diseases, fully a third of the patients prove, after detailed study, to have an unidentifiable disease.

In this chapter, we endeavor to share with the reader a distillate of our own clinical experiences with the main neurologic syndromes of childhood and adolescence, particularly with respect to the neonatal encephalopathies, cerebral palsies, states of mental retardation, states of cognitive and behavioral disturbances, and special neurologic syndromes such as ataxias, basal ganglia disorders, spastic paraplegia, hemiplegias, the epilepsies, polymyoclonus, peripheral nerve diseases, ocular abnormalities, and deafness.

In this didactic exposition, we have tried to extract practical rules of differential diagnoses that have been helpful and to draw attention to some of the pitfalls we have encountered. We have also given a brief description of the semiology and pathophysiology of the main symptoms and signs by which the diseases express themselves, as we believe that this information is always necessary for the proper interpretation of their significance.

DIFFERENTIAL DIAGNOSIS OF GENETIC NEUROMETABOLIC DISEASES IN THE NEONATAL PERIOD

Perinatal Hypoxia and Circulatory Insufficiency: Hypoxic-Ischemic Encephalopathy of the Newborn

Hypoxia and reduction of cerebral blood flow in the newborn may accompany a number of pathologic events: intrauterine asphyxia (caused by alteration of fetomaternal circulation and gas exchange); intrauterine hemorrhage; intrapartum complications such as traumatic, difficult, or prolonged labor, premature separation of placenta, or cord prolapse; asphyxia and circulatory failure at birth, as a consequence of congenital cardiopathies, apneic spells, and severe pulmonary disease, mostly in the premature baby. At least 20 percent of newborns with a hypoxic-ischemic encephalopathy have suffered from intrauterine asphyxia, which evokes changes in fetal activity and in cardiac function (slowing of the cardiac rate and irregularities of rhythm). Early detection of these signs by electronic monitoring and determination of acid-base balance and P_{O_2} from samples of fetal scalp blood should help in the recognition of impending hypoxic and ischemic injury and lead to the initiation of protective measures.

At birth and during the first 24 hours, the newborn, who has been injured by pre- or perinatal asphyxia and circulatory failure, is stuporous or comatose, markedly hypotonic with no spontaneous motility. There is an enfeeblement of all motor automatisms, including sucking and swallowing. Irregular or periodic breathing are frequent. Seizures occur in the majority of patients. Apneic spells and jitteriness usually appear after the 12th hour of life.[1] Later the infant becomes hypertonic. Eye movements may be disconjugate but pupillary responses are usually preserved. Fixed, dilated pupils

and the abolition of the doll's eye reaction occur if there is dysfunction of the neuraxis at the brain stem level and always presage an unfavorable prognosis. On ultrasound scans, characteristic echodensities in the periventricular white matter or in the basal ganglia, and possibly small hemorrhagic areas in the white matter, are usually demonstrable. Acidosis, hypoxemia and hypercarbia corroborate the clinical diagnosis. Occasionally there is hypoglycemia, hypocalcemia, and even transient hyperammonemia. If death does not occur in the first days of life, by the end of the first week the child's condition begins to improve. Some children recover completely. The more severely injured later develop diplegia, athetosis, quadriplegia, seizures, and various degrees of mental deficit.

To sum up, the important differences between a hereditary metabolic disorder and brain anoxia-ischemia in the newborn are as follows:

1. *In favor of a perinatal anoxic-ischemic encephalopathy* Evidence of intrauterine asphyxia; meconium-stained amniotic fluid, a stigmata of perinatal hypoxia; abnormalities of labor and delivery; prematurity; a maternal disorder that might impair fetomaternal circulation and transplacental gas exchanges (arterial hypertension, preeclampsia, toxemia gravidis, diabetes); twinning; the immediate appearance of neurologic signs after birth; and characteristic abnormalities on ultrasound brain scans.

2. *Findings supporting the diagnosis of an HMD* Findings include an uneventful pregnancy and the normal birth of a full-term infant (rarely, infants are born 2 or 3 weeks before term, and there may be intrauterine growth retardation); a free interval between birth and onset of the disease; certain types of facial dysmorphism (especially in lysosomol, mitochondrial and peroxisomal diseases); a peculiar odor of the urine; an enlarged liver; the presence of a cardiomyopathy; skeletal abnormalities or renal dysplasias; history of a familial disease; and characteristic biochemical abnormalities (see Chap. 2).

Intracranial Hemorrhage

Among the different types of intracranial hemorrhage, periventricular (matrix) hemorrhages with bleeding in the lateral ventricles and in the cerebral white matter are a very common cause of neonatal neurologic distress in the prematurely born infant. Intracerebral bleeding may also occur in association with periventricular leukomalacia. Occasionally a disorder of coagulation is the cause. Intracerebellar hemorrhage is a rare but serious condition in the premature infant. In cases of acute hydrocephalus and large intracerebral hemorrhages, the neurologic status deteriorates rapidly. Stupor or coma, hypotonia, decerebrate posturing, and respiratory abnormalities are usual manifestations. Intraventricular and intraparenchymal bleeding are readily demonstrated by ultrasound and demand urgent intercession. Chronic hydrocephalus, cerebral palsies, and developmental delay are frequent in survivors.

Kernicterus

High blood levels of unconjugated bilirubin—related to Rh or ABO blood incompatibility or to other causes—are toxic to the neonatal brain, both in children born at term and in prematures. Bilirubin anions cause neuronal injury in specific areas of the brain, particularly in the globus pallidus, certain thalamic nuclei, the subthalamic nucleus, substantia nigra, hippocampus, hypothalamus, VIIIth cranial nerve nuclei, inferior olives, and the dentate nuclei. The encephalopathy induced by bilirubin is referred to as kernicterus. (*Kern* is German for nucleus; some nuclear structures are colored yellow.)

Most infants with kernicterus develop, within 2 to 3 days postnatally, breathing difficulty, hypotonia, diminished responsivity, and poor sucking. After a few days, retrocollis and opisthotonus appear. Seizures are rare. There may be bouts of unexplained fever. Anoxia, hypercarbia, acidosis, and infections may complicate and aggravate bilirubin encephalopathy and may terminate the illness. In surviving infants, later sequelae may not be evident before the second year of life. They consist essentially in choreoathetosis, paralysis of vertical gaze, and deafness. Diagnosis of bilirubin encephalopathy or of children in danger of developing kernicterus is not difficult when blood concentrations of free bilirubin are very high. If not, identification of infants at risk may be difficult. Relatively low levels of bilirubin can result in kernicterus in prematures. Prevention of hemolytic disease in the newborn by various methods, including administration of anti-Rh immunoglobulins to prevent maternal sensitization in case of Rh incompatibility; intrauterine blood transfusion and exchange-transfusion or phototherapy in the treatment of hyperbilirubinemia in the neonate, have considerably diminished but not eradicated kernicterus in countries with well-developed medical facilities.

Prenatal Encephalitis; Neonatal Bacterial Meningitis

Cytomegalovirus (CMV), *rubella virus* and *toxoplasma* cross the placental barrier, invade the fetal organism, and produce lesions of the brain manifested at birth by lethargy, hypotonia, seizures, microcephaly, or hydrocephaly (in toxoplasmosis), chorioretinitis and other ocular abnormalities. Diagnosis is aided by finding pleiocytosis in the CSF and possibly brain calcifications in CT scans. Jaundice, hepatomegaly and purpura are other common features. The risk of fetal infection can be predicted by the systematic measurement of the antibodies against these infectious agents in the pregnant mother, and proof of the infection is obtained by examination of fetal blood samples and amniotic fluid in cases of toxoplasmosis and CMV infections. Transplacental infection of the fetal brain by the *varicella virus* is very rare, but it gives rise to a dramatic and distinctive syndrome with cutaneous scars, limb abnormalities, and severe neurologic deficits. Congenital infections by the spirochete of *syphilis* and the *human immunodeficiency virus (HIV)* usually do not produce clinical manifestations in the newborn. (Syphilis may cause stillbirth.) Neonatal infection by the *herpes virus* is nearly always acquired from the mother at the time of birth. Neurologic and other symptoms are seldom manifest before the end of the first week of life.

Neonatal *bacterial meningitis* may present with a clinical picture similar to that of the metabolic encephalopathies and is only reliably diagnosed by examination of the CSF, a procedure which should be carried out in every neonate with an obscure neurologic problem.

To be noted is the fact that any febrile neonatal infection may trigger the decompensation of an underlying metabolic disorder.

Prenatal Developmental Abnormalities of the Brain

Prenatal developmental defects of the central nervous system are numerous and still imperfectly classified and understood. Affected infants may present with evident abnormalities at birth, such as microcephaly, hydrocephalus or gross deformities of the face, eyes, limbs, and genitourinary tract. However, brain malformations cannot be anticipated on clinical grounds alone and their neurological expression, such as seizures and developmental delay, is nonspecific and may not be obvious in the first weeks of life. Most of them are now recognizable in MRI scans.

In the presence of developmental brain defects, the possibility of a metabolic disorder is remote and other, mostly genetic, abnormalities take priority. However, not to be overlooked are a few metabolic disorders, such as mitochondrial disorders, peroxisomal diseases, and aminoacidopathies, or the defect of cholesterol biosynthesis demonstrated in the Smith-Lemli-Opitz syndrome (Table 6.1).

Other Neonatal Conditions

These essentially include hypoglycemia, hypocalcemia, passive drug addiction, and the complications of respiratory distress. All may be the cause of postnatal seizures, stupor, irritability, hypotonia, and respiratory irregularities.

Transient hypoglycemia of the neonate (a much more common condition than the severe recurrent hypoglycemia of metabolic and endocrine disorders) is frequent in prematures, in infants who are small for gestational age, in children born to diabetic mothers, and in neonates with a hypoxic-ischemic encephalopathy or intracranial hemorrhage.

Hypocalcemia may cause neurologic signs in the newborn. It is most likely to develop towards the end of the first postnatal week and is expressed by jitteriness and seizures. The condition is relatively benign and responds to calcium medication.

Intoxication with local anesthetics results in a characteristic picture of bradycardia, hypotonia, apnea, tonic seizures, dilated pupils, and inhibition of the normal passive oculocephalic (doll's eye) maneuver.[1] The symptoms disappear in a few days.

Passive drug addiction of the newborn has become a frequent situation. The drug withdrawal syndromes in neonates born to mothers addicted to heroin, methadone, or cocaine are similar but not quite identical. In heroin addiction, the infant is very alert and hyperactive with stimulus-sensitive rhythmic tremors, frantic sucking and decreased sleep. Sweating, sneezing, tachypnea, and fever may be observed. Seizures are rare. The withdrawal syndrome of methadone addiction is similar, but seizures are probably more frequent. In children

Table 6-1

Prenatal developmental defects (and encephaloclastic lesions) of the brain in the hereditary neurometabolic diseases

Diseases	Type of defect
Zellweger disease	Constant characteristic disorder of cortical neuronal migration and dysplasia of inferior olives
Peroxisomal disorders with the Zellweger phenotype	Similar abnormalities, less constant, more limited
Pyruvate dehydrogenase (E_1) deficiency in boys and heterozygote girls	Heterotopias of inferior olives, periventricular heterotopias, fragmentation of dentate nucleus
	Defect of the corpus callosum (agenesis or extreme atrophy) absence of bulbar pyramids
	Widespread atrophy of the cerebral hemispheres. Cystic necrosis of white matter and basal ganglia.
Pyruvate carboxylase deficiency	Cystic necrosis of white matter; thin corpus callosum
Glutaric aciduria II	Cortical dysplasia; disorder of neuronal migration?
Nonketotic hyperglycinemia	"Agenesis" of the corpus callosum; cortical dysplasia
Molybdenum cofactor deficiency (sulfite oxidase deficiency)	Multicystic necrosis of white matter
3-Hydroxyisobutyric acidemia	Pachygyria; abnormalities of migration? "Agenesis" of the corpus callosum.
	Frontal and subependymal calcifications
3-Hydroxybutyryl-CoA deacylase deficiency	"Agenesis" of the corpus callosum and gyrus cingulus
Smith-Lemli-Opitz syndrome	Defects in the cerebellum and cerebral hemispheres
Carnitine palmitoyltransferase II deficiency	Cortical dysplasia
Maternal PKU (untreated)	Multiple cerebral anomalies

born to mothers addicted to cocaine, jitteriness is usually not present; brain malformations, congenital heart disease, abruptio placentae, and stillbirth have been reported.

In the *respiratory distress syndrome* in prematures and in other pulmonary disorders of the neonate, the infant may become unresponsive and hypotonic, and there may be seizures. P_{O_2} is low and P_{CO_2} elevated, but not when hyperventilation occurs in relation to metabolic acidosis or other mechanisms in the organo-acidopathies, mitochondrial disorders, and other HMDs.

Abnormal respiratory rhythms can also be observed in two rare syndromes, the congenital hypoventilation syndrome and Joubert syndrome. The congenital central hypoventilation syndrome (Ondine curse) is due to a decreased ventilatory drive, essentially during REM sleep, resulting in hypoventilation, periodic apnea, hypoxemia, and hypercarbia. Joubert syndrome is characterized by an extremely rapid panting respiration present at birth (more than 100 respirations per minute) and apneic pauses without modifications of the acid-base equilibrium. Abnormal eye movements are also present. There is an absence of the cerebellar vermis occasionally associated with an occipital ventriculocele. In surviving children, mental retardation and ataxia are usual.

In *Steinert myotonic dystrophy*, hypotonia, respiratory difficulties, and swallowing impairment may be striking. Diagnosis is based on a characteristic facial appearance, arthrogryposis, the presence of signs of the disease in the mother, and the EMG.

In the few cases of Werdnig-Hoffman disease with severe hypokinesia and respiratory insufficiency at birth, the mental state is normal. Some congenital myopathies are associated with malformation of the cerebral cortex and evidence of mental dysfunctions in the neonate.

DIFFERENTIATION OF HEREDITARY METABOLIC DISEASES FROM STATIC ENCEPHALOPATHIES AND DEVELOPMENTAL ABNORMALITIES IN INFANCY AND EARLY CHILDHOOD

Distinction between the progressive hereditary metabolic and degenerative brain disorders and static, acquired, or genetic encephalopathies of pre- or perinatal origin at later ages must be finely drawn for several reasons: (1) information about prenatal events is often lacking; (2) the clinical expressions of all types of brain damage tend to have been similar and unvaried in the neonate and young infant; (3) the neurologic consequences of fixed congenital lesions may be delayed for several months because of the immaturity of the nervous system; (4) some HMDs progress so slowly, at least during the initial phase of the disease, that marks of their clinical syndromes are occult and may be mistaken for cerebral palsies or simple psychomotor retardation.

Some of the problems in differential diagnosis between HMDs and fixed congenital encephalopathies are described under the following headings:

- Cerebral palsies
- Prenatal developmental brain disorders
- Psychomotor retardation
- Behavioral disorders

Cerebral Palsies and their Differentiation from HMDs

Brain damage acquired in the perinatal period and during the last weeks of pregnancy almost invariably results in various types of motor abnormalities. These are traditionally referred to as cerebral palsies.

Etiology and Pathogenesis According to the current terminology, the several clinical subtypes of cerebral palsy are spastic diplegia, congenital hemiplegia, dyskinetic (dystonic) cerebral palsy, tetraplegia, ataxic diplegia, and ataxic cerebral palsy (nonprogressive congenital cerebellar ataxia). Since the nineteenth century, the cerebral palsies were believed to result from "birth injury" in which anoxia and mechanical factors played a major role. Recent epidemiological studies, modern methods of neonatal and prenatal brain imaging, and neuropathological studies have provided new perspectives concerning the risk factors and mechanisms of brain lesions.

It has been shown that perinatal asphyxia (i.e., anoxia, hypercarbia, acidosis, and other metabolic changes) is found in only about 20 percent of children with cerebral palsy[2] when strict criteria are used. Twinning occurs in 10 percent of cases. Prematurity is statistically the most important risk factor. Even more remarkable has been the observation that pregnancy and birth are normal, in a substantial proportion of cases. Approximately 70 percent of congenital hemiplegias, 30 percent of spastic diplegias, 20 percent of dyskinetic cerebral palsies, many cases of ataxic diplegia, and practically all patients with congenital nonprogressive cerebellar ataxia have had a normal birth and perinatal period. Even when prematurity, asphyxia, or gemellarity have occurred, the brain lesions are not rarely of an age that indicates they happened some time before birth. This has also been amply confirmed by prenatal and neonatal ultrasonography and MRI. Therefore, in the differential diagnosis with HMD, an uneventful pregnancy and neonatal period cannot be held as a sufficient argument against cerebral palsy. While many cerebral palsies result from ischemic, anoxic, or hemorrhagic insults, genetic factors (particularly in congenital, non-progressive cerebellar ataxia), progressive hydrocephalus (in ataxic diplegia), prenatal infections, and developmental disorders also figure importantly. Kernicterus, once a common cause of choreoathetosis, deafness, and supranuclear oculomotor palsy, has almost been eliminated in developed countries.

Much remains to be learned about the *causes and mechanisms of pre- or perinatal disturbances of cerebral circulation* leading to these cerebral palsies. When severe asphyxia is present, anoxemia reduces systemic blood pressure and impairs the normal regulatory mechanisms of cerebral blood flow. When the cerebral blood flow falls below a certain level, ischemia occurs. Oxygen deprivation is believed to promote the accumulation of excitotoxic amino acids, which contribute to neuronal death. In prematures, even without notable asphyxia, the lability of arterial pressure, the pressure-passive cerebral blood flow, and the limited vasodilatory response to hypercarbia are thought to be important factors in the production of cerebral ischemia and hemorrhagic infarcts. Other mechanisms of ischemic or hemorrhagic lesions include fetofetal or fetomaternal transfusion, arterial occlusions by emboli or thrombosis and spontaneous, usually unilateral, hemispheric hematoma due to disorders of coagulation. The cause of ischemic brain necrosis in the *fetus* is frequently obscure. It may be induced by CMV infection in some cases.

Other mechanisms have been put forward to explain periventricular matrix hemorrhage.[1]

Notable also is the topography of the principal lesional patterns, which allows one properly to interpret radiological data. A generalized reduction of the cerebral blood flow below a critical level results in bilateral ischemic or hemorrhagic infarcts at sites of maximum vulnerability. These differ in prematures and term infants. In term infants, the zones of gray matter predominantly affected are the arterial borders between the territories of the middle and anterior cerebral arteries, producing bilateral parasagittal infarcts that cause spastic diplegia. Also, there is neuron loss, gliosis, and aberrant myelination in the basal ganglia, especially the

striatum (leading to status marmoratus) which may be the basis of dyskinetic cerebral palsy. In the premature, the ischemic lesions involve paraventricular hemispheric white matter (possibly because the cerebral blood flow is significantly lower in these areas in the premature or because of the abundance of meningeal and cortical anastomoses and the immaturity of cortical neurons at this age). By far the most frequent lesion is periventricular leukomalacia, an acknowledged cause of spastic diplegia. More diffuse multicystic leukomalacia usually results in tetraplegia. Unilateral cerebral lesions with hemiplegia are produced by occlusion of the middle cerebral artery, by spontaneous intracerebral hematoma, or more rarely by asymmetric periventricular leukomalacia.

Detection of these lesions on neuroimaging is an important element in the diagnosis of cerebral palsies and, when observed in the neonate, the subsequent occurrence of motor dysfunctions and other neurologic abnormalities can be predicted. However, in our experience, clinicopathologic correlations are often imprecise. In some patients with congenital hemiplegia, spastic diplegia, or dyskinesia, abnormalities in brain scanning are minimal and not explanatory; other radiologic features may be difficult to interpret. Periventricular leukomalacia can result in widespread resorption of the white matter, thus producing an "ex vacuo" enlargement of the lateral ventricles which may be difficult to differentiate from an incipient or stable hydrocephalus or from diffuse brain atrophy of which hereditary metabolic diseases may be a cause. Also, certain HMDs, such as sulfite oxidase deficiency, pyruvate dehydrogenase deficiency, and pyruvate carboxylase deficiency, which give rise to late fetal or neonatal destructive lesions of the white matter and basal ganglia, are difficult or impossible to distinguish from the much more frequent ischemic encephalopathies.

Clinical Features: The Progressive Emergence of the Neurologic Deficit
Motor disturbances which result from fixed peri- or prenatal brain damage cannot generally be detected by clinical examination at birth. Instead, they emerge progressively at a later age, after a *free interval*. The delayed appearance and gradual progression of cerebral palsies over a limited period of time is a function of normal brain maturation, not of progression of brain lesions. The free interval between the occurrence of a congenital brain lesion involving the motor system and its clinical expression in an infant is a cardinal characteristic of cerebral palsy. The mechanism of its relationship to brain maturation remains obscure. In our experience, the length of the free interval

is approximately 2 months in spastic diplegia, 4 to 6 months in congenital hemiplegia, 8 to 10 months in choreoathetosis, and 10 to 12 months for cerebellar incoordination.

During this period of latency, changes in muscle tone (hypotonia) and certain abnormal reactions to motor testing may be present, but specific motor deficits in relation to recognized brain damage are not discernible. The link between maturation of brain function and neurologic signs is particularly clear in congenital hemiplegia: weakness and spasticity first appear in the upper limb at 5 months, when voluntary prehension is being acquired, and become evident in the lower limb when the child starts to walk. Somatagnosia of the upper limb is not observed until age 18 months.

Although cerebral palsies in older children show a tendency to improve, especially when correctly managed, late additions to their symptomatology are possible. As time passes, sometimes even after several years, choreoathetosis and dystonic postures may appear or increase in congenital hemiplegia or become increasingly evident in the upper limbs of children affected with spastic diplegia. In rare instances, aggravation of a congenital hemiplegia is the result of a progressive expanding porencephaly, a condition caused by the diverticulation of one lateral ventricle following a periventricular destructive lesion.[3] After many years some children with choreoathetosis experience what is usually a transitory worsening of their motor handicap during infections, as a result of drug therapy (e.g., phenytoin) or for obscure reasons. We have also observed adolescents with mental retardation and a moderate spastic diplegia, apparently due to perinatal brain damage, who suddenly become incapable of walking, lose interest in their surroundings, and lose their capacity to speak and communicate. The possibility of an HMD was considered, but not confirmed. The mechanisms underlying these late changes in the symptomatology of a fixed congenital encephalopathy are indeterminate. They could possibly be the consequence of secondary neuronal degenerations, the progressive building of aberrant interneuronal connections, prolonged seizures, the effect of certain medications, or depression.

Differential Diagnosis of Cerebral Palsies   Cerebral palsies are easily recognized when anamnestic, clinical, and radiological features are typical. Problems in differential diagnosis from hereditary metabolic disorders may arise in children whose birth and pregnancy have been normal and in the milder forms of cerebral palsy. Minor forms of hemiplegic cerebral palsy often remain unsuspected for several years, and when discovered, the motor deficit may appear to be recent. In these cases, the existence of fine motor difficulties of the affected side since infancy, a relative hypoplasia of the affected hand (especially evident when the nails are examined), and typical neuroradiological abnormalities will attest to the congenital origin of the paresis.

Chronic forms of progressive paraplegias, due to hereditary metabolic or degenerative disorders (such as metachromatic or globoid cell leukodystrophy and the childhood form of familial spastic paraplegia), can be mistaken in late infancy for mild forms of congenital spastic diplegia, in which the bipyramidal syndrome only becomes evident at the end of the first year of life. One should be particularly cautious in making the diagnosis of congenital cerebral diplegia in the absence of prematurity (and other known pre- and perinatal abnormalities) and of typical lesions on MRI.

In a number of HMDs, *dysarthria* constitutes an early indication of a progressive encephalopathy. An isolated dysarthria can also be related to a congenital pseudobulbar syndrome due to the dysfunction of the corticobulbar tracts. A remarkable variety is the biopercular syndrome of Foix-Thevenard and Chavany which is produced by pre- or perinatal lesions of the lower perisylvian parts of the motor cortex. There are also other nonprogressive *faciobuccopharyngeal dyspraxias*, of more obscure origin.

The differential diagnosis between congenital nonprogressive cerebellar ataxias and the hereditary metabolic disorders with early-onset cerebellar ataxia is discussed further on.

Unexplained late changes and symptomatic modifications of cerebral palsies occasionally raise the question of a hereditary metabolic disorder.

The differential diagnosis of dyskinetic cerebral palsy in infants may be difficult when a slowly emerging dystonia has been due to Pelizaeus-Merzbacher disease, Leigh disease, bilateral striatal necrosis, glutaric aciduria type I, Lesch-Nyhan disease, and a few other HMDs listed in Table 6-5.

Prenatal Developmental Brain Defects

Etiology   The developmental fetal brain disorders stand as the most important terra incognita of neuropediatric research. It is clear that many cases of mental retardation and severe behavioral disturbances and, as noted above, a proportion of cerebral palsies are related to prenatal brain anomalies of obscure origin. Although some progress has been made in recent years, many of them have yet to be investigated.

Known Causes

(a) Nonlethal chromosomal aberrations. They were said to represent 6 percent of the congenital defects at birth in 1977, but they will certainly prove to be more frequent with the wider use of new cytogenetic and molecular biology techniques. Many arise as new mutations.

(b) Monogenic diseases, such as tuberous sclerosis and other neurocutaneous syndromes, or syndromes with multiple congenital anomalies and certain brain malformations. The causative gene of lissencephaly type I (Miller-Dieker syndrome) has been identified on chromosome 17 and cloned. It encodes for the brain platelet-activator factor, which possibly plays a role in neuronal development and function.[4] The gene for X-linked hydrocephalus on chromosome X encodes a cell adhesion molecule (CAML 1). A deletion of the KALIG-1 gene on chromosome X is related to the Kallman syndrome (absence of olfactory tracts and hypogonadism).

(c) Polygenic or multifactorial conditions thought to be at the origin of some congenital abnormalities, particularly neural tube defects.

(d) Fetal encephalites during the first trimester due to cytomegalovirus, toxoplasmosis, rubella, and congenital HIV infection.

(e) Intoxications, essentially the fetal alcohol syndrome and cocaine intoxication.

(f) Prenatal brain defects are observed in a few metabolic diseases (see Chap. 2, and Table 6-1).

(g) There are constellations of congenital anomalies that involve the nervous system and other body structures, face, oral cavity, eyes, limbs, spine, heart and genitourinary tract, which are parts of well-recognized, genetically determined, or sporadic polymalformative syndromes, such as de Lange syndrome and Rubinstein-Taybi syndrome. For some of them, the molecular defect has been identified. The list of these syndromes is available in several monographs and in computerized data banks. The vast majority of the syndromes caused by the hereditary metabolic diseases do not produce these types of somatic developmental defects. Major departures from normalcy, as seen in marked hypotelorism, hypertelorism, midline defects of nose and palate or major malformations of the ears and eyes, and defects of limbs and genitourinary tract, very

rarely occur in these conditions. There are a few exceptions to this rule. Abnormalities of the limbs, kidneys, and genitourinary tract have been observed in such metabolic disorders as glutaric aciduria type II and PDH deficiency (Table 7-8). Also, the Smith-Lemli-Opitz syndrome has been shown to be related to a disorder of cholesterol biosynthesis.[5,6]

Prenatal Malformations of the Brain   These deserve special attention because of their relative frequency as causes of mental retardation and the possibility of diagnosis by neuroimaging. A few generalizations are pertinent.

Prenatal brain malformations vary with respect to the different stages of development when the causative agency occurs—a basic teratologic axiom. The main anomalies of the different morphologic states in the organogenesis and histogenesis of the brain are: the failure of separation of the telencephalon into two hemispheres; the failure of formation of the interhemispheric commissures; agenesis of the olfactory tracts; lack of the normal number and size of neurons with resulting microcephaly; the failure of migration of neurons from the ventricular zone or their arrest en route to the cortical plate (heterotopias); and a variety of other malformations of the cortical plate.

Such defects, always attended by severe mental retardation, may be of genetic, toxic, viral, endocrine, or circulatory origin. Their causes frequently remain recondite. The formal nosology of these malformations is as follows:

• Holoprosencephaly (undivided brain) and the more minor forms of arrhinencephaly.

• Genetically determined hydrocephalus. X-linked hydrocephalus, first described by Bickers and Adams, accounts for as much as 25 percent of male patients with congenital hydrocephalus. A marked prenatal hydrocephalus with absence of the vermis and a smooth cortex is observed in autosomal recessive type II lissencephaly (Walker-Warburg syndrome).

• Agenesis of the corpus callosum with longitudinal Probst bundles (either isolated or associated with other defects); absence, hypoplasia or extreme atrophy of the corpus callosum.

• Septo-optic dysplasia.

• Primary diffuse disorders of migration, essentially represented by type I lissencephaly and the so-called double cortex. Type I lissencephaly associated with certain facial dysmorphic features constitutes the

Miller-Dieker syndrome. It is caused by a mutant gene located on chromosome 17 and may be familial.

• Complex and multifocal disorders of neuronal migration with other brain lesions, as in Zellweger disease.

• Postischemic polymicrogyria, a frequent condition dating approximately from the 20th fetal week. The defect may be diffuse or localized.

• Disorders probably related to inherited anomalies of the mesenchymal envelopes of the brain: type II lissencephaly, Fukuyama disease.

• Microcephaly vera, a genetically determined developmental microcephaly in which the gross morphology of the brain is not profoundly altered.

• Disorders of neuronal and glial specification, represented by tuberous sclerosis, hemimegalencephaly, and more localized cortical defects, all of which are highly epileptogenic.

All these abnormalities underlying mental retardation have been carefully described by neuropathologists and are detectable by MRI. But only now, with advances in molecular biology, is it becoming possible to explore their primary cause.

Practical Diagnostic Considerations   The diagnosis of *prenatal nonprogressive brain disorders* rests on clinical findings and data obtained by radiological investigations, serologic and virologic studies, cytogenetic studies and DNA analysis. The main clinical and radiological features of practical importance for the differential diagnosis of the static encephalopathies from HMDs are given below.

Family History   Family history and the clinical examination of parents and siblings may be informative. For instance, one parent may show evident, although occasionally minor, stigmata of dominantly inherited disorders such as tuberous sclerosis, arrhinencephaly, Steinert's disease, nonprogressive macrocephaly. The nonprogressive nature of a disease may be confirmed when examining an older sibling affected with the same condition. Also, one sibling may have more characteristic clinical features than another. (Obviously, examination of the family is also of paramount importance in the autosomal dominant, X-linked, and maternally inherited metabolic encephalopathies.)

Microcephaly   A microcephaly due to a fixed prenatal defect may be evident before birth, at birth, or

after birth. In our experience, stunting of fetal head growth in developmental (usually genetic) encephalopathies is not discernible on ultrasonic imaging before the 20th to 25th gestational week or later in cases of acquired brain disorders.

Although a moderate degree of reduction in head size is observed at birth or shortly afterwards in some HMDs, particularly in mitochondrial disorders, a frank congenital microcephaly with a head circumference at 3 standard deviations below the normal mean is not a feature of this category of disorders. Very important microcephalies at birth are usually the consequence of a genetically determined developmental encephalopathy. In some of these cases, the brain is very small, whereas the volume of the skull is only moderately reduced.

When a slowly progressive stunting of head growth is observed after several postnatal months, this may reflect a progressive brain destruction caused by a hereditary metabolic or degenerative encephalopathy or a chronic encephalitis (e.g., an HIV infection). In most instances, however, a delayed microcephaly is due to a failure of brain growth, not to radiologically or anatomically discernible destructive brain lesions. It is conceivable in these cases that a genetic or acquired disorder of maturation becomes perceptible long after birth, when the structures which require the action of a specific growth factor reach a critical stage.

Macrocephaly   A macrocephaly at birth or in the very young infant is related to an increase of brain volume or to the accumulation of cerebrospinal fluid in the cerebral ventricles or pericerebral spaces.

A *progressive* megalencephaly (enlargement of the brain) at that age is a characteristic feature of a few rare metabolic disorders (Table 6-2).

Nonprogressive congenital megaloencephalies are a heterogeneous group that includes familial megalencephalies of unknown origin, frequently autosomal dominant, with or without mental retardation. Large brains have occasionally been reported in tuberous sclerosis, neurofibromatosis, Sotos syndrome, and achondroplasia. We have observed two neonates born at term who died in the first days of life. Their brains weighed 650 g and 800 g. There were no discernible neuropathological changes. In the metabolic encephalopathies, a nonprogressive megalencephaly at birth has been occasionally observed (Table 6-2).

Much more frequently, a large head in a young infant is related to a hydrocephalus, a pericerebral hygroma (external hydrocephalus), a congenital arachnoidal cyst or a tumor. A progressive hydrocephalus is

Table 6-2
Macrocephaly in the hereditary neurometabolic diseases

Nonprogressive congenital macrocephaly (megalencephaly)
Glutaric aciduria type I
L-2-Hydroxyglutaric acidemia
Some cases of Alexander disease?

Progressive megalencephaly
Alexander disease
Canavan disease
G_{M2} gangliosidosis (late)

Hydrocephalus
Mucopolysaccharidoses (communicating H)
PDH E_1 deficiency (in some patients)

Subdural hematoma
Menkes disease

---

seen in Hurler disease and other mucopolysaccharidoses, as a consequence of the infiltration of the leptomeninges by macrophages containing mucopolysaccharides. (Even in the absence of hydrocephalus, the head circumference is somewhat large in Hurler disease and Hunter disease because of a dolichocephalic deformation related to a synostosis of the longitudinal suture.) A hydrocephalus also occurs in some cases of early-onset PDH E_1 deficiency.

Prematurity   Prematurity is not generally a feature of HMD, and a very low birth weight is quite rare in this category of diseases. Moderate degrees of prematurity and intrauterine growth retardation have been reported in mitochondrial disorders, homocystinuria and a few other conditions. A polyhydramnios strongly suggests a prenatal disorder; this anomaly may occur in a limited number of HMDs.

Short Stature   A short stature of prenatal onset is not found in HMDs, whereas it is an essential feature of certain well-defined conditions, such as Cornelia de Lange syndrome, Russell-Silver syndrome, Seckel syndrome, Apert syndrome, and various prenatal skeletal dysplasias. However, a postnatal stunting of body growth may be observed in HMDs. In Cockayne syndrome, growth deficiency with a loss of adipose tissue occurs by mid or late infancy and a short stature is an important sign in Hurler disease and in other conditions with dysostosis multiplex. A short stature is observed in the mitochondrial encephalomyopathies.

Polymalformative Syndromes   (see above)

Neuroimaging   Modern methods of neuroimaging provide considerable diagnostic help in the diagnosis of prenatal encephalopathies. Several of the various brain malformations are readily detected. However, the terminology employed to designate them remains confusing. Very different cortical defects underlie the gross modifications of the brain surface, referred to as pachyria, lissencephaly, and microgyria (see Chap. 8).

Indisputable evidence as to the origin of a congenital encephalopathy may be lacking. In what is still a high a proportion of young children with mental retardation, behavioral disturbances, and motor dysfunction, the prenatal origin of the disease is inferred only because of an early onset of symptoms, the absence of any significant perinatal or neonatal events, and a nonprogressive clinical course. In these circumstances, the possibility of an HMD—although very rare—must be considered (see end of Chap. 4 and Table 5-9).

Psychomotor Retardation, Developmental Delay, Mental Retardation

Prior to the onset of obvious neurologic deterioration in early or late childhood, patients with an HMD either develop normally or merely present a delay in psychomotor development for several months or years. During this period, the patient may be thought to have a fixed encephalopathy and such terms as psychomotor retardation, developmental delay, or mental retardation are applied to them. Because of these particularities in the clinical expression of neurometabolic disorders (already discussed in Chap. 4), when a young child does not reach developmental milestones at the expected age (with due allowance for the broad variations which naturally occur among children) and continues to make little progress at a slower pace than the normal referent, the clinician must keep in mind the possibility—in rare instances—of an underlying hereditary metabolic disorder. Repeated clinical evaluations will serve to distinguish a fixed developmental anomaly from a progressive metabolic disorder.

Assessment of Motor and Mental Development In evaluating the *purely motor aspects of development*, one must remember that some children may be slow to sit and walk, but will eventually attain a normal motor function; their slowness is not here clinical evidence of a lesion of the motor system. When walking is not achieved before the age of 2 to 3 years, the gait may remain abnormal because of a coxa vara, not a neurological abnormality. In other children, motor retardation is manifestly the consequence of a dysfunction of the central or peripheral nervous system, and only in this case can the possibility of an HMD be plausibly entertained. Clumsiness, motor instability, and poor coordination, observed in some children with a benign developmental delay, must not be mistaken for choreoathetosis or cerebellar ataxia.

Attention deficits and hyperkinesia are among the most common neuropsychological disorders of childhood and a major cause of learning disabilities. In the majority of cases, these deficits have not been traced to an organic brain disorder and they tend to improve considerably with time, if properly managed. There are, however, exceptions to this rule and some children referred with the diagnosis of learning disability have, in fact, on closer clinical analysis, an organic brain disorder. In our clinical experience, this has been the case in children with Sanfilippo disease, juvenile lipofuscinosis, adrenoleukodystrophy, PKU, Steinert disease, and a few other conditions.

A careful appraisal of cognitive functions and fine motor abilities is necessary in infants and young children suspected of having a delay in mental achievements. Some of the important milestones of cognitive development are relatively easy to assess in general practice.

In the first 6 to 8 months of life, the reaction to visual and auditory stimuli, the maintenance of attention to novel stimuli, and the social and affective reactions all provide important information. The progress of fine motor skills and mental development can be assessed after the age of 10 to 12 months with a set of blocks. At 10 months, infants are able to demonstrate an understanding of cause and effect, perhaps expressed by laughter. Later, such capacities as the understanding of size and shape of objects, the emergence of symbolic thought (particularly evident during play), and the recognition of pictures are early indications of the child's cognitive abilities. Formal developmental testing may be helpful, carried out by an experienced psychologist, using tests adapted to the clinical problem. Among the numerous available screening tests,[7] one of the most widely used is the Denver Developmental Screening Test III. Prelanguage and language skills can be assessed by specialized tests, e.g., the Early Language Milestone Test.[8] Repetition of cognitive testing at regular intervals may provide the first indication of intellectual deterioration.

Behavioral Syndromes: Autism and Rett Syndrome

Autism is a behavioral syndrome related to various brain disorders or occurring without any underlying cause (the so-called Kanner autism). Its main clinical characteristics are a severe impairment in reciprocal social interactions; disturbances in verbal and nonverbal communication; restricted, repetitive and stereotyped patterns of motor activities and interests; and possibly retention of certain mental functions. Mental retardation is usually present. Onset is before the age of 30 months. The first signs may be discernible in infancy. Minor forms occur, expressed by eccentricity of social behavior and highly developed single special abilities (idiot savant). There are no somatic or other neurologic abnormalities.[9] Rarely an autistic syndrome of unknown cause develops by the age of 4 or later (Heller syndrome).

In what is usually considered to be a minor form of autism, Asperger syndrome, impairment of social interaction, inappropriate, eccentric behavior, and narrow all-absorbing interests are associated with a formally perfect and pedantic language. Intelligence is usually normal.

The syndrome of autism is rarely associated with HMDs, but one may observe autistic traits in early infantile lipofuscinosis and in some patients with phenylketonuria, Sanfilippo disease, and adenylosuccinyl-lyase deficiency.

Rett syndrome is a specific, mostly sporadic clinical syndrome which is restricted to girls.[10] Onset is between 6 months and 18 months, after a usually normal initial development. The disease begins as an arrest or deterioration of motor and mental activities. Head circumference is normal at birth, but deceleration of head growth is evidenced in early childhood. There may be elements of autism. After having achieved normal motor activities, the patients rapidly lose the purposeful use of their hands, a prerequisite to the diagnosis. Typical manual stereotypies appear (washing, rubbing, and other automatisms). Hyperventilation is a common feature. Seizures are frequent. Truncal ataxia and spasticity appear several years later. After the age of 10 years, patients are wheelchair-bound, motility is much reduced and scoliosis is usual. The cause of the syndrome is unknown. The diagnosis of Rett syndrome is difficult or impossible before the age of 2 years. The initial phase of developmental arrest is uncharacteristic and the presence of autistic features may have led to the diagnosis of autism. By the time mental and motor deterioration are evident, the possibility of an HMD comes under consideration. Only when loss of purposeful hand movements and stereotypic movements become apparent does the strong possibility of Rett syndrome rest on a firm basis. The neuropathology of the condition is still not firmly established. (To be noted is the fact that washing movements of the hands occur in NCL1; we have also observed this automatism in a case of Tay-Sachs disease.)

There are a few other encephalopathies with more or less characteristic behavioral features; one of the most striking is *Angelman syndrome* (happy puppet syndrome) caused by a maternally inherited deletion of chromosome 15. In *Williams syndrome*, children develop apparently good language capacities, and are particularly talkative and friendly. Mental retardation is usually moderate. There are serious visuo-spatial defects. Hypersensitivity to sound has been noted. Periods of autistic behavior may occur. The disease is due to hemizygosity for a submicroscopic deletion in the region of the elastin gene locus on chromosome 7q11.23.

Concluding Remarks

Some hereditary metabolic encephalopathies evolve over a period of years under the mask of a nonprogressive congenital encephalopathy and may mimic a cerebral palsy, an unspecified delay in motor and mental achievements, or a pure mental retardation. To recognize in these circumstances an underlying metabolic disease, one should be aware both of the characteristic features of pre- or perinatal fixed encephalopathies and of the elements on which one might be led to suspect an HMD before undertaking confirmatory paraclinical investigations. This problem has already been discussed in detail in Chap. 5 and at the end of Chap. 4. The presence of special facial features, skeletal dysplasias, ocular abnormalities, and visceromegaly are among the best clinical indicators of an HMD. But sometimes no etiological clue can be obtained. A good rule, therefore, is to follow regularly any child with apparently cryptogenetic psychomotor retardation or mental retardation, looking for incipient signs of one or more of the neurologic syndromes indicative of these diseases. From this perspective, the current emphasis on early detection and intervention in developmental delays is helpful.[11]

Paraclinical investigations that are recommended when a suspicion of HMD arises are described in Chap. 4 and listed in Table 5-9. They must be interpreted in light of the clinical findings. A deficiency in the activity of a specific enzyme should not be accepted as a final proof, when the clinical features are at odds with the enzymologic results; the possibility of a pseudo-deficiency should be checked. Certainly, in the near future, the availability of specific methods for the detection of the mutant gene in an increasing number of diseases will greatly facilitate the solution of these problems.

DIFFERENTIAL DIAGNOSIS OF NEUROLOGIC SYNDROMES ENCOUNTERED IN THE HEREDITARY METABOLIC AND DEGENERATIVE ENCEPHALOPATHIES OF CHILDHOOD AND ADOLESCENCE

Ataxias

This term applies to special disorders of movement resulting from lesions in the cerebellum or cerebellar tracts in the brain stem and spinal cord. Incoordination of voluntary movements and unsteadiness of gait may also be due to impairment of position sense from interruption of afferent sensory fibers in the peripheral nerves, posterior roots, or spinal cord, or from destruction of large neurons in the spinal sensory ganglia. Action myoclonus can also disorganize volitional movements simulating an ataxia, as do irregular tremors and asterixis.

It is essential for clinical purposes to differentiate between these mechanisms. This is not always easy, for several of these mechanisms may be conjoined, as is the case when both ataxia and action myoclonus are present in cerebellar diseases.

Unquestionable signs of cerebellar ataxia can usually be recognized by the end of the first year, when the child attempts to maintain the sitting position, to stand, and to reach for objects. In some infants and young children, a cerebellar disorder should be suspected when there is marked hypotonia, weak tendon reflexes, and motor delay; actual ataxia is at first minimal or may be absent. Such patients may first be thought to have a neuromuscular disorder. We have considered the latter diagnosis in the early-onset form of neuroaxonal dystrophy.

It is in the older child and adolescent that cerebellar ataxia emerges most clearly. Then the motor dysfunction is essentially the same as that of the adult. The volitional movements of the limbs are manifestly uncoordinated because of a lack of harmonious enlistment of all the muscles needed in an act (dyssynergia). Rapid alternating movements are slowed and irregularly timed (dysdiadochokinesia). The gait is unsteady with a widened base, and steps are uneven and erratic. There is a tremor during voluntary movements which increases as the limb approaches its target, and there may be nystagmus. Speech is typically altered, both slow and uneven in volume. Muscle tone is generally unchanged or arguably reduced and tendon reflexes may be pendular.

Sensory (or tabetic) ataxia can be suspected in the first years of life in children with a severe peripheral neuropathy (Déjerine-Sottas disease), but its full clinical expression is not observed before late childhood or adolescence; it differs from cerebellar ataxia. Even at this age, one can see the ameliorating effect of vision, the lack of intention tremor, and the brusqueness of the incoordinated movements. When the eyes are closed, there are irregular movements of the outstretched fingers (pseudoathetosis) due to an unawareness of their position. When both legs and trunk are affected, as is usually the case, a Romberg sign is present (swaying when standing with feet together and eyes closed, but not when the eyes are open). The postural sense of hands and feet is impaired.

One should be cautious in the interpretation of minor imperfections in motor control. Small irregularities of movement and instability of posture are found in some normal children, particularly in those who are clumsy or suffer from motor delay and attention deficits. These benign and fluctuant peculiarities are sometimes inappropriately referred to as a minor chorea. Also, some degree of action tremor and motor instability may be observed in motor neuron disease (spinal muscular atrophy). Mild incoordination, due to a deficit of sensation, is combined with distal muscle weakness and action tremor in some of the chronic familial polyneuropathies.

Progressive Ataxias in Children and Adolescents

Again, it may be said that cerebellar ataxia is practically never an isolated phenomenon in the hereditary metabolic or neurodegenerative disorders. It is variably associated with sensory ataxia, pyramidal tract signs, polymyoclonus, epilepsy, and dementia.

The hereditary metabolic disorders in which ataxia is the dominant part of the neurologic syndrome are listed in Table 6-3. Their clinical features have been described in Chap. 5.

The nonmetabolic diseases with progressive ataxia, from which they must be differentiated, include tumors of the cerebellum and brain stem and, much more rarely, subacute encephalitis. Cerebellar tumors may be a source of confusion in some cases if the ataxia develops slowly in relatively pure form over a period of a year or more before the appearance of headache or papilledema. There is a tendency for the ataxia to be asymmetric or even unilateral, which is not seen in the HMD. In brain stem gliomas, asymmetric pyramidal signs and cranial nerve palsies, nystagmus, and oculomotor disturbances accompany the cerebellar signs. In the child with a neuroblastoma, ataxia, myoclonus and opsoclonus may occur, and in adults with any one of several types of systemic tumor, a subacute cerebellar degeneration may be the manifestation (paraneoplastic syndrome).

Subacute measles and rubella encephalites, an enterovirus infection in children with X-linked hypogammaglobulinemia, and HIV may cause a slowly progressive encephalopathy with ataxia. Serologic, virologic, and immunologic studies in blood and CSF and radiologic investigations, usually substantiate the diagnosis.

A long-standing congenital hydrocephalus may, after some years, cause an unsteady gait, which is alleviated by ventricular shunting. Cerebellar incoordination may also be due to type I Arnold-Chiari malformation, often in association with syringomyelia in an adult. It is revealed by radiologic scan procedures.

Nonprogressive Idiopathic Isolated Hereditary Cerebellar Ataxias

This is a heterogeneous group of congenital abnormalities, usually inherited as an autosomal recessive, much less frequently as an autosomal dominant or X-linked trait. In terms of cerebellar dysfunction, their clinical expression is variable. In some children, a cerebellar syndrome with an unsteady gait, dysmetria, and intention tremor is evident as soon as standing and walking are achieved, usually between the ages of 2 and 4 years. In others, there is mainly a "dysequilibrium syndrome,"[12] in which failure to develop postural control and an inability to maintain equilibrium when standing are the main features; dyssynergia and intention tremor are minimal. Standing is seldom achieved before 6 to 8 years and walking before 8 to 9 years. Regardless of whether the predominant feature is dyssynergia or dysequilibrium, cerebellar dysfunction tends to improve with time. By imaging techniques, a cerebellar hypoplasia (or atrophy) can be visualized. From all available data, including one personally observed case, with postmortem examination, the neuropathological basis of this syndrome corresponds to the "primary degeneration of granule cells" described by Norman in 1940,[13] and subsequently reported by several authors. The population of granule cells is considerably reduced with variable loss and den-

Table 6-3

Progressive cerebellar ataxia as a main sign in the hereditary metabolic and degenerative encephalopathies

Diseases	Other important neurological signs
Friedreich ataxia + + +	Proprioceptive sensory loss: tabetocerebellar ataxia (cardiomyopathy)
Early-onset ataxia with retained TR + + +	No proprioceptive sensory loss (no cardiomyopathy)
AD spinocerebellar and cerebellar ataxias + + +	Frequent ophthalmologic signs, other neurologic signs
Abetalipoproteinemia + + +	Friedreich phenotype
Hypobetalipoproteinemia + + +	Friedreich phenotype
Ataxia with vitamin E deficiency (AVED) + + +	Friedreich phenotype
Ataxia-telangiectasia + + +	Choreoathetosis; supranuclear ophthalmoplegia
Late infantile and juvenile sphingolipidoses	
$\quad$ G$_{M2}$ gangliosidosis	Lower motor neuron involvement
$\quad$ Niemann-Pick C disease	Supranuclear ophthalmoplegia
$\quad$ Metachromatic leukodystrophy	Neuropathy
$\quad$ Krabbe leukodystrophy	Neuropathy
$\quad$ Gaucher type III disease	Supranuclear ophthalmoplegia; seizures (splenomegaly)
Late infantile ceroid lipofuscinosis	Seizures; polymyoclonus
Leigh disease	Signs of brain stem involvement; dystonia; intermittent hyperventilation; fluctuating course
Pyruvate dehydrogenase deficiency	
MERRF	Polymyoclonus; epilepsy; proprioceptive sensory loss
Other mitochondrial encephalomyopathies	Ataxia usually less prominent
Ramsay Hunt syndrome	See text
Lafora disease	Polymyoclonus; seizures; dementia; rapid course
Unverricht-Lundborg type of myoclonus epilepsy	Polymyoclonus; seizures
Cholestanolosis	
Refsum disease	Polyneuropathy; deafness; ataxia infrequent
Pelizaeus-Merzbacher disease	Nystagmus
Intranuclear neuronal inclusion disease	Evidence of lower motor neuron disease
L-2OH glutaric acidemia	
Carbohydrate-deficient glycoprotein syndrome	Cerebellar atrophy
Succinic semialdehyde deficiency	
Juvenile neuroaxonal dystrophy	Polymyoclonus
Juvenile nonketotic hyperglycinemia	Very rare phenotype

Abbreviations and symbols: + + + = disease in which cerebellar ataxia is a practically constant sign; AD = autosomal dominant. Cerebellar ataxia may be difficult to ascertain in the presence of polymyoclonus and seizures.

dritic changes in Purkinje cells. There were no significant abnormalities in the telencephalon.

One of the most remarkable clinical features of nonprogressive congenital cerebellar ataxias is the presence of variable degrees of mental retardation and language disorder and occasionally seizures. The increased usage of neuroimaging techniques is calling attention to the many cases of unsuspected cerebellar atrophy (or aplasia) and normal cerebral morphology in children presenting with motor delay, mental retardation, and language disorders, but no significant or only a moderate ataxia. We have personally observed 15 cases in 12 families. These findings raise interesting questions about the role of the cerebellum in cognitive function. This possibility is strongly suggested by a number of clinical, anatomical, PET scan, and MRI studies. This matter has been reviewed recently.[14–16] Dow and Moruzzi had already noted in 1958[17] that practically all cases of congenital abnormalities of the cerebellum were mentally defective.

Some families have been reported in which non-progressive cerebellar ataxia, cerebellar atrophy, and mental retardation are combined with other physical signs, such as small stature and cataracts. This constellation conforms to the Marinesco-Sjögren syndrome, a condition of uncertain specificity. Other families have had abnormalities involving the eyes (cataracts, retinitis pigmentosa, aniridia, fixed mydriasis), muscle, kidneys and hematopoietic system. In another disease described by Norman,[18] there is an association of the typical lesions of Werdnig-Hoffmann disease and atrophy (hypoplasia) of the cerebellum, inferior olives, and pons.

Recently, a number of cases of childhood cerebellar atrophy have been reported under the name *olivopontocerebellar atrophy*, because on MRI the pons and occasionally the medulla appeared to be atrophic. While descriptively correct, we believe that the use of this term may be confusing because it has also been applied to at least five types of adult cerebellar degenerations. We prefer to reserve *olivopontocerebellar atrophy or degeneration* for the autosomal dominant disorders which occur in adults, but may occasionally start in adolescence.

The condition known as *congenital pontoneocerebellar aplasia* appears to be a different disorder. Described first by Brun in 1917, it is characterized by a massive reduction of neurons in the nucleus pontis, hypoplasia (i.e., underdevelopment) or atrophy of the cerebellar hemispheres (neocerebellum), and preservation of the vermis. Microcephaly and various types of cortical changes in the brain coexist. The condition is usually fatal in early life. Its origin is unknown. Some cases have been familial. We have observed three brothers affected with this condition. (For a review see Gadisseux et al.[19])

Acute and Episodic Ataxias

Metabolic Disorders A number of autosomal recessive, X-linked, or maternally transmitted hereditary *metabolic disorders* (see Table 6-4) may become manifest clinically in early or late childhood, with recurrent episodes of ataxia of acute onset, sometimes in a setting of fever and dietary irregularity. Frequently, there is an associated lethargy and vomiting. The ataxia may only become apparent during the recovery period and it persists for a week or more. This sequence should always arouse the suspicion of an HMD, but in the instance of a

first episode of acute ataxia, other possibilities must be considered.

Nonmetabolic Acute Ataxias The most frequent causes of nonmetabolic acute ataxias are infections and intoxications.

An *acute, isolated, self-limiting cerebellar ataxia syndrome* may appear abruptly during an infection or a few days after. There is generally pleiocytosis in the CSF. Usually, the patient improves after a few weeks or months and residual deficits are rare. Viruses, such as enteroviruses, Epstein-Barr virus, varicella, and occasionally measles, mumps, and herpes simplex virus may be the cause of this cerebellitis, but attempts to isolate the virus or to show rising titers of antibodies have occasionally failed. The organism of mycoplasma pneumonia has been isolated in a few cases.

Kinsbourne myoclonus-opsoclonus syndrome is another recognizable form of acute incoordination mimicking a cerebellar syndrome in infants and young children under the age of 3 years. It is characterized by large-range, erratic muscular jerks of the limbs upon attempted movement and by sudden, brusque, chaotic eye movements in all directions (dancing eyes) precipitated by changes in fixation, usually accompanied by palpebral flutter. The movement disorder is self-limiting in most instances, with possible recurrence or worsening during febrile illnesses. Residual mental and motor retardation are frequent. The syndrome may be related to viral infections and is relatively frequently associated with a neuroblastoma. Here, the primary tumor is located in the thorax, abdomen, or pelvis and may be very small. Varicella is a well-documented cause. In many cases, no cause has been found. Corticosteroids

Table 6-4
Main disorders with intermittent cerebellar ataxia[a]

Pyruvate dehydrogenase deficiency (E_1)
Pyruvate carboxylase deficiency
Leigh disease
Disorders of mitochondrial fatty acid oxidation
Leucinosis (maple syrup urine disease)
Other aminoacidopathies and organic acidopathies
Biotinidase deficiency
Fructose 1,6-bisphosphatase deficiency
Hartnup disease

[a] Intermittent cerebellar ataxias, with or without concomitant episodes of stupor and vomiting, occur mainly in the late infantile and juvenile, relatively benign, forms of the diseases listed in this table.

are often remarkably effective, as is removal of a neuro-blastoma.

Intoxications with benzodiazepines, barbiturates, phenytoin, carbamazepine, phenothiazines, and other drugs are well-known causes of acute ataxia, nystagmus, drowsiness, and vomiting.

Peripheral neuropathies, particularly the Miller-Fisher syndrome and an unusual form of the Guillain-Barré syndrome with weakness in the proximal segment of the lower limbs, may present as an ataxia, but on closer examination, muscle weakness, areflexia, and more or less evident distal sensory impairment will affirm the neuropathic nature of the condition. In diphtheric neuropathy there is often a tabetic type of ataxia related to selective demyelination of posterior spinal roots.

In nonconvulsive status epilepticus, a few random myoclonic jerks may cause incoordination of movements. Extreme hyperthermia, most often consequent to heat stroke (not a febrile infection), can destroy Purkinje cells and result in severe ataxia during recovery. Transitory ataxia may also occur as a sequel of bacterial meningitis.

Other causes of acute ataxia include basilar migraine, arterial occlusions or malformations in the vertebrobasilar arterial system, cerebellar hematoma, cerebellar abscess, multiple sclerosis, posterior fossa tumor, and severe head trauma (usually with hemorrhage or ischemia in posterior fossa structures).

Nonmetabolic Diseases with Episodic Ataxia One form of episodic ataxia is *familial periodic ataxia* which is inherited as an autosomal dominant trait. It is characterized by recurrent attacks of cerebellar ataxia and dysarthria, occasionally nystagmus, without disturbance of consciousness, lasting a few hours. Oral administration of acetazolamide suppresses the attacks. A few other reports of familial periodic cerebellar ataxia which do not conform exactly to this description have been reported by Bain.[20]

Episodic cerebellar ataxia should be differentiated from *benign paroxystic vertigo and paroxysmal choreo-athetosis*.

Various *acquired conditions* may occasionally give rise to several attacks of ataxia. We have observed a child with Guillain-Barré syndrome who experienced three episodes of unsteadiness of gait and dysequilibrium following a succession of infections. Post-infectious recurrence of the opsoclonus-myoclonus syndrome has been documented.

The *Münchausen syndrome by proxy* may be a source of considerable diagnostic difficulty. We have

observed two children who were surreptitiously given either benzodiazepine or phenothiazine by their mothers, resulting in numerous episodes of ataxia and drowsiness. Only after several months was it possible to elucidate the problem. Metabolic disorders were at first considered most likely.

Circulatory insufficiency in the vertebrobasilar arterial system may produce successive episodes of ataxia and other neurological signs in *basilar migraine*, and in arterial occlusions or arterial malformations, as was the case in one of our patients.

Basal Ganglia Disorders

The basal ganglia can be targeted by hereditary metabolic or degenerative diseases and by other conditions from which they must be differentiated. These disorders of movement are combined in several configurations. Best delineated are 4 to 6 per second tremors at rest associated with bradykinesia and rigidity, as in Parkinson disease; chorea, consisting of sudden, rapid arrhythmic movements of the limbs (frequently with a proximal limb and a facial predominance) associated usually with hypotonia and pendular reflexes; athetosis, characterized by slow, sinuous movements predominating in the fingers and toes, face and tongue; dystonia (or torsion dystonia) with slow, sustained twisting spasms and abnormal postures often interspersed with more rapid involuntary movements of muscle jerks; abrupt, wide-ranging movements of the limbs on one side of the body (hemiballismus); and other tremors. Dystonia and athetosis are closely allied and these terms are used almost indiscriminately in the medical literature. Involuntary movements often have a choreic as well as an athetotic component, hence the term choreoathetosis. One may observe many combinations of these movement disorders sometimes in association with pyramidal or cerebellar signs. The metabolic diseases expressed by progressive extrapyramidal syndromes were described in Chap. 5 and are listed in Table 6-5.

In this section we will consider successively (1) the differential diagnosis of extrapyramidal movements and (2) the nonmetabolic causes of basal ganglia disorders.

(1) Differential Diagnosis of Extrapyramidal Movement Disorders Even in the young child it is usually possible to separate the pyramidal syndromes characterized by paralysis, spasticity, hyperreflexia and Babinski signs from the extrapyramidal syndromes. In

Table 6-5
Hereditary progressive metabolic and degenerative encephalopathies with prominent extrapyramidal signs[a]

Hereditary disorders	Dystonia, athetosis, choreoathetosis	Chorea	Parkinsonian rigidity	Tremor	Mental deterioration, psychiatric signs	Other important neurological signs
Wilson disease	+		+++	++	+++	Kayser-Fleischer ring (liver cirrhosis)
Juvenile Huntington disease	+	+	+++	+	+++	Seizures
Juvenile Parkinson disease			+++		±	
Idiopathic torsion dystonia	+++		+	+	0	Myoclonus
Dopa-responsive torsion dystonia	+++		++	+	0	
Other primary dystonias	+++				0	See text
Hallervorden-Spatz disease	+++	±	++	+	++	Retinitis pigmentosa
Chorea-acanthocytosis	+	+++	+		++	Axonal neuropathy; tics
Familial striatal necrosis	+++				++	
Familial striatal necrosis and visual failure (Leber disease)	+++		++		0	Subacute visual failure; maternal inheritance
Dentatorubral pallidoluysian atrophy	++				+++	Polymyoclonus; seizures
Familial striatal calcifications	++		++		++	
Cockayne disease	++			++	+++	Leukodystrophy
MPS and keratan sulfaturia with athetosis	+++			+	+	
Ataxia-telangiectasia	++	±		++	++	Cerebellar ataxia; ocular signs
Glutaric aciduria type I	+++				+++	Episodic comas; striatal necrosis
Molybdenum cofactor (sulfate oxidase) deficiency	++				+++	Ectopia lentis
3-Methylglutaconic acidemia	+++				+++	Striatal necrosis; optic atrophy
Niemann-Pick C disease	++				+++	Supranuclear ophthalmoplegia
Juvenile ceroid lipofuscinosis			++		++	Retinal degeneration; vacuolated lymphocytes
Chronic G_{M2} gangliosidosis	++					Lower motor neuron disorder
Late-onset G_{M1} gangliosidosis	++					
Neuronal intranuclear inclusion disease						Ataxia; lower motor neuron disease
Spinocerebellar degeneration (Friedreich disease and others)	±			+++		Cerebellar and proprioceptive ataxia
Leigh syndrome	++			++	+++	Ocular, respiratory signs; cerebellar signs
Pelizaeus-Merzbacher disease	+++				++	Pendular nystagmus; leukodystrophy
Lesch-Nyhan disorder	+++	±			++	Automutilation

Symbols: +++ = constant or very frequent; ++ = frequent; + = occurs but not frequently; ± = rare or not well documented, or mild; 0 = absent; MPS = mucopolysaccharidosis.

[a] Nonprogressive benign chorea or choreoathetosis is described in the text. Other very rare extrapyramidal disorders, and other disorders which present exceptionally with extrapyramidal signs are mentioned in the text.

the extrapyramidal disorders there is slowness of movement without paralysis, muscle rigidity, and involuntary movements.

Clinical and electrophysiological features serve to differentiate extrapyramidal rigidity from myotonia congenita, paramyotonia, syndromes of continuous muscular activity (such as Isaac syndrome), the Schwarz-Jampel syndrome and other forms of neuromyotonia and myokymia. Some of these disorders start in infancy.

Involuntary movements due to basal ganglia disorders must be differentiated from a variety of other involuntary movements occurring in childhood or adolescence: tics, action myoclonus, cerebellar intention tremors and dysmetria, motor stereotypes, e.g., the automatisms of autism, Rett syndrome, and other behavioral disturbances; and hysteric gesticulation. In patients with proprioceptive sensory deficits (as in Friedreich ataxia and MERRF), there are irregular movements of outstretched fingers when the eyes are closed, sometimes referred to as pseudoathetosis.

Presently, the authors have had the most trouble not in the recognition of the fully developed extrapyramidal syndromes, but of their earliest expression. At this time, only an involuntary spasm or twitch or a newly appearing clumsiness and slowness of movements; a spasm of the foot; a change in facial appearance; modification of the voice; odd postures or mannerisms are the only expression of the incipient disease. We have seen inability to keep the eyes open, a mild torticollis, a writer's cramp, and a strained vocalization as the initial sign of a generalized or segmental dystonia.

One's first inclination may be to minimize these manifestations, to pass them off as "functional" or to relate them to familial or scholastic stress. Slowness and incoordination of movements have occasionally been mistaken for the "soft neurologic signs" of learning and attention disorders (and the reverse is also true). Some adolescents have been labeled hysteric, especially as psychological and behavioral disturbances may have coincided with the onset of a basal ganglia disorder, such as in Huntington disease and in Wilson disease. And psychological derangements may even antedate characteristic extrapyramidal symptoms by months or years, leading to the erroneous diagnosis of a psychiatric disorder.

In all such childhood conditions it is advisable always to begin the clinical inquiry by looking for subtle signs of one of the HMDs. If not present, it is best to temporize and recheck the findings in a succession of examinations without unduly alarming the family.

(2) Differential Diagnosis with Nonmetabolic Disorders of the Basal Ganglia

Progressive Extrapyramidal Symptoms   While a progressive extrapyramidal syndrome should, at any age, suggest the possibility of a hereditary metabolic or degenerative disease, there are a few notable exceptions to this rule. An infiltrating glioma of the basal ganglia may rarely give rise to unilateral dystonia. A parkinsonian syndrome, dyskinesia of the face and tongue, and dystonic movements of the trunk and limbs may arise as a complicaton of long-term antipsychotic treatment with phenothiazines or butyrophenones in adolescents and adults, and may persist indefinitely after withdrawal of the drug. This is called *tardive dyskinesia*. We have found this to be one of the troublesome problems in differential diagnosis encountered in a psychiatric hospital, where we have been asked to screen adolescents and adults for inherited metabolic and degenerative diseases.

Intermittent and Acute Extrapyramidal Dyskinesias   Extrapyramidal symptoms may at times be intermittent. In glutaric acidemia type I, dystonic spasms often appear after an infection and at least partially subside. More often, acute transient attacks of dystonia or rigidity are seen in certain acquired nonmetabolic conditions, particularly as side effects of drugs or after an infection. High levels of phenytoin, carbamazepine or, more exceptionally, phenobarbital may induce facial dyskinesia or choreoathetoid movements of the limbs. Phenothiazines (when used as antiemetics in children) may induce parkinsonian rigidity or involuntary movements of the facial muscles and tongue along with dysphagia, retrocollis, and oculogyric crises. These acute dystonic spasms respond remarkably to ethylbenzatropine (Ponalide®). Transitory or persistent extrapyramidal syndromes have also been reported after treatment with methylphenidate, amphetamines, and lithium.

Acute bilateral striatal necrosis related to viral diseases or infections by mycoplasma pneumonia[21,22] has been the source of a striking parkinsonian picture or dystonic syndromes from which recovery occurs slowly over a period of weeks or months. The radiological findings of this rare condition are typical. We have observed prolonged choreoathetosis as a sequela of an acute encephalitis of uncertain viral origin in two children who finally recovered from their motor abnormality. A choreic syndrome has been reported after cardiac surgery.[23] Chorea may be a complication of systemic lupus erythematosus. Also, chorea in Huntington disease, chorea-acanthocytosis, and a few other HMDs may initially be mistaken for Sydenham chorea, and the opposite also happens, as we have recently observed. A syndrome of acute coma with bursts of involuntary movements has recently been described. No cause was found. [23a]

Calcification of the Basal Ganglia in Hereditary Disorders Deposits of calcium in the basal ganglia and other brain structures, notably the dentate nuclei, are found in a few hereditary metabolic or degenerative encephalopathies as a constant or frequent feature. They are best seen on CT scans. This happens in Cockayne disease, Fahr syndrome (striatopallidodentate calcinosis) and MELAS. In these disorders, neuropathological studies show that calcium deposits are essentially perivascular and that surrounding neurons in gray structures are little affected (see Chaps. 5 and 8). Calcifications may also occur in biopterin deficiency and 3-hydroxyisobutyryl acidemia.

Another curious familial syndrome with basal ganglia calcifications and persistent lymphocytosis is the *Aicardi-Goutières syndrome*. This possibly autosomal recessive condition[27] starts in the very first weeks of life. Neurologic development remains very poor. There is marked hypotonia, opisthotonic spasms, and lack of mental development. Death occurs after a few years. The hallmark of the disease consists of calcifications of the basal ganglia, progressive brain atrophy with white matter lesions, and a persistent, mild CSF lymphocytosis (10 to 80 cells). The pathology of the disorder has not been adequately documented. HIV infection can also cause an encephalopathy with pleiocytosis in the CSF and basal ganglia calcifications.

The Diagnostic Problems in Infants Although the fully fledged clinical features of a basal ganglia type of movement disorder are not evident before the second or third year of life, the first indications of them, such as athetoid movements of hands and feet, abnormal movements of face and tongue, sialhorrea (an early sign in our patients), or dystonic posturing of neck or limbs, are not infrequently observed within the first year of life, sometimes as early as the fourth month. These symptoms are generally associated with or preceded by marked hypotonia, which may mimic a neuromuscular disorder. Such a precocious early infantile onset of involuntary movements occurs in some of the HMDs. It has been observed in glutaric acidemia type I, Lesch-Nyhan disease, Leigh syndrome, PDH deficiency, and familial

striatal necrosis. One of our young infants wth COX deficiency manifested athetoid movements of the extremities, hypotonia, lethargy, and cardiomyopathy at 3 months of age. At autopsy there were areas of necrosis in the basal ganglia.[24]

A few subtle peculiarities of movement in an infant may at times be falsely interpreted as signs of basal ganglia disease. Involuntary movements or vagrant posturing of the trunk or limbs may be seen in normal infants, and the distinction between normal and abnormal is uncertain. We have several times made the mistake of assuming them to be the first manifestation of a basal ganglia disorder. A transient or intermittent slight dystonic posture, such as hyperpronation of the forearm, a flexed wrist, external rotation of one leg, head hyperextension, or torticollis, may last several months or more in an otherwise normal child before "being outgrown."[25] Perlman and Volpe[26] have remarked upon fleeting choreiform movements and orolingual dyskinesia in prematures with bronchopulmonary dysplasia.

Differential Diagnosis with Dystonic Cerebral Palsy In chronic infantile choreoathetosis the essential problem is in differential diagnosis between an HMD and a dyskinetic cerebral palsy. After a pre- or perinatal ischemic/anoxic encephalopathy, involuntary movements tend to appear progressively at the age of 8 to 10 months and are associated with hypotonia and motor delay. A history of abnormal perinatal events can be elicited in only about two-thirds of these patients. Neuroimaging may reveal signs of hypoxic-ischemic lesions sometimes involving the lenticular nuclei, but the images are frequently uncharacteristic. Consequently, in any infant with choreoathetosis of uncertain origin, one should pursue the possibility of such metabolic disorders as Lesch-Nyhan disease, glutaric acidemia type I, and other organic acidurias, or a mitochondrial encephalopathy. These disorders should be investigated by measuring uric acid and organic acids in urine and lactic acid in blood and CSF. Pelizaeus-Merzbacher disease is another possibility.

Spastic Paraplegia

Spastic paraplegia and quadriplegia result from bilateral lesions of the corticospinal (pyramidal) tracts, which extend directly without synaptic interruption from the motor cortex to the brain stem motor nuclei and spinal cord.

In spastic paraplegia a slow and stiff gait with reduced motion of hip and knee, spasticity of calf and adductor muscles (scissor gait), weakness in the extensor muscles of the foot and flexors of the hip and thigh, exaggerated tendon reflexes, and a bilateral Babinski sign are the denominating features. They are easily distinguished from extrapyramidal rigidity. To be separated are certain myopathies and some lower motor neuron disorders, where weakness and atrophy are essentially proximal, and the more typical chronic polyneuropathies where there is a selective weakness and atrophy of the tibialis anterior and peroneal muscles, distal sensory deficits, and areflexia.

In mild forms of paraparesis, however, the spasticity may not at first be obvious and the extensor plantar response may be equivocal. Moreover, in incipient chronic polyneuropathies, sensory abnormalities may not be detectable and tendon reflexes are initially retained. In such instances, the distinction between these two conditions may be somewhat difficult. One important difference lies in the distribution of muscle weakness. In spastic paraplegias, weakness is not restricted to the anterolateral muscles of the legs, but always extends to the thigh. This results in a characteristic gait and in a genu recurvatum, which in our experience is not present in polyneuropathies of the common type of childhood and adolescence.

As stated in Chap. 5, a bipyramidal syndrome is found in many HMDs, but in most of them a spastic paraplegia is associated with other abnormalities, such as weakness of the arms, cerebellar ataxia, dysarthria, dystonia, a peripheral neuropathy, and mental retardation. But since an isolated or predominant bipyramidal syndrome is frequently observed early in the course of some of them, neurometabolic disorders must always be included in the differential diagnosis of a spastic paraplegia (see Chaps. 4 and 5 and Table 5-2).

The differential diagnosis of a slowly progressive spastic paraplegia in childhood includes mainly *congenital spastic diplegia*, which is one of the most frequent of the pediatric neurologic diseases. Hence the early-onset paraplegias of either metabolic or degenerative origin are not infrequently mistaken for mild forms of congenital diplegia which have not significantly delayed motor development. Two of our patients, one with metachromatic leukodystrophy and another with Strümpell-Lorrain hereditary spastic paraplegia, were at first thought to have congenital spastic diplegia. Neither was born prematurely. As was stated earlier, since 30 percent of spastic diplegias are probably of

prenatal origin, a diagnosis of cerebral palsy should not be made in a child born at term and with no radiological evidence of periventricular leukomalacia or parasagittal cortical necrosis, without due consideration being given to other possible etiologies.

A tumor invading or compressing the spinal cord may occur in a child. The paraparesis is usually asymmetric and there is spinal and radicular pain, evident sensory disturbances, and urinary incontinence. A clinical and radiologic examination of the spine and spinal cord are crucial for the diagnosis. Radiologic investigations should always be done in case of a paraparesis of uncertain origin before a lumbar puncture, which may aggravate the paralysis in case of a tumor. Defects of the vertebrae or spinal canal, including atlanto-axial dislocation, and congenital malformations of the spinal cord are possible causes of paraplegia or quadriplegia.

Approximately 3 percent of all cases of *multiple sclerosis* may begin with a transverse myelitis or, rarely, as a rapidly progressive myelopathy with a paraplegia plus sensory and sphincter disturbances. Suspicion of multiple sclerosis, occasionally a late childhood or adolescent disease, is supported by clinical and/or radiological and electrophysiological evidence of several successive demyelinating lesions in the brain stem, optic nerves, and spinal cord; oligoclonal IgG bands are found in the CSF. There is a spastic paraplegia associated with acquired cirrhosis and hyperammonemia.

A pure spastic paraplegia, due to an infection with *HTLV-1*, has been observed in tropical countries and southern Japan, but nearly always in adults. There is also a spinal form of *AIDS*.

A number of *hereditary syndromes* of unknown origin have been catalogued in which a relatively fixed or slowly progressive paraplegia has been associated with other signs (*complicated familial spastic paraplegia*). These conditions are very rare and some of them have only been reported in one family. Their mode of inheritance is generally autosomal recessive or more rarely autosomal dominant or X-linked. Concomitant abnormalities include amyotrophy, a sensory neuropathy, dystonia, mental retardation or dementia, deafness, retinal degeneration, optic atrophy, palmoplantar keratosis, ichthyosis and other cutaneous abnormalities, in various combinations. A list of these syndromes is to be found in a paper by Appleton et al.[28] Such diseases have no defined metabolic basis and are presently classified as degenerative (Chap. 5).

In summary, the main problem with these spastic paralyses is to separate the metabolic leukodystrophies and storage polioencephalopathies from the congenital cerebral palsies of infancy and childhood and from the familial "degenerative" spastic paraplegias.

Hemiplegias

Progressive Spastic Hemiplegia As stated in Chap. 5, this condition may stand alone for several months as the initial manifestation of juvenile metachromatic leukodystrophy, juvenile Krabbe disease, and adrenoleukodystrophy. Leigh disease is another possible cause. We have also observed two 10 to 12-year-old patients with a slowly progressive hemiplegia and bilateral striatal necrosis, without the usual clinical and radiological features of Leigh disease (see bilateral striatal necrosis, Chap. 5). In all these conditions, the possibility of a *tumor* may first come to mind and can be readily eliminated by MRI scanning. But CT scans do not always demonstrate lesions in the early phase of a leukodystrophy. This may also be true of an infiltrating glioma, even when neurological deficit is definite. We have found that some thalamocapsular gliomas may be radiologically mute for a relatively long period.

A progressive hemiplegia is also a feature of so-called *Schilder disease*. As is now generally conceded, the three patients reported by Schilder between 1912 and 1924 had three entirely different conditions.[29] One had a postinfectious encephalitis (probably a subacute sclerosing panencephalitis); another had most probably an adrenoleukodystrophy (this was also the case of many male patients later reported as Schilder disease before 1980); the third patient, described in 1912, was a 14-year-old girl with neurological deterioration, signs of raised intracranial pressure, and multifocal cerebral demyelination. The latter disease is now called *true Schilder disease*.

Schilder disease (inflammatory myelinoclastic diffuse sclerosis) is a sporadic subacute or chronic demyelinating disorder of unknown origin with a probable relationship to multiple sclerosis. Both sexes are affected, mostly children between 5 and 14 years of age; occasionally the disease is seen in adults. A progressive hemiplegia has been the first clinical manifestation in most cases. Headache, vomiting, and papilledema occur in some instances, suggesting at first a brain tumor. Even a brain biopsy showing widespread gliosis may be misinterpreted as an astrocytoma. Abnormal behavior, dysarthria and swallowing difficulties, and lethargy are other possible presenting signs. Pseudobulbar palsies and evidence of involvement of pyramidal tracts are usually present. Visual loss may also occur, due to the involvement of the optic radiations. The CT scan and MRI typically show one, two, or three large areas of hypodensity in the hemispheric white matter with enhancement in T2-weighted MRI images. These well-demarcated lesions predominate in the frontal regions. There are no other demyelinating plaques in the central nervous system in most cases, and the peripheral nervous system is spared. IgG oligoclonal bands are sometimes found in the CSF. Total protein may be moderately elevated and there may be an excess of white blood cells. The level of very long chain fatty acids in the plasma is normal, an absolute prerequisite to the diagnosis of Schilder disease. The brain lesions are remarkably sensitive to steroids, which cause their shrinkage and the disappearance of contrast enhancement. Clinical improvement is usual but sequelae may persist. The course of the disease is variable and its outcome is unpredictable. In five patients reported by Aicardi,[30] there was no recurrence during a period of 9 years. (In one of our cases of acute multiple sclerosis, there was no recurrence after 28 years). In other cases the disorder pursues a relapsing course reminiscent of chronic multiple sclerosis, with more or less complete remissions lasting months or years. In a child followed over a period of 10 years, we have observed four episodes of right or left hemiplegia with headache, vomiting, and lethargy, symptoms which first resembled hemiplegic migraine. The initial CT scan was not demonstrative, but later there were unmistakable foci of myelin destruction.

Sudden (Apoplectic) Hemiplegias Four neurometabolic disorders—homocystinuria, Fabry disease, MELAS, and methylenetetrafolate reductase deficiency—are apt to produce vasculopathies or arterial occlusions resulting in strokes, or possibly nonischemic foci of brain tissue necrosis, in children or adolescents. Menkes disease also causes multiple vascular occlusions in infancy. Low levels of high-density lipoprotein and/or high levels of triglycerides have been reported in children with acute hemiplegia.[31] Familial lipoprotein abnormalities might therefore predispose children to ischemic strokes. Also, in any HMD with a cardiopathy, a cerebral embolism may occur.

It is clear that these relatively infrequent HMDs must be differentiated from a number of genetically determined or acquired disorders, in which an acute hemiplegia is the consequence of a thromboembolic ischemia, a brain hemorrhage, or a hemorrhagic leukoencephalitis, i.e., the hemorrhagic encephalitis of Hurst (presumably a hyperacute form of postinfectious leukoencephalitis). These conditions are listed in Table 6-6.

The more common acute hemiplegias of childhood are acquired vascular occlusions, frequently of undetermined cause. Over a period of 20 years, we have observed more than 100 cases of *acute idiopathic ischemic strokes* in this age-group. Onset is sudden and unexpected in an otherwise healthy child. There may have been a benign febrile illness a few days before the attack. Occasionally there was a brief focal seizure at the onset. The severity of unilateral paralysis (with or without aphasia) and the degree of recovery are variable but often substantial. In some patients, dystonic movements (hemiathetosis) or tremor appear after several months in the affected limbs as the hemiplegia recedes. The mental status remains relatively normal and, along with others, we have not observed a recurrence of the stroke. Ischemic lesions are demonstrated by brain scanning; an occlusion of the middle cerebral artery, carotid artery, or a cerebral vein is substantiated in some patients, whereas others exhibit no significant abnormality by arteriography performed several days after the attack. A disintegrating embolus or a resolving venous thrombosis may have been the cause.

The acute ischemic strokes of childhood are a heterogeneous group of diseases and, in our series, not all the etiologies enumerated in Table 6-6 have been ruled out. The cryptogenetic group of acute hemiplegias in children will certainly diminish in the future. In particular, an increasing frequency of various coagulation defects is now established, sometimes leading to specific treatments.

Acute postconvulsive hemiplegia is also relatively frequent. It occurs mostly in the first three years of life as a consequence of unilateral or bilateral asymmetrical status epilepticus. The hemiparesis is at first flaccid with facial palsy; spasticity usually develops later. Mental impairment and epilepsy are the usual sequelae. These cases of definitive postconvulsive hemiplegias are to be distinguished from the transient hemiplegias that may be associated with seizures.

Rasmussen focal encephalitis is a cause of focal motor seizures and of hemiparesis.

Epilepsy

Since epilepsy as a major neurologic disorder has not been discussed in the previous chapters, it will be presented here in connection with metabolic and nonmetabolic conditions.

Epileptic seizures may occur in practically all of the hereditary metabolic or degenerative encephalopathies, but are a constant or major feature in only a few. They may constitute an early manifestation of most of the polioencephalopathies and are rare in the leukoencephalopathies. When present, they raise problems in the differential diagnosis with the much more frequent developmental and acquired encephalopathies and with primary epilepsy. Because of this, we shall give here a brief description and classification of both the epileptic seizures and epileptic syndromes before considering the relationship of epilepsy and HMDs.

Description and Classification of Childhood Seizures and Epileptic Syndromes   Seizures are more frequent and varied in childhood than in any other period of life. The child's nervous system appears to be more excitable and subject to a wider range of diseases that evoke seizures. The form which the seizure takes varies not only with the type and location of the pathologic process, but also with the stage of maturation of the nervous system.

Epileptic disorders are chronic and recurrent paroxysmal disorders resulting from the abnormal or excessive activity of cerebral neurons.

Beginning with Gastaut in 1969,[32,33] there have been several attempts to classify the many types of epilepsy, the last of which was published in 1989.[34] The value of an international classification is that it provides a common terminology by which clinicians can speak of the multiple and complex manifestations of epilepsy. It is now known that the different types of seizures may be related to specific causes and may require different treatments.

The Seizures States   Seizures are described as either partial or generalized (Table 6-7). In *simple partial seizures*, consciousness is not impaired. They may assume many forms: motor (including Jacksonian seizures and versive seizures), somatosensory, special sensory (e.g., visual, auditory, or olfactive hallucinations), or various psychic or affective symptoms. The EEG changes are focal. In *complex partial seizures*, consciousness is impaired initially or secondarily. Interruption or alteration of consciousness is frequently accompanied by characteristic motor automatisms and may be preceded by symptoms of "simple partial seizures," including psychosensorial phenomena (hallucinations, illusions), dysmnesic symptoms (déjà vu, feelings of strangeness), affective experiences (fear), and various other cognitive and psychic manifestations. Such a sequence of events

Table 6-6

Main causes of acute hemiplegia (stroke) in childhood and adolescence[a]

Hereditary disorders

Metabolic disorders

Homocystinuria (AR), Fabry disease (AR), MELAS (Mat), Menkes disease in infancy (AR), methylenetetrahydrofolate reductase deficiency (AR), hereditary dyslipoproteinemia (AD, AR),[b] phosphoglycerate kinase deficiency (X-linked recessive), amyloidosis* (AD). Cardiopathies in neurometabolic disorders may be a source of brain embolism.

Vascular dysplasias

Idiopathic Moya-Moya disease (AR)

Fibromuscular dysplasia (AD)

Neurofibromatosis (AD)

Connective tissue disorders*

Ehlers-Danlos IV disease (AD)

Pseudoxanthoma elasticum (AD, AR)

Progeria

Hematologic disorders

Sickle-cell anemia (AR)

Hereditary polycythemia (AD, AR)

Coagulopathies*

Heparin cofactor II deficiency (AD)

Protein C deficiency (AD)

Antithrombin III deficiency (AD)

Protein S deficiency (AD)

Deficiency in release of plasminogen activator (AD)

Platelet disorders

Cardiopathies (which may be sources of brain embolism)

Familial myxoma (AD)

Rhabdomyoma of tuberous sclerosis (AD)

Hereditary mitral valve prolapse (AD)

Hereditary conduction abnormalities (AD)

Hereditary cardiomyopathies (AD, AR)

Acquired disorders

Vascular dysplasias*

Angiomas and other vascular malformations, including cryptic vascular malformations

Cardiac disorders

Congenital heart disease, endocarditis, myocarditis, tumors, conduction defects

Vasculitis

Systemic lupus erythematosis, panarteritis

Infectious diseases

Bacterial meningitis, viral disease (herpes zoster)

Rasmussen encephalitis

HIV encephalitis

White matter disorders

Schilder disease, postinfectious leukoencephalitis, Hurst's hemorrhagic leukoencephalitis,* multiple sclerosis

Hematologic disorders*

Head trauma*

Arterial catheterization

Fat embolism

Acute idiopathic stroke

Abbreviations and symbols: AR = autosomal recessive; AD = autosomal dominant; Mat = maternal heredity; an asterisk (*) indicates a disease which may cause hemorrhagic strokes.

[a] With the exception of demyelinating disorders, the cause is usually a thromboembolic event.

[b] Including homozygous type II hyperlipoproteinemia (AD).

Table 6-7

Simplified classification of the epilepsies in childhood and adolescence[a]

Partial epilepsies (localization-related)
Idiopathic (or primary) epilepsies
  *Benign epilepsy with centrotemporal spikes (Rolandic epilepsy) (4–12 years)
  Childhood epilepsy with occipital spikes (childhood)
Symptomatic epilepsies
  *Partial seizures with simple or complex symptomatology; temporal lobe, frontal lobe, parietal lobe, occipital lobe epilepsies (after 4 years)

Generalized epilepsies
Idiopathic (or primary) generalized epilepsies
  *Typical absence epilepsy of childhood (4–8 years)
  Absence epilepsy of adolescence
  Benign myoclonic epilepsy of infancy
  *Juvenile myoclonic epilepsy
  *Grand mal epilepsy (generalized tonicoclonic seizures) of adolescence on awakening
Symptomatic generalized epilepsies: related to a specified lesion or cryptogenetic
  *Infantile spasms (West syndrome) (<1 year)[b]
  Early myoclonic encephalopathy (± burst-suppression EEG) (<3 months)[c]
  *A group of epilepsies starting between 1 and 6 years of age with sudden, brief seizures (tonic, atonic or myoclonic), atypical absence, frequent falls, mental retardation, and resistance to treatment. This group includes
    *Lennox-Gastaut syndrome[b]
    *Epilepsies with myoclonic-astatic seizures and with myoclonic absences

---

An asterisk (*) indicates the most frequent syndromes.

[a] See Refs. 33 to 35 for classification.

[b] May also be primary (occurring in a previously normal child).

[c] See Ref. 35.

---

occurs particularly in the temporal lobe epilepsies. Epilepsies originating in the frontal lobes also give rise to complex partial seizures. The EEG changes are variable and sometimes difficult to interpret. High quality MRI scans are now visualizing cortical dysgenesis and mesialtemporal sclerosis in an appreciable number of complex partial seizures.

In *generalized seizures*, initial motor symptoms and ictal EEG changes are bilateral. Consciousness is generally impaired and this may be the initial or only clinical expression of a seizure.

Generalized seizures include *absence seizures* which comprise the following:

• Typical absence seizures characterized by brief abrupt and numerous episodes of suspension of consciousness (occasionally accompanied by a minor motor phenomenon, by myoclonic contractions, or rarely, by automatisms) with bilateral symmetrical 3 Hz spike-wave discharges in the EEG. Occasionally there may be a prolonged petit mal status.

• Atypical absence seizures (less abrupt onset and cessation, more variable motor symptoms, and less typical EEG).

Other types of *generalized seizures* include clonic seizures, tonic seizures, tonico-clonic seizures (grand mal), atonic seizures, and myoclonic seizures with variable EEG changes.

Myoclonic seizures are characterized by sudden brief, shock-like muscular contractions lasting a fraction of a second. They may have a pattern that is either massive, bilateral and symmetrical, fragmentary, or random. Consciousness is usually retained. Myoclonic seizures are in general easily distinguished from action myoclonus (with which they may be associated in certain hereditary metabolic or degenerative diseases).

Neonatal seizures have been described in Chap. 2.

Epileptic Syndromes (*Table 6-7*)   A number of electroclinical epileptic syndromes have been delineated and tentatively classified on an etiological basis. Their classification has been difficult because of our imperfect knowledge of their pathophysiological mechanisms; the lack of any constant relationship between many epileptic syndromes and their etiology (i.e., the same syndrome may have several causes); and a variable importance given to one or another paroxysmal component. This accounts for some of the inconsistency in terminology, an ambiguity that is particularly evident in the so-called *myoclonic epilepsies.* Myoclonic jerks can occur in practically any type of epilepsy. Also, sudden and brief motor seizures may have different mechanisms and include not only myoclonus, but tonic or atonic phenomena as well. These differences may have prognostic and therapeutic implications. Generally speaking, in the severe myoclonic epilepsies of infancy and early childhood, the myoclonic seizures are usually associated with (and sometimes difficult to differentiate from) tonic seizures, atonic seizures, atypical absence, and possibly tonico-clonic or partial seizures. These complex "minor motor seizures," whatever their cause, generally have a bad prognosis. Conversely, there is a good prognosis for some of the epilepsies of late childhood with a predominant myoclonic component. This is true of benign juvenile myoclonic epilepsy, a well-defined and probably genetically determined entity.

In the classification of the epilepsies, a broad distinction is made between *primary* or *idiopathic* and *secondary* or *symptomatic* epilepsies. Primary epilepsies tend to be of genetic origin and generally have a benign self-limited course and a good response to treatment. Secondary epilepsies are symptomatic of known diseases (prenatal developmental defect, nonprogressive genetic disease, perinatal injury, metabolic disease) but may also be cryptogenic.

In general, it can be stated that the majority of epilepsies starting in infancy and early childhood before the age of 3 years are likely to be associated with a definitive brain disease and have a poor prognosis, whereas the primary epilepsies beginning in later childhood (after the age of 4 years) and in adolescence are more frequently benign.

A simplified presentation of the epilepsies and epileptic syndromes that we believe to be pertinent to our subject in this section is presented in Table 6-7. For further information the reader is referred to the *1989 Revised Classification of Epilepsies and Epileptic Syndromes,*[34] and related works.[33,35]

Epilepsy and the Hereditary Metabolic Disorders

In considering the possibility of a metabolic origin of seizures, (1) the type and pattern of seizures and (2)

the associated neurologic and visual abnormalities are of clinical importance.

(1) Types of Seizure Most types of generalized seizures, including infantile spasms, may be manifestations of a metabolic disease. However, typical absence seizures are an exception; they are not a feature of HMDs. A metabolic disease is only exceptionally the cause of typical Lennox-Gastaut syndrome. The same may be said of simple or complex partial seizures as isolated phenomena.

One pattern that should arouse suspicion of an underlying metabolic encephalopathy (among other causes), especially in infants and young children, is multiple myoclonic jerks involving all parts of the body in association with tonic seizures, atonic seizures, and atypical absences, usually referred to as *myoclonic epilepsy.* This seizure pattern frequently shows marked temporal variations. There are of course nonmetabolic causes of myoclonic epilepsies, and it must be concluded that there is no one seizure type and no epileptic syndrome which is specific for an HMD.

A special problem is posed by *isolated seizures.* In some of the slowly progressive HMDs, a few isolated generalized seizures may occur and continue for many months (or 1 or 2 years) before the other signs of an encephalopathy appear. This has been the case, in our experience, in patients with Lafora disease, the juvenile ceroid lipofuscinosis, and Sanfilippo mucopolysaccharidosis. The distinction between a primary and secondary epilepsy is for a time difficult or even impossible, especially when the EEG shows paroxysmal activities identical to those of a primary generalized epilepsy. Laboratory tests in search of an HMD are fully justified in patients with cryptogenic seizures only when there is a hint of cognitive deterioration (unrelated to status epilepticus or drug intoxication), or the development of some ocular, neurologic, or extraneurologic abnormalities (dysarthria, facial dysmorphism, changes in the eyegrounds), or when there is deterioration of the EEG background activity. In these cases paraclinical investigations include a search for vacuolated lymphocytes, x-rays of the skeleton, MRI, electroretinography and skin biopsy.

Nonconvulsive (absence) status epilepticus may occasionally have to be considered in the differential diagnosis of the intermittent hereditary metabolic disorders. Atypical absence status is relatively frequent in the Lennox-Gastaut syndrome; it is characterized by periods of apathy or stupor and erratic myoclonic jerks that cause incoordination of movements and an unsteady gait. This state lasts for several hours, a few days, or even weeks. A characteristic EEG tracing and an unu-sually rapid response to treatment help to differentiate it from metabolic disorders or an intoxication.

No EEG tracing is specific for any HMD with seizures, but the likelihood is greater with certain abnormalities. In Bielschowsky late infantile lipofusci-nosis, the high-amplitude occipital spikes induced by slow photic stimulaton are characteristic and help in diagnosis. A progressive flattening of the EEG over a relatively short period of time is seen in Alpers syndrome and in the Santavuori (early infantile) type of lipofusci-nosis. In the neonate and young infant, the tracing may be of the burst-suppression type, particularly in nonke-totic hyperglycinemia, but this pattern may have other causes, such as prenatal developmental defects of the brain. A progressive deterioration of the EEG back-ground activity (and possibly also a disruption of the sleep pattern) in a child with epileptic seizures should always suggest an underlying diffuse encephalopathy.

(2) Associated Neurologic and Visceral Abnormal-ities Indications of a metabolic origin of an encephalo-pathy producing epilepsy derive more importantly from other associated neurologic or visceral abnormalities than from the type and pattern of seizures. The follow-ing symptoms and signs are in favor of a progressive metabolic or degenerative disorder:

- Action myoclonus
- Progressive dysarthria and language difficulties
- Mental deterioration and/or behavioral distur-bances
- Characteristic dysmorphic, skeletal, or visceral abnormalities

The relationship between epilepsy and *cognitive derangement* is complex. A useful practical guideline, to which there are few exceptions, is that seizures per se usually do not cause relentless mental deterioration. We do not recognize the entity called epileptic demen-tia in idiopathic epilepsy. Nevertheless, cognitive dis-turbances do occur in the course of some epilepsies and they may be difficult to interpret. The mental sta-tus is not easy to assess in young patients with numer-ous subclinical seizures and heavy medication, both of which may interfere with mental processes. Some epi-lepsies, particularly West syndrome and Lennox-Gastaut syndrome, regularly are associated with an arrest in mental development and possibly a loss of previously acquired mental attainments as well. This deterioration is apparently self-limited. Serious changes

in behavior, particularly motor and mental inactivity, and aggressiveness are frequent features of the Lennox-Gastaut syndrome and of complex partial epilepsies. Psychotic signs may also occur in adolescents and adults with temporal lobe epilepsy, especially of the left side of the brain. In other complex types of epi-lepsy a striking defect in cognitive function sometimes improves with control of the epilepsy.[35a]

Because *language disturbances* may be an early sign in a number of HMDs, it is important to consider here the *Landau-Kleffner syndrome* of acquired aphasia with seizure disorder. This heterogeneous condition of unknown cause(s) starts usually between the ages of 4 and 7 years, either with aphasia or seizures. The lan-guage disorder develops over a short period of time. Verbal comprehension is severely affected along with elements of auditory agnosia. The child may appear to be deaf. Verbal expression is also abnormal. Seizures may or may not be present, but the EEG nearly always displays paroxysmal abnormalities. Hyperkinesia and violent behavior are frequent. The prognosis of the lan-guage defect is variable but, on the whole, it must be guarded. The pathologic basis of this syndrome has not been established. It may have more than one cause.

The Hereditary Metabolic Encephalopathies with Seizures Hereditary metabolic encephalopathies with seizures fall into three categories (see Table 6-8).

In some disorders, seizures are an obligatory sign. They include:

- Three conditions starting in the neonatal period or in infancy in which frequent seizures constitute the only or largely dominant neurologic manifestation (usually with an arrest of neurological development). One is pyridoxine dependency, a highly curable disease; another is the as yet incurable Alpers syndrome, in which there is also progressive brain atrophy, character-istic EEG pattern, and in many cases hepatic dysfunc-tion. Frequent and intractable seizures are also a feature of glucose transporter protein deficiency.

- The familial progressive myoclonic epilepsies of late childhood and adolescence, in which seizures of var-ious types and frequency are invariably associated with action myoclonus and other neurological signs. They include essentially three very different conditions: Unverricht-Lundborg disease (Baltic myoclonus) asso-ciated with nonspecific multifocal neuronal degenera-tion; Lafora disease in which specific intracytoplasmic inclusions arc found in neurons and other tissues; and

Table 0-0

Main hereditary metabolic and degenerative diseases with constant or frequent epileptic seizures[a]

Neonatal period and early infancy (<1 year of age)
Amino- and organoacidopathies including nonketotic hyperglycinemia +
Urea cycle disorders
Biotinidase deficiency +
Vitamin B_6 dependency + +
Alpers syndrome + +
Menkes disease +
Peroxisomal diseases
Mitochondrial diseases
Glucose transporter protein deficiency + +
Molybdenum cofactor deficiency +

Late infancy and early childhood (1 to 6 years)
Late infantile ceroid lipofuscinosis (NCL2)+
Sialidosis type II +
Other lysosomal storage disorders
Vitamin B_6 dependency + +
Biotinidase deficiency +
Alpers syndrome + +

Childhood and adolescence
Unverricht-Lundborg progressive myoclonic epilepsy (Baltic myoclonus) + +
Lafora disease + +
MERRF + +
Juvenile Gaucher disease +
Juvenile ceroid lipofuscinosis (NCL3)
Juvenile G_{M2} gangliosidosis
Acute intermittent porphyria
Mucopolysaccharidosis type III
Huntington disease

Abbreviations and symbols: + + = seizures are constant; + = seizures are very frequent.
[a] This table is not exhaustive.

MERRF, a disorder related to a defect in mitochondrial DNA.

There are other diseases in which seizures are a usual but inconstant clinical component. Seizures in this group are frequently described as myoclonic seizures, although they do not always conform to this somewhat elusive definition. But many patients do exhibit brief myoclonic, atonic, or tonic seizures, and atypical absence, possibly associated with intention myoclonus.

In the neonate and young infant the causes may be biotinidase deficiency, or one of the amino- or organoacidopathies (particularly nonketotic hyperglycinemia), Menkes disease, Zellweger disease, and neonatal adrenoleukodystrophy; in late infancy, NCL2 and other lysosomal diseases.

In late childhood and adolescence certain of the neuronal storage disorders, including juvenile Gaucher disease, juvenile ceroid lipofuscinosis, juvenile G_{M2} gangliosidosis, some cases of Sanfilippo disease, and Huntington disease are possible causes.

Interestingly, in some of the neuronal storage disorders the frequency of seizures is apparently a function of the age of onset of the disease. For instance, in the lipofuscinoses, seizures are much more prominent in the late infantile type than in the early infantile or juvenile forms. In early infantile G_{M2} gangliosidosis (Tay-Sachs disease), seizures are rare whereas they are relatively frequent in the juvenile variant. The reasons for these differences are not clear. As previously stated, there could be some relationship between brain maturation and seizure activity. Another tentative explanation is based on the rate of structural changes of affected neurons. Purpura[36] has shown that in the more chronic neuronal storage disorders there are progressive modifications of the cytoplasmic membranes of neurons, and the formation of new dendritic expansions, which may lead to aberrant intercellular connections. Changes in interneuronal circuitry could result in enhanced excitability of neurons.

Finally, in some HMD seizures are unusual. Only an occasional patient may be seen in whom frequent seizures are a major problem. Possibly in these patients the existence of an independent genetically determined epileptogenic factor reduces the seizure threshold.

Pathogenesis of Seizures The pathogenesis of seizures in the hereditary metabolic encephalopathies is not fully understood. How such abnormalities as the accumulation of organic acids or amino acids, or mitochondrial or peroxisomal deficiencies evoke seizure activity remains quite obscure. Hypoglycemia, electrolyte imbalance or hypoxia-ischemia are obvious factors in some cases. Some of the mitochondrial and peroxisomal disorders are known to produce prenatal cortical dysplasias, and these are known to be epileptogenic. As already stated, in the lysosomal storage diseases of childhood, progressive changes in interneuronal circuitry could have an epileptogenic effect.

In the late infantile and juvenile period it can be said that frequent seizures are essentially the consequence of gray matter lesions. White matter lesions are usually nonepileptic. But in some rare diseases presently classified as leukodystrophies (Alexander disease and Canavan disease) the cortex is also involved. A direct relationship between a biochemical abnormality and the occurrence of convulsions is most convincingly ascertained in vitamin B_6 dependency and in biotinidase deficiency, where supplementation with vitamin B_6 or with biotin eradicates seizures.

Summary

In a neonate or young infant with no immediate evidence of a perinatal or prenatal disorder or other possible etiologies, numerous intractable seizures or status epilepticus with major EEG changes and an abnormal neurologic development should always suggest the possibility of an HMD. Under these circumstances a systematic therapeutic trial with pyridoxine and with biotin is strongly recommended, and a search should be undertaken for an organoacidopathy or aminoacidopathy as well as a peroxisomal or a mitochondrial defect. In view of the relative frequency of aminoacidopathies and organoacidopathies, systematic protein restriction and administration of vitamins is warranted (see Chap. 2). If no cause is found, liver function should be assessed, especially in infants where brain atrophy has been documented by imaging techniques, since hepatic disorder is a usual feature of Alpers-Huttenlocher syndrome. Glucose levels in the CSF should be checked.

Nevertheless, intractable seizures during this period of life are far more often the consequence of prenatal events, such as a prenatal encephalitis, tuberous sclerosis, type I lissencephaly, and hemimegalencephaly, than of an HMD.

In children between the ages of 1 and 6 years, numerous brief epileptic phenomena, such as myoclonic or atonic seizures and atypical absence, usually associated with other seizure patterns, are a feature of a number of metabolic disorders, particularly neuronal storage disorders such as NCL2. The main disorder in differential diagnosis of this condition is the much more frequent Lennox-Gastaut syndrome, a cryptogenetic type of epilepsy characterized by axial tonic, atonic, and myoclonic seizures, atypical absence, and a failure of intellectual development. The EEG characteristically shows irregular 1–2 Hz slow spike-wave complexes and bursts of fast rhythms during sleep. In NCL2, slow spike-wave complexes are absent, but there is a remarkable response to slow photic stimulation in the EEG.

Seizures in late childhood and adolescence occasionally may be an early manifestation of an HMD, but they rarely remain for long as an isolated phenomenon. Progressive dysarthria, mental deterioration, action myoclonus ataxia, ophthalmologic signs, and nonneurologic abnormalities soon appear in various combinations.

Differential Diagnostic of Action Myoclonus (Polymyoclonus)

Action myoclonus (polymyoclonus), i.e., multiple, erratic, asynchronous muscle jerks precipitated by action, intentional movements, and emotional stimuli, is a sign of great diagnostic importance in a number of hereditary metabolic and degenerative diseases described mostly in Chap. 5 and listed in Table 5-6. In these diseases, polymyoclonus is always associated with other neurologic disturbances, essentially with cerebellar ataxia and seizures, frequently with dementia, and occasionally with extrapyramidal or ocular abnormalities. One must first distinguish polymyoclonus from other paroxystic phenomena.

Action myoclonus is relatively easy to distinguish from essential tremor, chorea, and tics. In *essential tremor*, the involuntary movement is usually the only sign. Rhythmic oscillations (with a frequency of 6–7 or 8–10 Hz) predominate in the distal part of the upper extremities. Absent at rest, they increase during maintenance of posture and voluntary movements. Myoclonus may be conjoined with tremor, particularly in benign essential myoclonus. *Chorea* consists of sudden, brusque, random, purposeless movements of the limbs slower than myoclonus (with a proximal predominance) as well as complex movements of the facial muscles. Hypotonia and pendular reflexes are usual. *Tics* are semipurposeful, repetitive, stereotyped contractions of functionally related muscle groups. Blinking, contraction of shoulder or neck muscles, sniffing, clearing the throat, and in some cases utterance of words, are usual manifestations. They may be briefly suppressed by an effort of will.

Startle disease (hyperexplexia) is an autosomal dominant condition starting in infancy. Auditory, visual, tactile, and proprioceptive stimuli evince a strikingly excessive involuntary contraction of trunk and limb muscles to which there is no habituation: the startle response. Some neonates also exhibit a persistent hypertonia (except during sleep), up to the age of 2 to 4 years. In these children, general stiffening of the body and loss of postural control may result in unprotected falls. As hypertonia decreases, myoclonic jerks of the limbs often appear, especially on falling asleep. Mutations have been identified in a subunit of the glycine receptor gene.

Differentiation with *cerebellar ataxia* and with *myoclonic seizures*, two conditions with which polymyoclonus is frequently associated, may sometimes be difficult. When multiple myoclonic jerks mar a volitional movement it may be mistaken for a cerebellar intention tremor. Sudden, brief, shock-like muscle contractions (associated with fast spike and waves or polyspikes on the EEG) occur in many types of seizures, particularly in the so-called myoclonic epilepsies of infancy or adolescence. This type of myoclonus may take many forms: brief bilateral and symmetric or unilateral contractions, massive spasms, and also erratic, asynchronous, segmental twitches which may be mistaken for polymyoclonus. In the myoclonic epilepsy of adolescence, for instance, single, segmental myoclonic shocks or serial jerks are manifest upon awakening. Massive myoclonic spasms are characteristic of West syndrome, and are also a feature of *benign myoclonus of early infancy* with a normal EEG, a condition which closely mimics West syndrome.

On the whole, myoclonic phenomena related to seizures occur usually at rest, are not enhanced by voluntary movements, and may be bilateral and symmetrical. These features are not encountered in polymyoclonus.

Pure polymyoclonus constitutes a striking and highly incapacitating symptom in two acquired disorders: *Kinsbourne myoclonus-opsoclonus syndrome*, and the *Lance and Adams syndrome*. Kinsbourne syndrome is encountered in infants and young children, and is usually related to a viral infection or a neuroblastoma. It is characterized by violent, erratic muscle jerks of the limbs at attempted movements, and brusque, chaotic eye movements and a palpebral flutter. The movement disorder is usually self-limited, with possible recurrence. Corticosteroids and removal of a neuroblastoma are generally effective.

In the Lance and Adams syndrome, a permanent and considerably incapacitating action myoclonus follows acute cerebral ischemia after cardiac arrest. There may be no other significant neurologic signs and intelligence is preserved. We have observed this type of myoclonus in infants, after accidental asphyxia, usually as a transitory phenomenon, and in some patients as a sequela of viral encephalitis. In subacute sclerosing panencephalitis (measles subacute or chronic encephalitis), muscle jerks are symmetrical, periodical, and usually less rapid and more complex than in other types of myoclonus. In the adult, disseminated myoclonus associated with dementia suggests Creutzfeld-Jacob disease. Rarely a segmental myoclonus may be a sign of a myelopathy. Benign essential familial myoclonus has been described in Chap. 5.

PRINCIPAL FEATURES AND DIFFERENTIAL DIAGNOSIS OF HEREDITARY METABOLIC AND DEGENERATIVE NEUROPATHIES

Diseases of the peripheral nervous system include the sensorimotor neuropathies, and the primary motor and sensory neuronopathies (by *neuronopathy* we refer to disease affecting the entire neuron, not just its axon or myelin sheath).

Most *neuropathies* give rise to various combinations of motor, sensory, and occasionally autonomic disturbances. Nerve conduction velocities (NCVs) and sensory nerve action potentials are abnormal. In disorders affecting *the lower motor neuron* (motor neuron disease, anterior horn cell disease, motor neuronopathies) the clinical manifestations are exclusively motor. NCVs are not significantly affected in most cases. Sensory changes alone typify the *hereditary sensory neuropathies and neuronopathies* due to a selective involvement of the primary sensory neurons.

Sensorimotor Neuropathies

General Features All the sensorimotor neuropathies are manifested by weakness, sensory loss, areflexia, denervation atrophy, and sometimes autonomic disturbances. In most chronic neuropathies there is segmental myelin degeneration or both axon and myelin degeneration. Sensory disturbances may involve all sensory modalities but are often restricted to certain types of loss because of a selective pattern of sensory fiber involvement. Demyelination and axonal degeneration restricted to large fibers result in loss of the proprioceptive input from muscle and disturbance of joint position and vibratory senses. The sensory symptoms resulting from selective degeneration of large sensory neurons in dorsal root ganglia, as in Friedreich ataxia, are similar. In most hereditary sensorimotor polyneuropathies there is mainly a defect of proprioceptive sensation. Small fiber lesions result in a selective loss of pain and temperature sensation (pseudosyringomyelic syndrome). The autonomic disturbances are the consequence of lesions of the sympathetic and the sacral parasympathetic ganglion cells. Their clinical expression includes abnormalities of pupillary function, orthostatic hypotension, gastrointestinal and genitourinary symptoms, and disorders of sweating. Dysautonomic symptoms are prominent in the amyloid polyneuropathies, in the Riley-Day syndrome, in Fabry disease, and in certain neuropathies of diabetes mellitus.

In terms of their *topography* (distribution), peripheral neuropathies can be divided into two categories: the bilateral generalized symmetric polyneuropathies and the focal or multifocal neuropathies (mononeuropathy and mononeuropathy multiplex). These patterns may guide one to etiological diagnosis.

In the symmetric polyneuropathies the lower limbs are predominantly affected and there is generally a distal distribution of muscle weakness, atrophy, and sensory deficit with sparing of the trunk. A proximal distribution of weakness is rare, but is occasionally seen in acute intermittent porphyria and Tangier disease. Upper limb predominance in symmetric polyneuropathies may be observed in Tangier disease, porphyria, and amyloid neuropathies.

Focal and multifocal neuropathies are rarely observed in the HMDs. One thinks, instead, of a nonfamilial disorder such as diabetes mellitus, panarteritis, or trauma, or of familial compressive mononeuropathy. However, entrapment of a single nerve, especially in the carpal tunnel syndrome, may accompany one of the mucopolysaccharidoses.

In terms of their *pathophysiology*, generalized polyneuropathies can be divided into those with primary segmental demyelination and those with primary neuroaxonal degeneration, but this distinction is not always valid. In primary segmental demyelination there is a reduction in motor and sensory nerve conduction velocities, whereas primary neuroaxonal degeneration produces motor NCVs that are only slightly diminished or normal; sensory nerve conduction velocities are generally reduced and the voltage of sensory nerve action potentials markedly depressed.

Diagnosis of a Peripheral Polyneuropathy In many cases the diagnosis of a peripheral neuropathy can be established on clinical grounds alone. Characteristic is a combination of muscle weakness, amyotrophy, sensory loss, and tendon areflexia in a distribution compatible with the involvement of peripheral nerves. The relative importance, type, and topography of motor, sensory, and autonomic phenomena, and the temporal course, may help in etiological diagnosis.

Confirmation of the diagnosis of a neuropathy and indications of its type are based on studies of *nerve conduction velocity and sensory action potential.* Early in the course of the disease or when tendon reflexes are not yet abolished, and sensory disturbances and weakness are uncertain (as may be the case in young children, and in the frequent *formes frustes* in adolescent and adult patients), diagnosis rests nearly entirely on electrophysiological data. But one must be cautious in interpreting minor changes in electrophysiological tests because they may only represent variations of normal.[37] Some researchers incorrectly report a modest decrease of nerve conduction velocity as proof of peripheral nerve dysfunction. Altered NCVs do not necessarily indicate a structural alteration of the peripheral nerves; phenytoin may induce a transient metabolic disturbance, and low body temperature at the time of the recording may temporarily impair nerve conduction. For all these reasons one should always interpret electrophysiological data with respect to the clinical status of the patient.

Quantitative structural assessment of a sural nerve biopsy specimen is sometimes necessary for the diagnosis of a neuropathy.

In some peripheral neuropathies, particularly Charcot-Marie-Tooth disease, unsteadiness of gait or tremor may be important signs. They may raise problems in clinical interpretation and in differential diagnosis. Unsteadiness of stance and gait may result from both a defect of proprioceptive sensation and muscle weakness. Unsteadiness caused by muscle weakness is usually more evident in standing and is not enhanced by eye-closure (absent Romberg sign). Postural tremor of the upper extremities is striking in some patients (Roussy-Levy variant of CMT disease). It may resemble action tremor.[37] In some instances it is probably the consequence of a defect in proprioceptive muscle afferents; in others it may represent an associated familial tremor. In either case, when there is a defect of proprioceptive sensation with tremor, one must first consider the diagnosis of Friedreich ataxia.

Diagnosis of Hereditary Metabolic and Degenerative Polyneuropathies During childhood and adolescence an HMD or a familial degenerative disease are the most frequent causes of chronic peripheral nerve disorders. In the adult the usual causes are diabetes, paraneoplastic polyneuropathies, angiopathies, dysproteinemias, paraproteinemias, alcoholism and other nutritional deficiencies, and occasionally HIV infection. The prevalence of diabetic polyneuropathy in childhood is low, estimated at less than 2 percent. In a series of 25 consecutive admissions of diabetic children under the age of 16 years, only four had clinical evidence of a neuropathy.[37] We observed a severe sensory neuropathy in a 16-year-old diabetic girl. The lesional pattern, topography, and clinical expression of polyneuropathies are quite variable in HMDs.

(1) In a Number of Hereditary Metabolic Disorders a Demyelinating Neuropathy is a Constant or Major Feature and Frequently the Presenting Clinical Sign Involvement of the peripheral nerves follows several patterns:

(a) In most diseases in this category, there is a *slowly progressive, predominantly motor and, to a lesser extent, sensory demyelinating* polyneuropathy. Charcot-Marie-Tooth type I (HMSN I) and Dejerine-Sottas disease (HMSN III) are notable in this group because of their relative frequency and the fact that they are caused by genetic defects that affect selectively peripheral myelin proteins. HMSN I represents the most typical example of an isolated distal, symmetrical, slowly progressive, demyelinating polyneuropathy. HMSN III starts usually in childhood or infancy

and has a more rapidly progressive course. Electrophysiological studies are necessary to differentiate HMSN I from the clinically similar HMSN II—an axonal disorder of genetic cause—and from *distal spinal muscular atrophy*, a disorder of the lower motor neuron (neuronopathy). Both conditions display the Charcot-Marie-Tooth phenotype (see Chap. 5). In HMSN I, motor and sensory nerve conduction velocities are decreased. In HMSN II, motor nerve conduction velocities are practically normal and sensory action potentials are depressed. In the spinal muscular atrophies, motor nerve conduction velocities are normal or slightly altered and sensory nerve conduction velocities and action potentials are normal.

An infantile or juvenile lower motor neuron disorder, *Wolfhart-Kugelberg-Welander syndrome*, is usually easy to differentiate from the hereditary motor and sensory neuropathies. Here, weakness predominates in the proximal muscles of the lower limbs, sensory nerve conduction velocities and action potentials are normal, motor nerve conduction velocities are not significantly altered, and there is denervation atrophy. Early in the course of HMSN I and HMSN II and other polyneuropathies, distinction between a peripheral neuropathy and motor difficulties of central origin may not be easy: tendon reflexes may be present, deformity of the feet and distal amyotrophy are not obvious, and sensory abnormalities are difficult to detect. In these cases also, as in the numerous "formes frustes" of the Charcot-Marie-Tooth syndrome, electrophysiologic studies are essential for diagnosis (see Chap. 5).

Severe late infantile cases of Déjerine-Sottas disease must be distinguished from late infantile metachromatic leukodystrophy. Enzyme assays of arylsulfatase A and measurements of sulfatides in the urine are recommended in all children with a progressive polyneuropathy starting in the second or third year of life. When HMSN III starts in early infancy (viz. congenital forms of hypomyelinative polyneuropathy), the differential diagnosis includes *Krabbe disease, Werdnig-Hoffmann disease and the congenital myopathies*. In Werdnig-Hoffmann disease, an autosomal recessive motor neuron disease, muscle weakness predominates in the proximal segment of the limbs; pronation of the forearms, early and severe paresis of the intercostal muscles, and lingual fasciculation are characteristic. Intelligence is normal. In the congenital myopathies and myotonic dystrophy, involvement of the facial and neck muscles and dysphagia, are typical when present. Mentation may be affected. In congenital muscular dystrophy, arthrogryposis may be present and cerebral defects are frequently associated.

In other metabolic disorders with a constant, symmetric, essentially motor demyelinating polyneuropathy, there are always associated abnormalities of the central nervous system or other organs. Refsum disease and late infantile metachromatic leukodystrophy are two examples (Table 6-9).

In most patients with early infantile Krabbe leukodystrophy and in many with late infantile metachromatic leukodystrophy, the demyelinating neuropathy—anatomically a constant feature—is largely subclinical and associated with evidence of corticospinal tract disturbance. Lesions of the peripheral nerves may be suspected if tendon reflexes are absent and/or conduction velocities are impaired.

(b) Signs of *sensory and autonomic systems* involvement are in the foreground in some HMDs. When a predominantly sensory polyneuropathy with dissociated pain and temperature sensory loss is present, amyloid polyneuropathy is the leading diagnosis, but Tangier disease and other rare conditions listed in Table 6-9 must be considered. Occasionally, the upper limbs are predominantly involved. Dysfunction of the autonomic nervous system is a prominent feature of amyloid polyneuropathy. Boys with Fabry disease have lesions in both the central and peripheral autonomic systems manifested by episodes of burning pain and paresthesias, especially during febrile illnesses and physical activity. These are frequently the first indications of the disorder. Some of the patients are mistakenly labeled hysteric. *The hereditary sensory and autonomic neuropathies* (HSAN) constitute another group. These are listed in Table 6-10 with their principal characteristics. This group includes (1) a dominantly inherited disorder with onset in the second decade or later and a progressive course, characterized by plantar ulcers and sensory loss in the distal part of the lower extremities (ulcerative and mutilating acropathy of Thevenard, HSAN I); and (2) a group of congenital, nonprogressive autosomal recessive sensory and autonomic polyneuropathies affecting all four limbs (HSAN II to V), the most frequent of which are familial dysautonomia (Riley-Day syndrome, HSAN III) and HSAN II. Sensory and autonomic symptoms are also features of *diabetic neuropathies.*

In Friedreich ataxia and other conditions with the Friedreich phenotype (see Chap. 5), involvement of the primary sensory neuron is an essential element of the lesional pattern. There is a selective degeneration of the larger neurons of dorsal root ganglia and loss of large myelinated fibers (which convey proprioception)

in the peripheral nerves, posterior roots, and posterior columns of the spinal cord. The lower motor neuron may be slightly involved later in the disease.

(c) A hereditary metabolic disorder may also give rise to *an acute or subacute peripheral nerve syndrome*. An acute, predominantly motor polyneuropathy, which may be most marked in either the lower or in the upper limbs, is a feature of acute intermittent porphyria and type II tyrosinemia. The main differential diagnoses of acute intermittent porphyria are the *Guillain-Barré syndrome, acute metal poisoning*, and *drug abuse*. The association with abdominal pain and psychiatric symptoms, and possibly the existence of a typical precipitating factor (e.g., ingestion of barbiturates), usually makes the distinction relatively easy. In some cases the conjunction of paresis and psychic manifestations may suggest hysteria. An apparently acute or subacute onset or acute exacerbations of a chronic sensorimotor neuropathy are frequently observed in Refsum disease. Then they must be differentiated from a *chronic relapsing demyelinating inflammatory polyneuropathy*, a more common disease. Nerve biopsy reveals focal inflammation and myelin destruction. There may be serum antibodies against myelin proteins. Steroids are usually an effective treatment. Acute or subacute recurrent episodes of focal neuropathies are also observed in two disorders with an autosomal dominant mode of inheritance: *inherited brachial plexus neuropathy* and *inherited tendency to develop pressure palsies*.

(2) In Other Metabolic Disorders a Demyelinating Polyneuropathy Is an Inconstant and Largely Subclinical Manifestation Segmental demyelination of peripheral nerves has been documented in sural nerve biopsies in a number of patients with Leigh disease, ataxia-telangiectasia, and the other metabolic disorders listed in Table 6-9. Here, involvement of the peripheral nervous system—which is not constant—is frequently subclinical or expressed only by tendon areflexia, slight sensory deficits, or muscular atrophy that exceeds that of disuse. Nerve conduction velocities are decreased.

(3) In many other HMDs, including Niemann-Pick type A disease, mucopolysaccharidoses, oligosaccharidoses, and sialidoses, a segmental demyelination or axonal loss has been reported in *an occasional patient*, or a neuropathy has been suspected because of a reduction of nerve conduction velocities. Some of the data, especially slight alterations of nerve conduction velocities, are difficult to interpret and there is a tendency to

Table 6-9

Involvement of the peripheral nerves and lower motor neuron in the hereditary metabolic and degenerative disorders

---

HMDs with a polyneuropathy (PN) as a constant or frequent component, may inaugurate the disease, or be detected only by NCV studies[a]

Sensorimotor (essentially motor) demyelinating PN
  Refsum disease
  Late infantile and, less constantly, juvenile metachromatic leukodystrophy
  Multiple sulfatase deficiency
  Early infantile and, less constantly, juvenile Krabbe disease
  Cockayne syndrome
  Long-chain 3-hydroxyacyl-CoA dehydrogenase deficiency
  Adult polyglucosan disease
  Rare juvenile peroxisomal disorder

Demyelinating PNs with predominantly sensory and/or autonomic dysfunction
  Familial amyloid neuropathies
  Fabry disease
  Tangier disease
  Neuropathy, ataxia, and retinitis pigmentosa (NARP)
  Neuroacanthyocytosis
  Friedreich ataxia[b]
  Hereditary folate malabsorption

Acute or subacute recurrent PNs
  Acute intermittent porphyria
  Tyrosinemia type I
  Refsum disease (acute exacerbations)

Axonal neuropathies
  Neuroaxonal dystrophy
  Schindler disease
  Giant axonal neuropathy
  Lowe syndrome?
  Tyrosinemia type I
  MPS III?
  Friedreich ataxia[b]
  Ataxia with vitamin E deficiency (AVED)[c]
  Adult polyglucosan disease

HMDs with documented PNs in some patients[d]

Leigh disease
Ataxia-telangiectasia
Xeroderma pigmentosum
Marinesco-Sjögren syndrome
Cholestanolosis
MPS III
Chediak-Higashi disease
Hyperoxaluria type I
Abetalipoproteinemia[e]
Adrenomyeloneuropathy
Neonatal adrenoleukodystrophy
Mitochondrial trifunctional enzyme deficiency

Entrapment mononeuropathies; carpal tunnel syndrome

Mucopolysaccharidoses; oligosaccharidoses

Table 6-9 (contd.)

Lower motor neuron dysfunction
Chronic form of G_{M2} gangliosidosis
Juvenile Sandhoff disease (1 case)
Neuronal nuclear inclusion disease
Glycogenesis II?
Farber disease?

Cranial nerves palsies (see also Table 6-12)
Abetalipoproteinemia
Tangier disease
Déjerine-Sottas disease
AI porphyria
Giant axonal neuropathy
Intranuclear neuronal inclusion disease

---

[a] HMSN I to III in which the peripheral neuropathy is the only disorder are not listed here (see text). Nerve biopsy studies are necessary or useful for diagnosis in: neuroaxonal dystrophy, giant axonal dystrophy, adult polyglucosan disease, familial amyloid neuropathy, Krabbe leukodystrophy, and metachromatic leukodystrophy (see also Table 8-1).

[b] In Friedreich ataxia there is essentially a loss of large primary neurons in dorsal root ganglia (explaining tabetic ataxia). Lower motor neurons may be slightly affected.

[c] Pathology probably as in Friedreich ataxia.

[d] Not cited here are HMDs in which a subclinical neuropathy has only been reported in an occasional patient or has not been sufficiently documented.

[e] Lesions are essentially those of Friedreich ataxia.

attach no clinical significance to these fortuitous findings.

Axonal Neuropathies in the HMDs   In a few infantile HMDs with marked hypotonia and hypomotility, absence of tendon reflexes, EMG evidence of denervation atrophy, and normal conduction velocities, the possibility of an axonal neuropathy has been assumed. In Lowe syndrome, denervation atrophy and mild slowing of nerve conduction velocities have been reported, but to our knowledge, there has been no pathological verification of such changes. In hereditary tyrosinemia, electrophysiologic and pathologic studies have shown the polyneuropathy to be of axonal type.

Hereditary degenerative sensorimotor axonal neuropathies with no established metabolic origin include neuroaxonal dystrophy, HMSN II, and giant axonal neuropathy.

Mononeuropathies   Deformity of joints and dysostosis may result in entrapment of individual nerve trunks in the mucopolysaccharidoses and oligosaccharidoses. In these conditions, a carpal tunnel syndrome with its painful paresthesias is the most common.

Lower Motor Neuronopathies in HMDs

In some patients with a chronic form of G_{M2} gangliosidosis and in the majority of cases of neuronal intranuclear inclusion disease, there are patent signs of lower motor neuron dysfunction: areflexia, muscle weakness, amyotrophy, fasciculations, electromyographic evidence of denervation atrophy, and relatively normal nerve conduction velocities. Although central nervous system lesions are always present, the clinical picture may mimic a spinal muscular atrophy. In glycogenosis type II, neuronal storage in anterior horn cells could partly explain the hypotonia and depressed tendon reflexes. EMG evidence of denervation atrophy has been reported in Farber disease (see Table 6-9).

Involvement of Cranial Nerves in HMDs

Progressive paralysis of cranial nerves is a rare event in HMDs with one notable exception: Kearns-Sayre syndrome and the syndrome of progressive external ophthalmoplegia seen in other mitochondrial disorders. Oculomotor and other cranial nerve palsies may also be observed in Leigh disease, in early infantile Gaucher disease, in some instances of maple syrup urine disease, and in a few other conditions (Tables 6-9 and 6-11).

Table 6-10
The hereditary sensory and autonomic neuropathies (HSANs)[a]

Classification	Heredity	Main symptoms and signs	Lesions of peripheral nerves
HSAN I	AD	Onset in second or third decade; slowly progressive; plantar ulcers; stress fractures; bone resorption in feet; burning or lancinating pain in feet; loss of pain and thermal sensation (± other modalities) in distal part of lower limbs; depressed ankle reflex (late); decreased sensory nerve action potentials; no muscle weakness or atrophy. *Variants:* with spastic paraplegia, with peroneal muscle atrophy, with deafness	Loss of fibers, predominantly small myelinated and unmyelinated fibers
HSAN II	AR	Onset at birth, not progressive; upper and lower limbs affected; sensory loss affecting all modalities; ulcers of fingers and feet; whitlows, paronychia, Charcot joints; sweating loss; absence of sensory nerve action potentials; no amyotrophy	Virtual absence of myelinated fibers; decreased numbers of unmyelinated fibers
HSAN III (familial dysautonomia, Riley-Day syndrome)	AR Ashkenazic Jews	Onset at birth; vomiting and swallowing difficulties; autonomic disturbances (defective lacrimation, defective temperature control, excessive perspiration, skin blotching, postural hypotension, etc.); insensitivity to pain; corneal insensitivity; automutilation (oral and other); areflexia; poor coordination; emotional lability; kyphoscoliosis; absence of fungiform papillae of the tongue; abnormality of catecholamine metabolism. *Main signs:* autonomic signs; absence of fungiform papillae; Jewish origin	Normal density of myelinated fibers; marked decrease in the number of unmyelinated fibers; decrease in number of neurons in autonomic and spinal ganglia; moderate involvement of the CNS
HSAN IV (familial sensory neuropathy with anhydrosis)	AR Rare	Congenital; insensitivity to pain leading to mutilations; anhydrosis; loss of temperature sensation; mild mental retardation	Virtual absence of unmyelinated fibers; myelinated fibers present; absence of small neurons in spinal ganglia
HSAN V	Rare, uncertain nosology	Congenital; selective loss of pain sensation (other modalities normal); sudomotor dysfunction; muscle strength and tendon reflexes normal; sensory nerve evoked potentials normal. *Differential diagnosis:* congenital indifference to pain	Decrease of small myelinated fibers and unmyelinated fibers

Abbreviations: AD = autosomal dominant; AR = autosomal recessive.

[a] Some cases of HSAN have been difficult to classify. In some kindreds HSAN has been associated with other neurologic, ocular, or skeletal manifestations. For further details on HSAN and their variants see Ref. 37.

Table 6-11
Ocular abnormalities[a]

Diseases	Retinal degeneration PDR	CRS macular degeneration	Early OA	Corneal clouding	Lenticular opacities (cataracts)	Early visual failure[b]		Other important ocular abnormalities
						Pre	Post	
Zellweger disease	++				++			Glaucoma; Brushfield spots
Other peroxisomal disorders with Zellweger phenotype	++							
X-linked adrenoleukodystrophy			+			++	++	
Early infantile G_{M2} gangliosidosis		+++CRS				++		
Late infantile or juvenile G_{M2} gangliosidosis	+	++	+					Possible CRS; oculomotor disorder
Early infantile G_{M1} gangliosidosis		++CRS						
Early infantile Niemann-Pick disease		++CRS						
Farber disease		++		+	+			CRS in late infantile form and occasionally in early form
Metachromatic leukodystrophy		++						Visual failure usually late in disease
Multiple sulfatase deficiency		++						
Late-onset Krabbe leukodystrophy			++			++	++	
Sudanophilic leukodystrophies			+					
Pelizaeus-Merzbacher disease			++					Pendular nystagmus
Cockayne syndrome	+++				++			
Canavan disease			+++					
Leigh disease			+					Oculomotor abnormalities
MILS	+++							
Kearns-Sayre syndrome and mitochondrial PEO syndrome	+++							Progressive external ophthalmoplegia
MERRF	+		+					
MELAS	+						++	Transient blindness or hemianopsia

(continued)

Table 6-11 (contd.)

Diseases	Retinal degeneration PDR	CRS macular degeneration	Early OA	Corneal clouding	Lenticular opacities (cataracts)	Early visual failure[b]		Other important ocular abnormalities
						Pre	Post	
NARP	+ + +							Neuropathy; ataxia
Leber optic neuropathy						+ + + subacute		Retrobulbar neuropathy Retinal edema
AD myopathy with deletions of mtDNA					+ +			Ophthalmoplegia (PEO)
Mitochondrial trifunctional enzyme deficiency	+ +							
LCHAD	+							
Galactosemia					+ + +			Intraocular hemorrhages ±
Lowe disease				+	+ + +			Glaucoma + + Megalocornea
Menkes disease	+							Microcyst of iris and pigmentary epithelium of retina
Alpers syndrome							+ +	
Neuroaxonal dystrophy			+ +					
Biotinidase deficiency			+					
Homocystinuria					+			Ectopia lentis + + + Myopia + + + Glaucoma Retinal detachment
Combined deficiency of MM and MHM (Cbl C group)	+ +							
Sulfite oxidase deficiency								Ectopia lentis + + +
Mevalonic acidemia					+			
3-Methylglutaconic acidemia	+							
Hyperornithinemia	+ + +							Gyrate atrophy of the retina
MPS I H; H/S; S	+ +			+ + +				
MPS II	+ +							
MPS III	+ +							
ML II	+			±				Corneal clouding very rare
ML III	+			+ + +				
ML IV	+ + +			+ + +				

Table 6-11 (contd.)

Diseases	Retinal degeneration PDR	CRS macular degeneration	Early OA	Corneal clouding	Lenticular opacities (cataracts)	Early visual failure[b] Pre	Early visual failure[b] Post	Other important ocular abnormalities
α-Mannosidosis				++	++			
β-Mannosidosis								Tortuosity of retinal vessels
Fucosidosis III	+							Tortuosity of retinal vessels
Aspartylglucosaminuria					+			
Sialidosis type I		+++CRS						
Sialidosis type II		++CRS						
CDG syndrome	++							
Lipofuscinoses (NCL)	+++					+++ juvenile NCL		
Refsum disease	+++				+			
Familial amyloid neuropathy								Vitreous amyloid deposits ++ Corneal lattice dystrophy
Tangier disease				++				
Fabry disease				+++	++			Tortuosity of conjunctival and retinal vessels
Giant axonal neuropathy			++					
Acute intermittent porphyria							++	Transient amaurosis
Cholestanolosis					+++			
Ataxia-telangiectasia								Conjunctival telangiectasia ++ Disorder of conjugate gaze ++
Wilson disease								Kayser-Fleisher corneal ring +++

(continued)

Table 6-11 (contd.)

Diseases	Retinal degeneration PDR	CRS macular degeneration	Early OA	Corneal clouding	Lenticular opacities (cataracts)	Early visual failure[b]		Other important ocular abnormalities
						Pre	Post	
Hallervorden-Spatz disease	++							
Friedreich disease			±					
AD spinocerebellar and cerebellar ataxias	++		++					
Abetalipoproteinemia	++							
Strümpell-Lorrain familial paraplegia	++							
Sjögren-Larsson syndrome	++							

Abbreviations and symbols: NARP = neuropathy, ataxia, and retinitis pigmentosa; LCHAD = long-chain 3-hydroxyacyl-CoA dehydrogenase deficiency; PDR = pigmentary degeneration of retina; OA = optic atrophy; CRS = cherry red spot; CDG = carbohydrate-deficient glycoprotein syndrome; AD = autosomal dominant; ML = mucolipidosis; MPS = mucopolysaccharidosis; MHM = methyltetrahydrofolate: homocysteine methyltransferase; MILS = maternally inherited Leigh syndrome; PEO = progressive external ophthalmoplegia; +++ = constant or very frequent and/or of major diagnostic value; ++ = frequent or important; + = occasional or less significant; ± = rare.

[a] Oculomotor disorders are listed in Table 6-10.

[b] Pre = pregeniculate; Post = postgeniculate.

Paralyses of oculomotor nerves are to be differentiated from supranuclear palsies (see below).

In childhood by far the most common cause of progressive paralysis of cranial nerves is an infiltrating tumor of the brain stem. Other causes include myasthenia gravis, sarcomas and lymphomas of the meninges, some cases of Arnold-Chiari malformation, and two rare familial disorders: progressive bulbar paralysis of Fazio-Londe and the Van Laere syndrome.

Fazio-Londe syndrome,[38] a progressive degeneration of cranial nerve nuclei, starts between ages 2 and 10, usually by a paralysis of the abductors of the vocal cords (Xth cranial nerves), followed by a progressive involvement of other cranial nerves. Death from asphyxia generally ensues within a few years. The disorder is inherited as an autosomal recessive trait. Some cases of progressive bulbar paralysis have been reported with a more prolonged course.

Van Laere syndrome,[39] also an autosomal recessive disorder, starts in adolescence or adulthood and has a protracted course. Progressive hearing loss precedes involvement of other cranial nerves.

OCULAR ABNORMALITIES

Visual failure; disturbances of oculomotricity; and abnormalities of the retina, lens, cornea, and conjunctiva have special significance in the diagnosis of HMD. Significant ocular abnormalities occur in approximately 45 of these conditions and are of major diagnostic importance in at least 25 disorders (see Tables 6-11 and 6-12).

Visual Failure

Amblyopia or blindness may result from lesions at different levels of the visual system: retina, optic nerves and tracts, retrogeniculate optic tracts, and visual cortex. Cataracts, corneal clouding, or glaucoma are other possible causes.

Lesions of the *retina* in HMDs involve either the ganglion cell layer, which comprises the output neurons of the retina whose axons form the optic nerve; or the sensory epithelium, which includes the photoreceptors (the rods and cones) and is apposed to the pigment epithelium. Storage of sphingolipids and possibly other substances (oligosaccharides) in *ganglion cells*, predominantly in the perimacular region, gives rise to the classic macular cherry red spot appearance of the retina. Other types of macular degeneration, probably related to lipid storage in ganglion cells, are also observed (Table 6-11).

Degeneration of the *sensory and pigmentary epithelium of the retina* is known as pigmentary degeneration of the retina, retinitis pigmentosa, or tapetoretinal degeneration. Its ophthalmoscopic appearance is characteristic, although somewhat variable, and there are constant and typical alterations of the electroretinogram (ERG) which often precede the fundoscopic changes. The first clinical manifestations of retinitis pigmentosa are night blindness, intolerance to bright light, and peripheral constriction of the visual fields, but these particularities are frequently overlooked. Pigmentary retinopathy is found in a wide variety of HMDs, including lysosomal, mitochondrial, and peroxisomal diseases. Visual failure may be the first clinical manifestation of these HMDs, so, initially, it can be very difficult to differentiate them from primary degeneration of the retina, in which the disease process is restricted to the eyes.

Primary degeneration of the retina, transmitted as an autosomal dominant, autosomal recessive, or X-linked trait, is the major cause of hereditary blindness. Its frequency, however, should not prevent the clinician from thinking about an HMD. Among the most common HMDs with early amblyopia due to retinitis pigmentosa are ceroid lipofuscinoses and Refsum disease.

Retinitis pigmentosa may also be a part of nonprogressive and nonmetabolic hereditary syndromes, not infrequently in combination with deafness (Leber's congenital amaurosis, Usher syndrome, Laurence-Moon syndrome, and Alström syndrome).

Lesions of the **optic nerves** with blindness and optic atrophy may occur early in the course of Canavan disease, neuroaxonal dystrophy, Lafora disease, Leigh disease, juvenile Krabbe leukodystrophy and adrenoleukodystrophy (in Krabbe leukodystrophy and adrenoleukodystrophy, blindness may also result from lesions of the retrogeniculate visual tracts). The ERG is always normal. The possibility of an HMD should therefore always be considered in a child with apparently isolated optic atrophy and no evidence of a tumor compressing or infiltrating the optic nerve chiasm. One should be cautious in interpreting the role of a subchiasmatic arachnoidal cyst or arachnoiditis. We have observed a patient with juvenile Krabbe disease in which optic atrophy was at first thought to result from the compression by a suprasellar cyst and who was subjected to needless craniotomy.

When an HMD causes progressive involvement of the retina and optic nerve, the first manifestations of

Table 6-12
Disorders of ocular movements

Disease	Supranuclear disturbance of conjugate gaze and saccades[a]	Nuclear ophthalmoplegia (oculomotor palsies)	Nystagmus[b]
Gaucher disease type II	+++	++	
Gaucher disease type III	+++ vertical gaze		
Niemann-Pick disease type C	+		+
Juvenile G_{M2} gangliosidosis	+	+	
Leigh disease	++		+
Ataxia-telangiectasia	+++		+
Huntington disease	+++		
Kearns-Sayre syndrome		+++ PEO	
Progressive external ophthalmoplegia[c]		+++	
Friedreich disease	+		+
Abetalipoproteinemia	+	+	
Tangier disease			++
AD spinocerebellar and cerebellar ataxias	++		
Pelizaeus-Merzbacher disease			+++ pendular
Maple syrup urine disease		+ fluctuating	
Dominant mitochondrial encephalomyopathy with multiple deletions of mtDNA		+++ PEO	
mtDNA depletion syndrome		+	
Familial amyloid polyneuropathy (FAP IV)		++	
Fumarate deficiency	+		
Neuronal intranuclear inclusion disease	++	++	

Abbreviations and symbols: PEO = progressive external ophthalmoplegia; AD = autosomal dominant; +++ = practically constant or of major importance; ++ = frequent or important; + = occasional or less significant.

[a] For a description of disorders of saccades see Leigh DS, *The Neurology of Eye Movements*. Philadelphia, FA Davis, 1991.

[b] Nystagmus of various types; frequently poorly described; nystagmus related to amblyopia excluded.

[c] Sporadic, maternally inherited, or autosomal dominant.

visual failure are often unnoticed in young children and loss of vision may then appear to have been abrupt. The differential diagnosis of such cases includes diseases with acute visual failure such as multiple sclerosis, postinfectious optic neuritis and pseudo-tumor cerebri. In these conditions, blindness occurs abruptly, may be unilateral, and the ophthalmoscopic features and clinical context are characteristic. Leber optic neuropathy, a disorder due to point mutations in mtDNA, may also have a subacute onset.

Lesions in the *retrogeniculate optic pathways and visual cortex* are rarely a cause of early loss of vision in HMDs. A notable exception is adrenoleukodystrophy. Here, the optic radiations are generally involved at an early stage by the parieto-occipital demyelinating process; the visual field defects may be accompanied by visual agnosia. This also may occur in the juvenile form of Krabbe leukodystrophy. In one 4-year-old child with this disease, who came to medical attention because of a visual deficit, the eyegrounds were normal but the periventricular optic pathways were manifestly demyelinated in MR images. In metachromatic leukodystrophy on the other hand, optic radiations are usually preserved for a long time and if visual failure occurs it generally results from retinal degeneration.

In MELAS, central blindness or hemianopsia are produced by bilateral or unilateral corticosubcortical areas of necrosis involving the central optic tracts and visual cortex.

In many diseases diffusely affecting the cerebral cortex, such as the neuronal storage disorders, failure of vision is clearly the result of concomitant retinal involvement, except perhaps at the final stage when the striate cortex is destroyed. In Alpers-Huttenlocher syndrome, the diffuse loss of cortical neurons usually predominates in the occipital regions; cortical blindness may be a relatively early sign.

Derangement of Ocular Movements

Abnormalities of ocular movements comprise oculomotor palsies resulting from direct lesions of the oculomotor nuclei or nerves, supranuclear paralysis of conjugate gaze due to the involvement of central pathways of oculomotricity, and abnormal eye movements (nystagmus) (Table 6-12).

Oculomotor Palsies   Oculomotor palsies are rare in the metabolic encephalopathies except in Kearns-Sayre syndrome. In this juvenile mitochondrial disorder and the other mitochondrial syndromes of progressive external ophthalmoplegia, progressive oculomotor palsies stand as an obligatory sign. In a few others HMDs (Table 6-12) ocular palsies, although inconstant, always constitute a valuable diagnostic clue.

Comments on disturbances of ocular movements in the neonatal periods are to be found in Chap. 2.

HMDs represent a relatively rare cause of oculomotor palsies, and in a child or adolescent with progressive paralysis of ocular muscles, one should first consider the possibility of *myasthenia gravis* or *an infiltrating glioma of the brain stem* (paralytic mydriasis may then be present). *Tumors* of the optic chiasma and nerves, meningeal sarcomas, arterial or arteriovenous malformations are other possibilities.

Supranuclear Paralyses of Conjugate Gaze   These occur in a limited number of neurometabolic disorders as a constant or frequent abnormality of great diagnostic importance. Their pathogenesis is generally not clear. Highly characteristic signs are, without doubt, a disorder of horizontal gaze with abnormal saccades in ataxia-telangiectasia, a defect of vertical gaze in juvenile Niemann-Pick type C disease, and a paralysis of lateral and vertical conjugate gaze in juvenile Gaucher disease. Supranuclear palsies of conjugate gaze may also occur in Leigh disease, Huntington disease, G_{M2} gangliosidosis, and a few other conditions (Table 6-12).

Cogan's congenital oculomotor apraxia is a nonmetabolic, probably autosomal recessive disorder in which imperfections of horizontal saccades result in peculiar movements of the eyes and head (especially brusque head thrusts) upon attempted lateral gaze. Oculomotor apraxia is also a feature of the ataxia-oculomotor apraxia syndrome (and of ataxia-telangiectasia).

Other common causes of supranuclear ophthalmoplegia are *tumors of the brain stem, brain stem encephalitis* and, in the adolescent and young adult, *multiple sclerosis*.

Nuclear oculomotor palsies and supranuclear ophthalmoplegias produce squints and deviations of the eyes which should not be mistaken for the squints and the anomalous upward, downward, or oblique positioning of the ocular globes in children with congenital blindness.

Nystagmus   Clinical descriptions of many HMDs often remark upon a nystagmus, but exact description and precise qualification of the abnormal eye movements are all too often lacking. Typical vestibular jerk nystagmus with slow and quick phases is, in fact, very rare in the metabolic encephalopathies. It is observed occasionally in Leigh disease and Friedreich ataxia. A different type of jerk nystagmus is associated with a derangement of ocular gaze and with neuromuscular insufficiency. A bilateral pendular nystagmus due to visual loss from involvement of the anterior visual pathway is the most common form of nystagmus observed in the metabolic encephalopathies. It is one of the most obvious indications of amblyopia in young children. The ocular movements consist of pendular oscillations on which quick phases and saccades may be superimposed. There are horizontal, vertical, oblique or torsional components to the movement of the globes, and characteristically there are changes in direction every few seconds or minutes. The amplitude varies from small oscillations, only detected by close scrutiny, to the large, irregular, abrupt excursions of the eyes in children with severe visual deficits. A pendular nystagmus is among the first manifestations of Pelizaeus-Merzbacher disease in young infants. There may also be abnormal head movements. The relationship to a loss of central vision is uncertain.

The pendular nystagmus of early visual failure must be distinguished from congenital nystagmus (with or without head movements) and spasmus nutans, a rare and benign condition in which ocular oscillations are frequently unilateral.

Characteristic Morphological Changes of the Eyes

Careful examination of the eyes by clinical means and with the help of the ophthalmoscope and slit-lamp (to explore the corneas and lenses) may detect the following pathognomonic or highly characteristic abnormalities (Table 6-9):

• The Kayser-Fleischer corneal ring, a unique feature of Wilson disease.

• The conjunctival telangiectasies in ataxia-telangiectasia, composed of vessels that run horizontally at the equator of the ocular bulbs and stop abruptly at the border of the cornea. These unique characteristics help to differentiate them from conjunctival vessel dilatations in conjunctivitis, from other types of telangiectasias, and from the peculiar tortuosities of vessels seen in Fabry disease.

• A macular cherry red spot with its typical white or grayish perimacular ring. This is an essential element

in the diagnosis of a number of sphingolipidoses (essentially G_{M2} gangliosidosis) and sialidoses.

• Corneal clouding encountered in various mucopolysaccharidoses (with the notable exception of Hunter disease), oligosaccharidoses, mucolipidosis IV and a few other conditions. This is easily differentiated from keratitis and other corneal disorders. Whorl-like corneal opacities are typical of Fabry disease in affected males and in some female heterozygotes (a similar corneal dystrophy is observed in lengthy chloroquine or amiodarone therapy).

• Dislocation of the lens observed in homocystinuria and also in sulfite oxidase deficiency. It is a major sign in Marfan disease.

• Cataracts. These are encountered in HMDs, but their prevalence limits their diagnostic value. A high incidence of cataracts is notable in galactosemia, Lowe disease, and cholestanolosis. Characteristic lenticular changes are found in Fabry disease and myotonic dystrophy.

Microphthalmia and small orbits very rarely are caused by an HMD. Buphthalmos is a feature of Lowe disease.

DEAFNESS

Neurosensory (and/or conduction) deafness is an important and, at times, early feature of Refsum disease, mucopolysaccharidoses, multiple sulfatase deficiency, mannosidosis, Cockayne syndrome, and a few other conditions listed in Table 6-13. In the mucopolysaccharidoses, hearing loss may contribute to the important behavioral disturbances of some patients.

Central deafness, resulting from the involvement of axons extending from the medial geniculate nucleus to the auditory cortex of the superior temporal gyrus, occurs as a result of demyelination of the posterior part of the cerebral hemispheres in adrenoleukodystrophy. Central deafness, resulting from lesions in the brain stem, may be observed in Leigh disease.

Deafness is frequently discussed but rarely proved in many of the early infantile encephalopathies with diffuse brain involvement. The condition is most difficult to detect when there is a severe mental retardation. The child appears to have lost all interest in the sounds of the outer world, but on closer observation tends not to heed visual or contactual stimuli as well. The study of the cochleopalpebral reflex is too variable in normal

Table 6-13
Early deafness in the hereditary neurometabolic disorders[a]

MPS IH, IH-S, II, III	+ + +
Mannosidosis	+ + +
Multiple sulfatase deficiency	+ +
I-cell disease	+
Sialidosis II	+
Other mucolipidoses and diseases of glycoprotein degradation	+
Kearns-Sayre disease	+ +
MERRF	+ +
MELAS	+ +
Other defects of mtDNA	+
Refsum disease	+ + +
X-linked ALD	+ +
Zellweger disease	+ +
Other peroxisomal disorders with the Zellweger phenotype	+ +
Leigh disease	+
Biotinidase deficiency	+ +
Methylglutaconic acidemia	+
Cockayne syndrome	+ +
Xeroderma pigmentosum	+ +
Friedreich ataxia	±
Autosomal dominant SCA	+
Lafora disease	+

Abbreviations and symbols: ALD = adrenoleukodystrophy; SCA = spinocerebellar ataxia; + + + = very frequent or of major diagnostic importance; + + = frequent; + = occurs in some patients; ± = rare.

[a] The exact mechanism of deafness is not always clear. In most HMDs it appears to be of the neurosensory type. A conduction defect probably also occurs in the mucopolysaccharidoses. Lesions of the central auditory pathways are the cause of deafness in X-linked ALD and in Leigh disease.

children to be of much value. The recording of auditory evoked potentials provides the best evidence of an auditory defect, under these circumstances.

On the whole, metabolic disorders represent only a small proportion of cases of hereditary deafness. There are numerous other nonprogressive genetic neurologic syndromes associated with deafness which are described in specialized textbooks.[40,41] In any case, an ear infection, the most common cause of hearing deficits in young children, must be ruled out.

REFERENCES

1. Volpe JJ: *Neurology of the Newborn*, 3d ed. Philadelphia, Saunders, 1995.

2. Nelson KB, Ellenberg JH: Antecedents of cerebral palsy: multivariate analysis of risk. *New Engl J Med* 315: 81–86, 1986.

3. Tardieu M, Evrard P, Lyon G: Progressive expanding porencephalies: a treatable cause of progressive encephalopathy. *Pediatrics* 68: 198–202, 1981.

4. Hattori M, Adachi H, Tsujimoto M, et al.: Miller-Dieker lissencephaly gene encodes a subunit of brain platelet-activating factor. *Nature* 370: 216–218, 1994.

5. Tint GS, Irons M, Elias ER, et al.: Defective cholesterol biosynthesis associated with Smith-Lemli-Opitz syndrome. *New Engl J Med* 330: 107–113, 1994.

6. Wallace M, Zori RT, Alley T, et al.: Smith-Lemli-Opitz syndrome in a female with a de novo balanced translocation involving 7q32: probable disruption of an *SLOS* gene. *Am J Med Genet* 50: 368–374, 1994.

7. Glascoe FP, Martin ED, Humphrey S: A comparative review of developmental screening tests. *Pediatrics* 86: 547–554, 1990.

8. Caplan S: *ELM Scale (Early Language Milestone Scale)*. Tulsa Okla., Modern Educational Corporation, 1983.

9. Gillberg C: Autism and autistic-like conditions, in Aicardi J (ed): *Diseases of the Nervous System in Childhood*. Oxford, Blackwell, 1992, pp. 1295–1320.

10. Hagberg B, Aicardi J, Dias K, et al.: A progressive syndrome of autism, dementia, ataxia and loss of purposeful hand movements in girls: Rett syndrome. *Ann Neurol* 14: 471–479, 1983.

11. First LR, Palfrey JS: The infant and young child with developmental delay. *New Engl J Med* 330: 478–483, 1994.

12. Hagberg B, Sanner G, Steen M: The dysequilibrium syndrome in cerebral palsy. *Acta Pediatr Scand* 65: 403–408, 1972.

13. Norman RM: Primary degeneration of the granular layer of the cerebellum: an unusual form of familial cerebellar atrophy occurring in early life. *Brain* 63: 365–379, 1940.

14. Leiner CH, Leiner AL, Dow RS: The human cerebro-cerebellar system: its computing, cognitive and language skills. *Behav Brain Res* 44: 113–128, 1991.

15. Middeton FA, Strick PL: Anatomical evidence for cerebellar and basal ganglia involvement in higher cognitive function. *Science* 266: 458–461, 1994.

16. Kim SG, Ugurbil K, Strick PL: Activation of a cerebellar output nucleus during cognitive processing. *Science* 265: 949–951, 1994.

17. Dow RZ, Moruzzi G: *The Physiology and Pathology of the Cerebellum*. University of Minnesota Press, 1958.

18. Norman RM, Urich H: Cerebellar hypoplasia associated with systemic degeneration in early life. *J Neurol Neurosurg Psychiatr* 21: 159–166, 1958.

19. Gadisseux JF, Rodriguez J, Lyon G: Pontoneocerebellar hypoplasia. *Ann Neurol* 3: 160–167, 1984.

20. Bain PG, O'Brien MD, Keevil SF, et al.: Familial periodic cerebellar ataxia: a problem of cerebellar intracellular homeostasis. *Ann Neurol* 31: 147–154, 1992.

21. Goutieres F, Aicardi J: Acute neurological dysfunction associated with destructive lesions of basal ganglia. *Ann Neurol* 12: 328–332, 1982.

22. Rosemberg S, Amaral LC, Klieman E, et al.: Acute encephalopathy with bilateral striatal necrosis. A distinctive clinicopathological condition. *Neuropediatrics* 23: 310–315, 1992.

23. Robinson RO, Samuels M, Pohl KR: Choreic syndrome after cardiac surgery. *Arch Dis Child* 63: 1466–1469, 1988.

23a. Sébire G, Devictor D, Huault G, et al.: Coma associated with intense bursts of abnormal movements and long-lasting cognitive disturbances: an acute encephalopathy of obscure origin. *J Pediatr* 121: 845–851, 1992.

24. Scalais E: Personal communication, 1994.

25. Deonna T, Ziegler AI, Nielsen J: Transient idiopathic dystonia in infancy. *Neuropediatrics* 22: 220–224, 1991.

26. Perlman JM, Volpe JJ: Movement disorders of premature infants with severe bronchopulmonary dysplasia. A new syndrome. *Pediatrics* 84: 215–218, 1989.

27. Aicardi J, Goutieres F: A progressive familial encephalopathy in infancy with calcifications of the basal ganglia and persistent lymphocytosis. *Ann Neurol* 15: 49–54, 1984.

28. Appleton RE, Farell K, Dunn HG: "Pure" and "complicated" forms of hereditary spastic paraplegia presenting in childhood. *Dev Med Child Neurol* 33: 304–312, 1991.

29. Poser CM: Myelinoclastic diffuse and transitional sclerosis, in Vinken PJ, Bruyn GW (eds): *Handbook of Clinical Neurology*. Amsterdam, Elsevier-North-Holland, 1970, vol. 9, pp. 469–484.

30. Aicardi J: *Diseases of the Nervous System in Childhood*. Oxford, Blackwell Scientific, 1992.

31. Glueck CJ, Daniels SR, Bates S, et al.: Pediatric victims of unexplained strokes and their families: familial lipid and lipoprotein abnormalities. *Pediatrics* 69: 308–316, 1982.

32. Gastaut H: Clinical and electroencephalographical classification of epileptic seizures. *Epilepsia* 11: 102–113, 1969.

33. Gastaut H: A proposed completion of the current international classification of the epilepsies, in Clifford-Rose (ed): *Research Progress in Epilepsy*. London, Pitman, 1983, pp. 8–13.

34. Commission on Classification and Terminology of the International League against Epilepsy: Proposal for revised classification of epilepsies and epileptic syndromes. *Epilepsia* 30: 389–399, 1989.

35. Aircardi J: *Epilepsy in Children*. New York, Raven, 1994, pp. 79–17.

35a. Deonna Th. Personnal communication, 1994.

36. Purpura D: Ectopic dendritic growth in mature pyramidal neurons in human ganglioside storage disease. *Nature* 276: 520–521, 1978.

37. Thomas PK, Ochoa J: Clinical features and differential diagnosis, in Dick PJ, Thomas PK (eds): *Peripheral Neuropathy*. Philadelphia, Saunders, 1993, pp. 749–774.

38. Albers JW, Zimnovodski S, Lowrey CM, et al.: Juvenile progressive bulbar palsy. *Arch Neurol* 40: 351–353, 1983.

39. Summers BA, Swash M, Schwartz MS, et al.: Juvenile onset bulbo-spinal muscular atrophy with deafness: Violetto-Van Laere syndrome. *J Neurol* 23: 440–442, 1987.

40. Fraser GR: *The Causes of Profound Deafness*. London, Baillière Tindall, 1976.

41. Konigsmark BW: Hereditary deafness in man. *New Engl J Med* 281: 713–720; 774–778; 827–832, 1969.

Chapter 7

VISCERAL AND OTHER TISSUE ABNORMALITIES THAT ARE ASSOCIATED WITH THE HEREDITARY METABOLIC ENCEPHALOPATHIES

LIVER AND SPLEEN

CARDIOVASCULAR SYSTEM

KIDNEYS

ADRENAL INSUFFICIENCY

DIABETES MELLITUS

SKELETAL SYSTEM

ALTERATIONS OF SKIN AND HAIR

HEMATOLOGIC CHANGES

FACIAL DYSMORPHIAS. SOMATIC MALFORMATIONS

RESPIRATORY TRACT

GASTROINTESTINAL SIGNS, MALNUTRITION, AND GROWTH FAILURE

In a notable proportion of the metabolic encephalopathies, the disease is not restricted to the nervous system; it also involves other organs and tissues. In some conditions, the pathogenesis of visceral involvement is understood. This is the case, for instance, when a metabolic block results in the infiltration of reticuloendothelial or nonneural parenchymal cells (as in the neurovisceral lipidoses, the mucopolysaccharidoses and oligosacchar-idoses) or when the accumulation of a metabolite causes nonspecific changes of the parenchyma (such as copper-induced cirrhosis in Wilson disease). The relationship between arylsulfatase C and ichthyosis in multiple sulfatase deficiency is another example. In other diseases, the cause of nonneurologic lesions remains obscure, as in the cardiomyopathy of Friedreich ataxia, the renal involvement in Lowe disease and the liver dysfunction in Alpers syndrome.

Whatever the mechanism, nonneurologic abnormalities accompanying metabolic encephalopathies are of great diagnostic value. They may be clinically demonstrable, as an enlargement of viscera, abnormalities of skin and hair, or facial dysmorphia, and they may be detected by relatively simple laboratory procedures, such as x-ray films of the skeleton and chest; ultrasound scans of the abdomen and thorax; electrocardiogram; bone marrow aspiration; and laboratory tests of hepatic, renal, adrenal, or cardiac function.

Ultrastructural analyses of the stored substances may often provide indispensable clues to diagnosis in biopsy specimens from a variety of tissues (conjunctiva, skin, liver, nerve, rectum, appendix) (see Chap. 8 and Table 8.1).

Although the clinical manifestations of visceral and neurologic diseases usually coincide, visceral abnormalities may, for a time, be more obvious than neurologic dysfunction. In some of the mucopolysaccharidoses, for instance, facial and skeletal changes are the first to alert the clinician to the disease, being so typical as to make the diagnosis evident at a glance. Visceral abnormalities can be misinterpreted, as sometimes happens in early infantile metabolic disorders. Here, the neurologic examination of a very sick child is problematic and the infant may, at first, be thought to have a primary gastrointestinal disease, hepatic disease, pulmonary infection, or malnutrition; the malnutrition is secondary to anorexia, vomiting, or diarrhea or an inadequate diet. Actually, the clinical evidence of visceral disease may antedate signs of involvement of the nervous system by several years. This is true of splenomegaly in Gaucher III disease, of signs of hepatic dysfunction in hepatolenticular degeneration and in some patients with Niemann-Pick type C disease; and of signs of adrenal insufficiency in patients with adrenoleukodystrophy. Also, there may be purely visceral forms of an HMD. There is, for instance, a purely hepatic form of Wilson disease and an adrenal form of adrenoleukodystrophy.

Involvement of the visceral organs may affect their function and may cause or contribute to the nervous system disorder (for instance, in hepatocerebral degeneration and in abetalipoproteinemia). Also, hepatic failure, renal insufficiency, cardiac failure and dysrhythmia, or adrenal insufficiency eventually contribute to a fatal outcome.

Tables 7-1 to 7-10, list the nonneurologic accompaniments of the various metabolic disorders under consideration.

LIVER AND SPLEEN (TABLE 7-1)

Enlargement or dysfunction of the liver and enlargement of the spleen in a child with a neurologic disorder strongly suggests a metabolic disease, although such a combination may occasionally be observed in hematologic and infectious disorders or malnutrition.

Hepatomegaly and/or splenomegaly without notable functional alterations of these organs are major features of the lysosomal storage disorders and occur more or less frequently in many other neurometabolic disorders. In infants, the visceral involvement may initially overshadow the neurologic signs, as in Niemann-Pick disease. In type III Gaucher disease an isolated splenomegaly may be present before neurologic symptoms appear; eventually there may be hematologic signs of hypersplenism and the spleen may become so voluminous as to warrant its removal.

Cirrhosis and/or evidence of liver dysfunction are present and of great diagnostic importance in Wilson disease, infantile Niemann-Pick disease, Niemann-Pick type C disease, Zellweger disease, Alpers syndrome and a few other conditions listed in Table 7-1.

Hepatic dysfunction always precedes the neurologic signs in Wilson disease and may play a role in its pathogenesis. Also, patients with type C Niemann-Pick disease have often presented self-limited episodes of jaundice in early infancy. Finally, infants with Wilson disease and Niemann-Pick type C disease may have a purely hepatic form of their condition.

The metabolic disorders in which hydrops fetalis may occur are listed in Table 7-2.

CARDIOVASCULAR SYSTEM (TABLE 7-3)

A *cardiopathy* occurs in a number of different metabolic encephalopathies and is the usual cause of death. Involvement of the heart sometimes assumes considerable diagnostic importance, as for glycogenosis type II, Friedreich ataxia, disorders of mitochondrial fatty acid oxidation, and Kearns-Sayre syndrome.

The pathogenesis and clinical expression of cardiac disorders are variable.

In the usual type of glycogenosis type II, infiltration of the heart leads to a significant degree of cardiomegaly, eventually ending in heart failure. In other storage disorders (mucopolysaccharidoses, mucolipidoses, Fabry disease, familial amyloid neuropathy, and some cases of Refsum disease), an infiltration of the endocardium, the myocardium, the bundles of His, and the coronary arteries leads to various degrees of valvular insufficiency, cardiomegaly, arrhythmia, myocardial ischemia, and congestive heart failure. A hypertrophic cardiomyopathy is a feature of several HMDs, including Friedreich disease ("nonmetabolic" cardiomyopathies are genetic disorders). In Friedreich ataxia, degenerative changes in the cardiac muscle and conduction system also result in valvular defects, dysrhythmia, and sometimes heart failure. Patients affected with these various disorders are in danger of sudden death and may require insertion of an artificial pacemaker. Cerebral embolisms and strokes are potential complications of some of the metabolic cardiopathies.

Table 7-1

Involvement of liver and spleen in the metabolic encephalopathies[a]

*Hepatomegaly and/or splenomegaly, usually without evidence of
functional failure[b]*

The neurovisceral sphingolipidoses
Mucopolysaccharidoses, mucolipidoses, and glycoprotein
  degradation disorders
Peroxisomal disorders
Refsum disease
Mitochondrial disorders
Disorders of amino and organic acid metabolism
Pompe disease
Galactosemia
Tangier disease (splenomegaly)

Cirrhosis, jaundice, and liver failure

Wilson disease	Progressive cirrhosis is a constant (preneurologic) feature; portal hypertension; purely hepatic forms, including acute liver failure
Niemann-Pick C disease	Transient neonatal or infantile jaundice; prenatal ascites; fatal liver failure in some early-onset cases
Alpers syndrome	Various degrees of hepatic lesions and liver failure
Zellweger disease and other peroxisomal disorders	Cirrhosis
Early infantile Niemann-Pick disease	Neonatal ascites and jaundice in some patients
Mitochondrial disorders	
Galactosemia	

[a] This table is not exhaustive.

[b] Present in many neurometabolic disorders.

Table 7-2

Possible occurrence of hydrops fetalis in the hereditary metabolic diseases

I-cell disease (ML II)
Sly disease (MPS VII)
α-Mannosidosis
Gaucher disease
Sialidosis II
Galactosialidosis
Sialic acid storage disease

Abbreviations: MPS = mucopolysaccharidosis, ML = mucolipidosis.

Cardiac congenital malformations are not a feature of metabolic disorders. The very few exceptions to this rule are indicated in Table 7-3.

Alterations of the *systemic and cerebral arteries*, which may cause strokes or visceral infarctions, are seen in a limited number of diseases; including homocystinuria, Fabry disease, Menkes disease, and MELAS. This has already been discussed in Chap. 6 (see Table 6-6).

KIDNEYS (TABLE 7-4)

In the neurovisceral lysosomal disorders, the stored substances infiltrate the kidneys, usually without notable disturbances of renal function. An important exception is Fabry disease, where deposition of glycosphingolipids affects predominantly the glomeruli and results in progressive renal failure. Severe renal involvement also

Table 7-3

Cardiopathy in the hereditary neurometabolic diseases[a]

Disease		Type of cardiopathy
Neonatal and early infantile mitochondrial disorders (glutaric aciduria type II, LCAD, trifunctional enzyme, CPT II, primary generalized carnitine, and carnitine-acylcarnitine translocase deficiencies; deficiency of complex I and complex IV)	+ +	Cardiomyopathy; dysrhythmia (CPT II deficiency)
Zellweger disease	+ +	Septal and aortic defects
G_{M1} gangliosidosis 1	+	Cardiac failure; dysrhythmia; endocardial fibroelastosis
Farber disease	+ +	Granulomatous deposits
Gycogenosis 2	+ + +	Cardiomegaly; typical ECG
Sialic acid storage disease	+ +	Cardiomegaly
Friedreich disease	+ + +	Valvular defects; conduction defects Hypertrophic obstructive cardiomyopathy
Abetalipoproteinemia	+	Cardiomyopathy (as in Friedreich disease)
AVED	+	Cardiomyopathy (as in Friedreich disease)
Refsum disease	+ + +	Atrioventricular conduction impairment; heart failure
Hereditary amyloid neuropathy	+ +	Conduction defects
Kearns-Sayre syndrome	+ + +	Conduction defects; propensity to complete heart block
Fabry disease	+ + +	Valvular defects; conduction defects; myocardial ischemia; heart failure; cardiopathy in some heterozygotes
Tangier disease		Foam cells in heart valves
Cholestanolosis	+ +	Atherosclerotic cardiovascular disease
Mucopolysaccharidoses (MPS), mucolipidoses (ML), and disorders of glycoprotein degradation	+ + +	Myocardial thickening; valvular dysfunction; coronary arterial stenosis; pulmonary hypertension
MPS I H	+ + +	
MPS I H/S	+ + +	
MPS I S	+ +	Aortic valve defect
MPS II	+ + +	
MPS III	+	
ML II	+ + +	
ML III	+	Aortic valve defect
Fucosidosis	+ +	
Aspartylglucosaminuria	+	
CDG syndrome	+ +	Heart failure; pericardial effusions
Homocystinuria	+ +	Myocardial infarction
Combined deficiencies of MCoAM and MHM	+	Congestive heart failure
3-β-hydroxyisobutyryl-CoA deacylase deficiency	+	Cardiac malformations
Tyrosinemia type I	+	Cardiomyopathy

Abbreviations and symbols: CPT = carnitine palmitoyl transferase; LCAD = long-chain acyl-CoA dehydrogenase; AVED = ataxia with vitamin E deficiency; CDG = carbohydrate-deficient glycoprotein; MCoAM = methylmalonyl-CoA mutase; HMM = methyltetrahydrofolate: homocysteine melthyltransferase; + + + = cardiopathy constant or very frequent and/or severe; + + = cardiopathy frequent and/or of diagnostic importance; + = cardiopathy infrequent or mild, not well documented, or in rare disease.

[a] A cardiopathy is always a serious complication of an HMD, and possibly a cause of cerebral embolism. It is a usual cause of death, occasionally of sudden, unexpected death.

occurs in one form of type II sialidosis. In familial amyloid neuropathy, a nephrotic syndrome and subsequent renal failure are feared complications of the disease. In the neurovisceral lipidoses, lipid storage in the kidneys may begin during the fetal period of life.

Renal tubular dysfunction, with a Fanconi syndrome and rickets, is an obligatory element of Lowe syndrome and occurs as an accessory abnormality in a few other disorders, including Wilson disease, galactosemia and fructose 1,6-bisphosphatase deficiency.

Nephrolithiasis and an obstructive nephropathy are major components of Lesch-Nyhan disease. Renal stones may occasionally be observed in Wilson disease.

Renal cysts and dysplastic changes are a feature of Zellweger disease and glutaric acidemia type II. In the latter, the kidneys may be enlarged and palpable.

Table 7-4

Nephropathy in the hereditary metabolic encephalopathies

Disease		Type of nephropathy	Urine color/odor
Lowe oculocerebrorenal syndrome	+ + +	Tubular, later glomerular, dysfunction	
Zellweger hepatocerebrorenal disease	+ + +	Renal cysts	
Other neonatal peroxisomal disorders	+ +	Renal cysts	
Glutaric aciduria II	+ +	Renal cysts, dysplasias	Odor
Fabry disease	+ + +	Late renal failure (glomerular and tubular dysfunction)	
Lesch-Nyhan disease	+ + +	Nephrolithiasis; obstructive nephropathy	Uric acid crystals; hematuria
Familial amyloid neuropathy	+ +	Nephrotic syndrome (FAP III); bladder dysfunction	
Menkes disease	+ +	Hydronephrosis; bladder diverticuli	
Nephrosialidosis	+ + +	Renal failure	
Wilson disease		Tubular dysfunction	Possible hematuria
Fructose 1,6-bisphosphate deficiency		Tubular dysfunction	
Galactosemia	+ +	Generalized aminoaciduria; albuminuria	
Pompe disease, late form		Enlargement of bladder	
Sialic acid storage disease		Nephrotic syndrome	
CPT I deficiency		Tubular dysfunction	
Complex IV deficiency		Tubular dysfunction	
Homocystinuria		Renal infarcts	
Acute intermittent porphyria	+ +		Red color
CPT II deficiency			Myoglobinuria
LCHD deficiency			Myoglobinuria
Mitochondrial trifunctional enzyme deficiency			Myoglobinuria
MSUD	+ + +		Odor
Isovaleric acidemia	+ + +		Odor
HS deficiency			Odor

Abbreviations and symbols: CPT = carnitine palmitoyltransferase; LCHD = long-chain 3-hydroxyacyl-CoA dehydrogenase; MSUD = maple syrup urine disease; HS = holocarboxylase synthetase; + + + = constant or very frequent; + + = frequent or of diagnostic importance.

ADRENAL INSUFFICIENCY

Adrenal insufficiency is a major element within X-linked adrenoleukodystrophy, varying in degree of clinical expression, and often remaining subclinical. A purely Addisonian form of the disease exists. Typical lesions of the adrenal glands and subclinical functional disturbances are also found in Zellweger disease and in neonatal adrenoleukodystrophy.

DIABETES MELLITUS

Diabetes may occur in Friedreich ataxia, Kearns-Sayre syndrome and other juvenile mitochondrial disorders, and ataxia-telangiectasia.

SKELETAL SYSTEM (TABLE 7-5)

A characteristic pattern of skeletal deformities, involving essentially the spine, hips, metacarpals, and the long bones—called *dysostosis multiplex*—is associated with the different varieties of mucopolysaccharidoses, mucolipidoses, disorders of glycoprotein degradation, multiple sulfatase deficiency, and early infantile G_{M1} gangliosidosis. The abnormalities are of varying degree and may be so slight that only careful examination of skeletal x-ray films will disclose their presence, as for instance in Sanfilippo disease. No skeletal abnormalities are found in mucolipidosis type IV.

The early skeletal changes in this category of diseases (for instance, in G_{M1} gangliosidosis type 1, α-mannosidosis and I-cell disease) may resemble rickets (osteomalacia, epiphyseal changes, and periosteal shafting). The vertebral alterations must not be confused with those seen in hypothyroidism.

Other metabolic encephalopathies, in which there are characteristic osteoarticular changes, include Farber disease, Zellweger disease, Lowe syndrome, homocystinuria, Fabry disease, and Refsum disease. In two unrelated patients, a progressive neurologic disorder, with a bipyramidal syndrome and progressive intellectual regression, was associated with skeletal abnormalities resembling those of Pyle disease.

ALTERATIONS OF SKIN AND HAIR (TABLE 7-6)

Alterations of skin and hair can be of diagnostic value in a few of the metabolic diseases, and sometimes the clin-

ical diagnosis may not be possible in their absence. This is true of Menkes disease, Hartnup disease, Farber disease, Sjögren-Larsson disease, xeroderma pigmentosum, cerebrotendinous xanthomatosis and giant axonal neuropathy.

Angiokeratoma in Fabry disease, fucosidosis sialidoses and a few other disorders, ichthyosis in multiple sulfatase deficiency and Refsum disease, a photosensitive dermatitis in Cockayne syndrome, skin rashes in biotinidase deficiency or holocarboxylase deficiency, and melanoderma in X-linked adrenoleukodystrophy also assume great diagnostic value. The hair shafts are characteristically altered in a number of diseases, such as Menkes disease, argininosuccinic aciduria, and giant axonal neuropathy. Alopecia may occur in disorders of biotin metabolism. Cholesterol deposits on the tonsils are specific to Tangier disease.

Finally, the characteristic microscopic deposits may be verified in the skin and its adnexae by the ultrastructural analysis of biopsy specimens. They may be of considerable diagnostic value (see Chap. 8).

HEMATOLOGIC CHANGES (TABLE 7-7)

Hematologic abnormalities are necessary for the diagnosis of a few neurometabolic disorders: acanthocytosis of red blood cells in neuroacanthocytosis; vacuolated lymphocytes in the juvenile form of ceroid lipofuscinosis; Gaucher cells; megaloblastosis in cobalamin and folate deficiency disorders; and sea-blue histiocytes in the bone marrow of Niemann-Pick type C disease. Other abnormalities in peripheral blood and bone marrow are listed in Table 7-7 (see also Chap. 8).

FACIAL DYSMORPHIAS. SOMATIC MALFORMATIONS (TABLE 7-8)

Changes in physiognomy occur in a variety of metabolic encephalopathies at all ages. Some are highly characteristic of a given disorder or class of disorders, such as is the case in mucopolysaccharidoses, oligosaccharidoses, and related conditions (Table 7-8A). In other metabolic diseases, morphologic changes of the face are characteristic, as in Lowe disease or Zellweger disease (Table 7-8B) or are less obvious and not really specific. Slight deviations from normality are of dubious value. The clinician should nevertheless pay attention to coarseness of facial features, thick lips, gingival hypertrophy, frontal bossing or a high forehead, heavy eyebrows, a thick

Table 7-5

Skeletal changes in the hereditary neurometabolic disorders

Disease	Degree of dysostosis multiplex on x-ray films[a]
Mucopolyssacharidoses (MPS), mucolipidoses (ML) and other lysosomal disorders with various degrees of dysostosis multiplex	
MPS I	Marked
MPS II	Marked
MPS III	Moderate: vertebrae, femoral heads, and acetabula
ML II (I-cell disease)	Marked
ML III	Marked (reminiscent of Morquio disease)
α-Mannosidosis	Moderate to marked
Fucosidosis	Moderate to marked
Aspartylglucosaminuria	Slight to moderate
Sialidosis II	Marked
Multiple sulfatase deficiency	Moderate
G_{M1} gangliosidosis type II	Moderate
Infants with G_{M1} gangliosidosis, fucosidosis, I-cell disease and other mucopolysaccharidoses, oligosaccharidoses	Rickets-like changes: demineralization, periosteal new-bone formation, broad irregular metaphyses
Other metabolic disorders	*Type of abnormality*
Zellweger disease	Patellar calcifications (typical)
Farber disease	Arthropathy (limbs, larynx); juxta-articular bone destruction
Lowe disease	Rachitic deformation; demineralization
Menkes disease	Scurvylike change
Homocystinuria	Osteoporosis (vertebrae); susceptibility to fractures; biconcave vertebrae; metaphyseal spicules; scoliosis
Fabry disease	Arthritis and calcification of distal interphalangeal joints; necrosis of femoral heads and other bones
Refsum disease	Short metacarpal and metatarsal bones; epiphyseal dysplasia; osteochondritis dissecans
Friedreich disease	Scoliosis
Abetalipoproteinemia	Scoliosis
AVED	Scoliosis
Giant axonal neuropathy	Scoliosis
CDGS	Scoliosis
Lysinuric protein intolerance	Osteoporosis
Wilson disease	Arthropathy; osteoporosis; fractures
MPS with athetosis and keratan sulfaturia	Abnormalities of vertebrae, femoral heads, and acetabula
Progressive encephalopathy with osteopathy resembling Pyle disease[b]	Condensing osteopathy

Abbreviations: MPS = mucopolysaccharidosis; ML = mucolipidosis; AVED = ataxia with vitamin E deficiency; CDGS = carbohydrate-deficient glycoprotein syndrome.

[a] Skeletal changes are progressive; they may be minimal during early childhood and become evident in late adolescence, as changes to the vertebrae, acetabula, hands, etc.

[b] Diament AJ, et al.: *Arquivos de Neuropsiquiatria* 29: 43–102, 1971; Roy C, et al.: *Arch. Fr. Pediatr.* 25: 893–905, 1968.

Table 7-6

Abnormalities of skin and hair in the hereditary neurometabolic disorders

Disease		Skin	Hair
MPS, ML II, fucosidosis	+ +	Thick skin	Coarse hair and eyebrows; hirsutism
MPS II		Whitish macular lesions on back and shoulders	
Fucosidosis II		Excessive sweating	
Fucosidosis III		Angiokeratoma	
β-Mannosidosis		Angiokeratoma	
Sialidosis II, congenital form		Telangiectasic skin rash	
Aspartylglucosaminuria		Photosensitivity; large nevi	
CDGS	+ +	Skin pads; focal atrophy	
Multiple sulfatase deficiency		Ichthyosis	
Ataxia-telangiectasia	+ +	Telangiectasia (ears, cheek, limbs) and atrophy; café au lait spots	Graying
Biotinidase deficiency	+ +	Skin rash (seborrheic or atopic dermatitis)	Alopecia
Holocarboxylase synthetase deficiency	+ +	Skin rash	Alopecia (rare)
G_{M1} gangliosidosis type I		Edema of hands and feet	
Niemann-Pick type A		Brownish pigmentation (rare)	
Adrenoleukodystrophy	+ +	Addisonian melanoderma	
Fabry disease	+ +	Angiokeratoma (between umbilicus and knee)	
Refsum disease		Ichthyosis	
Giant axonal neuropathy			Curled
Lesch-Nyhan disease	+ +	Oral automutilations	
Riley-Day disease		Oral automutilations	
Menkes disease		Pale	Typically pale, wiry, and friable; pili torti + + +
Menkes disease, heterozygotes		Patchy abnormalities	
Farber disease	+ + +	Subcutaneous nodules containing ceramide	
ASL and ASS deficiency			Brittle hair; trichorexis nodosa + +
Isovaleric acidemia			Alopecia
3-Methylcrotonyl-CoA carboxylase deficiency			Alopecia
Homocystinuria		Malar flush; livedo reticularis	Graying
Propionic, methylmalonic aciduria		Erythematous rash	
Cobalamin C deficiency		Erythematous rash	
Hartnup disease	+ + +	Pellagra-like skin rash	
Cockayne syndrome	+ +	Photosensitivity; atrophic pigmented skin; loss of subcutaneous fat	
Xeroderma pigmentosum	+ + +	Severe photosensitivity; skin carcinoma	
Cerebrotendinous xanthomatosis	+ + +	Xanthoma of Achilles tendons	

Abbreviations and symbols: MPS = mucopolysaccharidoses; ML = mucolipidosis; CGDS = carbohydrate-deficient glycoprotein syndrome; ASL = argininosuccinate lyase; ASS = argininosuccinate synthetase; + + + = pathognomonic; + + = of diagnostic importance.

Table 7-7

Hematological abnormalities in the hereditary neurometabolic diseases

Disease	Bone marrow	Peripheral blood
Gaucher disease	Gaucher cell + + +	Anemia; leukopenia; thrombopenia ±
Niemann-Pick A disease	Foam cells	
Niemann-Pick C disease	Sea-blue histiocytes + + +; foam cells	
G_{M1} gangliosidosis type I	Foam cells	Vacuolated lymphocytes
G_{M1} gangliosidosis type II	Vacuoles and fibrillary inclusions in histiocytes	
Sandhoff disease	Foam cells	
Fabry disease	Foam cells	Anemia
Juvenile ceroid lipofuscinosis		Vacuolated lymphocytes + + +
MPS I, II, III	Typical inclusions (metachromatic or not) in plasmocytes, monocytes	Typical inclusions in leukocytes
I-cell disease	Vacuoles in leukocytes	Vacuoles in lymphocytes
Fucosidosis	Vacuoles; inclusions in leukocytes; histiocytes	Vacuolated lymphocytes; occasional inclusions
α-Mannosidosis	Foam cells ±	
Aspartylglucosaminuria	Foam cells	Vacuolated lymphocytes; anemia
Sialidosis II	Foam cells	Vacuolated lymphocytes
Sialic acid storage disease	Vacuolated histiocytes with granulofilamentous material	Vacuolated lymphocytes
Multiple sulfatase deficiency	Inclusions in WBC as in the MPS	Inclusions in WBC as in MPS
Choreoacanthocytosis		Acanthocytosis + + +
Abetalipoproteinemia		Acanthocytosis + + +
Hypobetalipoproteinemia		Acanthocytosis ±
HARP syndrome		Acanthocytosis + + +
McLeod syndrome[a]		Acanthocytosis + + +
Wilson disease		Hemolytic anemia; leukopenia; thrombopenia ±
Galactosemia		Bleeding ±
Isovaleric acidemia		Thrombocytopenia; leukopenia; anemia
Propionic acidemia		Thrombocytopenia; leukopenia; anemia
Methylmalonic acidemia		Thrombocytopenia; leukopenia; anemia
Combined MCoAM and MHM deficiencies (defects in cobalamin metabolism)		Macrocytic anemia, megaloblastosis + + +; thrombocytopenia; hypersegmented polymorphic leukocytes; hemolytic episodes
Methyltetrahydrofolate: homocysteine methyltransferase deficiency		Megaloblastic anemia + + +
Hereditary folate malabsorption		Megaloblastic anemia + + +

Abbreviations and symbols: MCoAM = methylmalonyl-CoA mutase; MHM = methyltetrahydrofolate: homocysteine methyl transferase; MPS = mucopolysaccharidosis; + + + = of great diagnostic importance, constant or very frequent; ± = rare.

[a] See Ref. 131, Chap. 5.

Table 7-8A

Craniofacial deformities in the hereditary neurometabolic diseases: gargoyle-like facial features[a]

Disease	Degree of gargoyle-like facial features in late infancy and early childhood
MPS I H	Marked
MPS I H/S	Moderate to marked; micrognathia
MPS II	Marked to moderate
MPS III	Minimal to moderate
ML II (I-cell disease)	Marked; gingival hypertrophy
ML III	Moderate
Fucosidosis	Mild to moderate
α-Mannosidosis	Moderate to marked
Aspartylglucosaminuria	Mild to moderate
Sialidosis II	Marked
Multiple sulfatase deficiency	Mild
G_{M1} gangliosidosis type I	Moderate; puffy eyelids; underslung jaw; gingival hypertrophy; long upper lip

Abbreviations: MPS = mucopolysaccharidosis; ML = mucolipidosis.

[a] Gargoyle-like features include coarse facial features, depressed nasal bridge, frontal bossing, scaphocephaly, thick lips, protruding tongue, thick eyebrows, puffy eyelids, short neck.

skin and the form of the nose and chin: such changes as may be related to a metabolic disorder. One must also be aware of, and be able to recognize, the most frequent dysmorphic changes occurring in chromosomal abnormalities (such as the Miller-Dieker syndrome), polymalformative syndromes and those related to chronic medication (Phenytoin).

Frank malformations of the face (midline changes, such as major hypertelorism and hypotelorism, midfacial hypoplasia, cleft palate) or anomalies of the limbs and genitourinary tracts generally do not occur in the metabolic encephalopathies. The few exceptions are listed in Table 7-8 and in Chap. 6.

RESPIRATORY TRACT (TABLE 7-9)

In the mucopolysaccharide storage diseases, mucolipidoses, and glycoprotein degradation diseases, infiltration of the mucosa of the upper respiratory tract and lungs by the stored substance is the cause of early and persistent nasal discharge and infections. This may constitute an early and significant diagnostic feature. Obstructive pulmonary insufficiency eventually develops. Scoliosis and thoracic deformities may also contribute to chronic repiratory failure.

Infiltration of the lungs with recurrent pulmonary infections, and chronic respiratory failure, may also be observed in Gaucher disease, Niemann-Pick disease and in the early infantile form of G_{M1} gangliosidosis. Repeated bronchopulmonary infections are an important feature of ataxia-telangiectasia. Asthma is observed occasionally in adrenoleukodystrophy and homocystinuria, and chronic pulmonary insufficiency may occur in Fabry disease and cerebrotendinous xanthomatosis.

Unexplained hyperpnea is a highly characteristic sign of Leigh disease and may sometimes be among the first manifestations of this disease. Respiratory distress in the young infant occurs in disorders that cause a metabolic acidosis, as in the congenital lactic acidoses and in some of the aminoacidopathies. Laryngeal stridor is observed in a number of HMDs.

GASTROINTESTINAL SIGNS, MALNUTRITION, AND GROWTH FAILURE (TABLE 7-10)

Anorexia and vomiting (more rarely, diarrhea) are among the first clinical manifestations in many early infantile metabolic encephalopathies, such as the lipidoses, Leigh disease, and other mitochondrial diseases. They may be misinterpreted as a primary disorder of the digestive tract. These infants fail to thrive. Their weight tends to reach a plateau and their growth remains stationary.

Table 7-8B
Craniofacial deformities in the hereditary metabolic disorders: other types of facial deformities

Disease	Type of deformity	Associated developmental defects[a]
Zellweger disease	Typically high forehead; wide-set eyes; shallow orbital ridges; broad root of nose; retrognathism	Brain
Other neonatal peroxisomal disorders	Less constant; less marked	Brain
PDH deficiency	Variable; mild	Short fingers and arms; hypospadias; anteriorly placed anus; brain
Glutaric aciduria II	High forehead; hypertelorism; low-set ears	Defects of abdominal wall and feet; hypospadias; brain
Molybdenum cofactor (sulfite oxidase) deficiency	Large head; upturned nose; triangular face; enophthalmos and telecanthus; cleft palate; broad nasal bridge	
Mevalonic aciduria	Uncharacteristic: broad nasal bridge; micrognathia; low-set ears	
3-Hydroxyisobutyric acidemia	Microcephaly; short, sloped forehead; narrow bitemporal diameter; hypoplastic orbital ridges; epicanthus; prominent philtrum; micrognathia	Brain
3-Hydroxyisobutyryl-CoA deacylase deficiency	Undefined (1 case)	Vertebra; heart; brain
Lowe disease	Prominent frontal bone; sunken eyes; large, low-set ears	
Cockayne disease	Loss of subcutaneous fat; thin, atrophic skin; prominent nose; large ears; retrognathism (or prognathism) "progeric" appearance	
2,4-Dienoyl-CoA reductase deficiency		Short arms, fingers, feet, and trunk
Smith-Lemli-Opitz syndrome	Ptosis, anteverted nares, abnormal ears, micrognathia	Hypospadias; multiple other congenital defects; brain

[a]For brain defects see Table 6-1.

Episodes of vomiting are also a feature of MELAS. The causes of vomiting, anorexia and malnutrition have not been satisfactorily explained.

Difficulty in swallowing, as part of the pseudobulbar syndrome, may contribute to the undernourishment. The trouble with feeding these infants frequently results in the selection of inappropriate diets. When the intestinal tract is infiltrated, as in some of the storage diseases, malabsorption could be an explanation, but this has not yet been substantiated except for abetalipoproteinemia and familial amyloid neuropathy in which intestinal malabsorption is one of the major signs. In abetalipoproteinemia a decrease in vitamin E absorption is responsible for the neurologic syndrome. Constipation due to an inadequate diet, immobility, and intestinal atonia may be very troublesome. Diarrhea occurs in Fabry disease and other disorders with dysfunction of the autonomic nervous system. Increased catabolism due to sustained rigidity and frequent spasms, may be another factor of malnutrition.

Attacks of abdominal pain are features of acute intermittent porphyria and Fabry disease.

Stunting of growth, unrelated to malnutrition, is a feature in Cockayne syndrome, the mitochondrial encephalomyopathies, the mucopolysaccharidoses, and other conditions. We are aware of a young child with glutaconic aciduria who first came to medical attention for growth failure.

Table 7-9

Chronic respiratory abnormalities in the hereditary neurometabolic disorders[a]

Infiltration of lung, trachea, larynx, pharynx, and a large tongue lead to repeated upper respiratory tract infections and to severe obstructive airway insufficiency

The mucopolysaccharidoses[b]

Some patients with mucolipidoses and disorders of glycoprotein
  degradation

Infiltration of lung by sphingolipids in the early infantile neurovisceral lipidoses

Farber disease	Respiratory insufficiency, possibly of the obstructive type
G_{M1} gangliosidosis	Minimal or moderate clinical consequence
Niemann-Pick disease	Minimal or moderate clinical consequence
Gaucher disease	Minimal or moderate clinical consequence

Other neurometabolic diseases

Fabry disease	Bronchitis; dyspnea (alveolar capillary block)
Ataxia-telangiectasia	Sinopulmonary infections
Menkes disease	Emphysema
Homocystinuria	Asthma
Adrenoleukodystrophy	Asthma
Cerebrotendinous xanthomatosis	Chronic pulmonary fibrosis
Glycogenosis II	Respiratory insufficiency; atelectasia (infiltration of lung)
Biotinidase deficiency	Laryngeal stridor
Gaucher disease	Laryngeal stridor
Idiopathic dystonia	Laryngeal stridor
Pelizaeus-Merzbacher disease	Laryngeal stridor
Familial lysinuric protein intolerance	Interstitial pneumonia

---

[a] Not mentioned here are intermittent episodes of respiratory dysrhythmia related to acute episodes of metabolic decompensation (for example, in disorders of amino acids and organic acids, and in mitochondrial disorders).

[b] A serious complication which may necessitate major therapeutic measures (see text) and is greatly relieved after bone marrow transplantation.

Table 7-10

Gastrointestinal symptoms in the hereditary metabolic encephalopathies[a]

Early infantile HMDs with anorexia, vomiting, and feeding difficulties as early manifestations which may mask neurologic signs

The early infantile neurovisceral sphingolipidoses
Krabbe leukodystrophy
Leigh disease
PDH E_1 deficiency

HMDs with acute, often remitting neurologic episodes: anorexia and vomiting may accompany neurologic signs; fasting, vomiting, and fever may trigger metabolic decompensation

Disorders of pyruvate metabolism
Disorders of the mitochondrial respiratory chain
Disorders of mitochondrial fatty acid oxidation
Leigh disease
Inherited disorders of amino acid and organic acid metabolism
Fructose 1,6-bisphosphate deficiency

Other disorders

Familial amyloid neuropathy	Celiac syndrome; diarrhea
Abetalipoproteinemia	Celiac syndrome
MELAS	Vomiting
Fabry disease	Abdominal pain; diarrhea; intestinal diverticuli
Acute intermittent porphyria	Abdominal pain
Metachromatic leukodystrophy	Exclusion of gall bladder
Fucosidosis	Exclusion of gall bladder
Lysinuric protein intolerance	Abdominal pain
GM2 gangliosidosis and all HMDs, especially if bedridden	Constipation; gastrointestinal reflux; dental caries

---

[a] This table is not exhaustive.

Chapter 8

LABORATORY TESTS FOR THE DIAGNOSIS OF HEREDITARY METABOLIC ENCEPHALOPATHIES

BIOCHEMISTRY AND MOLECULAR BIOLOGY
    Common Clinical Tests in Urine, Blood, and CSF
    Enzyme Assays
    DNA Studies

RADIOLOGY AND NEUROIMAGING
    Conventional X-rays
    Ultrasonography
    Neuroimaging

ELECTROPHYSIOLOGICAL METHODS

HEMATOLOGIC TESTS

EXAMINATION OF BIOPSIED TISSUE

PRACTICAL CONSIDERATIONS FOR THE COLLECTION OF SPECIMENS

For the physician concerned with the diagnosis of the diseases discussed in the preceding chapters, the matter of selecting the appropriate laboratory tests will doubtless arise. The clinician should be informed as to the reliability and validity of the many different tests, as well as the likely sources of artifact and error.

Included in this chapter are a number of laboratory tests and ancillary procedures that have proved useful in diagnosis. Many of them can be performed in any laboratory with standard equipment. But even the simplest test results may be difficult to interpret without some special knowledge. Every clinician appreciates that laboratory results never have full meaning unless viewed in a clinical context.

Recently, the extraordinary developments of biochemistry, molecular biology, and neuroimaging have added a new dimension to our diagnostic possibilities.

Clinicians will have to renew their efforts to understand these highly specialized techniques, in deciding when to apply them and how to interpret their findings.

The competent physician must know the laboratory tests that have been developed for each disease, the laboratories that are available in the community, and the relative reliability, validity, and cost of each test procedure.

This chapter discusses the following laboratory procedures:

- Biochemistry and molecular biology
- Radiologic testing and neuroimaging
- Electrophysiology
- Hematology
- Tissue biopsy

BIOCHEMISTRY AND MOLECULAR BIOLOGY

Common Clinical Tests in Urine, Blood, and CSF

A number of standard clinical procedures adapted to urine, blood, and CSF remain of great diagnostic importance and some of them should be performed systematically whenever a hereditary metabolic disorder is suspected in infants and children.

In the urine, testing for the following substances can be revealing, with due consideration of the clinical context: ketone bodies, glucose and galactose, lactic acid (in 24-hour urine specimen), orotic acid (in the hyperammonemias), copper (in Wilson disease), uric acid (in Lesch-Nyhan disease), sialic acid (in sialic acid storage diseases), *N*-acetylaspartic acid (in Canavan disease). Evidence of renal tubular dysfunction should be searched for especially when Lowe disease or Hartnup disease is suspected.

Various methods of *chromatography* are employed to detect amino acids, organic acids (by GC/MS), sulfatides, mucopolysaccharides, oligosaccharides, and purines (for adenylosuccinyl lyase deficiency).

As reliable biochemical tests have now been standardized and simplified, they can be carried out rapidly in most medical centers. There is little need for classical screening tests of PKU and other aminoacidopathies such as: acetest, dinitrophenylhydrazine (DPNH), $FeCl_2$ (Phenistix), the cyanide prusside reaction (for homocystinuria), and the clinitest (Benedict reaction) in the urine. All these screening tests may give false negative and false positive results.

In the blood, measurements of glucose, ketone bodies, acid-base balance, ammonia, urea, pyruvic acid, lactic acid, electrolytes, and in certain clinical contexts, tests for liver function, cholesterol, triglycerides, lipoproteins, vitamin E, copper, ceruloplasmin, and very long chain fatty acids (by GC/MS) usually yield essential information.

In the cerebrospinal fluid, evaluation of the levels of total protein, gamma globulins, glucose, lactic acid, GABA and other organic acids, and β-crystallin are of great diagnostic value. Most of these tests are performed routinely in any hospital laboratory. However, gas chromatography and mass spectroscopy are usually performed in more specialized, but usually easily accessible, centers.

Examples of the diagnostic importance of common biochemical tests *for neonates and young infants*, are given in Tables 2-2 to 2-8 and for the *acute intermittent encephalopathies* in Table 3-7.

In *older children* with a chronic neurologic disorder, the following tests are of significance:

1. Increase in urinary mucopolysaccharides in the mucopolysaccharidoses, and of urinary oligosaccharides in mucolipidoses and disorders of glycoprotein degradation.

2. Elevated concentration of lactate in CSF (and blood) in the mitochondrial encephalomyopathies.

3. Marked elevation of total protein in the CSF in metachromatic leukodystrophy, X-linked adrenoleukodystrophy, some cases of juvenile Krabbe disease, and a few other conditions. In several patients with MLD starting with psychiatric symptoms or in patients with MLD presenting as a slowly advancing paraparesis, the discovery of elevated total CSF protein has been a major orienting finding in our experience. Quantitative and qualitative evaluation of gamma globulin have been helpful in differentiating late infantile and juvenile metabolic encephalopathies from subacute sclerosing panencephalitis and chronic rubella encephalitis. In these conditions, total CSF proteins are usually not elevated.

4. High levels of blood VLCFAs in peroxisomal diseases.

5. Hyperuricuria and hyperuricemia in Lesch-Nyhan disease.

6. Low levels of cholesterol in cholestanolosis, abetalipoproteinemia, and Smith-Lemli-Opitz syndrome.

7. Presence of β-crystallin in the CSF of Alexander disease.

8. High levels of GABA and homocarnosine in disorders of GABA metabolism.

9. Low concentrations of CSF glucose in De Vivo disease.

10. Low levels of the thyroxine-binding protein in serum in the carbohydrate-deficient glycoprotein syndrome; serum electrophoresis for transferrin isoforms is also a useful test for this disease.

Enzyme Assays

For many neurometabolic disorders, the specific enzymatic defect is known and enzyme assays will help to confirm the diagnosis.

A few methodological requirements and problems in interpretation of results, are of practical importance for the clinician.

a Requests for specific enzyme assays should always be determined within the context of the clinical, radiological, and other biochemical findings. A systematic screening without any clinical justification is pointless, wastes time, and consumes expensive resources.

b For the most meaningful results, the type of cell or tissue on which the tests are performed should be carefully selected as it can vary according to the disease. In most neurometabolic disorders, enzymatic tests can be carried out on either plasma, leukocytes, or cultured fibroblasts. Some disorders require the use of muscle or liver biopsy specimens or red blood cells. Tears and blood on a blotting paper can be of practical use when a great distance separates the clinical hospital from the biochemical laboratory.

Some conditions (such as defects of the mitochondrial respiratory chain or PDH deficiency) may require assays on more than one tissue (e.g. muscle and cultured skin fibroblasts) because of tissue specificity or variability of isoenzymes. This may complicate prenatal diagnosis.

c When an enzymatic deficiency is suspected, the parents and other family members should be tested for diagnostic confirmation and for the purpose of genetic counseling.

d The interpretation of the results of enzymatic assays and the need to undertake further tests are influenced by clinical data.

Difficulties in interpretation arise when there is a discrepancy between a given enzymatic defect and the clinical picture. The clinical features may be typical, but the testing of the activity of the corresponding enzyme is, paradoxically, normal. This can occur when the right substrate for enzyme testing is not used or when the disorder is related to deficiency of a protein cofactor of the enzyme. For example, for the diagnosis of the B_1 variant of G_{M2} gangliosidosis, a sulfated substrate or the natural substrate must be used. To take another example, there are rare cases of juvenile metachromatic leukodystrophy which are due to a deficiency of an activator protein.

Contrariwise, the activity of an enzyme may be very low in a totally uncharacteristic clinical syndrome or in a normal individual. This is the situation encountered in cases of pseudo-deficiency of MLD and a few other disorders (see Chap. 4). Not to be aware of this could lead to errors in genetic counseling or treatment. Screening for specific metabolites in urine, enzymatic studies of the family, and DNA analysis will assure the correct diagnosis.

DNA Studies

The mutant gene responsible for an ever increasing number of neurometabolic disorders is known.

For diagnostic purposes, molecular biology techniques are essential for the diagnostic confirmation and genetic counseling of hereditary diseases, mainly diseases in which there is a failure to form the gene product or when the protein product of the gene is not easily accessible. Here, diagnosis is more easily achieved by examining the gene itself. Examples include myelin formation disorders, such as Pelizaeus-Merzbacher disease

and CMT disease, trinucleotide repeat disorders such as Huntington disease, and defects of mt DNA. When the approximate genetic locus is known, but the gene itself has not been cloned, linkage analysis in informative families can aid in the diagnosis of an affected individual. DNA studies are also of considerable help when the result of the measurements of the catalytic activity of the enzyme are not convincing, as may happen in some cases of PDH deficiency and defects of the respiratory chain. They are increasingly important in heterozygote detection (in families or population-based tests); in prediction of the severity of a disease on the basis of the mutation present; in presymptomatic diagnosis, and prenatal diagnosis when sufficient information is available from testing of other family members.

The interpretation of the result of these DNA studies must also be integrated into the general clinical and biochemical context, as it is known that many different mutations can be associated with the same disease and, apparently, an identical mutation may give rise to different clinical phenotypes.

Some familial disorders, such as Huntington disease, are currently without treatment, so DNA screening of apparently unaffected, but possibly presymptomatic, family members may raise serious ethical problems.

RADIOLOGY AND NEUROIMAGING

Conventional X-rays

Conventional x-ray films of the skeleton—spine, hips, limbs, and cranium—remain essential for the diagnosis of the mucopolysaccharidoses, oligosaccharidoses, mucolipidoses, amd multiple sulfatase deficiency, in which there is a characteristic pattern of bone alteration known as *dysostosis multiplex*. There may be various degrees of this condition. Changes may be subtle, although revealing in the absence of obvious facial dysmorphia, as in Sanfilippo disease.

There are many other metabolic encephalopathies, with characteristic bone alterations; they are listed in Table 7-5. X-rays of the thorax may reveal a cardiomegaly or pulmonary lesions.

On the whole, it can be said that conventional x-rays retains an important place among routine diagnostic laboratory tests in the metabolic encephalopathies.

Ultrasonography

Ultrasound scanning is a useful method for detecting a cardiomegaly, the enlargement of liver and spleen and cystic changes in the kidneys. These are important features of a number of metabolic disorders (Chap. 7).

Pre- or perinatal echographies are useful for detecting developmental abnormalities or destructive lesions of the brain of acquired or genetic origin. Only a minority of prenatal lesions are the result of a metabolic disease (Table 6-1).

Neuroimaging

Brief Descriptions of Imaging Techniques

Computed Tomography   In computed tomography (CT), an x-ray source and a detector are rotated around the head of the patient and the image is generated from differences in radiodensity. The CT scan provides successive images of a single plane of tissue. Bone, brain, CSF, blood vessels, and calcifications can be visualized.

Magnetic Resonance Imaging   Magnetic resonance imaging (MRI) provides images that localize atomic nuclei and enable different brain components to be distinguished according to their individual chemical and cellular composition. When placed in a strong magnetic field, the protons of water and fat behave like small bar-magnets and align along the applied external field. Individual magnetic moments from these protons precess around the applied magnetic field with a certain rotational speed called the resonance frequency. Application of brief radio frequency pulses at the resonance frequency disturbs this equilibrium. The spins will try to regain their equilibrium by emitting radio signals which can be detected and processed into an image. In MRI, with the use of magnetic field gradients in different directions, it is possible to separate the signals coming from different locations. The spins absorb energy from the externally applied radio waves and are converted to an excited state. As they return to a lower state, they release energy in a process called relaxation. The rate of relaxation can be described as an exponential decay. Two fundamental time parameters are used to describe this decay of MRI signals: T1 (longitudinal or spin-lattice relaxation) and T2 (transverse or spin-spin relaxation). Differences in T1 and T2 of tissues are the primary basis of contrast in clinical MRI.

With MRI, the precise structure of the brain is revealed in three planes. Gray matter, white matter, CSF, meninges, and blood vessels are distinguished. Bone and calcifications (which have a very low content of free water) do not generate any signal. Intravascular injection of gadolinium compounds (a paramagnetic substance) will outline brain vasculature, intracranial structures that have no blood-brain barrier (such as meninges, choroid plexuses, pituitary and pineal glands), and brain tissues in which the blood-brain barrier is altered. MRI can also detect the motion of water molecules; MR angiography selectively images the flow of blood in blood vessels and may be used to measure brain perfusion.

Magnetic Resonance Spectroscopy   Now within the reach of modern clinical instruments, magnetic resonance spectroscopy (MRS) allows various metabolites to be studied in the brain (and in muscle).

N-acetylaspartate (NAA), creatine (Cr), choline (Cho) compounds, lactic acid and several amino acids can be studied with proton MRS. With phosphorous (^{31}P) MRS, regional energy metabolism can be studied.

Various other new techniques for mapping brain function derived from MRI are currently being developed.

Positron Emission Tomography (PET) Scan   PET scanning provides images of brain function that reflect the distribution in the tissues of an injected or inhaled isotope that emits radiation. Information on the functional activity of the brain can be obtained by mapping glucose metabolism of neurons. This metabolic parameter is studied using deoxyglucose, an analog of glucose that is taken up by neurons in the same manner as glucose but is not metabolized in the cell. In injecting deoxyglucose bound to the positron-emitting isotope of fluorine 18 (^{18}F-deoxyglucose), it is possible to disclose the pattern of regional metabolic activity and to detect areas of impaired metabolic activity. It is also possible to evaluate the density of transmitter receptors in administering radiolabeled neurotransmitters. Unfortunately, the resolution of PET scans remains low.

Clinical Use of Neuroimaging: Practical Considerations
Because of the vastly superior contrast resolution of MRI, CT scanning has been largely replaced, except for the visualization of bone structures and brain calcifications which are not detected by MRI. Hereditary metabolic or neurodegenerative disorders with brain calcifications are indicated in Chap. 6. The precise nature

of brain calcification is not revealed on CT scans. It should be remembered that at autopsy, calcium deposits appear either as confluent, seemingly extracellular aggregates, as incrustations of degenerated neurons and glial cells and their expansions, or as minute, discrete perivascular concretions without notable alteration of surrounding tissues. This is the case in Cockayne syndrome and we have found it in MELAS, too. The actual extent of brain calcifications may be much enhanced on CT scans (personal observation of an autopsied case).

MRI is now used as the method of choice to explore the "in vivo" anatomy of the brain. This method is free from radiation hazards, and the time required for this procedure has been shortened. However, the equipment used for MRI may seem quite frightening to children (and some adults) and sedation may be necessary. Therefore, in some cases, the clinician may decide to use the CT scan, at least as the initial test.

MRI may confirm a clinical hypothesis or may reveal the clinically unsuspected nature and location of a neurologic disorder. This method should therefore be widely used in chronic progressive or apparently nonprogressive neurologic disorders.

Judicious modulation of the different methods of imaging requires the radiologist to be guided by precise clinical indications. Both T1- and T2-weighted images are employed on all occasions, but will vary with the clinical problem, whether a polioencephalopathy or a leukoencephalopathy. The best definition of gray matter structures, especially the cerebral cortex, is obtained with a thin section of T1-weighted images or with *inversion recovery*. Abnormal signals in the white matter are best seen with T2-weighted images and appropriate measurements of proton density.

Changes in *the cerebral cortex* that can readily be detected by MRI in such encephalopathies include cortical-subcortical areas of necrosis (e.g. in MELAS) and diffuse cortical atrophy or degeneration (in Alpers syndrome and early infantile lipofuscinosis). Cortical malformations are revealed. Cortical dysplasias (some of which may be observed in a few metabolic encephalopathies) alter the surface markings of the brain. One can visualize changes in size and thickness of convolutions (pachygyria, microgyria), the absence of convolutions (lissencephaly); and subcortical or periventricular heterotopias of neurons. Recent methods make it possible to visualize the cytoarchitectony of the cortex.

The anomalies of *subcortical gray structures* in the metabolic encephalopathies include striatal (essentially putaminal) lucencies seen in Leigh disease, in related mitochondrial encephalopathies, and in other conditions (see Chap. 5). Atrophy of the caudate nucleus is an early sign in Huntington disease, and there are characteristic changes of the globus pallidus in Hallervorden-Spatz disease

Cerebellar atrophy as an isolated or predominant abnormality may be seen in a variety of metabolic or degenerative disorders and is also a feature of a familial, nonprogressive syndrome, combining slow motor development, moderate ataxia, mental retardation, and language disorder (Chap. 6).

The detection of abnormalities in the *cerebral white matter* is one of the major contributions of MRI. Certainly, the diagnosis of a leukodystrophy can no longer be made in the absence of abnormal white matter signals on MRI on T2-weighted images. Although diagnosis requires typical clinical and biochemical features, certain morphologic characteristics are important for the differential diagnosis of this group of diseases. Bilateral and symmetrical abnormalities in the vicinity of the posterior segment of the lateral ventricle suggest either metachromatic leukodystrophy or Krabbe leukodystrophy at their earliest stages. Asymmetric or unilateral occipital (or frontal) areas of alteration with peripheral enhancement after injection of gadolinium compounds are characteristic of adrenoleukodystrophy (and can also be seen in MS and Schilder disease).

White matter abnormalities of other leukodystrophies, such as Pelizaeus-Merzbacher disease, Canavan disease, and Alexander disease, are less characteristic. Extensive white matter lesions may also occur in Leigh disease, Cockayne syndrome, Sjögren-Larsson syndrome, Zellweger disease and polyglucosan disease). Occasionally striking white matter changes are found which seem out of context and have no explanation. The so-called familial white matter hypoplasia may be related to a primary axonal disorder (G. Lyon, *Ann. Neurol.* 27: 193, 1990). Prenatal defects of the corpus callosum in the HMD are listed in Table 6-1.

A reduced amount of myelin, as visualized by MRI, may reflect a failure of myelin development due to a primary metabolic disturbance in the synthesis of a myelin protein, i.e., proteolipid protein in Pelizaeus-Merzbacher disease; a secondary effect of a metabolic error, as in phenylketonuria; or a breakdown in myelin, as in the genetic leukodystrophies. The characteristic signal given by myelin on MRI makes it possible to appreciate the level of myelination in young infants and to evaluate degrees of delay of myelination. The exact significance of such findings, however, and their relationship to a precise disease are now under scrutiny.

Summary

• MRI yields information about a few disorders which are presently defined solely on a clinicoanatomical basis: Leigh disease, Hallervorden-Spatz disease, Alexander disease, Alpers syndrome, and some of the white matter disorders.

• MRI may lead to an unsuspected diagnosis when the clinical picture is unrevealing or atypical. This has occurred, in our experience, in patients with late-onset Leigh disease, Krabbe leukodystrophy, metachromatic leukodystrophy, and Hallervorden-Spatz disease.

• MRI may reveal typical alterations of the brain at a preclinical stage. By permitting the extent of brain damage to be evaluated before the onset of clinical signs it provides an opportunity to consider bone marrow tranplantation or gene therapy. Also, it allows the effects of these and other treatments to be objectively addressed.

• Nuclear magnetic resonance spectroscopy will probably enter the field of diagnostic neuroimaging in the near future.

• PET scanning, using ^{18}F-deoxyglucose, has proven useful to us in the early detection of Huntington disease and in monitoring the effect of the treatment of Wilson disease. Future development in the mapping of receptors of neurotransmitters could prove useful to the diagnosis of basal ganglia disorders when MRI is not specific.

• MRI is thus an indispensable tool in the exploration of neurologic diseases, including neurometabolic disorders. Technical advances in neuroimaging are proceeding at an extraordinary pace, and remarkable refinements in morphologic and functional analysis of the brain are predictable even before this monograph goes to press.

ELECTROPHYSIOLOGICAL METHODS

The *EEG* is of relatively little help in diagnosing metabolic disorders. However, in the late infantile type of ceroid lipofuscinosis, low-frequency photic stimulation induces very characteristic high-amplitude occipital spikes. And in early infantile lipofuscinosis, a flattening of the tracing occurs early in the disease and is a notable peculiarity. Progressive deterioration of background activity in a child with cognitive or psychiatric abnormalities or seizures may constitute an important indication of a progressive organic pathologic process. It is an oversimplification to say that the EEG reveals generalized high-voltage slow waves in leukodystrophies, whereas it features a paroxysmal pattern in a gray matter disorders. There are too many exceptions to this rule for it to be of much help in diagnosis. The problem of the EEG in neurometabolic disorders has also been considered in detail in Chap 6.

Data supplied by *electromyography, measurement of nerve conduction velocity, somato-sensory evoked potentials, auditory* and *visual evoked potentials,* and *electroretinogram* all have their place in verifying the lesional topography of a metabolic disorder. Certain anatomical patterns are highly characteristic if viewed in a given context.

The *measurement of peripheral nerve motor and sensory conduction velocities, sensory evoked potentials* and the *EMG* are important diagnostic tools in revealing the involvement of the peripheral nervous system in a disease process. Measurement of motor and sensory nerve conduction velocity should be undertaken in most patients with a neurometabolic encephalopathy, especially in the first two years of life, when clinical evidence of peripheral nerve disease may be difficult to ascertain or is entirely lacking. There are established standards of normal conduction rates for each age period. It should be realized that these are difficult techniques which necessitate expertise. Much attention should be given to skin temperature in performing the test, and to drugs taken by the patient.

The EMG is a painful test which should be reserved to detect or confirm denervation only when motor nerve conduction velocities are normal or slightly reduced, as is the case in motor neuron disease and type II Charcot-Marie-Tooth disease.

Evaluation of these electrophysiologic methods in exploration of peripheral nerves, and their results in the different metabolic encephalopathies, have been discussed in Chap. 6. Notable is the fact that a significant slowing of nerve conduction velocities is a constant characteristic of early infantile metachromatic leukodystrophy, Krabbe leukodystrophy, and of types I and III HMS neuropathies. A normal motor nerve conduction velocity and reduced sensory evoked potentials are characteristic of Friedreich ataxia and type II HMS neuropathy. A denervation pattern with normal motor conduction velocities occurs in neuroaxonal dystrophy, in juvenile or adult G_{M2} gangliosidosis and neuronal intranuclear inclusion disease. Myotonic-like discharges of the EMG in severely hypotonic infants suggests Pompe disease (Table 6-9).

Auditory evoked potentials are useful in detecting loss of hearing and may be the only way of doing so in infants and young children. In our experience, abnormalities in auditory evoked potentials may be an early sign of a leukodystrophy. *Visual* evoked potentials may be of some value in detecting the site of a lesion in the central or peripheral pathways of the visual system. They disappear early in the course of the infantile form of neuronal ceroid lipofuscinosis.

Extinction of the *electroretinogram* indicates a degeneration of the sensory epithelium of the retina, which is found in pigmentary degeneration of the retina, even before obvious ophthalmoscopic signs are present. Pigmentary degeneration of the retina is a nearly constant feature of the lipofuscinoses and is found in many other metabolic encephalopathies (Table 6-11).

Somato-sensory evoked potentials can be helpful in confirming the presence of long tract lesions in the spinal cord.

Finally, the *ECG* is helpful in detecting or specifying the nature of a cardiopathy, for instance in Friedreich disease, the mucopolysaccharidoses, or familial amyloid neuropathy.

HEMATOLOGIC TESTS

The study of peripheral blood cells and bone marrow aspirates may yield important information about the metabolic encephalopathies listed in Table 7-7.

Abnormalities of blood or bone marrow cells are essential to the diagnosis of at least six categories of disorders: neuronal ceroid lipofuscinosis type 3 (vacuoles in circulating lymphocytes); Gaucher disease (Gaucher cells in bone marrow); Niemann-Pick disease type C (sea-blue histiocytes in bone marrow); abetalipoproteinemia (acanthocytes); chorea-

acanthocytosis (acanthocytes); disorders of cobalamin and folate metabolism (megaloblastic anemia). Inclusions in peripheral leukocytes are found in several lysosomal disorders; their presence is of diagnostic importance.

Acanthocytes are characteristic spiky or thorny red blood cells that are best shown in preparation of fresh blood suspended in Dacie solution. Acanthocytes should be searched for in all chronic cases of chorea.

The typical Gaucher cell is a large histiocyte, 20 to 100 μm in diameter, with a homogeneous, slightly crumpled cytoplasm, as visualized in Giemsa stains. In electron micrographs, its cytoplasm is shown to contain twisted membranous bilayers composed of glucocerobroside. Other diseases with rapid turnover of white blood cells, such as the leukemias, may occasionally display Gaucher cells.

Sea-blue histiocytes are revealed in Giemsa or Wright stains. They are large, measuring up to 60 μm in diameter with homogeneous granules colored intensely in blue. In electron micrographs, these granules appear as lamellar, amorphous or granular cytosomes that contain phospholipids and glycolipids. Foam cells are interspersed with the sea-blue histiocytes.

In atypical or uncharacteristic forms of juvenile Niemann-Pick disease type C; Gaucher disease; in the Sandhoff variant of G_{M2} gangliosidosis; in mucopolysaccharidoses, oligosaccharidoses, and the mucolipidoses, examination of bone marrow smears has sometimes permitted an initial diagnosis of congenital nonprogressive encephalopathy, later changed to that of an inherited metabolic disorder.

EXAMINATION OF BIOPSIED TISSUE

Examination of biopsied tissue remains an indispensable diagnostic procedure in a small number of "metabolic" or "degenerative" disorders in which specific abnormalities are known to exist outside the CNS in peripheral nerves, skin, conjunctiva, or skeletal muscle. This is

---

Figure 8-1
A. Sural nerve biopsy. (Top) Krabbe leukodystrophy: electron microscopy shows typical membrane profiles in Schwann cell cytoplasm (arrow). (Bottom) Metachromatic leucodystrophy: light microscopy using toluidine blue reveals metachromatic granular inclusions. **B**. Sural nerve biopsy. Metachromatic leukodystrophy: electron microscopy shows characteristic inclusion in macrophage (arrow) (inclusions in Schwann cells and segmental demyelination present at other levels). **C**. Late infantile ceroid lipofuscinosis, skin biopsy: electron microscopy shows curvilinear inclusions in fibroblast. **D**. MERRF, muscle biopsy: Giemsa stain reveals ragged red fibers. Note dense subsarcolemmal mitochondrial aggregates (arrows).

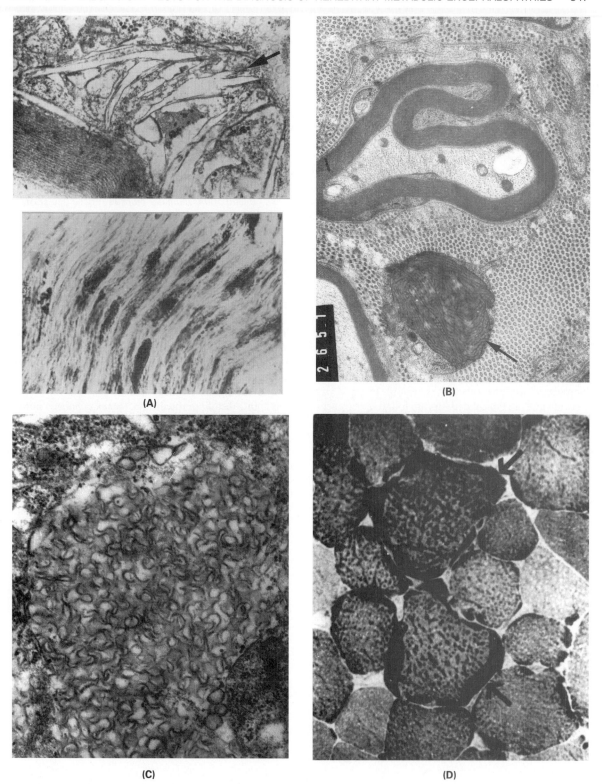

(A)

(B)

(C)

(D)

most valuable in diseases where no specific biochemical abnormalities are known. Biopsies must be resorted to for diagnosis of the following disorders (Table 8-1, Fig. 8-1).

In *neuroaxonal dystrophy*, where specific membranous aggregates accumulate in the distal part of peripheral nerve axons, especially at the neuromuscular junction.

In *giant axonal neuropathy*, where abnormal fibrils are found in peripheral nerve axons and also in other tissues.

In *familial amyloid neuropathy* a nerve biopsy is also essential.

In the *lipofuscinoses*, where deposits of ceroid lipofuscin with special ultrastructural features are found in lysosomes of fibroblasts and other cells in biopsy specimens of the skin or conjunctiva. (We now prefer skin biopsies because they are less traumatic for the child.) Each variety of lipofuscinosis has a predominant type of inclusion: curvilinear bodies in the late infantile form (Fig. 8-1), fingerprint-like deposits in the juvenile type, and granular material in the early infantile form.

In *Lafora disease*, where typical polyglucosan inclusions can be detected in sweat gland cells (in skin biopsies, especially in the axillary region). In *adult polyglucosan disease*, typical deposits are found in peripheral nerves.

In *mucolipidosis IV* in which the detection of intralysosomal membranous inclusions in mesenchymal cells is necessary for diagnosis.

In primary or secondary *defects in mitochondrial DNA*, particularly the juvenile encephalomyopathies, where the detection of abnormal accumulations of mitochondria at the sarcolemmal border in muscle biopsy specimens treated with Gomori trichome stain (*ragged red fibers*) constitutes an essential element of the diagnosis.

In addition, morphological studies of biopsied tissue may complement or affirm a diagnosis when biochemical results are uncertain, when a discrepancy exists between clinical and biochemical data (for instance, in cases of pseudo-deficiency or when an activator protein is defective) or when long delays are anticipated in obtaining the result of specialized laboratory tests. This may be the case in metachromatic leukodystrophy and Krabbe disease, in which typical inclusions accumulate in Schwann cells and macrophages in peripheral nerves that can be readily detected in a sural nerve biopsy specimen. The electron microscope is necessary to finalize the diagnosis of Krabbe globoid

leukodystrophy or to reveal the characteristic pattern of sulfatide deposits in MLD (Fig. 8-1). But in MLD, light microscopic studies of frozen sections of nerve stained with 1% acid cresyl violet or toluidine blue will be sufficient to disclose the characteristic metachromatic inclusions (Fig. 8-1). In fact, before the enzymatic defect was known, a sural nerve biopsy was our only means of confirming the diagnosis of metachromatic leukodystrophy during life.

Abnormal inclusions in Schwann cells also occur in X-linked ALD and a few other metabolic disorders but are of little value to diagnosis.

Rectal or appendicular biopsies for the detection of typical inclusions in neurons of the Meissner and Auerbach plexuses may allow the diagnosis of *intranuclear neuronal inclusion disease*. They have been used occasionally in the past to detect atypical forms of G_{M2} gangliosidosis (especially the B_1 variant), and in cases of neuronal ceroid lipofuscinosis in which skin biopsy findings were inconclusive.

Liver biopsies. Microchemical measurement of liver copper is necessary for the preclinical diagnosis of Wilson disease or its variants. In the Niemann-Pick disease type C, an infant with otherwise unexplained jaundice several weeks or months after birth, the liver biopsy will reveal a giant cell hepatitis.

In abetalipoproteinemia, *jejunal biopsy* shows typical alteration of the intestinal mucosa.

Also, the *demonstration of enzyme deficiencies and gene defects* are made on cultured fibroblasts from skin biopsy specimens, on liver biopsies (urea cycle disorders), and on muscle biopsies (some mitochondrial disorders).

Brain biopsies are no longer justified for the diagnosis of metabolic encephalopathies. For the great majority of HMDs, specific biochemical or molecular defects are now available. When this is not the case, the characteristic brain lesions can be demonstrated during life with MRI. In the few conditions where biochemistry and neuroimaging are not specific a cortical biopsy would be of little help. Only in the case of a child in an advanced stage of disease, whose family asked that all possibilities of diagnosis be explored for genetic purposes, have we agreed, very exceptionally, to a biopsy of cerebral tissue.

Table 8-1

Morphological diagnosis

	Specific lesions in CNS	Characteristic MRI	Peripheral nerve	Skin or muscle	Rectal biopsy
Leigh syndrome	+ +	+ +			
Alpers syndrome	+ +	+ +			
Hallervorden-Spatz disease	+ +	+ +			
Leukodystrophies (MLD, KL, ALD)	+ +	+ +	+ +		
Canavan disease	+ +				
Alexander disease	+ +	+ +			
Neuroaxonal dystrophy	+ +		+ +	+ M[a]	
Giant axonal neuropathy	+ +		+ +	+	
Familial amyloid neuropathy			+ +		
Adult polyglucosan disease		+	+ +		
Lipofuscinoses	+ +			+ + S	
Lafora disease	+ +			+ + SM	
Defects in mtDNA	+	+		+ + M	
Neuronal intranuclear inclusion disease	+ +	+			+ +
Mucolipidosis IV				+ + S	

Symbols: + + = essential for diagnosis; + = frequent or important, but not specific; S = skin; M = muscle. (S, M indicate the usual site for a diagnostic biopsy.)

[a]Neuromuscular junction.

PRACTICAL CONSIDERATIONS FOR THE COLLECTION OF SPECIMENS

To collect urine from a very young child, a Hollister U-bag or similar collection device should be placed over the child's clitoris or penis and securely fixed to the perineum by its gummed edges. The child can be left overnight with the bag held in place by a diaper. When removing the bag in the morning, the parent should hold the child in a vertical position, using gravity to ensure that the collected urine remains in the bottom of the bag and does not flow out of its opening. The bag containing the urine can be placed into a plastic jar with a lid or the urine can be transferred to a clean plastic container from which all cleaning solutions and other contents have been thoroughly rinsed. The use of a plastic container with a secure fitting cap will permit the specimen to be preserved frozen until it can be transported to the laboratory. For the child who is able to cooperate for a specimen collection, an early morning specimen is most desirable, as it is likely to be more concentrated than a specimen obtained at any other time of day. When transferring a urine specimen from one container to another, it is necessary to include all the sediment; a small amount of water may need to be added to harvest any sediment that remains behind.

While it is often possible to test urine present in a diaper, either by squeezing the diaper to extract the urine or by performing the test directly on the diaper, we do not advocate the use of diaper urine for metabolic disease testing. The reason is that diapers, especially disposable diapers, may contain substances that interfere with the assays needed, causing false negative or false positive results.

Blood specimens for enzyme analysis are usually collected in heparinized tubes and refrigerated immediately at 4°C. They must not be frozen, since freezing will release intracellular contents and will prevent subsequent separation of leukocytes, platelets, or lymphocytes from the red blood cells. This separation should be done as soon as possible, certainly within the same day that the blood is drawn, while the cellular elements are still intact.

Blood for DNA analyses should be collected in EDTA-coated tubes, not in heparinized tubes, since heparin will interfere with amplification of the DNA by polymerase chain reaction (PCR). Blood obtained for DNA isolation should be refrigerated. However, refrigeration may be delayed, if necessary, for one or two days. The DNA isolated from whole blood is in the form of genomic DNA and is only useful for molecular diagnoses, when the gene structure is known and PCR primers have been constructed that allow amplification of the region of interest. If only the cDNA sequence is known, then it is usually necessary to obtain a skin biopsy for fibroblast culture and isolation of mRNA from which the cDNA can be prepared. Alternatively, lymphoblasts can be prepared by transformation of blood lymphocytes in tissue culture.

Specimens of blood drawn for enzyme analyses and DNA isolation should also be obtained from parents and other close relatives and treated in an identical manner. This is necessary to show the presence of reduced enzyme activity, indicative of the carrier state for an autosomal recessive condition in a parent or sibling, and to search for the putative mutation in other family members.

In seeking evidence of a storage disease, the peripheral blood smear should first be examined, as the presence of vacuoles or other types of inclusions may obviate the need for a bone marrow examination or skin biopsy. Should a bone marrow study be performed, both a marrow aspirate for smears and a biopsy with formalin fixation of the specimen should be done. Sectioning of the fixed specimen will permit a more detailed examination than smears of marrow alone.

In securing a skin biopsy, our preferred site is the inner aspect of the upper arm near the axilla. This region has a high density of sensory nerve endings and sweat glands, and a scar in this area will rarely be noticed. A 70% solution of isopropyl alcohol may be used to prepare the skin. Iodine preparations should be avoided, as iodine can interfere with the growth of the cells in tissue culture. Analgesia is achieved wth 1% lidocaine, with instillation in a circle around the area to be biopsied, so that the specimens will not be deformed in any way by the injection of the anesthetic agent. We use a disposal skin punch to obtain two adjacent 3 mm circular specimens, being careful to handle each specimen at its edge only, using tiny sawtooth forceps to avoid crushing the tissue.

One specimen is placed in fresh sterile tissue culture media and immediately refrigerated. The second is deposited into glutaraldehyde fixative for electron microscopy. If the sole purpose of the biopsy is to obtain tissue for enzymatic assays and morphologic studies are not needed (as for example to analyze cholesterol esterification in a case of suspected Niemann-Pick disease type C), then only a single specimen is obtained. The wound, which generally involves only the upper skin layer, may be closed with Steri-strips. Skin biopsy samples can also be obtained from the anterior abdominal wall, on the occasion of the placement of a G-tube as a feeding assist or from the incision line during a muscle biopsy procedure.

A muscle biopsy should be performed in an area not previously used during electrodiagnostic procedures. Local or general anesthesia is used, depending on the age of the child. Sufficient tissue must be obtained so that adequate amounts are available for frozen sections, for paraffin embedding, for electron microscopy, and for assays of mitochondrial or other muscle-specific enzymes or for immunochemistry of muscle proteins. While still in the operating room, the specimens must be processed immediately with the appropriate fixative and a separate piece is stored in liquid nitrogen for biochemical determination.

If a rectal biopsy is to be done, a transmural incision is made to secure the ganglionic plexuses in the muscularis layer and an end-to-end anastomosis performed to restore the integrity of the colon.

Chapter 9

TREATMENT AND PREVENTION OF NEUROMETABOLIC DISORDERS

CORRECTION OF THE GENETIC METABOLIC
DEFECT
     Counteracting the Offending Metabolite
     Acting on the Dysfunctional Enzyme
     Vitamin Therapy
     Enzyme Replacement Therapy

SYMPTOMATIC TREATMENT

PREVENTION

In the first edition of this book, we wrote that any comment on treatment and prophylaxis in relation to the hereditary metabolic diseases comes "more as an apology than an epilogue." Twelve years later, while many of these diseases remain incurable, prospects are certainly brighter.

It is obvious that effective treatment and prevention of hereditary metabolic disorders require accurate diagnosis and early intervention, preferably before neurologic symptoms have developed.

Early therapeutic intervention is now possible for many disorders because of technical advances that allow rapid and accurate biochemical enzymatic and DNA analysis of a patient's cells and body fluids even before birth. Some of these methods are incorporated in statewide neonatal screening programs for such conditions as PKU, galactosemia, maple syrup urine disease, homocystinuria, and biotinidase deficiency as well as thyroid deficiency.

Therapeutic attempts have been hampered by our incomplete understanding of the pathophysiologic mechanisms leading to the alterations of the nervous system. We are still ignorant of the ways by which specific molecular and enzymatic defects produce lesions.

These shortcomings underscore the value of preventive measures based on genetic screening, genetic counseling, and prenatal diagnosis.

Nevertheless, some diseases have recently become amenable to treatment (Table 9-1), and new approaches are being contemplated. Although still at an experimental stage, they might prove effective in the near future.

We will deal here with general aspects of current therapeutic approaches for the metabolic encephalopathies. More detailed treatments of individual diseases have been described in previous chapters. Treatment is directed essentially at (a) correcting the biochemical or DNA defect, i.e., the cause of the disease (etiological treatment); (b) alleviating the symptoms of disease (symptomatic treatment); and (c) helping families as they try to cope with the personal and social effects.

CORRECTION OF THE GENETIC METABOLIC DEFECT

Attempts at correcting the metabolic defect include various strategies. The target may be (1) the offending metabolite or (2) the dysfunctional enzyme.[20]

Counteracting the Offending Metabolite

When a large quantity of potentially toxic metabolites accumulate in body fluids (essentially in inborn errors of amino acids, organic acids, and ureagenesis), their reduction is obtained essentially by dietary means, sometimes including vitamin therapy (see below). In the acute phase, urgent elimination of all protein intake is needed, especially in neonates and infants with disorders affecting organic acid metabolism or urea cycle intermediates. Assuming the child survives, or when the disease is detected by neonatal screening, correction of the metabolic imbalance is accomplished by removal from the diet of the offending metabolite. In PKU this involves restricting phenylalanine intake; in galactosemia it involves removal of galactose from the diet; and in maple syrup urine disease and classic homocystinuria, the use of special diets low in specific metabolites is required. Feeding infants adapted commercialized formulas, monitoring the diet in older children, and deciding when to abandon or liberalize the diet (if possible) raise many problems and frequently necessitate consultation with a nutritionist. Galactosemia requires lifelong adherence to a galactose-restricted diet. A minimum amount of the offending substrate must be present and the diet must be sufficiently balanced to allow for normal growth to occur. Episodes of protein catabolism, related to intercurrent infections or trauma, may result in the accumulation of large amounts of a toxic metabolite of endogenous origin and require urgent therapeutic measures, including peritoneal dialysis or exchange transfusion. Mothers afflicted with PKU and galactosemia should be on an appropriate diet throughout pregnancy.

The metabolic block that causes a substrate to accumulate can also result in reduced amounts of products distal to the enzymatic step which is blocked. Accordingly, tyrosine may be reduced in PKU, leading to lowered levels of tyrosine-derived catecholamine neurotransmitters. Tyrosine supplementation has therefore been advocated in PKU to correct abnormalities in CSF monoamine levels. Similarly, cysteine supplementation may be beneficial in homocystinuria, citrulline and arginine in the urea cycle disorders, and uridine in galactosemia to restore UDP galactose levels to normal.

Yet another approach in correcting the metabolic abnormality is to stimulate an alternative pathway. Betaine is used in this way in homocystinuria to promote homocysteine methylation and a substantial reduction of homocysteine in affected patients. It also has the effect of preventing thromboembolic complications. Similarly, the clinical appearance of adrenoleukodystrophy may sometimes be transitorily modified by the use of glycerol trioleate and glycerol trierucate oil. These monounsaturated fatty acids compete with the long-chain saturated fatty acids for the same microsomal elongation system. In conjunction with dietary restrictions, the accumulation of VLCFAs is reduced.

It is also possible in the case of certain disorders to detoxify the toxic metabolite by binding it to another substance which converts it into a nontoxic and readily eliminated conjugate. This mechanism is the basis of the use of benzoate and phenylbutyrate in the hyperammonemias; benzoate in nonketotic hyperglycinemia; glycine in isovaleric acidemia; carnitine in defects of fatty acid oxidation and some organic acidurias; and penicillamine to remove copper in Wilson disease.

Though their results may be remarkable, these dietary manipulations do not always allow patients to escape without any mental impairment or behavioral abnormalities, especially if treatment has been delayed. This again reflects our inadequate knowledge of the pathophysiology of these conditions.

In some disorders the enzymatic block results not in an accumulation but in the loss of an essential substance: for example, glucose or biotin. Severe intermittent hypoglycemia occurs, along with other biochemical abnormalities, in disorders of mitochondrial fatty acid oxidation and some of the organic acidopathies, in fructose 1,6-bisphosphate deficiency and von Gierke disease. Maintaining a normal level of blood glucose is lifesaving here and may prevent severe sequelae. Ingestion of fructose-containing substances should be avoided in fructose 1,6-bisphosphate deficiency (as well as in hereditary fructose intolerance) and, for that matter, in all neonates. Avoidance of long periods of fasting and fractioning of glucose-rich meals will help to prevent the recurrence of hypoglycemic episodes.

Acting on the Dysfunctional Enzyme

If a coenzyme, such as a vitamin, is involved, supplementation by the coenzyme, or a precursor to the coenzyme, may be effective in activating the dysfunctional enzyme. When poor binding of the coenzyme to the mutant enzyme is at fault, then pharmacologic, rather than physiologic, quantities of the coenzyme are required. In cases of coenzyme deficiency due to defects in production, then supplementation of the diet by large amounts of the cofactor is necessary.

Another alternative is to replace the mutant enzyme by a normal enzyme (enzyme replacement therapy), a procedure still in a preliminary stage.

Vitamin Therapy (see Table 9-1)

About 50 percent of patients with homocystinuria due to the deficiency of cystathionine β-synthase benefit from the administration of large doses of vitamin B_6 (50 to 500 mg/day). Some cases of maple syrup urine disease and $PDHE_1$ deficiency respond to large quantities of

Table 9-1

Specific treatments of the hereditary neurometabolic diseases[a]

Disease	Effective in preventing or alleviating neurologic signs			Generally recommended (variable results)
	Substances restricted	Products supplemented	Other treatments	
Urea cycle disorders*	Reduction of hyperammonemia (1) Acute phase Hemodialysis I/V Sodium benzoate (250 mg/kg/d), phenylacetate (250–500 mg/kg/d) or phenylbutyrate; arginine (2) Long-term treatment Oral sodium benzoate (250 mg/kg/d) Phenylacetate (250–500 mg/kg/d) or phenylbutyrate (500 mg/kg/d)	Citrulline (OTC, CPS) L-Arginine (400–800 mg/kg/d) (ASS, ASL)		
Arginase deficiency*	Arginine			
HHH syndrome*				Ornithine supplement
Familial lysinuric protein intolerance*				Supplement Citrulline (300 mg/kg/d) Lysine (150 mg/kg/d)
MSUD*	BCAA: leucine, isoleucine, valine	Thiamine	Hemodialysis	
Isovaleric acidemia*				Supplement Glycine L-Carnitine
Propionic acidemia*				Supplement Biotin L-Carnitine Metronidazole
Methylmalonic acidemia*	Isoleucine, valine, methionine, threonine	Hydroxycobalamin (1 mg i/m 2/week) (Cbl A +++, Cbl B ++)		L-Carnitine (100 mg/kg/d) Metronidazole
Combined deficiencies of methylmalonyl-CoA mutase and methyltetrahydrofolate: homocysteine methyltransferase		Hydroxycobalamin Betain (250 mg/kg/d)		

Table 9-1 (contd.)

	Effective in preventing or alleviating neurologic signs			Generally recommended (variable results)
Disease	Substances restricted	Products supplemented	Other treatments	
Methyltetrahydrofolate: homocysteine methyltransferase deficiency		Hydroxycobalamin		
Hereditary folate malabsorption		Folates		
Methylenetetrahydrofolate reductase deficiency				Betaine Folic acid, vitamins B_6 and B_{12} Methionine
3-Methylcrotonyl-CoA carboxylase deficiency				Leucine restriction L-Carnitine supplement
3-Hydroxy-3-Methylglutaryl-CoA deficiency			Avoid fasting	Fat, leucine restriction L-Carnitine supplement

Glutaric aciduria type I				Restriction of lysine and tryptophan
				Supplement
				  L-Carnitine
				  Riboflavin
				  Baclofen

Homocystinuria	(1) Children, adolescents Methionine (±) (2) Neonates Methionine	Pyridoxine (150–1000 mg/d) L-Cysteine Pyridoxine		Betaine
Histidinemia				Histidine restriction (clinically effective?)
Phenylketonuria	Phenylalanine (250–500 mg/d) 0.25 mM < plasma levels < 1 mM			
Tetrahydrobiopterin (BH_4) deficiency	Phenylalanine	Levodopa (5–10 mg/kg/d) + carbidopa 5-Hydroxytryptophan (5–10 mg/kg/d) BH_4		Folinic acid supplement
Galactosemia (transferase deficiency)	Galactose-free diet			

(continued)

355

Table 9-1 (contd.)

Disease	Effective in preventing or alleviating neurologic signs			Generally recommended (variable results)
	Substances restricted	Products supplemented	Other treatments	
Fructose 1,6-bisphosphatase deficiency	Avoidance of fructose, sucrose	Acute episodes I/V glucose and bicarbonate	Maintain normal levels of glucose	
Glycogenosis type II			Maintain normal levels of glucose	
Succinic semialdehyde dehydrogenase deficiency		γ-Vinyl-GABA, orally		
Holocarboxylase synthetase deficiency		Biotin (10–20 mg/d)		
Biotinidase deficiency		Biotin (5–10 mg/d)		
PDH E$_1$ deficiency (neonatal or early infantile form)				High-fat, low-carbohydrate diet L-Carnitine, thiamine, dichloroacetate, lipoic acid
PDH E$_1$ deficiency (late infantile and juvenile form)		Thiamine (400–800 mg) effective in some patients		Ketogenic diet
PC deficiency (neonates)				Aspartic acid supplement
Acyl-CoA dehydrogenase deficiencies (defects in mitochondrial fatty acid β oxidation)			Avoid fasting	Low-fat diet L-Carnitine
Glutaric acidemia type II		Riboflavin (100–300 mg/d) effective in milder, later-onset forms		
Primary generalized carnitine deficiency (defect in carnitine transport)		L-Carnitine		
CPT I deficiency				Medium-chain triglycerides
Complex I deficiency				Nicotinamide, riboflavin, carnitine
Complex III deficiency				CoQ, menadione, ascorbate
MELAS, MERRF, KS				Nicotinamide, riboflavin, dichloroacetate, carnitine CoQ10 (KS)

Table 9-1 (contd.)

Disease	Effective in preventing or alleviating neurologic signs			Generally recommended (variable results)
	Substances restricted	Products supplemented	Other treatments	
Wilson disease			(1) D-Penicillamine 1000 mg/d or more (according to urinary excretion of copper); 500 mg/day in young children (2) Trientine 400–900 mg/d (3) Zinc acetate 50–150 mg/d or zinc sulfate 660–1320 mg/d	
Huntington chorea				Baclofen (glutamate antagonist) Diltiazem (calcium blocker) Phenothiazines and butyrophenones (dopamine blockers) Cysteamine (blocks release of somatostatin)
Dopamine-responsive dystonias			Levodopa + carbidopa (25 mg 2/day up to 250 mg/d)	
Juvenile neuronal ceroid lipofuscinosis				Antioxidants Polyunsaturated fatty acid supplement
X-linked adrenoleukodystrophy			Steroids for adrenal insufficiency	Dietary VLCFAs and 4:1 mixture of glyceryl trioleate and glyceryl trierucate (lowers VLCFA levels without significant clinical effect)
Cerebrotendinous xanthomatosis		Chenodeoxycholic acid (chenodiol 750 mg/d)	Mevinoline	
Abetalipoproteinemia		Vitamin E (1000–2000 mg/d in infants; 5000–10,000 mg/d in older patients)		Vitamin A Vitamin K
AVED		Vitamin E (5–10 mg/kg/d)		
Refsum disease	Drastic reduction of phytanic acid intake			
AI porphyria	Acute episode I/V Hematin Glucose		Avoid illicit drugs	

(continued)

Table 9-1 (contd.)

Disease	Effective in preventing or alleviating neurologic signs			Generally recommended (variable results)
	Substances restricted	Products supplemented	Other treatments	
Giant axonal neuropathy				Penicillamine
Lesch-Nyhan disease			Allopurinol for hyperuricemia	
Hartnup disease		Nicotinamide (200–400 mg/d) High-protein diet		
Glucose transporter protein deficiency		Ketogenic diet		
Smith-Lemli-Opitz syndrome		High-cholesterol diet		

Abbreviations and symbols: HHH = hyperornithinemia-hyperammonemia-hypercitrullinuria; MSUD = maple syrup urine disease; BCAA = branched-chain amino acids; PDH = pyruvate dehydrogenase; PC = pyruvate carboxylase; CPT = carnitine palmitoyltransferase; an asterisk (*) indicates that in inborn errors of amino acid and organic acid metabolism, protein intake should be restricted to 0.8–2 g/kg/d; lower levels could induce protein catabolism and interfere with normal growth; caloric intake must be sufficient.

ᵃ Symptomatic treatment; corrections of acidosis, hypoglycemia, circulatory collapse, etc., during acute metabolic episodes; organ transplantation and gene therapy are not mentioned in this table (see text).

thiamine. Riboflavin has been used in certain forms of lactic acidosis and in glutaric aciduria II. Also, the epileptic encephalopathy of vitamin B_6 dependency, if detected early enough, may be cured by lifelong administration of large doses of vitamin B_6. Other vitamin B_6 responsive disorders are cystathionuria, hyperornithinemia with gyrate atrophy of the retina and xanthurenic aciduria.

Biotinidase deficiency results in losses of biotin and impairment of the biotin-dependent carboxylases. Administration of biotin has remarkable effects. Certainly, the replacement therapy with vitamin B_6 and biotin, respectively in vitamin B_6 dependency and biotinidase deficiency represent two of the most successful therapies of neurometabolic disorders. In Hartnup disease, nicotinamide therapy alleviates some of the symptoms. Cobalamin and folate are effective in some disorders.

Enzyme Replacement Therapy

Bone Marrow Transplantation The concept of enzyme replacement therapy as a means of treating children with lysosomal storage diseases stems from the observation by Neufeld[1] of "in vitro" correction of fibroblasts of patients with Hurler disease when cocultured with fibroblasts of Hunter disease or normal fibroblasts.

A potential method for enzyme replacement is allogeneic bone marrow transplantation (BMT), which provides an exogenous source of normal enzyme. This technique has been evaluated in animal mutants with lysosomal storage diseases involving the CNS, including mucopolysaccharidoses, fucosidosis, Krabbe leukodystrophy, and the mannosidoses.[2,3] In most cases there is an increase in normal enzymatic activity in cells of the recipient, including brain cells, a reduction of the accumulated substrate, and sometimes a stabilization of the disease. One model for Krabbe leukodystrophy is the twitcher mouse; when it undergoes BMT there is the appearance of galactocerebrosidase and a decrease of psychosine in the brain.

Since 1981[4] allogeneic BMT has been used in selected cases for therapeutic trials of human lysosomal storage disorders and a few other genetic neurometabolic diseases. The largest series available are those obtained by the Minnesota Bone Marrow Transplant Group,[5] the Westminster Bone Marrow Team,[2,3] and the European Group for Bone Marrow transplantation.[6] For reviews, see also Parkman[7] and Weinberg et al.[8]

Transplant mortality is approximately 10 percent when the donor is an HLA identical sibling, and 2 to 3 times higher if this is not the case.[6] The availability of an HLA identical sibling donor has therefore to be considered in the decision to perform BMT in patients who could possibly benefit from this treatment.

The majority of patients treated with BMT had Hurler disease or some other form of *mucopolysaccharidis* (MPS), especially Hunter disease, Sanfilippo disease, and Maroteaux-Lamy disease. Biological parameters were improved. Enzyme levels in circulating leukocytes corresponded to those of the donors' leukocytes. In one patient with Hurler disease, levels of glycosaminoglycans in the CSF were normalized 48 months posttransplant.[3] In another patient with Hurler disease, examined postmortem 15 months after BMT, the brain contained 40 percent of the normal content of α-iduronidase, whereas brains from nontransplanted patients contained no detectable activity.

Clinical improvement was evident in upper airway obstruction and sleep apneas, hepatosplenomegaly, cardiac hypertrophy, and growth. Resolution of corneal clouding was obtained in some patients. The effect on skeletal lesions was much less obvious, although they usually appeared to have stabilized and joint motility was occasionally improved. Also noted was a beneficial action on intracranial hypertension, due to obstructive hydrocephalus, possibly with a favorable effect on intellectual capacity.[9] Stabilization of cognitive functions was obtained in some patients whose IQ was above 80 before BMT, but mental deterioration was not halted when the initial intellectual quotient was below this level.[2] Behavioral disturbances, when present, were unchanged.

It can be concluded that BMT in MPS may have a favorable effect on the quality of life by its action on the visceral abnormalities, but its effect on mental and neurological dysfunction is much less obvious. Definitive statements on the long-term effects of transplantation on the central nervous system must await longer follow-ups.

Results of BMT *with late infantile and juvenile MLD* have been variable. In three patients [2,10] a stabilization of the mental and neurological status was reported. In one girl whose disease started at $2\frac{1}{2}$ years, BMT was performed at age 5 years and its effects followed beyond the age of 10 years. Dysarthria, pyramidal and cerebellar signs remained unchanged. No mental deterioration occurred and she was able to advance scholastically. CT studies showed no progression of white matter lesions. In six other patients with MLD, including three with the juvenile form, BMT was without clinical effect.[6] In all cases, levels of arylsulfatase A in circulating leukocytes was that of the donor, or exceeded this level 3 to 5 months after engraftment.[6] Urinary excretion of sulfatides decreased. In one patient it was shown that cells cultured from the CSF were of donor origin.[10]

To our knowledge, BMT did not alter the clinical course of the following lysosomal disorders with involvement of the CNS: G_{M2} gangliosidosis, G_{M1} gangliosidosis, Niemann-Pick disease, Farber disease, Pompe disease, and neuropathic Gaucher disease. We are aware of a child with *late infantile Krabbe disease* who has now been stabilized for a period of 5 years.[11] Other Krabbe disease patients with the onset of symptoms in childhood have also benefited from BMT. One girl who was 12 years old at the time of BMT has progressed in all areas involving language and academic performance. Ataxia and tremor have disappeared and neurophysiological parameters stabilized or improved.[12] (In non-neuropathic Gaucher disease, successful engraftment leads to complete disappearance of symptoms. Patients are usually splenectomized. An alternative and innocuous treatment is lifelong infusion of macrophage-targeted human glucocerebrosidase. This should certainly be seriously considered when no HLA identical donor is available.)

Treatment by the way of BMT has also been tried in nonlysosomal disorders. Stabilization of neurologic function has been observed in several patients *with X-linked adrenoleukodystrophy*.[13,14,14a] In *Lesch-Nyhan disease* there has been no evidence of clinical improvement.[15]

Therapeutic use of BMT in neurologic disorders is based on the assumption that the normal enzyme will penetrate the nervous system by circumventing the blood-brain barrier. That this may happen has been demonstrated in experimental animals with lysosomal disorders.[2,3] The mechanism by which the exogenous enzyme reaches the brain is not fully understood. In experimental animals, hematopoietic cells (bone marrow cells) of donor origin are found in the CNS, where they may enter through capillaries by diapedesis. (It has been shown that normal microglial cells in the CNS may be of bone marrow origin.[16]) Enzyme uptake could occur by cell-to-cell contact or by endocytosis. It is also possible that the circulating enzyme released by blood leukocytes directly enters the brain.

To summarize, in lysosomal neurovisceral storage disorders (particularly the MPS), favorable results have been obtained on visceral abnormalities by replacement of the patient's reticuloendothelial cells by cells of donor origin. Results of engraftments on long-term intellectual

and neurologic function remain uncertain Stabilization of neurologic deficits and mental status has been observed in some patients with MPS, MLD, late-onset Krabbe disease, and X-linked adrenoleukodystrophy. Further CNS deterioration may possibly be prevented, but it is not expected that a successful engraftment will reverse preexisting damage. BMT should therefore be performed as early as possible in the course of the disease. Although a few remissions of more than 5 years have been obtained, the long-term effects of BMT on mental and neurologic function need further evaluation.

A child affected with a hereditary metabolic disorder has the best chances to benefit from BMT if the following criteria are met:

1. An HLA identical sibling should be available.

2. The neurologic disorder should be at a preclinical or early stage. A delay of 4 to 8 months has been observed in experimental animals[3] before donor monocytes gain access to the CNS. One must therefore anticipate a long delay before the clinical effects are realized. The results of BMT on a rapidly evolving neurologic disorder are therefore very improbable.

A significant mortality (9 to 25 percent) and morbidity of BMT (nausea and vomiting of immunosuppressive procedures, temporary bone marrow aplasia, acute and chronic graft-versus-host disease, loss of engraftment) and cost-effectiveness must also be considered in the final decision to resort to BMT.

A limitation of the use of BMT is that only 20 to 25 percent of patients who could benefit from this treatment have a histocompatible donor. In neurometabolic disorders in which the gene has been cloned, patients without a histocompatible donor may possibly benefit in the future from autologous BMT following insertion of the cloned DNA for the missing enzyme, i.e., gene therapy.

Gene Therapy for Neurometabolic Diseases   Gene therapy for genetic diseases can be defined as the correction of a patient's cells by the addition of a normal copy of the defective gene.[3] This method can only be used when the gene responsible for the disease has been identified.

Gene therapy is still in a preliminary experimental stage, and only a very limited number of clinical trials have been undertaken. In the usual "ex vivo" technique, the normal exogenous gene is transferred into cells obtained from and returned to the patient. Gene transplant into target cells is commonly achieved by inserting the exogenous gene into a viral vector, usually a retrovirus, which has been rendered replication-defective and innocuous. The retroviral vector integrates into the host cell genome, resulting in permanent expression of the therapeutic gene. In most instances, gene transfer is performed on the patient's own bone marrow cells, which are then returned to the patient by way of the "autologous" bone marrow transplantation. Hepatocytes, fibroblasts, lymphocytes, and other cell types have also been employed.

Direct "in vivo" gene delivery has also been tested experimentally, using viral and nonviral methods. Among the latter, receptor-mediated gene transfer and liposome-mediated gene transfer are apparently the closest to clinical application.

To date, a limited number of genetic diseases have been approved for clinical trials (using bone marrow or other target cells): severe combined immunodeficiency due to adenosine deaminase deficiency (using T lymphocytes or bone marrow cells), hemophilia (using fibroblasts) and familial hypercholesterolemia (using hepatocytes). Other hereditary metabolic disorders which have been tested experimentally include Lesch-Nyhan disease (although allogeneic BMT has not resulted in clinical improvement), nonneuropathic Gaucher disease, ornithine transcarbamylase deficiency (using hepatocytes), and possibly a few other lysosomal disorders.[17,18] Gene therapy may also offer interesting prospects for Huntington chorea.

The use of gene therapy in neurometabolic disorders by way of autologous BMT or other "ex vivo" techniques will have the same problem as allogeneic transplantation: success will depend on whether the hematopoietic derived enzymes can gain access to cells of the nervous system. The results of gene therapy may be inferior to those of allogeneic BMT because of the lack of insertion of the normal gene into all transplanted stem cells and because of a lower level of gene expression. Another possible complication is the potential development of an immune reaction to the gene-carrying vector. The potential advantages of transfected autologous bone marrow transplantation reside in the fact that there is neither risk of immunologically mediated rejection of the graft nor the need of a histocompatible donor.

Liver Transplantation   Liver transplantation has been achieved with apparently good clinical results in a few patients with Wilson disease. Indications for liver transplantation in hepatolenticular degeneration are limited to patients with fulminating liver disease or severe progressive hepatic decompensation unrelieved by D-penicillamine.[19] Liver transplantation also has achieved good results in a nonneuropathic Gaucher disease patient with cirrhosis. This procedure has also been considered in OTC deficiency.

Agents Acting at the Neurotransmitter Pathways
In a limited number of genetic "metabolic" or "degenerative" disorders involving the basal ganglia, striking results have been obtained by drugs which act as neurotransmitters (e.g., dopa in some dystonias) or are thought to interfere with neurotransmitter circuits. Certainly, this therapeutic field offers promising advantages as more is learned about the pathogenesis of basal ganglia disorders. In Huntington disease the possible use of agents blocking endogenous excitotoxic products has also been proposed.

SYMPTOMATIC TREATMENT

The lack of a specific therapy does not relieve the physician of personal responsibility for the patient and troubled family. There are many ways in which the patient can be helped and the family supported.

In some diseases, especially those that appear during late childhood and adolescence, there are long periods of time when the patient's condition is relatively stable. For example, the late forms of Gaucher disease, Niemann-Pick disease, metachromatic leukodystrophy, ceroid lipofuscinosis, mucopolysaccharidoses, mucolipidoses, and mitochondrial encephalomyopathies can progress so slowly that little change is observed over a year. Being disabled in special ways, the patient and the family need advice as to a suitable program for the patient's care, schooling, and social, physical, and emotional adjustment. A board containing small pictures of common objects and actions may assist the nonverbal child to communicate wants and feelings. Personality peculiarities and emotional instability may necessitate psychiatric advice and a trial of behavior-modifying drugs. Anticonvulsant medication may be useful if seizures are part of the illness.

Physiotherapy and drugs, such as Lioresal or diazepam, may also relieve spasticity, improve motility of the limbs, and combat pain. The grave inconvenience of chronic respiratory insufficiency, particularly in the mucopolysaccharidoses, can be alleviated by treating intercurrent infections and by using a positive-pressure inhalation device at night. Treating respiratory infections is also useful in ataxia-telangiectasia. Should a child with a mucopolysaccharidosis require general anesthesia, the diameter of the endotracheal tube used must be smaller than normal, to accommodate the child's narrowed trachea, and the anesthesiologist must be alert to the possibility of postintubation airway obstruction from laryngeal edema.

There may be nutritional difficulties because of dysphagia, vomiting, regurgitation, and rumination. Metoclopromide may help the regurgitation and glycopyrrolate is useful to reduce drooling. Poor oral intake and failure to gain weight often lead to the placement of a G-tube in the stomach. When this is done, it is usually advisable to do a fundal plication to avoid constant regurgitation of gastric contents. A nutritionist may be consulted to prepare diets that are palatable, balanced, and appropriate for the child's specific metabolic deficiencies. Orthopedic advice may be needed for progressive kyphoscoliosis, atlanto-axial instability and carpal tunnel syndrome. A neurosurgeon may be enlisted to perform a ventriculoperitoneal shunt in   tension hydrocephalus in mucopolysaccharidoses. Glaucomas must be dealt with by an ophthalmologist.

In bedridden and mentally retarded children, attention should be given to the presence of esophagitis, constipation, renal stones, and dental caries, which may cause much discomfort and pain.

In metabolic disorders with a remitting course, the parents and older patients must be instructed to take simple precautions to prevent the recurrence of a serious, sometimes life-threatening, metabolic crisis. Patients and families must be warned to avoid the dangers of certain drugs in acute intermittent porphyria. Avoidance of prolonged fasting and fractioning of meals will prevent neurological attacks in disorders of fatty acid oxidation and carbohydrate metabolism. Inborn errors of organic acid and amino acid metabolism require a strict metabolic surveillance during intercurrent infections, trauma, or surgery. In newborns and infants with fructose intolerance, fructose-containing substances should never be administered (and as a necessary precaution fructose is prohibited in all newborns). Avoidance of sun exposure is necessary in Hartnup disease, De Sanctis-Cacchione syndrome (xeroderma pigmentosum) and in Cockayne syndrome.

PREVENTION

One way to prevent genetic disorders is by medical intervention at a preclinical stage. Systematic neonatal screening or early application of biochemical methods of diagnosis (including prenatal testing) makes this increasingly attainable.

Some couples or individuals are at risk of transmitting a metabolic disease; prevention offers them a better chance of giving birth to a normal child. This can be achieved by screening of heterozygotes in affected families or in populations with a high carrier frequency of a given disease, and by applying biochemical and molecular diagnostic tests to fetal cells recovered by amniocentesis or chorionic biopsy. A mother may terminate her pregnancy if the fetus is homozygous for a disease.

Heterozygote detection is now possible for a great number of autosomal and X-linked disorders and has become much more secure as molecular tests have become increasingly reliable and available. Investigations based only on enzyme determination do not always provide definitive proof.

Population-based screening for Tay-Sachs disease in major centers of the Jewish population has significantly reduced the incidence of the disorder. Extensive population screening, resulting in the systematic search for carriers of mutant genes in apparently normal individuals, can be of interest for the prevention of genetic diseases, but it also carries risks and raises serious questions. The detection of an incurable genetic abnormality in a person before occurrence of any symptoms raises problems of morality and ethics, and becomes a source of anxiety and despair for the future patient and the patient's family. This is especially true for later-onset forms of neurodegenerative diseases, such as Huntington chorea, in which an affected person may live a normal life until mid-adulthood. If testing is decided by a duly informed individual, it should remain strictly confidential.

Prenatal diagnosis allows parents to give birth to a normal child. This is now feasible in a considerable number of neurometabolic disorders by applying enzymatic tests or molecular genetic analysis to cultured amniotic cells (at 18 to 20 weeks' gestation) or by similar tests on chorionic villus samples (at approximately 10 weeks' gestation) (or possibly by testing an early embryo resulting from in vitro fertilization before uterine reimplantation). Results of these tests are only reliable if the enzyme abnormality or the DNA defect are known through studies made on a previously affected child, obligate heterozygotes, and other family members.

The foregoing statements imply that there are several reproductive options available for carrier-carrier couples who have given birth to an affected child or for individuals who have been found to be carriers by family or population screening. Medical information may influence the parents' choice about future pregnancies. Critical to their decision will be the severity of the disease, its pace and age of onset, the possibility of a satisfactory response to treatment (i.e. administration of vitamin B_6, biotin, dietary prescriptions, use of D-penicillamine), and new prospects for future therapeutics. Many couples accept selective abortion after prenatal diagnosis of an affected fetus. Others choose to adopt a child or to seek insemination with a noncarrier donor. They may prefer to avoid future pregnancies or may elect to give birth to an affected child, which may be treated effectively from birth. Other couples accept the responsibility of giving birth to a seriously ill child for religious reasons. In all these difficult choices, parents need guidance and attention from their physician.

REFERENCES

1. Neufeld EF: Replacement of genotype specific proteins in mucopolysaccharidosis, in Desnick RJ, Bernlohr RW, Krivit W (eds): *Enzyme Therapy in Genetic Disease, Birth Defects, March of Dimes Original Series,* vol. IX, no. 2. New York, Alan R. Liss, 1973, pp. 27–30.
2. Krivit W, Whitley CB, Chang PN, et al.: Lysosomal storage diseases treated by bone marrow transplantation: review of 21 patients, in Johnson FL, Pochedly C (eds): *Bone Marrow Transplantation in Children.* New York, Raven, 1990, pp. 261–287.
3. Lenarsky C, Kohn DB, Weinberg KI, et al.: Bone marrow transplantation for genetic diseases. *Hematology/Oncology Clinics of North America* 4(3): 589–602, 1990.
4. Hobbs JR, Hugh-Jones K, Barrett AJ, et al.: Reversal of clinical features of Hurler's disease and biochemical improvement after treatment by bone marrow transplantation. *Lancet,* 2: 709–712, 1981.
5. Krivit W, Whitley CB, Chang PN, et al.: Lysosomal storage diseases treated by bone marrow transplantation: a report from the University of Minnesota Variety Club Children's Hospital, in Gale RP, Champlin RE (eds): *Bone Marrow Transplantation: Current Controversies.* New York, Alan R. Liss, 1989, pp. 367–378.
6. Hoogerbrugge PM, Brouwer OF, Bordigoni P, et al.: Allogenic bone marrow transplantation for lysosomal storage diseases. *Lancet* 345: 1398–1402, 1995.
7. Parkman R: The application of bone marrow transplantation to the treatment of genetic diseases. *Science* 232: 1373–1378, 1986.
8. Weinberg KI, Parkman R: Bone transplantation for genetic disease, in Johnson FL, Pochedly C (eds): *Bone Marrow Transplantation in Children.* New York, Raven, 1990, pp. 243–260.
9. Whitley CB, Belani KG, Chang PN, et al.: Long-term outcome of Hurler syndrome following bone marrow transplantation. *Am J Med Genet* 46: 209–218, 1993.
10. Bayever E, Ladisch M, Philippart M, et al.: Bone marrow transplantation for metachromatic leukodystrophy. *Lancet* 1: 471–473, 1985.
11. Van Coster R, Cornu G. Personal communication, 1995.
12. Desnick RG: *Treatment of Genetic Disorders.* New York, Churchill-Livingstone, 1991.
13. Weinberg KI, Moser A, Watkins P, et al.: Bone marrow transplantation for adrenoleukodystrophy. *Pediatr Res* 23: 334A, 1988.
14. Aubourg P, Blanche S, Jambaque I, et al.: Reversal of early neurologic and neuroradiologic manifestations of X-linked adrenoleukodystrophy by bone marrow transplantation. *New Engl J Med* 322: 1860–1866, 1990.
14a. Krivit W, Sung JH, Lockman LA, et al.: Bone marrow transplantation for treatment of lysosomal and peroxisomal diseases, in Rich RR, Fleisher TA., Schwartz BD, Shearer WT, Stroler W (eds): *Principles of Clinical Immunology.* St. Louis, Mosby, 1995, pp. 1852–1864.
15. Nyhan WL, Page T, Truber AB, et al.: Bone marrow transplantation in Lesch-Nyhan disease, in Krivit W, Paul NW (eds): *Bone Marrow Transplantation for Treatment of Lysosomal Storage Disorders.* New York, Alan R. Liss, 1986, pp. 41–53.
16. Hickey WF, Kimura H: Perivascular microglial cells of the CNS are bone-marrow-derived and present antigen in vivo. *Science* 239: 290–292, 1988.
17. Morgan RA, Anderson WF: Human gene therapy. *Ann Rev Biochem* 62: 191–217, 1993.
18. Morsy MS, Mitani K, Clemens P, et al.: Progress toward gene therapy. *JAMA* 270: 2338–2345, 1993.
19. Hefter H, Rautenberg W, Kreuzpaintner G, et al.: Does orthotopic liver transplantation heal Wilson disease? Clinical follow-up of two transplanted patients. *Acta Neurol Scand* 84: 192–196, 1991.
20. Beaudet AL, Scriver CR, Sly WS, et al.: Genetics, biochemistry and molecular basis of variant human phenotypes, in Scriver CR Beaudet AL, Sly WS, Valle D (eds): *The Metabolic and Molecular Bases of Inherited Metabolic Disease.* New York, McGraw-Hill, 1995, pp. 102–110.

INDEX

Note: f following a page number indicates a figure and t indicates a table.

Abdominal pain, 337
Abetalipoproteinemia:
 clinical features, 190–191
 diagnostic laboratory tests, 191
 differential diagnosis, 191
 pathogenesis and physiopathology, 191
 pathologic findings, 191
 treatment, 191–192
Acanthocytes, 332, 335t, 346
α-N-Acetylgalactosaminidase deficiency (*see* Schindler disease)
N-Acetylglutamate synthetase (NAGS), 12, 14
Acid α-glucosidase deficiency (*see* Glycogenosis, type II)
Acousticomotor response, 50
Action myoclonus, 145–150, 182t, 192–199, 193t, 309–310
Acute intermittent porphyria, 226–229, 311
 clinical features, 227
 diagnostic laboratory tests, 227–228
 differential diagnosis, 228
 genetics, 228
 pathologic findings, 228
 treatment, 228
Acyl-CoA dehydrogenase deficiencies, 28–29, 101
Adenylosuccinate lyase (ASL) deficiency, 262, 292
Addison disease with spastic paraplegia, 250
Adolescent hereditary metabolic disorders, 177–281
Adrenal insufficiency, 249, 332
Adrenoleukodystrophy:
 neonatal, 37
 X-linked, 248–251, 249f, 258, 360
Adrenomyeloneuropathy, 179, 248–249, 250, 258
Adult polyglucosan disease, 196, 348
Aicardi-Goutières syndrome, 300
Aldehyde oxidase deficiency, 21

Alertness, impaired, 7
Alexander disease, 66, 74–76, 309, 344
 adult variant, 75
 clinical features, 74–76, 75t
 diagnosis, 76
 MRI, 76f
 neuroimaging, 76
 pathologic findings, 76
Alpers syndrome, 48, 81–84, 145, 307, 327, 328
 clinicopathologic correlations, 83–84
 diagnosis, 82–83
 etiology, 83
 MRI, 83f
 without liver disease, 82
Alpers-Huttenlocher syndrome, 82
Alpha-L-fucosidosis deficiency (*see* Fucosidosis)
Amaurotic idiocy, 48
Amino acids
 inherited disorders of metabolism, 12–14, 86–91
α-Aminolevulinic acid dehydrase deficiency, 229
Amyloid neuropathies (*See* Familial amyloid neuropathy)
Angelman syndrome, 293
Angiokeratoma, 332, 334t
Appendicular biopsy, 348
Arginase deficiency, 12, 14, 186
Argininosuccinate lyase deficiency, 12–14, 107
Argininosuccinate synthetase deficiency, 12–14, 107
Aspartylglucosaminuria, 169–170
 clinical features, 169–170
 diagnostic laboratory tests, 170
 prenatal diagnosis, 170
Asperger syndrome, 292
Ataxia:
 and action myoclonus, 192–196
 acute cerebellar metabolic, 296, 296t

Ataxia (*cont.*)
  acute cerebellar nonmetabolic, 296, 297
  amino acids, organic acids disorders with cerebellar, 86
  autosomal dominant progressive cerebellar, with retinal degeneration and opthlamoplegia (ADCA, types I and II), 190
  autosomal dominant spino-cerebellar (SCA type I–V), 190
  description of, in HMD, 293–294
  early onset cerebellar, with retained tendon reflexes, 189–190
  episodic (*see* intermittent)
  familial periodic cerebellar, 297
  intermittent, 296, 296t, 297
  Marie hereditary cerebellar, 190
  nonmetabolic, 294–297
  nonprogressive idiopathic cerebellar, 294–296
  progressive cerebral, 142, 181t, 186–192, 295t
  with vitamin E deficiency (AVED), 192
Ataxia-oculomotor apraxia syndrome, 323
Ataxia-telangiectasia (AT), 142–145, 295t, 313
  cancer risk, 143
  clinical course and life profile, 142f
  clinical features, 142–145
  diagnosis, 145
  diagnostic laboratory tests, 144
  genetics, 144
  mutant gene, 142
  pathologic findings, 144–145
  physiopathology, 145
  prenatal diagnosis, 144
  treatment, 145
Ataxia diplegia with deficient cellular immunity, 145
Athetosis (*see* dystonia, extrapyramidal diseases, basal ganglia diseases)
Attention deficits, 292
Auditory evoked potentials, 346
Austin disease (*see* Multiple sulfatase deficiency (MSD))
Autism, 292
Automatisms of trunk and limbs, 8–9
Autonomic disturbances, 311
Autosomal dominant conditions, 4
Autosomal recessive disorders, 3–4
Axonal neuropathies, 315

Baclofen in Huntington disease, 208
Bacterial meningitis, 284
Baltic myoclonus, 194

Basal ganglia:
  metabolic hereditary disorders of, 297–299
  nonmetabolic disorders of, 299–300
Basilar migraine, 297
Bassen-Kornzweig disease:
  clinical features, 190–191
  diagnostic laboratory tests, 191
  differential diagnosis, 191
  pathogenesis and physiopathology, 191
  pathologic findings, 191
  treatment, 191–192
Batten disease:
  early-onset, 148
  late-onset, 241
Behavioral abnormalities, 86–91, 184t, 270–272, 271t
Behavioral syndromes, 292
Benign essential familial myoclonus, 197–198
Benign nonprogressive familial chorea, 216
Benign paroxystic vertigo, 297
Bifunctional protein deficiency, 38, 38f
Bilateral striatal necrosis
  familial, 216–217, 288, 300
  acute, postinfectious, 299
Biochemical tests, 341
Biopercular syndrome, 288
Biopsied tissue, 346–348, 348f
Biotin metabolism, disorders of, 30, 76–77
Biotinidase deficiency, 30, 77, 308t, 359
  clinical features, 77
  genetics, 77
  laboratory findings, 77
  patholology, 77
  treatment, 77
  variants, 77
Bipyramidal syndromes, 180t, 301
Blood specimens, 350
Blood tests, 341
Bone marrow transplantation, 359–360
Brain:
  calcifications, 217–218, 262–263, 300, 343–344
  prenatal developmental defects, 91, 284–285, 285t, 288–291
  prenatal malformations, 289–290
Branched chain amino acids disorders of (*see* maple syrup urine disease)
Branched chain α-keto acid dehydrogenase, 16
Branching enzyme deficiency, 196
Butyrophenones in Huntington disease, 208

Calcifications (*see* Brain)
Canavan-Van Bogaert-Bertrand disease, 73–74, 266
   clinical features, 73
   diagnostic laboratory tests, 74
   differential diagnosis, 74
   genetics, 74
   pathologic findings, 74
   pathophysiology, 74
   prenatal diagnosis, 74
Carbamylphosphate synthetase (CPS), 12
Carbamylphosphate synthetase deficiency (CPSD), 12,
   13, 14, 107
Carbohydrate-deficient glycoprotein (CDG) syndrome:
   clinical features, 170
   diagnostic laboratory tests, 170–171
Carbohydrate metabolism, disorders of, 39–40, 90–91
Cardiovascular system, 328–329, 330t
Carnitine-acylcarnitine translocase deficiency, 28, 101
Carnitine cycle defects, 27, 28, 100–101
Carnitine palmitoyltransferase I (CPT I) deficiency, 101
Carnitine palmitoyltransferase II (CPT II) deficiency,
   27–28, 101
Carnitine transport system deficiency, 100–101
Cataracts, (*see* Ocular abnormalities)
Ceramide deficiency, 60
Cerebellar ataxia (*see* Ataxia)
Cerebral embolisms, 328
Cerebral palsies, 286–288
   clinical features, 287–288
   differential diagnosis, 288
   etiology, 286–287
   free interval, 287
   pathogenesis, 286–287
Cerebral white matter changes
   Neuroimaging, 344
   Hypoplasia of, 344
Cerebrohepatorenal disease (*see* Zellweger disease)
Cerebrospinal fluid tests, 341
Cerebrotendinous xanthomotosis, 252–253
Ceroid lipofuscinosis (*see* neuronal ceroid
   lipofuscinoses)
Charcot-Marie-Tooth disease (CMT), 220, 229, 312
Charcot-Marie-Tooth disease (CMT I), 229–231, 312
Charcot-Marie-Tooth disease (CMT II), 231–232, 312,
   315
Cherry red spot-myoclonus syndrome, 197
Childhood and adolescence hereditary metabolic
   disorders, 177–281
Cholestanolosis, 252–253, 258
Chorea:
   clinical features, 199, 310

   hereditary, 215–216
Chorea-acanthocytosis, 215–216, 300
Choreoamyotrophy, 191
Choreoathetosis, 4, 85–86, 142–145, 209, 214–215, 218,
   297 (*see also* dystonia)
Choreaathetosis and pallidal atrophy, 218
Chromosomal aberrations, 289
Chronic relapsing demyelinating inflammatory
   polyneuropathy, 313
Citrullinemia, 12
Claude Bernard-Horner syndrome, 8
Cobalamin, treatment with, 20, 21
Cockayne syndrome, 71, 262–263, 337, 344, 362
Cogan oculomotor apraxia 323
Cognitive abnormalities, 86–91, 270–272, 271t, 307
Cognitive functions, appraisal of, 292
Coma
   differential diagnosis of, 108, 109
   recurrent, 92, 150
Computed tomography (CT), 343–344
Congenital amaurosis, 31
Congenital hypomyelination polyneuropathy, 232
Congenital myopathies, 312
Congenital pontoneocerebellar aplasia, 296
Congenital spastic diplegia, 301
Conjunctival telangiectasia, 144f, 319t, 324
Corneal clouding, 318t, 319t, 324
Corpus callosum defects (*see* Brain developmental
   defects)
Corpus Luysi degeneration, 218
Cranial nerves, 315, 321, 322t, 323
Craniofacial deformities, 336t, 337t
Creutzfeld-Jacob disease, 310
Cystathionine β-synthase deficiency (CSD), 264–268,
   265t, 266t, 302, 353
   clinical features, 264–265
   clinicopathologic correlation, 267
   diagnosis, 266
   genetics, 267
   laboratory tests, 266
   pathologic findings, 267
   treatment, 267–268
Cysteamine in Huntington disease, 208
Cytochrome-*c* oxidase (COX) deficiency, 27, 93, 94, 97,
   140, 300
Cytomegalovirus, prenatal infection with (CMV), 284

Deafness, 324–325, 325t
Déjerine-Sottas disease, 125, 139, 220, 232–233, 294, 312
Dementia, 270–272

Demyelinating neuropathy, 312
Dentatorubral pallidoluysian atrophy, 197
Denver Developmental Screening Test III, 292
DeSanctis-Cacchione syndrome, 263–264, 362
De Toni-Debré-Fanconi syndrome, 27, 84, 331t
Developmental abnormalities (see Brain)
Developmental regression, 4–5
Developmental delay, 4, 291–292
DeVivo disease, 84
Diabetes mellitus, 332
Diabetic neuropathies, 311, 312, 313
2,4-Dienoyl-CoA reductase deficiency, 41
Differential diagnosis of HMDs, 282–326
Dihydrolipoyl dehydrogenase (E$_3$) deficiency, 26, 93
Dihydropterine reductase (DHPR) deficiency, 89
Dihydroxyacetone phosphate acyltransferase (DHAP-
    AT) deficiency, 39
Dimercaprol in Wilson's disease, 204
DNA studies, 2, 342, 350
Dopa-responsive dystonia, 211–212
Drug addiction, 285, 313
Dysarthria, 288
Dysmorphic facial features, 332, 336t, 337t
Dysostosis multiplex, 53, 150, 154, 332, 333t, 342
Dyssynergia cerebellaris myoclonica, 196
Dystonia:
    alcohol-responsive, 212
    in ataxia-telangiectasia, 142–143
    clinical features of, 199, 209, 297
    dopa-responsive, 208, 211–212
    in early infantile HMDs, 85–86
    focal, 211
    hereditary, 209–212
    hypnogenic, 215
    kinesigenic, 214–215
    Leber optic atrophy with, 217
    Leigh disease with, 96, 251
    nonkinesigenic, 215
    Parkinsonism in, 208, 211, 212
    paroxysmal, 214–215
    primary idiopathic, 209–212
    with putaminal hypodensity, 216–217, 300
    rare forms of idiopathic, 218–219
    secondary dystonias, 212
    with striatal necrosis, 216–217, 217t, 300
    torsion dystonia, idiopathic, 210–211
    X-linked with Parkinsonism, 212
Dystonia musculorum deformans, 210–211
Dystonia-Parkinsonian syndrome, 212
Dystonic cerebral palsy, 286, 300

Early infantile progressive metabolic encephalopathies,
    45–123, 111–115t
Early Language Milestone Test, 292
Early-onset multiple carboxylase deficiency, 30, 78
Electrocardiogram (ECG), 64, 64f, 346
Electroencephalogram (EEG), 345
Electron transfer of flavoprotein (ETF) deficiency, 28,
    103
Electrophysiological methods, 311, 345–346
Electroretinogram (ERG), 37, 346
Enzyme assays, 341–342
Enzyme deficiencies, 348, 353
Enzyme replacement therapy, 359–361
Epilepsy, 303, 305–309 (see also Seizures)
    cognitive defects in, 307
    description and classification, 303, 305, 306, 305t
    and hereditary metabolic disorders, 306–309, 308t
    progressive myoclonic, 192–196
Essential tremor, 216, 310
Ethanolaminosis, 66
ETF-ubiquinone oxidoreductase (ETF-QO) deficiency,
    28, 103
Extrapyramidal disorders, 183t, 200t, 297–300, 298t
    of late childhood and adolescence, 199–219
    summarizing remarks, 219
Eyes, morphological changes in HMDs, 324 (see also
    ocular abnormalities)

Fabry disease, 224–226, 264, 302, 311, 328, 329
    atypical variants, 225
    clinical features, 224–225
    clinicopathologic correlations, 226
    diagnostic laboratory tests, 225
    differential diagnosis, 226
    genetics, 225–226
    mild forms, 225
    pathologic findings, 226
    treatment, 226
Facial dysmorphias, 47, 332, 336, 336t, 337t
Faciobuccopharyngeal dyspraxias, 288
Fahr disease, 217–218
Familial amyloid neuropathies, 221–223, 311, 346
    clinical diagnosis, 222
    clinical features, 222
    genetics, 222
    laboratory tests, 222–223
    pathology, 223
    treatment, 223
    variants, 223
Familial bilateral striopallidodentate calcinosis, 217–

218, 300
Familial dystonias with putaminal hypodensities, 216–217
Familial Fahr disease, 217–218
Familial hepatolenticular degeneration (*see* Wilson disease)
Familial high-density lipoprotein deficiency, 223–224
Familial lysinuric protein intolerance, 107–108
Familial nonprogressive athetosis, 218
Familial polyneuropathies, 219–234
Familial progressive myoclonic epilepsy with Lafora bodies, 195–196
Familial spastic ataxia of childhood, 190
Familial spastic paraplegia (FSP), 179, 185, 301
  complicated forms, 185
  X-linked, 179, 185, 301
Familial striatal necrosis (*see* Bilateral familial striatal necrosis)
Fanconi syndrome, 27, 84, 331, 331t
Farber disease, 60–61, 60f, 258, 360
  clinical features, 60–61
  clinical variants, 61
  diagnostic laboratory tests, 61
  genetics, 61
  late-onset, 61, 240
  pathological findings, 61
  treatment, 61
Fazio-Londe syndrome, 321
Flavoprotein, electron transfer (ETF) deficiency of, 28, 103
Folate transport and metabolism disorders, 105
Friedreich ataxia (FA), 186, 313, 324, 327, 328
  clinical features, 187–188
  diagnosis, 189
  diagnostic paraclinical tests, 188
  genetics, 188
  pathologic findings, 188
  physiopathology and clinicopathologic correlations, 188
Fructose 1,6-bisphosphatase aldolase deficiency, 39
Fructose 1,6-bisphosphatase deficiency, 39, 331
  late-onset intermittent form, 107
Fructose intolerance, hereditary, 39
Fucosidosis, 167–169, 168f
  biochemical pathology, 169
  clinical features, 167–168
  diagnostic laboratory tests, 168
  pathologic findings, 169
  prenatal diagnosis, 169
  treatment, 169

Fumarase deficiency, 93–94

GABA metabolism disorders of, 86
GABA transaminase deficiency, 86
Galactokinase deficiency, 91
Galactose-1-phosphate uridyltransferase (GALT) deficiency, 40, 87, 90–91
Galactosemia (*see* GALT deficiency)
Galactosialidosis, 62, 170, 243–244, 258
  laboratory tests, 244
α-Galactosidase deficiency (*see* Fabry disease)
Galactosylceramide lipidosis (*see* Krabbe leukodystrophy)
Gargoyle-like facial features, 336t
Gastrointestinal symptoms, 336–337, 339t
Gaucher cells, 346
  in bone marrow smear, 59f
Gaucher disease, 47, 55, 57–60, 315, 346, 360, 361
  subacute neuropathic (juvenile), 240
  Type I, 57, 360
  Type II, 57–60
    clinical course and life profile, 58f
    clinical features, 58
    diagnostic biochemical tests, 59
    differential diagnosis, 59–60
    genetics, 59
    paraclinical features, 58
    pathologic findings, 59
    pathophysiology, 59
    prenatal diagnosis, 59
    treatment, 60
  Type III, 57, 240, 258, 328
Gene therapy for neurometabolic diseases, 360–361
Giant axonal neuropathy, 233, 348
Glaucomas, 317t, 318t, 321, 362
Globoid cell leukodystrophy (*see* Krabbe leukodystrophy)
Glucose 6-phosphatase deficiency, 107
Glucose transporter protein deficiency, 84
Glutamate formininotransferase deficiency, 105
Glutamic acid decarboxylase (GAD), 40
Glutaric aciduria:
  type I, 85, 106–107, 288
    biochemical findings, 106
    genetics, 106
    neuropathology, 107
    physiopathology, 107
    treatment, 107
  type II, 28–29, 103, 118
    ultrasound scan, 29f

Glutaryl-CoA dehydrogenase deficiency (*see* Glutaric ociduria type I)

Glycogen storage disease, 39–40
  type I, 40, 107, 262
  type II, 64–66, 64f, 360
    adult form, 65
    clinical features, 64
    diagnostic laboratory tests, 66
    differential diagnosis, 66
    genetics, 66
    pathologic findings, 66
    variants, 65
  type VII, 39

Glycoprotein degradation, disorders of, 161, 162–163t, 165–171

G_{M1} gangliosidosis, 53, 258, 360
  adult/chronic (type 3), 54, 237–238
  chronic form (type 3), 237–238, 258
  clinical course and life profile, 53f
  early infantile (Type 1), 53–55
    clinical features, 53
    diagnostic biochemical tests, 54
    differential diagnosis, 55
    genetics, 54
    laboratory findings, 53
    pathologic findings, 54
    pathophysiology, 55
    treatment, 55
  facial dysmorphism, 54f
  late infantile (Type 2), 140–141
    clinical course and life profile, 140f
    clinical features, 140
    diagnostic laboratory tests, 140–141
    differential diagnosis, 141
    pathological and biochemical changes, 141
  late-onset chronic form, 237–238, 258

G_{M2} gangliosidosis, 49, 145, 258, 308, 315, 360, (*see also* Tay-Sachs disease, Sandhoff disease)
  activator deficiency, 52
  adult-onset, 237
  β_1 Variants, 237
  chronic, 236
  early infantile, 49–52
  late infantile, 141
  late-onset, 235–237, 236f
  subacute, 235

Growth failure, 336, 337

Guanine triphosphate cyclohydrolase (GPT-CH) deficiency, 89

Guillain-Barré syndrome, 297, 313

Gyrate atrophy of choroid, 14, 185

Hair, 332, 334t

Hallervorden-Spatz disease, 138, 212–214, 214f
  age of onset and duration, 213f
  chemical pathogenesis, 213–214
  clinical features, 212–213
  diagnostic laboratory tests, 213
  differential diagnosis, 214
  pathologic findings, 213–214
  treatment, 214
  variants, 213

HARP syndrome, 213, 218

Hartnup disease, 268–270, 269f, 359, 362

Haw River syndrome, 197

Hearing, impaired, 32

Hematological abnormalities, 332, 335t

Hematological tests, 346

Hemiplegias, 302–303
  acute postconvulsive, 303
  cause of, 302, 303, 304t
  sudden (apoplectic), 302–303

Hemorrhage, intracranial, 283–284

Hepatolenticular degeneration (*see* Wilson disease)

Heredity in HMDs, 3–4

Hereditary coproporphyria (HCP), 228

Hereditary dentatorubral-pallidoluysian atrophy (DRPLA), 197

Hereditary folate malabsorption, 105

Hereditary metabolic neuropathies, 312–316, 314t (*see also* Peripheral neuropathies)

Hereditary motor and sensory neuropathies (HMSN):
  type I and II (*see* Charcot-Marie-Tooth disease)
  type III (*see* Déjerine-Sottas disease)

Hereditary sensory and autonomic neuropathies (HSANs), 313, 316t

Hereditary tyrosinemia I, 229

Heredopathia atactica polyneuritiformis (*see* Refsum disease)

Herpes virus prenatal infection, 284

Hexosaminidase A deficiency (*see* Tay-Sachs disease, Sandhoff disease)

Hexosaminidase B deficiency (*see* Sandhoff disease)

Hexosaminidase α subunit deficiency (*see* Tay-Sachs disease; G_{M2} gangliosidoses)

Hexosaminidase β subunit deficiency (*see* Sandhoff disease, G_{M2} gangliosidoses)

High-density lipoprotein deficiency, 223-224

Histidinemia, 87, 89–90

Histidinuria, 90

Holocarboxylase synthetase (HS) deficiency, 30, 78

Homocysteine methyltransferase deficiency, 20, 21, 105

Homocystinuria, 264, (*see* Cysthationine β-synthase

deficiency)
HTLV-1 virus, 179, 301
Human immunodeficiency virus (HIV), 284, 294, 301, 312
Hunter disease (MPS II), 156–157, 157f, 359
Huntington disease, 3, 205–208, 300, 308, 361
   clinical features, 205–206
   clinicopathologic correlation, 207–208
   diagnosis, 207
   genetics, 206
   pathogenesis, 207–208
   pathology, 207
   prediction, 207
   profile and key signs, 205f
   treatment, 208
Hurler disease (MPS I H), 151–156, 154f, 155f, 359
   diagnostic laboratory tests, 156
   pathology, 156
   prenatal diagnosis, 156
   treatment, 156, 359
Hurler phenotype, disorders with, 161–172, 162–163t
Hurler-Scheie syndrome (MPS I H/S), 151, 154, 156
Hydrops fetalis, 328, 329t
L-2-Hydroxyglutaric acidemia, 86, 192
3-Hydroxyisobutyric acidemia, 91
3-Hydroxyisobutyryl-CoA deacylase deficiency, 92
3-Hydroxy-3-methylglutaric aciduria, 29–30, 105–106
3-Hydroxy-3-methylglutaryl-CoA lyase deficiency, 29–30, 105–106
Hyperammonemias, 11t
   in aminoacidopathies, osganoacidopathies, 13, 14, 104, 105, 107
   in mitochondrial disorders, 26–28, 80, 101–103
   in ucea-cycle disorders, 12–14, 107
   transient, neonatal, 13
Hyper-β-alalinemia, 84
Hyperglycinemia, (see Nonketotic hyperglycinemia)
Hyperkinesia, 292, 307
Hyperornithinemia, 14, 185
Hyperornithinemia-hyperammonemia-homocitrullinuria (HHH) syndrome, 14, 108
Hyperphenylalaninemia, 86, 89
Hyperpipecolic aciduria, 37–38
Hyperplexia, 310
Hyperuricemia (see Lesch-Nyhan disease)
Hypnogenic paroxysmal choreoathetosis, 215
Hypobetalipoproteinemia, 192
Hypocalcemia, 285
Hypoglycemia, nonketotic, 100–104
Hypoprebetalipoproteinemia, 218
Hypoxanthine-guanine-phosphoribosyltransferase

(HPRT) deficiency, 258–262 (see Lesch-Nyhan disease)
Hypoxic-ischemic encephalopathy of the newborn, 283–284

I-cell disease (see Mucolipidosis II)
Idiopathic focal dystonias, 211
Idiopathic recurrent stupor, 109
Idiopathic torsion dystonia, 210–211
Infantile neuronal ceroid lipofuscinosis (INCL), 146–148
   clinical features, 146–147
   diagnostic laboratory tests, 147–148
   differential diagnosis, 148
Infantile neuronal ceroid lipofuscinosis (cont.)
   pathologic findings, 148
   prenatal diagnosis, 148
Inherited brachial plexus neuropathy, 313
Inherited tendency to develop pressure palsies, 313
Intention myoclonus, (see Action myoclonus)
Intergenomic signaling defects, 251
Intracranial hemorrhage, 283–284
Intranuclear neuronal inclusion disease, 348
Isolated complex I deficiency, 26–27, 93
Isolated complex II deficiency, 93
Isolated complex III deficiency, 27, 93
Isolated complex IV deficiency, 27, 93
Isovaleric acidemia (see Isovaleryl-CoA dehydrogenase deficiency)
Isovaleryl-CoA dehydrogenase deficiency, 17–18, 105
   biochemical abnormalities, 18
   diagnosis, 18
   genetics, 18, 105
   phenotypic variations, 18
   treatment, 18

Jansky-Bielschowsky disease, 148
Jejunal biopsy, 348
Juvenile (childhood and adolescence) HMDs, 177–272
Juvenile neuroaxonal dystrophy, 258
Juvenile neuronal ceroid lipofuscinosis, 241–243, 241f, 242f

Kayser-Fleischer corneal ring, 201f, 202, 324
Kearns-Sayre syndrome, 255, 315, 328
Kernicterus, 284
Ketoacidosis, intermittent episodes of, 104–107
α-Ketoglutarate dehydrogenase deficiency, 94

β-Ketothiolase deficiency, 41, 106
Kidney abnormalities, 329–331, 331t
Kinky hair disease (see Menkes disease)
Kinsbourne syndrome, 297, 310
Kjellin syndrome, 185
Krabbe leukodystrophy, 66, 258, 312, 321
    adult forms, 248
    chemical pathology, 69, 247
    clinical course and life profile, 67f, 68f, 246f
    clinical features, 67–68, 245–246
    diagnostic laboratory tests, 68–69
    differential diagnosis, 70
    early infantile, 67–70
    genetics, 69, 247
    late-onset, 245–248, 246f, 247f
    mechanism of deranged brain funciton, 69
    molecular biology, 69, 247
    nerve biopsy, 347f
    pathology, 69, 247
    treatment, 70, 360
    variants, 68, 246
Krebs cycle, defects of, 26, 93–94
Krebs-Henseleit cycle, 12
Kufs adult type of neuronal ceroid lipofuscinosis, 243

Laboratory tests of diagnostic importance, 11t, 47–48,
        172–173, 184t, 271t, 340–351
Lactic acidosis, 9, 11t (see also mitochondrial disorders,
        Krebs cycle disorders, Leigh disease)
Lafora disease, 195–196, 195f, 307, 348
Lance and Adams syndrome, 310
Landau-Kleffner syndrome, 307
Late infantile metabolic encephalopathies, 124–176,
        126–127t
Late infantile neuronal ceroid lipofuscinosis (LINCL),
        148–150
    clinical features, 148–149, 148f
    diagnostic laboratory tests, 149
    differential diagnosis, 150
    EEG, 149f
    pathologic findings, 149–150
    variants, 149
Leber hereditary optic neuropathy, 217, 257
Leigh disease, 27, 66, 92, 125, 258, 288, 300, 313, 315,
        324, 344
    age at onset and duration, 96t
    biology, 94, 140
    clinical findings, 94–97, 95t, 96t
    clinicopathologic correlations, 99
    course of, 96–97

diagnosis, 97–98
early infantile, 94–100
genetics, 97
intrafamilial variations, 97
juvenile, 251, 270
laboratory findings, 97
late infantile, 139–140, 139f
limits of, 98–99
main site of lesions, 100t
maternally inherited (MILS), 97, 257
MRI, 98f
pathologic findings, 99, 100t
treatment, 99
Leigh syndrome, (see Leigh disease)
Lennox-Gastaut syndrome, 306, 307
Lens, dislocation, 264, 266f, 318, 324
Lesch-Nyhan disease, 258–262, 260f, 288, 300, 331, 360
    biochemical pathology, 261
    clinical features, 258–259
    diagnosis, 261
    genetics, 261
    laboratory tests, 260
    neuropathologic changes, 261
    partial 4PRT deficiency, 260
    pathophysiology, 261
    treatment, 261–262
Leukodystrophies, 66, 67–76, 186, 344–345
Leukodystrophy with Rosenthal fiber formation (see
        Alexander disease)
Levine-Critchley syndrome, 215–216
Lipofuscinoses (see Neuronal ceroid lipofuscinoses)
Lipogranulomatosis (see Farber disease)
Lissencephaly type I, 289
Lissencephaly type II, 290
Liver, 328, 329t
    biopsies, 348
    transplantation, 361
Long-chain acyl-CoA dehydrogenase (LCAD)
        deficiency, 28, 102
Long-chain 3-hydroxyacyl-CoA dehydrogenase
        (LCHAD) deficiency, 102–103
Lowe disease, 84–85, 327, 331, 332
    biochemical findings, 84–85
    clinical features, 84
    facial appearance, 85f
    genetics, 85
    treatment, 85
Lower motor neuronopathies, 315, 315t
Lysinuric protein intolerance, 41, 107–108

Machado-Joseph syndrome, 190
McLeod syndrome, 216, 335t
Macrocephaly, 290, 291t
Macular cherry red spot, 49, 50, 51t, 317, 319t, 321, 324
Magnetic resonance imaging, 343–345, 349t
Magnetic resonance spectroscopy (MRS), 343
Malnutrition, 47, 336, 337
α-Mannosidosis, 166–167, 166f
  diagnostic laboratory tests, 167
  pathology, 167
  treatment, 167
β-Mannosidosis, 167
Maple syrup urine disease (MSUD), 315, 353
  clinical presentation, 16
  genetics, 16
  intermediate form, 104
  intermittent form, 104
  mechanism of brain lesions, 17
  neonatal screening, 17
  neuropathology, 17
  oculomotor palsies, 17, 315
  pathophysiology, 17
  prenatal diagnosis, 17
  specific biochemical abnormalities, 16
  thiamine responsive, 104
  treatment, 17
  variants, 17, 104
Marfan disease, 266, 266f
Marie hereditary cerebellar ataxia, 190
Marinesco-Sjögren syndrome, 296
Maroteaux-Lamy disease (MPS VI), 160, 359
Maternal (mitochondrial) inheritance, 4
Maternal mode of inheritance, diseases with a, 254–257
Maternally inherited Leigh syndrome (MILS), 97, 257
Medium-chain acyl-CoA dehydrogenase (MCAD) deficiency, 101–102
Mendelian mode of inheritance, 3–4
Meningitis, bacterial, 284
Menkes disease, 9, 78–81, 80–81f, 264, 308, 329
  clinical features, 78
  clinicopathologic correlations, 79–80
  genetics, 79
  laboratory findings of diagnostic importance, 78–79
  mild, 81
  pathology, 79
  pathophysiology, 79–80
  treatment, 80–81
  variants, 81
Mental development:
  assessment of, 291–292
  delay in, 272

Mental retardation and motor delay, 150–172, 184t, 218, 291–292
Metachromatic leukodystrophy (MLD), 66, 128–132, 258, 348, 347f, 359–360
  biochemical analysis, 132
  clinical course and life profile, 129f
  clinical features, 128–129
  diagnostic biochemical tests, 129–130
  differential diagnosis, 129–130, 131
  genetics, 131
  late infantile, 128–132
  late-onset, 128, 132, 244–245
  MRI, 130f
  pathological and chemical findings, 132
  physiopathology, 132
  preclinical, 131
  pseudo-deficiency, 128, 129, 130–131, 131t
  treatment and prevention, 132, 359–360
  variant forms, 132
2-Methylacetoacetyl-CoA thiolase deficiency, 41, 106
3-Methylcrotonyl-CoA carboxylase deficiency, 18, 106
Methylenetetrahydrofolate reductase deficiency, 105, 304t
3-Methylglutaconic acidemia:
  with 3-methylglutaconyl-CoA hydratase deficiency, 86
  without 3-methylglutaconyl-CoA hydrolase deficiency, 85–86
Methylmalonate metabolism, disorders of, 18, 19
Methylmalonic acidemia, 19–20, 104
  biochemical characteristics, 19–20, 104
  clinical features, 19, 104
Methylmalonyl-CoA mutase deficiency (see Methylmalonic acidemia)
Methylmalonyl-CoA mutase and tetrahydrofolate: homocysteine methyltransferase deficiency, 20–21, 105
Methylmalonyl-CoA racemase deficiency, 19
Methyltetrahydrofolate: homocysteine methyltransferase deficiency, 21
Metoclopromide, 362
Mevalonate kinase deficiency, 21–22
Mevalonic aciduria, 21–22
Microcephaly, 290
Microphthalmia, 324
Miller-Dieker syndrome, 289, 290, 336
Miller-Fisher syndrome, 297
Mitochondrial ATPase 6 gene point mutations, 94, 97
Mitochondrial DNA (mtDNA), 3
  defects in, 254–257, 348
  depletion syndrome, 27, 252

Mitochondrial encephalomyopathies
  juvenile, 254–257
  with lactic acidosis and stroke-like episodes
    (MELAS), 99, 256, 264, 302, 323, 329, 337
Mitochondrial encephalopathies, neonatal, 22–29, 23t,
    24t
Mitochondrial fatty acid oxidation defects, 27–29,
    100–103
Mitochondrial trifunctional enzyme deficiency, 103–104
Molybdenum cofactor deficiency, 21, 287, 324
Mononeuropathies, 315
Morphological diagnosis, 346–348, 349t
Morquio disease (MPS IV), 160
Motor development:
  assessment of, 291–292
  delay in, 46, 272
Mucolipidoses, 161–165, 162–163t, 361
  Type I (ML I), 62
  Type II (ML II), 161–164, 164f
    clinical features, 161–164
    diagnostic laboratory tests, 164
    pathologic findings, 164
    prenatal diagnosis, 164
    treatment, 164
  Type III (ML III), 164–165
  Type IV (ML IV), 165, 165f
Mucopolysaccharidoses (MPS), 150, 151–161, 359, 361
  classification and main characteristics, 151–152t
Mucosulfatidosis (see Multiple sulfatase deficiency
    (MSD))
Multiple acyl-CoA dehydrogenase deficiency, 28, 103
Multiple carboxylase deficiency (see disorders of biotin
    metabolism)
Multiple deletions of DNA, 251–252
Multiple sclerosis, 301
Multiple sulfatase deficiency (MSD), 132–135, 134f, 161
  chemical pathology, 135
  clinical course and life profile, 133f
  clinical features, 133
  diagnostic laboratory findings, 133–135
  pathological findings, 135
  variants, 135
Münchausen syndrome by proxy, 109, 297
Muscle biopsy, 351
Myasthenia gravis, 323
Mycoplasma pneumonia, 299
Myelin basic protein defects, leukodystrophy with, 72
Myoclonic epilepsy, 99, 305, 306, 307, 308, 309, 310
  familial, progressive, 192–196
  with ragged red fibers (MERRF), 196, 256–257, 308
Myoclonus (see action myoclonus, epilepsy, myoclonic

epilepsy)
  benign essential, 197, 198
  palatal, essential, 198
Myoclonus-opsoclonus syndrome, 297, 310

NADH-ubiquinone oxidoreductase deficiency, 26–27,
    93
Necrosis of the putamen and pallidum, 217t
Neonatal adrenoleukodystrophy, 37
Neonatal bacterial meningitis, 284
Neonatal HMDs, 9–44
  clinical and radiological characteristics, 9
  diagnostic laboratory tests, 9–12
  diagnostic plan, 11t
  distinctive features, 10t
Neonatal neurology
  general symptomatology, 7–9
Nephrolithiasis, 331
Nephrosialidosis, 62
Neuroacanthocytosis, 215–216, 300
Neuroaxonal dystrophy (NAD), 135–138, 213, 253, 346
  clinical course and life profile, 135f
  clinical features, 136
  clinicopathologic correlations, 138
  diagnosis, 137
  genetics, 136
  juvenile, 253
  laboratory tests, 136
  mechanisms of derangements of nervous system
    function, 138
  nosology and limits of, 137–138
  pathologic findings, 136–137
  sural nerve biopsy, 137f
Neuroimaging techniques, 343–345
Neurological regression, evidence of, 46
Neuronal ceroid lipofuscinoses (NCL), 146 (see also
    Infantile, late infantile, Juvenile neuronal ceroid
    lipofuscinosis)
  NCL$_1$ (infantile), 146–148
  NCL$_2$ (late infantile) 148–150
    variant of, 149
  NCL$_3$ (juvenile), 241–243
  NCL$_4$ (adult) (Kufs type), 243
  NCL$_5$, 149
Neuronal intranuclear inclusion disease, 253–254, 258
Neuropathy, ataxia and retinitis pigmentosa (NARP)
    syndrome, 257
Neuroradiologic imaging, 342–345
Neurotransmitter pathways, agents acting at, 361
Niemann-Pick disease, 47, 55, 328, 360, 361

Type A, 55–57, 313
  clinical course and life profile, 56f
  clinical features, 56
  diagnostic laboratory tests, 57
  differential diagnosis, 57
  genetics, 57
  pathological findings, 57
  prenatal diagnosis, 57
  treatment, 57
  variants, 56
Type B, 55, 56
Type C, 55, 141, 238–240, 239f, 258, 328, 332, 346
  chemical pathology, 239
  clinical features, 238
  diagnosis, 238
  laboratory tests, 238–239
  pathology, 239
  treatment, 239–240
Nonketotic hyperglycinemia (NKH), 14–16, 308
  biochemical findings, 15
  diagnosis, 15
  genetics, 15–16
  neuropathology, 15
  physiopathology, 15
  treatment, 16
  ultrasound scans, 15f
Nonneurologic abnormalities, 327–336
Nystagmus, 323–324

Ocular abnormalities 32, 46, 317–320t, 321–324, 322t
  in HMDs, 321–324
  differential diagnosis, 321–324
  in neonates, 8
Occipital horn syndrome, 78, 81
Ocular movements, 8
  derangement of, 323–324, 322t
Oculocerebrorenal syndrome, 84–85
Oculomotor palsies, 323
Olivopontocerebellar atrophy, 170, 296
Optic nerves, lesions of, 321, 322
Ornithine transcarbamylase (OTC) deficiency, 12–14, 107
5-Oxoprolinuria (glutathione synthetase deficiency), 41

Palatal myoclonus, 198
Pallidal atrophy, 218
Paralysis agitans, juvenile, 208
Paramyoclonus multiplex, 197
Parkinson disease, 199
  juvenile, 208
Paroxysmal choreoathetosis, 297
  (see also dystonias)
Paroxysmal dystonias, 214–215
Paroxysmal kinesigenic choreoathetosis, 214–215
Paroxysmal nonkinesigenic choreoathetosis, 215
Pearson syndrome, 255
Pelizaeus-Merzbacher disease, 66, 70, 71–72, 185, 288, 300, 324, 344
  animal models, 72
  clinical features, 71–72
  diagnosis, 72
  genetics, 72
  molecular biology, 72
  pathological findings, 72
  pathophysiology, 72
Penicillamine in Wilson's disease, 204
Perinatal hypoxia, 283–286
Peripheral myelin protein defects, 230, 232
Peripheral neuropathy, 125–142, 126–127t, 297
  differential diagnosis, 311–313
  general features, 311–312
  HMDs causing, 128–140, 314t
Peroxisomal acyl-CoA oxidase deficiency, 38
Peroxisomal disorders, neonatal, 30–39, 31t, 32t, 33t, 35f, 38f
Peroxisomal 3-oxoacyl-CoA thiolase deficiency, 38
Personality changes, 270–272
Phenylketonuria (PKU), 87–89, 353
  clinical features, 87
  diagnostic biochemical findings, 87–88
  genetics, 88
  maternal, 89
  neonatal screening, 88
  phenotypes, 87–88
  treatment, 88
Phosphoenolpyruvate carboxykinase deficiency, 93
Phosphofluctokinase deficiency, 66
Phosphoribosylpyrophosphatase (PP-ribose-P) synthetase deficiency, 262
Phytanic acid storage disease, 220–221
  (see also Refsum disease)
Polyglucosan disease, adult, 196, 348
Polyhydramnios, 291
Polymyoclonus (see Action myoclonus)
Polyneuropathy (see peripheral neuropathy)
Pompe disease (see Glycogenosis, type II)
Pontoneocerebellar atrophy, congenital, 296
Porphobilinogen (PBG) deaminase deficiency, 226–228
Porphyria (see Acute intermittent porphyria)
Positron emission tomography (PET), 48, 343, 345

Postprandial hyperammonemia, 107–108
Prematurity, 291
Prenatal encephalitis, 284
Prevention of HMD, 362–363
Primary degeneration of corpus luysi, 218
Primary degeneration of granule cells, 294
Primary idiopathic hereditary dystonias, 209–212
Progressive external ophthalmoplegia, 251, 252, 254, 255, 257, 323
Progressive myoclonic epilepsy, 192–196
  with RRF, 196, 255–257
Progressive spastic hemiplegia, 302
Propionic acidemia, 18–19, 104
  biochemical characteristics, 18–19
  course and treatment, 19, 104
  genetics, 19
  neuropathology, 19
  prenatal diagnosis, 19
Propionyl-CoA carboxylase deficiency (see Propionic acidemia)
Proteolipid protein (PLP) deficiency, 71, 72, 185
Protoporphyrinogen oxidase (PROTO) deficiency, 228–229
Pseudo-Hurler polydystrophy (see Mucolipidosis Type III (ML III))
Pseudo-neonatal adrenoleukodystrophy, 38
Pseudo-syringomyelic syndrome, 311
Pseudo-Zellweger syndrome, 38
Psychic function, arrest of, 172–173
Psychomotor retardation, 172–173, 291–292
Pupillary size, alterations of, 8
Purine nucleoside phosphorylase deficiency, 145
Purkinje cells, 295, 297
Pyle disease, 332
Pyridoxine dependency, 40–41
Pyruvate carboxylase (PC) deficiency, benign variant, 26, 93
  early infantile (North American type), 92–93
  neonatal, 26
  other forms, 26
Pyruvate dehydrogenase (PDHE$_{1\alpha}$) deficiency, 6, 140, 251, 300
  benign form, 92
  biochemistry, 25
  E$_2$ and E$_3$ deficiency, 26, 93
  early infantile, 92, 94–99
  late infantile, 139–140
  in Leigh disease, 94–99, 251
  molecular biology, 25
  neonatal, 22–26
  neuroimaging, 25f
  neuropathology, 23–26
  thiamine responsive, 92
  treatment, 26
  variants, 26
Pyruvate metabolism, disorders of, 22–30, 92–93
6-Pyruvoyltetrahydropterin synthase (6PTS) deficiency, 89

78Q syndrome, 72

Ragged red fibers (RRF), 27, 93, 348
  (see also defects in Mt DNA)
Ramsey Hunt disease (see juvenile Parkinson disease)
Ramsay Hunt syndrome, 194, 196
Rasmussen focal encephalitis, 303
Rectal biopsy, 348, 351
Refsum disease, 220–221, 313, 328
  infantile, 37, 31t, 33t
Renal cysts, 32, 331t
Renal tubular dysfunction, 331t
Respiratory alkalosis, 107–108
Respiratory chain defects, 26–27, 93
  (see also Leigh disease, juvenile mitochondrial encephalomyopathies)
  complex I deficiency, 27, 93, 255, 256
  complex II deficiency, 93
  complex III deficiency, 27, 93, 255, 256
  complex IV deficiency, 27, 93, 255, 256
Respiratory distress syndrome, 285, 286
Respiratory tract, abnormalities of, 47, 336, 338t
Retina:
  gyrate atrophy of, 185
  lesions of, 321, 317–320t
  primary degeneration, 321
Retinal degeneration, 317–320t, 321
Retinitis pigmentosa, (see Retinal degeneration)
Retrogeniculate optic pathways lesions of, 323, 317–320t
Rett syndrome, 292–293
Reye-like syndromes, 108–109
Riboflavin in glutaric aciduria II, 29, 103
Riley-Day syndrome, 311
Romberg sign, 294, 312
Rosenthal fibers in Alexander disease, 74–76
Roussy-Levy syndrome, 189, 231, 312
Rubella virus, prenatal infection with, 284

Salla disease, 63–64

Sandhoff disease, 52, 237
Sanfilippo disease (MPS III), 157–159, 159f, 308, 359
  diagnosis, 158
  neurologic signs, 158
  nonneurologic signs, 158
  pathology, 159
  prenatal diagnosis, 158
  subtype A, 158
  subtype B, 158
  subtype C, 158
  treatment, 159
Santavuori-Haltia-Hagberg disease,
  146–148
SAP 1 deficiency, 128, 130
Scheie disease (MPS I S), 159, 160f
Schilder disease, 67, 302
Schindler disease, 138
  clinical variants, 139
  laboratory investigations, 138
Segawa disease, 211–212
Seitelberger disease (see Neuroaxonal dystrophy (NAD))
Seizures (see also Epilepsy)
  early infantile syndrome with, 81–84
  HMDs with seizures, 307–309, 308t
  neonatal, 7
  seizure states, 303–305, 308t
Sensorimotor neuropathies, 311–315
Sensory ataxia, 187, 286, 294
Short-chain acyl-CoA dehydrogenase (SCAD)
  deficiency, 28, 102
Short-chain 3-hydroxyacyl-CoA dehydrogenase
  (SCHAD) deficiency, 103
Short stature, 291
Sialic acid storage disorders, 62–64, 63f
  biochemical characteristics, 63
  clinical features, 63
  morphologic characteristics, 63
  variants, 63
Sialidosis:
  type I, 197
  type II, 62, 145, 170, 243–244, 258
Single proton emission computed tomography
  (SPECT), 2, 48
Sjögren-Larsson disease, 67, 179,
  185–186, 344
Skeletal changes, 154, 155f, 168f, 332, 333t
Skin, 332, 334t
  biopsy, 350
Sly disease (MPS VII), 160
Smith-Lemli-Opitz (SLO) syndrome, 22, 109, 118, 289
Somatic malformations, 332, 336, 337t

Somatosensory evoked potentials, 346
Spastic paraplegia, 126–127t
  differential diagnosis, 300–302
  HMDs causing, 125–142
  X-linked, 72
Sphingolipidoses generalities, 48–49
Spielmeyer-Vogt disease, 241, 258
Spinal muscular atrophy, distal, 231, 312
Spleen, 328, 329t
Spongy degeneration of the nervous system (see
  Canavan-Van Bogaert-Bertrand disease)
Startle disease, 310
Static encephalopathies, 286–293
Status dysmyelinisatus of Vogt, 219
Status epilepticus, non convulsive, 297, 306–307
Steely hair disease (see Menkes disease)
Steinert myotonic dystrophy, 286
Striatal necrosis (see bilateral striatal necrosis, Leigh
  disease)
Stroke, 264–268, 302, 303, 304t, 328
Stroke-like episodes, 256
Strümpell-Lorrain familial spastic paralysis, 179, 185,
  301
Subacute necrotizing encephalomyelopathy (see Leigh
  disease)
Succinate-ubiquinone oxidoreductase deficiency, 27, 93
Succinic semialdehyde dehydrogenase deficiency, 86
Sudanophilic leukodystrophy, 66, 70–71
Sudden infant death syndrome (SIDS), 109, 118
Sulfatidosis (see Metachromatic leukodystrophy)
Sulfite oxidase deficiency, 21, 287, 324
Supranuclear paralyses of conjugate gaze, 323
Sural nerve biopsy, 347f, 348
Sydenham chorea, 206, 300
Symptomatic treatment, 361–362
Syphilis, congenital, 284

Tangier disease, 223–224, 311
Tardive dyskinesia, 299
Tay-Sachs disease, 49–52, 308, 362
  biochemical diagnosis, 51
  clinical course and life profile, 50f
  clinical features, 49–51
  clinicopathological correlations, 52
  differential diagnosis, 52
  genetics, 51
  neuropathology, 51–52
  prenatal diagnosis, 51
  retinal cherry red spot, 51f
Tay-Sachs disease (cont.)

treatment, 52
Tetrahydrobiopterin deficiency, 89
Tetrathiomolybdate in Wilson disease, 204
Thiamin, treatment with, 17, 92, 104
Toxoplasmosis, congenital, 284
Transferase deficiency galactosemia, 40, 90–91
Transient hyperammonemia of the newborn, 13
Transient hypoglycemia, 285
Treatment and prevention, 352–363, 354–358t
Triethylene tetramine in Wilson disease, 204
Trifunctional enzyme deficiency, 29
Tumors, 301, 323
Tyrosinemia type I, 229

Ubiquinol-cytochrome-*c* oxidoreductase deficiency, 27, 93
UDP-galactose-4-epimerase deficiency, 91
Ultrasonography, 343
Unverricht-Lundborg progressive familial myoclonic epilepsy, 194–195, 307
Urea cycle disorders, 12–14, 14t
  late-onset, 107
Urocanic aciduria, 90

Valine catabolism, disorders of, 91
Van Laere syndrome, 321
Varicella virus, prenatal infection by, 284
Variegate porphyria, 228–229
Very long chain acyl-CoA dehydrogenase (VLCAD) deficiency, 28, 103
Very long chain fatty acids (VLCFAs) in peroxisomal defects, 31, 31t, 32t
Visceral and other tissues, abnormalities, 327–339
Visual failure, 321, 323, 317–320t
(*see also* Macular CRS, Retinal degeneration, Retrogeniculate optic pathways)
Visual loss as an initial symptom in juvenile hereditary metabolic disorders, 234
Vitamin B$_6$ deficiency, 40
Vitamin B$_6$ dependency, 40–41, 359
Vitamin B^6, treatment in homocystinuria, 267
Vitamin E deficiency, 138, 190, 191, 192
Vitamin therapy, 353, 359, 354–358t
  (*see also* biotin, cobalamin, riboflavin, thiamin)
Vomiting, 336–337
Von Gierke disease, 40, 107, 262

Walking difficulties, 125–142, 126–127t
Werdnig-Hoffmann disease, 66, 296, 312
West syndrome, 305t, 310
Westphal-Strümpell pseudosclerosis, (*see* Wilson disease)
Williams syndrome, 293
Wilson disease, 199–205, 324, 328, 331, 353
  clinical features, 201
  clinical profile and key signs, 201f
  clinicopathologic correlations, 204
  counseling, 203
  diagnosis, 203
  diagnostic laboratory tests, 202–203
  genetics, 203
  liver disease in, 201
  neurologic signs, 201–202
  pathologic findings, 203–204
  pathophysiology, 204
  PET scans, 205f
  treatment, 204–205
Wolfhart-Kugelberg-Welander syndrome, 312
Wolfram syndrome, 257

Xanthine dehydrogenase deficiency, 21
Xeroderma pigmentosum, 263–264, 362
X-linked adrenoleukodystrophy, 248–251, 258, 360
X-linked diseases, 4
X-rays, 342

Zellweger disease (ZD), 31, 31–33t, 34–36, 35f, 66, 308, 328, 331, 332, 344
  biochemical abnormalities, 34–36
  clinical features, 34
  diagnostic laboratory tests, 36
  differential diagnosis, 36
  genetics, 36
  molecular biology, 36
  pathological findings, 36
  prenatal diagnosis, 36
  related disorders, 36–39
  treatment, 36
Zellweger phenotype, diseases with, 36–39
Zellweger-like syndrome, 31, 39
Zellweger syndrome, 6, 9
Zinc acetate in Wilson disease, 204
Zinc sulphate in Wilson disease, 204

ISBN 0-07-000389-0

9 780070 003897

90000>